Gastrointestinal and Liver Tumors

Springer

Berlin
Heidelberg
New York
Hong Kong
London
Milan
Paris
Tokyo

W. Scheppach · R.S. Bresalier · G.N.J. Tytgat (eds.)

Gastrointestinal and Liver Tumors

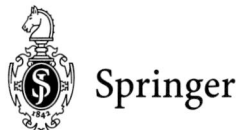

Springer

Cataloging-in-Publication Data applied for
A catalog record for this book is available from the Library of Congress.

Bibliographic information published by Die Deutsche Bibliothek
Die Deutsche Bibliothek lists this publication in the Deutsche Nationalbibliografie;
detailed bibliographic data is available in the Internet at http://dnb.ddb.de

ISBN 3-540-43462-3   Springer-Verlag Berlin Heidelberg New York

Springer-Verlag Berlin Heidelberg New York
a member of BertelsmannSpringer Science+Business Media GmbH

http://www.springer.de/medizin

© Springer-Verlag Berlin Heidelberg 2004
Printed in Germany

Cover Design: Frido Steinen, Spanien
Typesetting: Hilger VerlagsService, Heidelberg
Production Editor: Frank Krabbes, Heidelberg

SPIN 10843442   21/3109 – 5 4 3 2 1 0   Printed on acid-free paper

Foreword

Cancer of the digestive system, which includes the gastrointestinal tract, liver, pancreas and gall bladder, represents a major cause of cancer morbidity and mortality worldwide. In the year 2000, these malignancies were responsible for 30% of all cancers and 36% of all cancer-associated deaths (Parkin DM, Bray FI, Devesa SS, Cancer burden in the year 2000. The global picture. Eur J Cancer 2001; 37: S4-66).

This book provides a concise, but more than adequate overview of these malignancies and their premalignant states. It gives updated information on etiology – whether genetic or environmental, pathology, clinical features and treatments. It also gives information on screening, prevention and chemoprevention, where available. Understanding these latter features are of prime importance as we clinicians are moving from treatment of endstage disease, to prevention, chemoprevention and early diagnosis in order to reduce the cancer burden, to try and delay or at least modulate its manifestations and cure it by diagnosing in the earliest and curable stage.

As physicians, we are used to emphasizing diagnosis and treatment of disease. Today we already have some of the tools needed to *prevent* several important prevalent gastrointestinal malignancies. These include: immunization against hepatitis B, which will significantly reduce the incidence of hepatoma; improved hygiene and nutrition to decrease the prevalence and duration of exposure and severity of infection from *Helicobacter pylori* so as to decrease the occurrence of gastric cancer; colon cancer incidence can be reduced in the long-term by lifestyle modulation and morbidity reduced immediately by population screening, preventive polypectomy and early cancer diagnosis.

The chapter authors are authorities in their fields and have produced a text for the practicing physician who needs an easy to read and complete source of information on Digestive Cancers. This book will be an excellent source of information for the treating clinician, whether gastroenterologist, surgeon or oncologist.

PAUL ROZEN, MB.BS
Dept. of Gastroenterology, Tel Aviv Medical Center
and Professor of Medicine, Tel Aviv University

Preface

What can be a rationale to produce a medical textbook in the era of electronic multimedia? In the view of the editors the acquisition of information and knowledge by reading a book is still more delightful for most of us than by manoevering through PC menues. However, in order to keep up with the rapid progress in gastroenterology and hepatology, a short lag time between the writing of the individual chapters and the release of the book has to be assured.

The goal of this book is to present the diagnosis and treatment of gastrointestinal and liver tumors to medical doctors in hospitals or private practices, residents and libraries with interest in high-standard education in clinical oncology. On the one hand the book should provide comprehensive in-depth information on the entire clinical management of alimentary tract tumors; the text is enriched by high-quality illustrations and artwork. On the other hand the structure of chapters should allow quick reference to a topic. Therefore, text elements such as summaries, tables and treatment algorithms were introduced to make selective reading possible. The homogeneity of the individual chapters was assured by presenting all aspects in the same order (epidemiology, screening where appropriate, symptoms and clinical signs, diagnostic studies, staging and classification, treatment, prognosis, follow-up, future perspectives). The presentation of imaging techniques was integrated into those organ chapters where they are mostly applied. A paragraph on future perspectives was added to every chapter in order to point at new diagnostic and therapeutic tools that have not yet entered the clinical stage.

The final chapter of the book deals with the supportive care of cancer patients. In many of them there will be a stage when tumor-targeted therapies fail to control malignant growth. In these circumstances gastroenterologists should reassure their patients that best supportive care can be highly effective in alleviating symptoms.

Authors from more than one country with a high reputation within their respective areas reflect the international standard of the content. It was also our goal to demonstrate the interdisciplinary approach to patient care and to open new ways of cooperation between the classical disciplines of clinical medicine. With contributions by many authors, redundancy of information is unavoidable. We have not eliminated background information required to comprehend a complex topic even if it may appear in another chapter. Medical textbooks are usually not read from cover to cover like a novel; therefore we hope that remaining repetitions are not disturbing the general impression.

The book is dedicated to our cancer patients in the hope for further improvements in the management of their diseases.

Würzburg, Houston, Amsterdam, January 2003

WOLFGANG SCHEPPACH, ROBERT S. BRESALIER, GUIDO N.J. TYTGAT

Contents

X   Appendix

XI   Addendum

      Calculation of Body Surface Area

List of Contributors

ARNOLD, R., Philipps-Universität Marburg, Klinik für Innere Medizin, Abteilung für Gastroenterologie und Endokrinologie, Baldingerstraße, 35043 Marburg, Germany

AXON, A.T.R., The General Infirmary, The Leeds Teaching Hospitals, Gastroenterology Unit, Great George Street, Leeds, LS1 3EX West Yorkshire, UK

BEGER, H.G., Universität Ulm, Chirurgische Universitätsklinik u. Poliklinik, Steinhoevelstraße 9, 89075 Ulm, Germany

BEHR, T., Philipps-Universität Marburg, Klinik für Innere Medizin, Abteilung für Gastroenterologie und Endokrinologie, Abteilung für Nuklearmedizin, Baldingerstraße, 35043 Marburg, Germany

BIECKER, E., Rheinische Friedrich-Wilhelms-Universität, Zentrum für Innere Medizin, Sigmund-Freud-Straße 25, 53127 Bonn, Germany

BOND, J.H., University of Minnesota, VA Medical Center, Minneapolis, MN 55417, USA

BRAMBS, H.-J., Universität Ulm, Radiologische Universitätsklinik, Abteilung für Diagnostische Radiologie, Steinhövelstraße 9, 89075 Ulm, Germany

BRESALIER, R.S., M.D. Anderson Cancer Center, 1515 Holcombe Boulevard – Unit 436, Houston, TX 77030, USA

CACA, K., Universitätsklinikum Leipzig, Medizinische Klinik und Poliklinik II, Philipp-Rosenthal-Straße 27, 04103 Leipzig, Germany

CARETHERS, J.M., VA San Diego Healthcare System, GI Section, MC 9-111D, 3350 La Jolla Village Drive, San Diego, CA 92161, USA

CROOG, V., Mount Sinai School of Medicine, The Dr. Henry D. Janowitz Division of Gastroenterology, One Gustave Levy Place, New York, NY 10029, USA

DE WOLF-PEETERS, C., University Hospital KUL, Dpt. of Morphology and Molecular Pathology, Minderbroedersstraat 12, B-3000, Leuven, Belgium

DIXON, M.F., University of Leeds, Academic Unit of Pathological Sciences, LS2 9JT Leeds, UK

DRAGOSICS, B.A., Wiener Gebietskrankenkasse, Gesundheitszentrum Wien Süd, Wienerbergstrasse 13, 1100 Wien, Austria

EGGENBERGER. J.C., Henry Ford Hospital, Division of Colon & Rectal Surgery, Detroit, Michigan 48202, USA

ELL, C., HSK Dr.-Horst-Schmidt-Kliniken GmbH, Klinik Innere Medizin II, Ludwig-Erhard-Str. 100, 65199 Wiesbaden, Germany

FISCHER, H.P., Rheinische Friedrich-Wilhelms-Universität, Pathologisches Institut, Sigmund-Freud-Straße 25, 53127 Bonn, Germany

GASSEL, H.-J., Bayerische Julius-Maximilians-Universität, Chirurgische Universitätsklinik, Josef-Schneider-Straße 2, 97080 Würzburg, Germany

GASSER, M., Bayerische Julius-Maximilians-Universität, Chirurgische Universitätsklinik, Josef-Schneider-Straße 2, 97080 Würzburg, Germany

GEBOES, K., Universitaire Ziekenhuizen Leuven, Pathologische Ontleedkunde II, Minderbroedersstraat 12, 3000 Leuven, Belgium

GÖKE, R., Philipps-Universität Marburg, Klinik für Innere Medizin, Abteilung für Gastroenterologie und Endokrinologie, Baldingerstraße, 35043 Marburg, Germany

GOSSNER, L., HSK Dr.-Horst-Schmidt-Kliniken GmbH, Klinik Innere Medizin II, Ludwig-Erhard-Str. 100, 65199 Wiesbaden, Germany

Ho, S.B., VA Medical Center, GI Section (111D), 1 Veterans Drive, Minneapolis, MN 55417, USA

Itzkowitz, S.H., Mount Sinai School of Medicine, The Dr. Henry D. Janowitz Division of Gastroenterology, One Gustave Levy Place, New York, NY 10029, USA

Kellersmann, R., Bayerische Julius-Maximilians-Universität, Klinik und Poliklinik für Chirurgie, Josef-Schneider-Straße 2, 97080 Würzburg, Germany

Kuipers, E.J., Erasmus MC University Medical Center, Department of Gastroenterology and Hepatology, Burgemeester Oudlaan 50, NL-3062 PA Rotterdam, The Netherlands

Lambert, R., International Agency for Research on Cancer, 150 Cours Albert Thomas, Lyon, 69008, France

Lynch, H.T., Creighton University, Hereditary Cancer Institute, Dpt. of Preventive Medicine and Public Health, 2500 California Plaza, Omaha, Nebraska 68178, USA

May, A., HSK Dr.-Horst-Schmidt-Kliniken GmbH, Klinik Innere Medizin II, Ludwig-Erhard-Straße 100, 65199 Wiesbaden, Germany

Meijer, G.A., VU Medical Center, Dpt. of Pathology, De Boelelaan 1117, 1081 HV Amsterdam, The Netherlands

Mössner, J., Universitätsklinikum Leipzig, Medizinische Klinik und Poliklinik II, Philipp-Rosenthal-Straße 27, 04103 Leipzig, Germany

Mueller, J.G., Bayerische Julius-Maximilians-Universität, Pathologisches Institut, Josef-Schneider-Straße 2, 97080 Würzburg, Germany

Pech, O., HSK Dr.-Horst-Schmidt-Kliniken GmbH, Klinik Innere Medizin II, Ludwig-Erhard-Straße 100, 65199 Wiesbaden, Germany

Sauerbruch, T., Rheinische Friedrich-Wilhelms-Universität, Zentrum für Innere Medizin, Abt. für Innere Medizin I, Sigmund-Freud-Straße 25, 53127 Bonn, Germany

Scheppach, W., Bayerische Julius-Maximilians-Universität, Medizinische Universitätsklinik, Schwerpunkt Gastroenterologie, Josef-Schneider Straße 2, 97080 Würzburg, Germany

Scheurlen, M., Bayerische Julius-Maximilians-Universität, Medizinische Poliklinik, Klinikstraße 8, 97070 Würzburg, Germany

Schoppmeyer, K., Universitätsklinikum Leipzig, Medizinische Klinik und Poliklinik II, Philipp-Rosenthal-Straße 27, 04103 Leipzig, Germany

Scoazec, J.Y., Hospital E. Herriot, Dpt. of Pathology, Place d'Arsonval, F-Lyon 69003, France

Siech, M., Universität Ulm, Chirurgische Universitätsklinik und Poliklinik, Steinhoevelstraße 9, 89075 Ulm, Germany

Spechler, S.J., The University of Texas, Dallas Veterans Affairs Medical Center, Dpt. of Internal Medicine, Gastroenterology Section (111.B1), Division of Digestive and Liver Diseases, 4500 S. Lancaster Road, Texas 75216, USA

Strunk, H., Rheinische Friedrich-Wilhelms-Universität, Radiologische Klinik, Sigmund-Freud-Str. 25, 53127 Bonn, Germany

Sue-Ling, H.M., The General Infirmary, Division of Surgery and Centre for Digestive Diseases, Leeds LS1 3EX, UK

Timmermann, W., Bayerische Julius-Maximilians-Universität, Chirurgische Universitätsklinik, Josef-Schneider-Straße 2, 97070 Würzburg, Germany

van Grieken, N.C.T., VU Medical Center, Dpt. of Gastroenterology, De Boelelaan 1117, 1081 HV Amsterdam, The Netherlands

Waaga-Gasser, A.M., Bayerische Julius-Maximilians-Universität, Chirurgische Universitätsklinik, Abt. für Molekulare Onkologie and Immunologie, Josef-Schneider-Straße 2, 97080 Würzburg, Germany

Wied, M., Philipps-Universität Marburg, Klinik für Innere Medizin, Abteilung für Gastroenterologie und Endokrinologie, Baldingerstraße, 35043 Marburg, Germany

Esophagus

1 Squamous Cell Carcinoma of the Esophagus

S.J. SPECHLER

Summary

Squamous cell carcinoma of the esophagus is among the world's 10 most frequent malignancies.

Cigarette smoking and alcoholism are the major recognized risk factors, and there are dramatic geographic variations in the incidence of the tumor. There are no early warning symptoms for esophageal cancer, and most symptomatic patients have advanced disease. The diagnosis is established by barium swallow and endoscopy. Staging involves endosonography and computed tomographic scanning of the chest and abdomen. The tumors often exhibit genetic alterations in genes that regulate the transition from the G1 to the S phase of the cell cycle, a key step in cellular proliferation. Overall 5-year survival rates for patients with squamous cell carcinoma of the esophagus remain below 10%. Whereas the optimal treatment for this cancer has not been established, patients should be treated according to well-designed research protocols whenever possible.

Epidemiology

There are two major histologic types of esophageal cancer – squamous cell carcinoma and adenocarcinoma. Worldwide, >90% of all esophageal cancers are squamous cell carcinomas, and this tumor ranks among the world's 10 most frequent malignancies. One of the most striking epidemiological features of esophageal squamous cell carcinoma is the profound variation in its incidence among different geographic regions. Exceptionally high incidence rates are found in the Transkei region of South Africa, in Southern Brazil, in parts of Northern France and Italy, and throughout an esophageal cancer "belt" that extends from the shores of the Caspian Sea in Iran across northern China. In parts of China's Henan Province, the incidence of esophageal squamous cell carcinoma exceeds 100 per 100,000. In the United States, in contrast, the incidence of the tumor

in the general population is less than 4 per 100,000. In most countries, squamous cell carcinoma of the esophagus affects men two to four times more often than women and, within countries, there can be substantial differences in incidence rates among different ethnic groups. In the United States, for example, the incidence of squamous cell carcinoma of the esophagus in African-Americans is six times greater than that in Caucasians. These intriguing epidemiological features suggest that there are important cultural, dietary, environmental, and genetic risk factors for squamous cell carcinoma of the esophagus.

Etiology

In the United States and Europe, cigarette smoking and alcoholism are the major recognized risk factors for squamous cell carcinoma of the esophagus. Cigarette smoke contains a number of nitrosamines, polycyclic aromatic hydrocarbons, aromatic amines, aldehydes, and phenols that may contribute to carcinogenesis. The combination of cigarette smoking and alcoholism appears to have a synergistic (rather than merely additive) effect in esophageal carcinogenesis, but the mechanism of this synergy is not known. A variety of nutritional deficiencies have been associated with the tumor, including deficiencies in vitamins A and C, and in magnesium, selenium, and zinc. The esophagus is one of the first organs exposed to ingested carcinogens including N-nitroso compounds that can be formed from the nitrates and amines in pickled vegetables and cured meats. Regional practices such as opium smoking, and the chronic ingestion of very hot foods and beverages may play a role in esophageal carcinogenesis, and some high-incidence areas have soils that are poor in certain elements such as molybdenum and zinc.

There is evidence that certain microorganisms can contribute to esophageal carcinogenesis, and that local differences in endemic microflora might underlie some of the dramatic regional variations in the incidence of esophageal squamous cell carcinoma. The food and water in some high-incidence areas are contaminated with fungi and bacteria that promote the formation of carcinogenic N-nitroso compounds from dietary nitrates. The human papillomavirus (HPV) can infect squamous epithelial cells, and HPV infection has been implicated in the development of squamous cell carcinoma of the esophagus. The protein products of the E6 and E7 genes of HPV can interfere with normal tumor suppressor genes like p53 and retinoblastoma, and such interference might promote hyperproliferation and carcinogenesis. In high-incidence regions for esophageal cancer such as China and South Africa, researchers have found HPV DNA in > 20% of squamous cell carcinomas. In low-incidence areas like the United States, however, esophageal tumors generally do not show evidence of HPV infection.

There are a number of medical conditions that predispose to the development of esophageal squamous cell carcinoma. Tylosis, a rare heritable disorder characterized by hyperkeratosis of the palms and soles, is associated with a very high risk of developing esophageal cancer. Patients with tylosis have mutations in the tylosis esophageal cancer gene, a putative tumor suppressor located on the long arm of chromosome 17. Loss of heterozygosity for the tylosis esophageal cancer gene can be found frequently in sporadic esophageal cancers as well. Achalasia, lye stricture of the esophagus and Plummer-Vinson/Paterson-Kelly syndrome are risk factors for squamous cell cancers, perhaps because these conditions are associated with stasis of esophageal contents that leads to chronic inflammation of the mucosa. There is a strong association between cancer of the esophagus and malignancies of the head, neck, and lungs, presumably because these tumors share the strong risk factor of cigarette smoking. Celiac sprue (gluten sensitive enteropathy) has also been associated with esophageal cancer for reasons that are not clear.

Symptoms and Clinical Signs

The large majority of patients with squamous cell carcinoma of the esophagus present with the symptoms of dysphagia and weight loss. The dysphagia usually involves solid foods only, and the symptom progresses rapidly in severity (over a period of weeks to months). Patients typically perceive that swallowed material sticks at a point that is either above or at (but not below) the level of the obstructing tumor. Tumors of the proximal esophagus can invade the recurrent laryngeal nerve, causing vocal cord paralysis with hoarseness. Invasion into the airway with esophago-bronchial fistula causes coughing that is exacerbated by swallowing. Ulcerated tumors can cause odynophagia (pain with swallowing), and tumor necrosis occasionally causes esophageal hemorrhage. Local tumor invasion can cause chest pain, and metastatic disease can cause bone pain.

The physical examination is important for assessing the patient's nutritional status and ability to tolerate the invasive procedures that may be proposed for treatment, but only infrequently does the physical examination provide specific information about the esophageal cancer. Occasionally, the examiner may palpate a left supraclavicular (Virchow's) lymph node indicating that the tumor has metastasized.

Symptoms and signs of esophageal cancer generally develop only when the tumor has grown to the extent that it has narrowed the lumen of the esophagus substantially, has invaded local structures, or has metastasized. Therefore, the presence of symptoms is usually associated with disseminated disease, a feature that contributes to the poor prognosis of patients with squamous cell carcinoma of the esophagus.

Diagnostics

Synopsis

Standard imaging techniques for detection and staging of squamous cell carcinoma of the esophagus

▸ Barium swallow
▸ Endoscopy
▸ Computed tomography of the chest and abdomen
▸ Endoscopic ultrasonography

For patients with dysphagia, there is an unresolved debate whether to perform a barium swallow early in the evaluation, or whether it is more cost-effective to bypass the radiographic study and to proceed directly to endo-

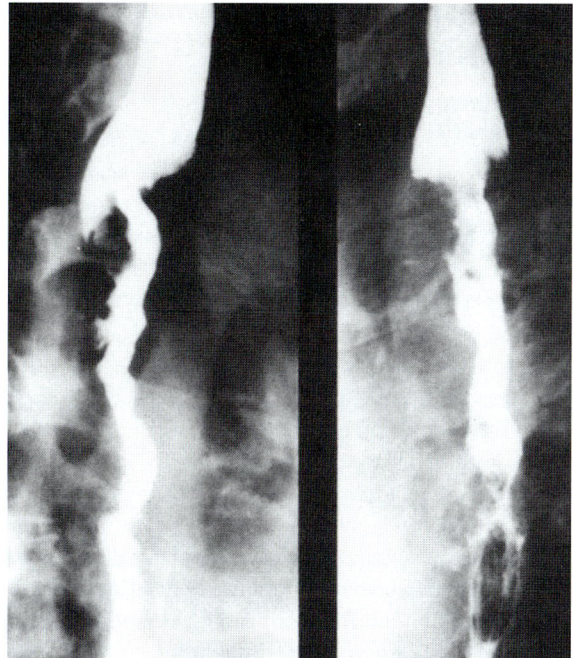

Figure 1
Barium swallow showing an advanced esophageal cancer. Not that the proximal edge of the ulcerated tumor forms an abrupt shelf that gives the lesion the appearance of an apple core. (Reprinted, with permission, from Spechler SJ, Esophageal disorders. Unit 9 of the Clinical Teaching Project of the American Gastroenterological Association)

proach, this debate will continue. Nevertheless, most authorities recommend both barium swallow and endoscopy for the evaluation of patients with esophageal cancer.

When a barium swallow demonstrates an esophageal lesion, features that suggest malignancy include irregular borders and sharp angles (Fig. 1). Unless contraindicated by serious comorbidity, endoscopic evaluation is recommended for virtually all patients with dysphagia irrespective of the radiographic findings. Unlike the radiologist, the endoscopist can obtain biopsy and brush cytology specimens to establish a specific diagnosis of esophageal cancer. Endoscopically, squamous cell carcinomas of the esophagus typically appear as nodular lesions that protrude into the lumen of the esophagus (Fig. 2). In Asian countries where there is a high incidence of esophageal cancer, physicians have described the endoscopic characteristics of early esophageal cancers. These superficial lesions cause either slight elevations or shallow depressions in the mucosal surface, and they have been categorized into flat, polyploid, or

scopic evaluation of the esophagus. Those who advocate early radiology contend that the barium swallow provides valuable anatomic information that may help to prevent procedural complications and to direct therapy. Also, an initial barium swallow provides an objective baseline record of the esophageal tumor that can be useful in assessing the response to therapy or progression of disease. Proponents of early endoscopy argue that this procedure is virtually always required in the evaluation of dysphagia, regardless of the radiographic findings, and that a barium swallow usually does not provide sufficient additional information to justify its added expense and inconvenience. Furthermore, no study has yet shown that performance of a barium swallow prior to endoscopy decreases complications or improves outcomes for patients with dysphagia. In the absence of meaningful studies validating the benefits of either ap-

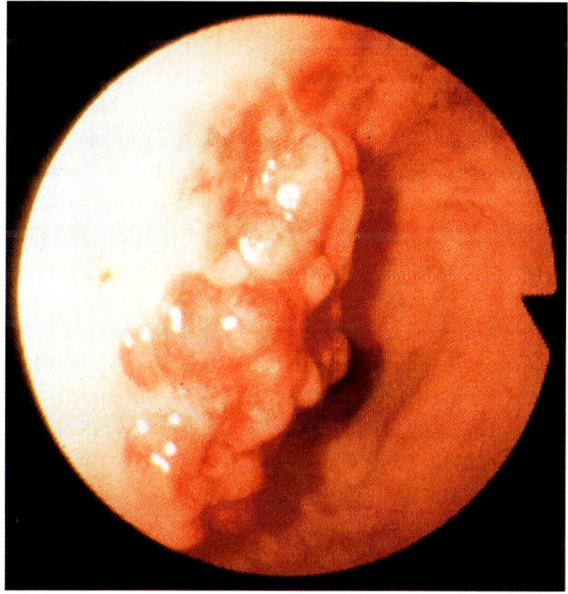

Figure 2
Endoscopic photograph of a nodular squamous cell carcinoma of the mid-esophagus. (Reprinted, with permission, from Spechler SJ, Esophageal disorders. Unit 9 of the Clinical Teaching Project of the American Gastroenterological Association)

ulcerated types. Staining of the esophagus with vital dyes such as toluidine blue or Lugol's iodine (chromo-endoscopy) can be useful for finding such early lesions during endoscopic evaluation. Superficial esophageal cancers are diagnosed infrequently in western countries.

For patients found to have squamous cell carcinoma by endoscopic evaluation, computed tomography (CT) of the chest and abdomen is recommended to assess the extent of disease within the chest, and to look for metastases. Similar information can be obtained with magnetic resonance imaging (MRI), but CT usually is recommended because it is more readily available, more familiar to clinicians, and less expensive than MRI. The sensitivity and specificity of CT for determining the extent of esophageal wall involvement and the presence of regional lymph node metastases is poor, however. Limited studies suggest that positron emission tomography (PET) may be more sensitive than CT for detecting metastases, but further studies are needed before PET scanning can be recommended for general clinical application in esophageal cancer.

Endoscopic ultrasonography (EUS) uses high frequency ultrasonic waves to provide detailed images of the esophageal wall and its adjacent structures. A number of studies have shown that EUS is more accurate than CT for assessing the depth of esophageal tumor penetration (the T-level) and for detecting tumor involvement in regional lymph nodes (the N-status). EUS correctly predicts the T and N status in approximately 70% to 80% of cases of squamous cell carcinoma of the esophagus. The accuracy of the test is dependent on the skill of the operator, however. Although EUS generally is recommended for patients with squamous cell carcinoma of the esophagus, there is no proof that the procedure has improved clinical outcomes.

Invasive diagnostic modalities that are sometimes used for the staging of esophageal cancer include bronchoscopy, laparoscopy, thoracotomy, and thoracoscopy. There is little consensus regarding the need for these procedures in the routine evaluation of patients with esophageal cancer, and usage of the procedures varies widely among different institutions.

Histological Classification and Molecular Genetics

Synopsis

Squamous cell carcinoma of the esophagus evolves through a sequence of genetic alterations that activate proto-oncogenes and disable tumor suppressor genes. Before the affected cells become malignant, the genetic alterations often cause morphological changes in the tissue that are recognizable histologically as dysplasia. Genetic abnormalities found in squamous cell carcinoma of the esophagus frequently involve genes that regulate the transition from the G1 to the S phase of the cell cycle including retinoblastoma, cyclin, and p53 genes. Aberrant telomerase expression is found in virtually all cases.

Histologically, squamous cell carcinoma of the esophagus is characterized by the presence of keratinocyte-like cells that exhibit intercellular bridges, keratinization, or both (Fig. 3). The tumors are thought to evolve through a sequence of genetic alterations, which endow the affected cells with growth advantages. With the accumulation of mutations that activate proto-oncogenes and disable tumor suppressor genes, the advantaged cells lose their responsiveness to normal growth controls (i.e. they become neoplastic). When neoplastic cells acquire

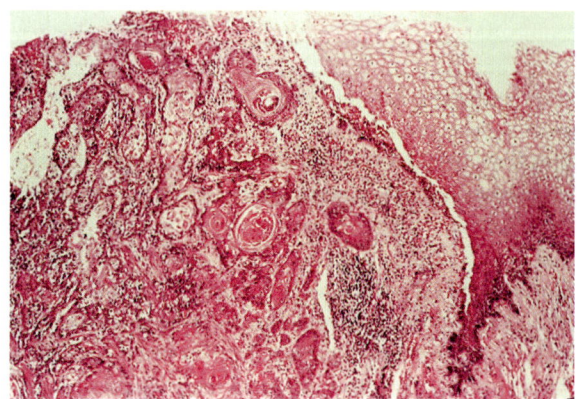

Figure 3
Photomicrograph of a well-differentiated squamous cell carcinoma of the esophagus. Note the keratin pearls and irregular configuration of the nests of malignant squamous cells. (Reprinted, with permission, from Spechler SJ, Esophageal disorders. Unit 9 of the Clinical Teaching Project of the American Gastroenterological Association)

some critical combination of DNA abnormalities, there emerges a clone of malignant cells that can invade adjacent tissues and proliferate in unnatural locations. Before the neoplastic cells become malignant, genetic alterations underlying the growth abnormalities may cause morphological changes in the tissue that are recognizable histologically as dysplasia (also called intra-epithelial neoplasia). Dysplasia is a histological diagnosis, which suggests that one or more clones of epithelial cells have acquired genetic alterations causing inappropriate proliferation, abnormal differentiation, and a predisposition to malignancy. Dysplasia is categorized as low or high grade depending on the extent of cytological and architectural changes.

The genetic alterations found in squamous cell carcinoma of the esophagus frequently involve genes that regulate the transition from the G1 to the S phase of the cell cycle, a key step in cellular proliferation. Retinoblastoma (Rb) protein functions as the molecular switch that ultimately controls the transition from G1 to S. Rb protein that is not sufficiently phosphorylated normally functions to block this transition. Phosphorylation inactivates the Rb protein, and thereby allows the cell cycle to advance from G1 to S.

Cyclins are intracellular proteins that complex with cyclin-dependent kinases (cdks), and these complexes effect the phosphorylation that inactivates Rb protein. The tumor suppressor gene p53 inhibits the phosphorylation of Rb protein, and thereby blocks progression from G1 to S. Abnormalities of the Rb gene have been found in up to 70% of esophageal squamous cell carcinomas. Abnormalities in cyclin expression have been observed in 40% to 60%, and mutations in p53 have been detected in 50% to 80% of cases.

Telomeres are tandem repeat nucleotide sequences found at the ends of chromosomes that prevent the ends from fusing, a process that can be lethal to the cell. As cells age, telomeric repeats are lost with each cell cycle until a critical point is reached at which the cell can no longer divide, and instead becomes senescent. Telomerase is an enzyme that adds telomeric repeat units to the ends of chromosomes. Aberrant expression of telomerase can induce the immortality that characterizes cancer cells, and aberrant telomerase expression has been found in virtually all squamous cell carcinomas tested.

Other potentially important genetic alterations that have been found in squamous cell carcinomas include abnormalities of the tylosis esophageal cancer gene, the DLC1 gene, the FHIT gene, the epidermal growth factor receptor gene, and the erbB2 gene.

Staging

Synopsis

TNM classification of squamous cell carcinoma of the esophagus

T	**Primary tumor**
TX	Primary tumor cannot be assessed
T0	No evidence of primary tumor
Tis	Carcinoma in situ
T1	Tumor invades lamina propria or submucosa
T2	Tumor invades muscularis propria
T3	Tumor invades adventitia
T4	Tumor invades adjacent structures
N	**Regional lymph nodes**
NX	Regional lymph nodes cannot be assessed
N0	No regional lymph node metastases
N1	Regional lymph node metastases
M	**Distant metastases**
MX	Distant metastases cannot be assessed
M0	No distant metastases
M1	Distant metastases

Stage groupings	T	N	M
Stage 0	Tis	N0	M0
Stage I	T1	N0	M0
Stage IIA	T2	N0	M0
	T3	N0	M0
Stage IIB	T1	N1	M0
	T3	N1	M0
Stage III	T3	N1	M0
	T4	Any N	M0
Stage IV	Any T	Any N	M1

The preoperative staging of squamous cell carcinoma is discussed in the Diagnostics section. Definitive staging is established postoperatively after the pathologist has evaluated resected tissue. Most authorities agree on the use of the TNM staging system for squamous cell carcinoma of the esophagus, but usage of the stage grouping system shown above varies among institutions.

Treatment

Synopsis

Treatment algorithm for squamous cell carcinoma of the esophagus. Entry into controlled therapeutic trials is the preferred management strategy for virtually all patients. The following algorithm is proposed as a general guide if trials are not available. This strategy assumes that patients have had staging that includes at least a CT scan of the chest and abdomen, and EUS. CRT = chemoradiation therapy.

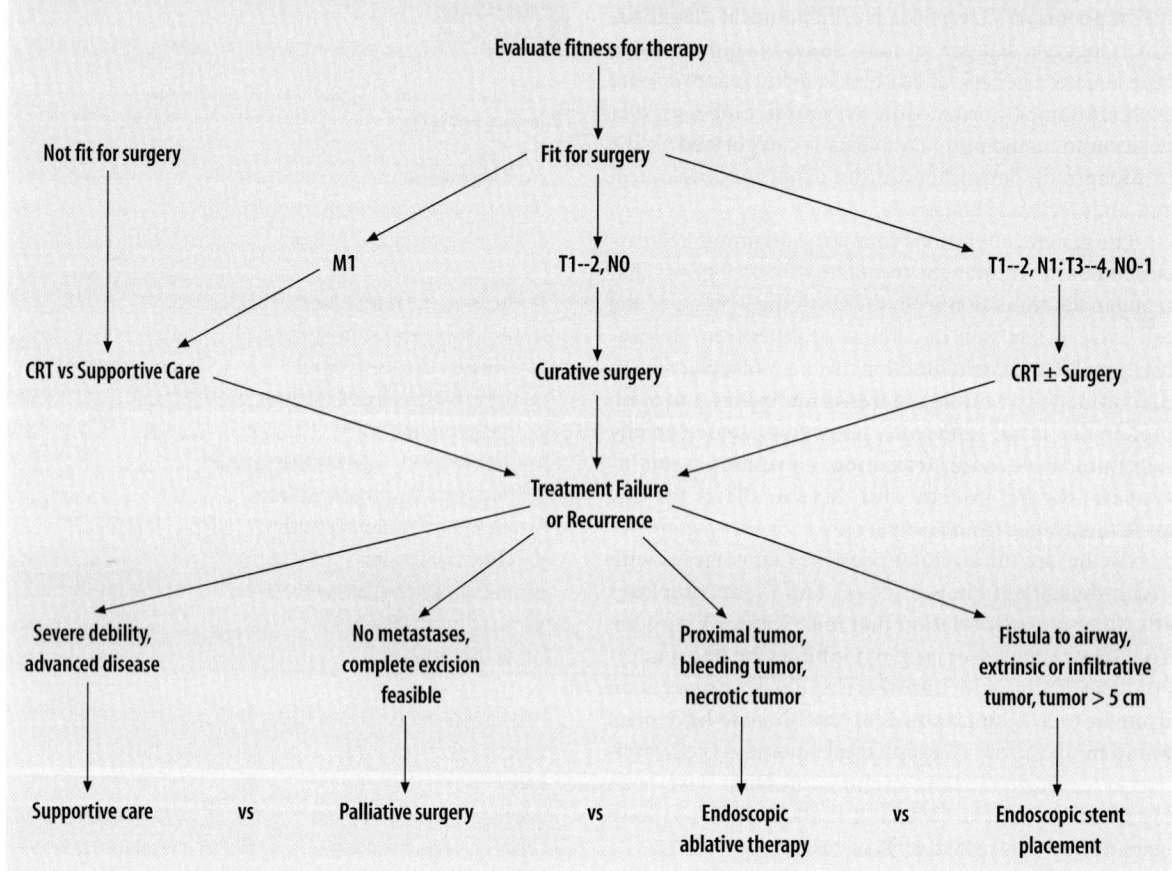

In designing therapies for esophageal cancer, the clinician should consider the extensive lymphatic system of the esophagus that serves as a ready conduit for tumor dissemination. Small lymphatic vessels in the esophageal mucosa drain into larger submucosal vessels that extend throughout the length of the organ. Similarly, small lymphatics in the muscularis propria drain into larger vessels that traverse the muscular layers and adventitia of the esophagus. These two major groups of esophageal lymphatics intercommunicate with one another and with vessels supplying adjacent lymph nodes, thereby providing the means for both longitudinal and lateral spread of esophageal cancer. Tumor cells often enter these lymphatic channels as evidenced by the common finding of metastases in the wall of the esophagus widely separated from the primary cancer, and by the frequent finding of metastases in abdominal lymph nodes of patients with tumors in the mid- and proximal esophagus.

Squamous cell carcinoma of the esophagus is usually disseminated at the time of diagnosis and, because there is no treatment that reliably eradicates metastatic disease, cure is not possible in most cases. Furthermore, patients are often elderly, alcoholic smokers with severe comorbidities (e.g. malnutrition; pulmonary, cardiac, liver disease) that further limit their treatment options. Initial treatment usually involves a choice among surgery, radiation therapy, chemotherapy, or some combination of these three modalities. When used in combination with surgery, radiation and chemotherapy have been used both pre- and postoperatively, alone or in combination. Despite recent advances in therapeutic options, however, overall cure rates for squamous cell carcinoma of the esophagus remain below 10%. For patients with localized, early lesions (Tis or T1, N0, M0), endoscopic therapies (endoscopic mucosal resection, photodynamic therapy) have been used with promising results in uncontrolled studies from Asia. These early lesions are seen rarely in western countries, however.

Surgery

Surgery (esophagectomy ± lymphadenectomy) can provide immediate palliation of symptoms and, arguably, the best potential for cure of squamous cell carcinoma. Mortality rates for esophagectomy vary significantly among institutions according to the frequency with which the operation is performed. In a recent study of 340 esophagectomies performed at 25 different hospitals, the mortality rate was 3.0% for patients treated at institutions that did 5 or more esophagectomies per year, compared to 12.2% for patients treated at institutions where the operation was performed less frequently. Esophagectomy also entails substantial morbidity. Common, serious complications of the operation include respiratory problems (e.g. pneumonia, atelectasis), cardiovascular problems (e.g. arrhythmias, myocardial infarction, heart failure), wound infections, and anastomotic leaks. One or more such complications can be expected in 30% to 50% of patients, and the average hospital stay for open esophagectomy is approximately two weeks. Available data on minimally invasive techniques for esophagectomy are promising but limited, and it is not yet clear that these techniques offer important advantages over the standard, open procedures. Cure rates vary widely among institutions, and with prognostic factors that include tumor stage and the number of positive lymph nodes. Surgery is not recommended for patients who have metastatic disease.

The acute mortality of radiation therapy is low, and radiation can cover a wider treatment area than is practical with surgery (to eradicate locoregional disease). However, radiotherapy usually takes 2 to 8 weeks to complete, palliation can be delayed for weeks, there can be substantial radiation damage to surrounding normal tissues, and the overall cure rate is low. Trials of radiation therapy as the sole treatment modality for squamous cell carcinoma of the esophagus have included primarily patients with advanced disease and tumors that were deemed unresectable. Results appear to be comparable to surgery, nevertheless, although there are no randomized trials directly comparing radiation therapy alone with surgery alone.

Chemotherapy

Chemotherapy has the potential to reach the disseminated disease that is usually present in symptomatic patients. Unfortunately, chemotherapy is associated with substantial morbidity and considerable mortality, is often ineffective, and the tumor response (if any) is often brief. Studies of chemotherapy as the sole treatment modality have included primarily patients with unresectable tumors. Modern studies have used cisplatin-based regimens, and response rates appear to be better with combination regimens than with single agents. Chemotherapy alone does not appear to improve survival, however.

Radiochemotherapy

A number of studies have explored the role of radiation or chemotherapy used either before (neoadjuvant) or after (adjuvant) definitive surgery for squamous cell carcinoma of the esophagus. Unfortunately, a number of randomized, controlled trials have shown no convincing benefit for adjuvant or neoadjuvant treatment with either radiation or chemotherapy for patients with potentially resectable tumors.

Much recent interest has focused on the role of combining chemotherapy with radiation therapy (chemoradiotherapy) for esophageal cancer. In some studies of patients treated with chemoradiotherapy followed by esophagectomy, complete histologic response (defined as no histologic evidence of tumor in the resected specimen) has been observed in almost 30% of cases. Complete histologic response is not tantamount to cure, however, and even complete responders frequently succumb to recurrent disease. Furthermore, chemoradiotherapy is associated with serious toxicity. Some randomized trials of chemoradiotherapy for patients with potentially resectable tumors have shown significant improvements in survival, whereas others have not. Consequently, the role of chemoradiotherapy remains unclear. Preliminary studies suggest that patients who have locally advanced tumors might benefit from preoperative chemoradiotherapy, especially if the tumors are located at or above the bifurcation of the trachea. The proximity of such tumors to the airway makes adequate surgical resection difficult, and "downsizing" the tumors with preoperative chemoradiotherapy may convert an unresectable tumor into a resectable one.

Endoscopic Palliation

Purely palliative therapies include esophageal dilatation and the placement of intraluminal stents. There also are palliative techniques designed to ablate the portion of the neoplasm that obstructs the esophageal lumen. These ablative therapies include endoscopic laser irradiation, the application of tumor probes that burn the neoplasm directly, the injection of caustic chemicals directly into the tumor body, and photodynamic therapy that uses photochemical energy to destroy the tumor. Other experimental therapies include the placement of radioactive materials within the esophageal lumen (brachytherapy) and the use of local hyperthermia to enhance the efficacy of radiation and chemotherapy.

Whereas the optimal treatment for cancer of the esophagus is not clear, patients should be treated according to well designed, established research protocols whenever possible. This approach eliminates anguish in choosing among treatments of dubious value, provides clear guidelines for patient management, and offers an opportunity to evaluate the efficacy of the experimental therapy in a systematic and meaningful fashion. If the initial use of research protocols is not feasible, an alternative approach is outlined above. After staging of the tumor that includes at least EUS and a CT scan of the chest and abdomen, the next step is to decide if the patient is fit enough to undergo surgery. If surgery is not a viable option because of advanced age or comorbidity, then primary therapy might include chemoradiation or supportive care alone. In general, surgery is not in-

dicated for patients with metastatic disease. Primary therapy for such patients might include chemoradiation or supportive care alone. For tumors that do not invade beyond the muscularis propria, and do not involve local lymph nodes, surgery appears to offer the best hope for cure. For lesions that are more advanced due to lymph node involvement or invasion to the adventitia and beyond, the choices for primary therapy include chemoradiation with or without surgery. If these primary treatments fail, or if the tumor recurs, there are a number of palliative treatment options. For a patient who is severely debilitated and who has advanced disease, the most humane option may be only supportive care with careful attention to pain control. If there are no apparent metastases, and complete excision of the tumor is possible, then surgery can be considered for palliation. The other options are ablative therapies or stents. Stents may not provide good palliation for patients with proximal tumors, bleeding tumors, and necrotic tumors, and ablative therapy may be preferable in these circumstances. On the other hand, ablative therapy has little to offer for a patient with an esophago-bronchial fistula, or for a patient with a tumor that is extrinsic or infiltrative. Moreover, ablative therapy may be difficult and time-consuming for patients with very long tumors, and stenting may be preferable in these circumstances.

Prognosis and Follow-Up

As discussed, patients who have symptoms of squamous cell cancer of the esophagus generally have advanced disease and a poor prognosis. Overall 5-year survival rates are below 10%. Among patients who are treated with esophagectomy, survival correlates with the number of positive lymph nodes in the resected tissue. Although prognosis clearly correlates with the stage of disease at presentation, reported survival rates within stages vary widely among institutions. For stage 0 and I tumors, which are rarely seen in western countries, 5-year survivals exceeding 60% can be anticipated with appropriate treatment. Five-year survival rates are approximately 10% to 15% for patients with stage III disease, and < 5% for those with stage IV tumors. Especially wide ranges of survivals have been reported for patients with stage II cancers, but a survival rate of 15% to 25% at 5 years seems a realistic overall estimate for this group.

There is no clear consensus regarding what constitutes appropriate follow-up of patients who have had treatment for esophageal cancer. Some authorities advocate periodic follow-up with endoscopy and CT scans for patients who have had curative resections of esophageal tumors, but there is little evidence that early detection of tumor recurrences and spread influences outcome.

Screening, Surveillance, Prevention

In most western countries, the incidence of squamous cell carcinoma of the esophagus is too low to warrant screening programs for the general population. In some high-incidence areas of Asia, high-risk populations have been screened for the tumor using either brush cytology (in which individuals swallow a balloon that is dragged through the esophagus to scrape off cells for cytologic examination) or with endoscopy. Although it is clear that these techniques can identify some individuals with early tumors, no published data document that screening programs for squamous cell carcinoma of the esophagus have decreased morbidity or mortality from the tumor. Also, there are no data that document the efficacy of surveillance programs for patients found to have high-risk lesions like dysplasia in esophageal squamous epithelium.

Dietary supplementation with β-carotene, selenium, and α-tocopherol was found to decrease mortality from esophageal cancer in a large, randomized trial of individuals living in a high-incidence area of China. No beneficial effect for dietary supplements was found in another large trial of Chinese patients who already had esophageal dysplasia, however. The chronic ingestion of green tea, which contains potentially protective compounds like phenols, was found to be associated with a decreased risk of esophageal cancer in study in Shanghai. Some studies suggest that it may be possible to reduce the risk of developing esophageal cancer by taking aspirin. In one study of 13,300 Americans who were followed for 12 to 16 years, the incidence of esophageal cancer among subjects who reported that they had used aspirin was found to be 80% to 90% lower than that for subjects who denied aspirin use. There are also data to suggest that abstinence from alcohol and cigarette smoking may decrease the risk of developing squamous cell carcinoma of the esophagus.

Future Perspectives

At least three factors contribute importantly to the dismal prognosis for patients with squamous cell carcinoma of the esophagus: 1) there are no early warning symptoms, 2) the tumor has a strong propensity to metastasize and 3) patients are often elderly and debilitated by alcoholism, cigarette smoking, and comorbid illnesses. In this setting, research directed at refining surgical techniques to eradicate local disease is important, but unlikely to result in major improvements in survival. Efforts directed at prevention in high-risk populations (e.g. avoidance of cigarette smoking and alcohol consumption), and at eradicating metastatic disease seem more likely to reduce morbidity and mortality from this lethal tumor. Recent data suggest that defects in the genes that regulate the transition from the G1 to the S phase of the cell cycle underlie the development of squamous cell carcinoma. Research efforts directed at correcting those defects could conceivably lead to the development of agents that could prevent or even reverse carcinogenesis in the esophagus.

References

1. Blot WJ, Li JY, Taylor PR, Guo W, Dawsey SM, Li B. The Linxian trials: mortality rates by vitamin-mineral intervention group. Am J Clin Nutr 1995; 62 (Suppl):1424S–1426S.
2. Blot WJ, McLaughlin JK. The changing epidemiology of esophageal cancer. Semin Oncol 1999; 26 (Suppl 15):2–8.
3. Bosset JF, Gignoux M, Triboulet JP, Tiret E, Mantion G, Elias D, Lozach P, Ollier JC, Pavy JJ, Mercier M, Sahmoud T. Chemoradiotherapy followed by surgery compared with surgery alone in squamous-cell cancer of the esophagus. N Engl J Med 1997; 337: 161–167.
4. Fleisher AS, Meltzer SJ. Esophageal cancer: molecular biology and genetics. In: Kelsen D, Daly JM, Kern SE, Levin B, Tepper JE, eds. Gastrointestinal oncology: principles and practice. Philadelphia: Lippincott Williams & Wilkins. 2002: 211–225.
5. Funkhouser EM, Sharp GB. Aspirin and reduced risk of esophageal carcinoma. Cancer 1995; 76: 1116–1119.
6. Nakagawa H, Zukerberg L, Togawa K, Meltzer SJ, Nishihara T, Rustgi AK. Human cyclin D1 oncogene and esophageal squamous cell carcinoma. Cancer 1995; 76: 541–549.
7. O'Sullivan GC, Sheehan D, Clarke A, Stuart R, Kelly J, Kiely MD, Walsh T, Collins JK, Shanahan F. Micrometastases in esophagogastric cancer: high detection rate in resected rib segments. Gastroenterology 1999; 116: 543–548.
8. Sibille A, Lambert R, Souquet JC, Sabben G, Descos F. Long-term survival after photodynamic therapy for esophageal cancer. Gastroenterology 1995; 108: 337–344.
9. Siewert JR, Stein HJ, Sendler A, Molls M, Find U. Esophageal cancer: clinical management. In: Kelsen D, Daly JM, Kern SE, Levin B, Tepper JE, eds. Gastrointestinal oncology: principles and practice. Philadelphia: Lippincott Williams & Wilkins. 2002:261–287.
10. Stoner G, Gupta A. Etiology and chemoprevention of esophageal squamous cell carcinoma. Carcinogenesis 2001; 22: 1737–1746.

2 Adenocarcinoma of the Esophagus

O. PECH, A. MAY, L. GOSSNER, C. ELL

Summary

As a result of the increase in its incidence, Barrett's carcinoma has increasingly become a focus of interest in recent years. If the lesion represents intraepithelial high-grade neoplasia or mucosal Barrett's carcinoma, then after a careful staging examination, local endoscopic therapy is the treatment of choice. If more advanced tumor stages are present, radical esophageal resection is the only curative procedure. In locally inoperable tumors, neoadjuvant chemoradiotherapy can be carried out to reduce the tumor volume. Otherwise, attention should concentrate on palliative treatment aimed at maintaining or restoring the esophageal passage.

Epidemiology

An increase in the incidence of adenocarcinoma of the esophagogastric junction occurred in the early 1990s. Among other reasons, this increase is due to better training of endoscopists and pathologists, the further development of endoscopic technology with the introduction of high-resolution video endoscopes, and not least due to a certain enthusiasm on the part of pathologists and gastroenterologists. The proportion of adenocarcinomas among esophageal carcinomas was only ca. 5% 20 years ago, but it has now become the most frequent malignant tumor of the esophagus in Western countries.

In Barrett's esophagus, a distinction needs to be made according to the length of the lesion between short-segment Barrett's esophagus (SSBE; <3 cm) and long-segment Barrett's esophagus (LSBE; ≥3 cm). The term "micro-Barrett's" refers to macroscopically invisible but histologically evident Barrett's mucosa.

A diagnosis of Barrett's esophagus is made in ca. 10% of esophagogastroscopies in patients with GERD. The risk of developing an adenocarcinoma is 30–125 times higher in patients with Barrett's esophagus than in the normal population. The frequency of carcinoma appears to correlate with the period and intensity of reflux symptoms. Patients with nocturnal reflux have an 11-fold increased risk, and patients with severe long-term reflux have a 44-fold increased risk of adenocarcinoma. The risk of developing Barrett's carcinoma also appears to correlate with the body mass index (BMI). It has been shown that patients with a BMI >30 kg/m^2 have a 16.2-fold increased risk in comparison with the normal population.

Although the data are not yet clear, SSBE must also be regarded as a precancerous condition, and it requires the same monitoring strategy as that used with LSBE [1].

Etiology and Pathogenesis

Barrett's esophagus is defined as the presence of specialized intestinal metaplastic columnar epithelium in the tubular esophagus. It represents a complication of chronic gastroesophageal reflux disease [2]. Patients frequently report heartburn that has persisted for several years, and in almost every case an axial hiatus hernia is found at esophagogastroduodenoscopy (EGD).

The chronic inflammatory irritation leads to tissue damage and chronic inflammation in the area of squamous epithelium. The process through which intestinal metaplasia develops during the course has not yet been fully clarified. The development passes from simple Barrett's metaplasia via the intermediate stages of low-grade intraepithelial neoplasia (LGIN) and high-grade intraepithelial neoplasia (HGIN) to reach the stage of adenocarcinoma.

Symptoms and Clinical Signs

Most patients with Barrett's carcinoma have a history of several years of heartburn. With the growing awareness of this pathogenetic link, patients with heartburn are undergoing upper gastrointestinal endoscopy increasingly earlier. It is during these endoscopic examinations that most intraepithelial neoplasias or early carcinomas are diagnosed.

There are no early symptoms of carcinoma as such. Advanced esophageal carcinomas mainly cause dysphagia; invasion of the recurrent laryngeal nerve leads to hoarseness, and invasion of the trachea often causes coughing.

Diagnosis

Synopsis

Techniques for detecting and staging Barrett's adeno-carcinoma:

▸ Upper endoscopy with four-quadrant biopsies
▸ Chromoendoscopy
▸ Endoscopic ultrasound
▸ Computed tomography
▸ Transabdominal ultrasound.

EGD should always be carried out in patients with chronic reflux symptoms. If the examination produces evidence of Barrett's esophagus, four-quadrant biopsies every 2 cm over the entire Barrett's segment are obligatory. If there is no dysplasia, an endoscopic check-up examination with biopsy every 2 years is sufficient. If LGIN is identified in the biopsies, further check-up endoscopies should be carried out twice at 6-month intervals, and thereafter annually. If HGIN is identified, the diagnosis should be confirmed by a reference pathologist. A tight check-up schedule every 3 months, or treatment, should then follow [3].

In addition to the obligatory blind four-quadrant biopsies, all abnormal areas in the Barrett's esophagus should be biopsied. The use of high-resolution video endoscopy should be standard. In addition, procedures such as chromoendoscopy or photodynamic diagnosis (PDD) are available.

Methylene blue staining using a special spraying catheter can stain specialized columnar epithelium with a sensitivity of ca. 90%. The dye is actively taken up by goblet cells of the intestinal mucosa, and produces reversible staining of the Barrett's mucosa. Inhomogeneous and weaker staining suggests the presence of intraepithelial neoplasia or early carcinoma.

Early malignant changes can be identified using PDD after oral administration of 5-aminolevulinic acid. A xenon gas lamp, an incoherent light source, selectively stimulates the protoporphyrin IX that forms in the blue wavelength range in malignant tissue. Areas with LGIN, HGIN or early adenocarcinoma ideally shine in red.

Both chromoendoscopy and PDD allow targeted biopsy of very discrete changes, thereby improving early diagnosis of neoplastic areas in Barrett's epithelium (Figs. 1–5).

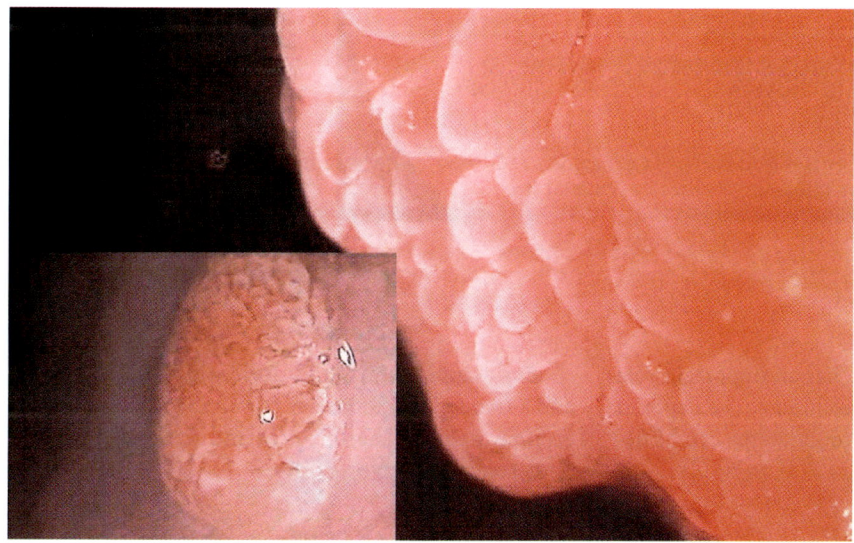

Figure 1
Early Barrett's carcinoma after acetic acid instillation

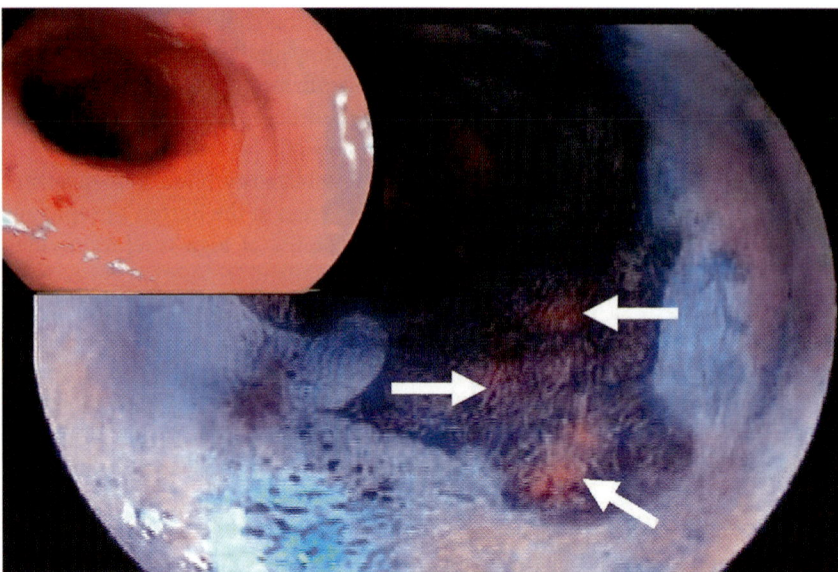

Figure 2
Early Barrett's carcinoma Type IIb
after methylene blue staining

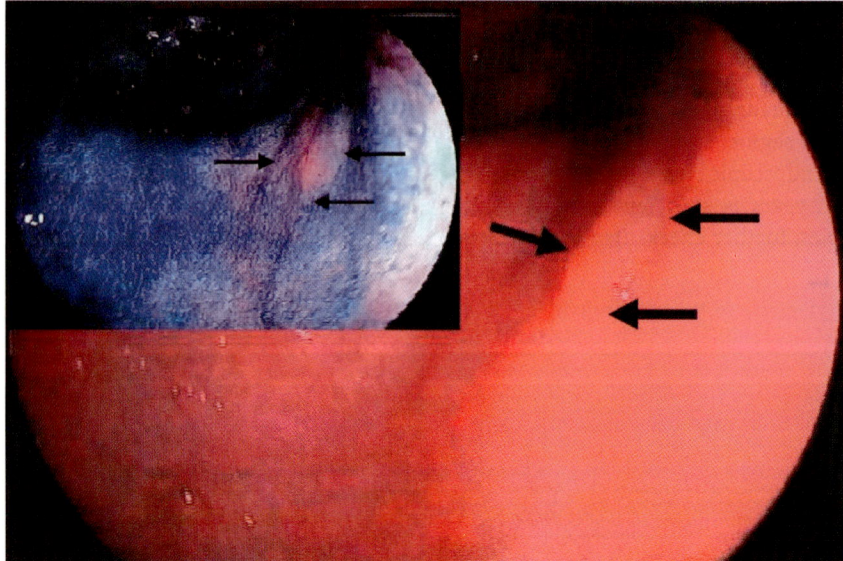

Figure 3
Early Barrett's carcinoma Type IIa
after methylene blue staining

Endoscopic ultrasonography has an important role in the diagnosis of esophageal carcinoma. The depth of tumor invasion and local lymph-node status can be determined using this method.

Endoscopic ultrasound devices with a 360° sector and a frequency of between 7.5 and 12 MHz have a penetration depth of up to 10 cm and are used to detect paraesophageal lymph nodes.

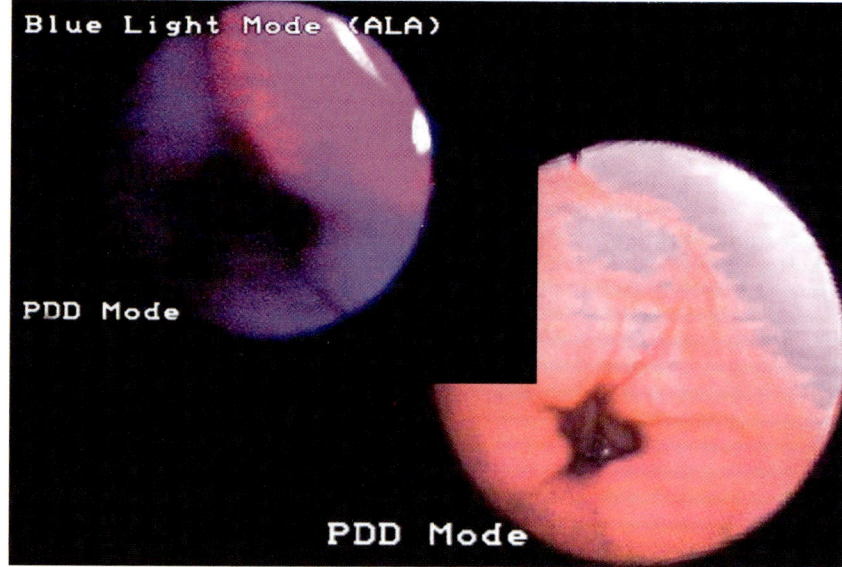

Figure 4
Early Barrett's carcinoma in PDD mode

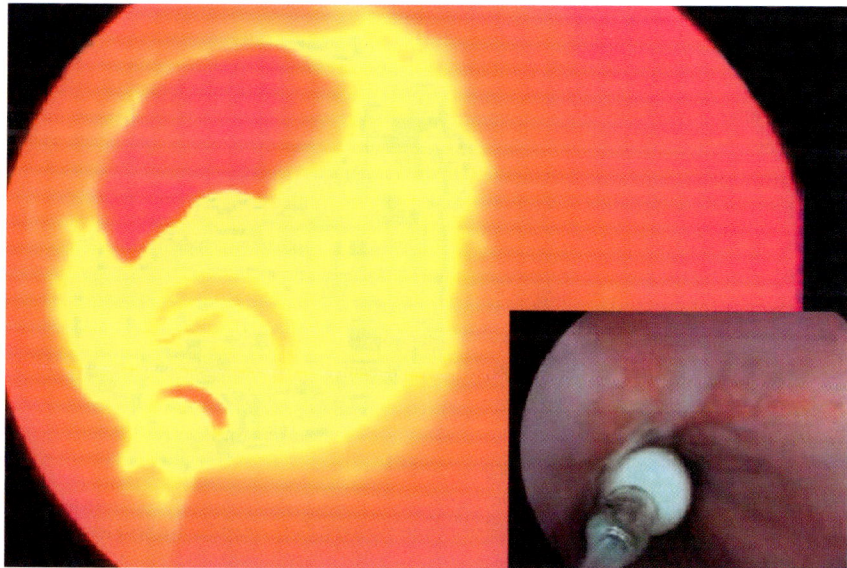

Figure 5
PDT of early Barrett's carcinoma

Miniature probes with a frequency of 15–20 MHz offer higher resolution, with a reduced depth of penetration. These probes make it possible to distinguish a mucosal carcinoma from a submucosal one, for example. This distinction is decisive particularly in relation to local endoscopic therapy, since the risk of lymph-node metastases in mucosal carcinomas is almost nonexistent. It is only with more advanced submucosal invasion (T1sm2–3) that positive lymph nodes can be expected in 20–25% of cases.

Computed tomography of the chest and upper abdomen should also be carried out in patients with adenocarcinoma of the esophagogastric junction. This method can detect distant metastases, in addition to local lymph-node metastases.

Histological Classification and Molecular Genetics

Synopsis

Metaplasia–dysplasia–adenocarcinoma sequence

Barrett's metaplasia – intraepithelial low-grade neoplasia – intraepithelial high-grade neoplasia – adenocarcinoma.

Macroscopic types:
▶ Type I polypoid lesions
▶ Type IIa slightly elevated
▶ Type IIb at the mucosal level
▶ Type IIc depressed
▶ Type III ulcerated.

Barrett's esophagus is defined as the replacement of the squamous epithelium lining the lower esophagus by specialized metaplastic columnar epithelium. Hence, "columnar epithelial-lined lower esophagus" is an alternative term for Barrett's esophagus. The specialized epithelium shows a distinctive villous-like pattern and consists mostly of columnar cells, with fewer interspersed goblet cells. Additional histological criteria for Barrett's metaplasia include pre-goblet cells and a newly formed muscularis mucosae.

Barrett's carcinoma has to be distinguished from adenocarcinoma of the distal esophagus, which is not associated with Barrett's mucosa. The various grades of differentiation range from well differentiated (G1) to poorly differentiated (G3). LGIN and HGIN are regarded as preliminary stages of carcinoma.

The adenoma-carcinoma sequence is an accepted model in the development of colorectal carcinoma. On analogy with this model, a metaplasia-dysplasia-adenocarcinoma sequence is currently described in Barrett's carcinoma. This process leads step by step, after the loss of cycle checkpoints and genomic instability, to clonal expansion as a result of increased proliferation. Important events in carcinogenesis include mutation of p16, p53 and cyclin D, aneuploidy and microsatellite instability.

Increased cyclin D1 expression, hypermethylated or mutated p16, increased telomerase RNA, and mobilization of cells from G0 to G1 with subsequent accumulation in the G2 phase, are frequently observed in dysplastic tissue. The mutation of p53 appears to take place only late in the development into adenocarcinoma. Sixty-five percent of LGINs, 75% of HGINs, and 50–90% of Barrett's carcinomas show p53 mutation [4].

In adenocarcinomas of the esophagus, loss of heterozygosity of the following tumor-suppressor gene loci is frequently found: CDKN2, retinoblastoma gene, APC and VHL. Ubiquitous microsatellite instability occurs in 5–15% of Barrett's carcinoma cell populations.

Staging

Synopsis

TNM classification of esophageal cancers

T	Primary tumor
TX	Minimum requirements for assessing the primary tumor cannot be met
T0	No evidence of primary tumor
T1a	Tumor is limited to the mucosa (T1 m)
T1b	Tumor limited to the submucosa (T1sm)
T2	Tumor invading the tunica muscularis propria
T3	Tumor invading the tunica adventitia
T4	Tumor invading other organs
N	Regional lymph nodes
NX	Minimum requirements for assessing the lymph-node status cannot be met
N0	No metastases in the regional lymph nodes
N1	Regional lymph-node metastases
M	Distant metastasis
MX	Minimum requirements for assessing distant metastases cannot be met
M0	No distant metastases
M1	Distant metastases

Stage groupings	T	N	M	5-year survival [%]
Stage I	1	0	0	67
Stage IIa	2–3	0	0	43
Stage IIb	1–2	1	0	26
Stage III	3–4	0–1	0	16
Stage IV	1–4	0–1	1	3

The examinations required for the staging of esophageal carcinoma (transabdominal ultrasound, endoscopic ultrasound, helical computed tomography) are mentioned above. The definitive tumor stage with regard to local extension and lymph-node involvement can only be determined by the pathologist, following surgical resection of the tumor.

Treatment

Synopsis

Treatment of Barrett's adenocarcinoma

▶ HGIN/T1 m: Local endoscopic therapy (Endoscopic mucosal resection (EMR) and/or Photodynamic therapy (PDT))
▶ T1sm, stage II + III: Esophagectomy/chemoradiotherapy
▶ Stage IV: Palliative treatment.

Surgery

Radical esophageal resection continues to be the gold standard in the treatment of esophageal carcinoma [5]. Candidates for surgical treatment are principally patients with a tumor stage of 1 or 2. If there is a mucosal carcinoma, however, esophageal resection, with its high mortality and morbidity rates, does not appear to be justified, in view of the current data regarding endoscopic therapy. If the tumor has already invaded the final two-thirds of the submucosa, or if lymph-node metastases are found during preoperative staging, esophageal resection is the only curative procedure.

Surgical treatment consists of subtotal removal of the esophagus and restoration of the alimentary passage by transposing the stomach or interposing colon (a long vascular pedicle is possible here), or in rare cases jejunum (often with the mesocolon being left too short). Anastomosis is usually made in an extrathoracic location in the throat (collar anastomosis), since any anastomotic insufficiency that occurs usually has the mildest course here.

In tumors of the lower quarter of the esophagus, blunt dissection of the esophagus can be carried out through the diaphragmatic aperture and the upper thoracic aperture without a thoracotomy (transhiatal esophagectomy with en-bloc lymphadenectomy). In this tumor location, adequate lymph-node removal can also be achieved with this surgical technique.

Due to the high mortality and morbidity associated with radical esophageal resection, various less invasive surgical techniques have been developed in recent years. Currently, laparoscopic esophageal resection with or without thoracoscopy, and limited resection of the distal esophagus and cardia with regional lymphadenectomy and reconstruction with an isoperistaltic jejunal interposition graft (the modified Merendino operation) are being evaluated [6]. The advantage of all the surgical procedures is the opportunity for complete removal of the Barrett's mucosa, which makes the metachronous carcinomas that often occur with local endoscopic treatment highly unlikely.

Endoscopy

Endoscopic Mucosal Resection

The reasons for carrying out local endoscopic therapy in cases of intraepithelial high-grade neoplasia and mucosal Barrett's carcinoma are, on the one hand, the high rates of morbidity (30–50%) and mortality (> 3%) associated with radical esophageal resection; and on the other, the reduction in quality of life that results with surgery. These factors contrast with the low risk of lymph-node metastases from mucosal Barrett's carcinomas, which is less than the mortality rate with esophageal resection, and the absence of lymph-node metastases in intraepithelial neoplasia [7].

EMR is an endoscopic procedure for resecting superficial premalignant and malignant lesions in the gastrointestinal tract, for therapeutic and diagnostic purposes. In our experience, it can be carried out with the patient under conscious sedation with midazolam and/or pethidine. The conventional loop resection, with or without injection under the target lesion, is the simplest variant of the endoscopic mucosal resection technique. The "suck-and-cut" technique, with or without prior ligation, allows extensive ablation including the submucosa, even in the most difficult conditions in the esophagus. The technique of suction mucosectomy is carried out either with ligation, or using a cap attached to the proximal end of the endoscope (the Inoue cap). The choice of which technique to use is guided by the anatomical conditions, the macroscopic type of the lesion, and the endoscopist's personal experience and preferences. Our own studies have not shown any significant differences between the two procedures with regard to the size of the resection specimen or the complication rate. The "suck-and-cut" technique only appears to be slightly superior in patients who have previously undergone local endoscopic treatment (Figs. 6 and 7).

The largest study published to date on EMR in patients with early Barrett's carcinoma and HGIN (n = 64), by our own group, confirmed the efficacy and safety of the technique. Complete remission was achieved in 82.5% of cases (97% in the low-risk group, 59% in the high-risk one). During a mean follow-up period of 12 months, recurrences or metachronous carcinomas occurred in 14% of the patients, and were again successfully treated. The rate of severe and mild complications in the study was 12.5%. Despite these initially good results, a definitive assessment of this technique will only be possible after a longer follow-up period [8].

In experienced hands, EMR is a safe method of resecting dysplastic lesions and early carcinomas, and it offers decisive advantages over other local endoscopic treatment procedures (e.g., thermal destruction, PDT): the histological processing of the specimen provides information about the depth of infiltration of the individual wall layers and regarding the completeness of removal with healthy margins. Patients with submucosal invasion that has not been detected before treatment, in whom a high rate of lymph-node metastases must be expected, can thus still receive surgical therapy.

PDT (Photodynamic Therapy)

PDT is an endoscopically guided, athermal, minimally invasive treatment procedure that has been successfully used to treat intraepithelial neoplasias and early carcinomas of the esophagus. Again, the method only requires conscious sedation.

Numerous photosensitizing agents are available for PDT, but the ones most frequently used are dihematoporphyrin (DHE, e.g. Photofrin®), a first-generation photosensitizer; *meso*-tetrahydroxyphenylchlorin (mTHPC), and protoporphyrin IX induced by 5-aminolevulinic acid (ALA-PpIX).

The principle of photodynamic therapy is based on semiselective photosensitization of the target lesion by a photosensitizing agent, which is administered either intravenously or orally and subsequently activated by endoscopically applied light at a specific wavelength. The oxygen radicals this releases lead to destruction of the treated tissue.

PDT is now being successfully used at many centers throughout the world to treat early carcinomas and dysplastic changes in the esophagus. The procedure has advantages over EMR in lesions that are multilocular, extensive, or not clearly demarcated, and it is mainly used in cases of this type.

Photofrin, the agent so far used most often in clinical cases, is a highly potent photosensitizer, but it is associated with considerable side effects. Esophageal stenoses often occur as a result of deep necrosis formation. Overholt's group reported high stenosis rates of 58% and 34%. In addition, long-lasting photosensitization of the skin can lead to substantial phototoxic side effects.

Despite the higher potency of photosensitizers of the first and second generations, ALA-PpIX is increasingly being used for photodynamic therapy. In addition to the possibility of oral administration, 5-aminolevulinic acid has greater mucosal and tumor specificity, as well as much faster degradation kinetics, so that phototoxic side effects in the skin occur extremely rarely. The lack of complications is achieved at the cost of reduced depth effectiveness and thus inadequate efficacy with carcinomas that are thicker than 2 mm. With dysplasias, the use of ALA-PpIX can achieve complete remission in 100% of cases without any method-related morbidity or mortality [9]. With early carcinomas, complete remission is possible in 50–80% of cases, depending on the thickness of the lesion. In these cases, better results can be achieved with first- and second-generation photosensitizers such as DHE and mTHPC.

The basic disadvantages of PDT lie in the limited availability of the procedure, its high costs, and methodological problems that have not yet been fully resolved. These concern dosimetry, the various photosensitizers that are still undergoing testing, and homogeneous light application. As the target lesion is destroyed, histological processing is not possible.

Only a few studies have so far been published concerning thermal destruction of Barrett's esophagus with intraepithelial high-grade neoplasia and/or adenocarcinoma. Several publications, although with extremely small numbers of cases, have documented successful treatment of early Barrett's carcinoma using argon plasma coagulation (APC) or potassium titanyl phosphate and neodymium–yttrium aluminum garnet laser. De-

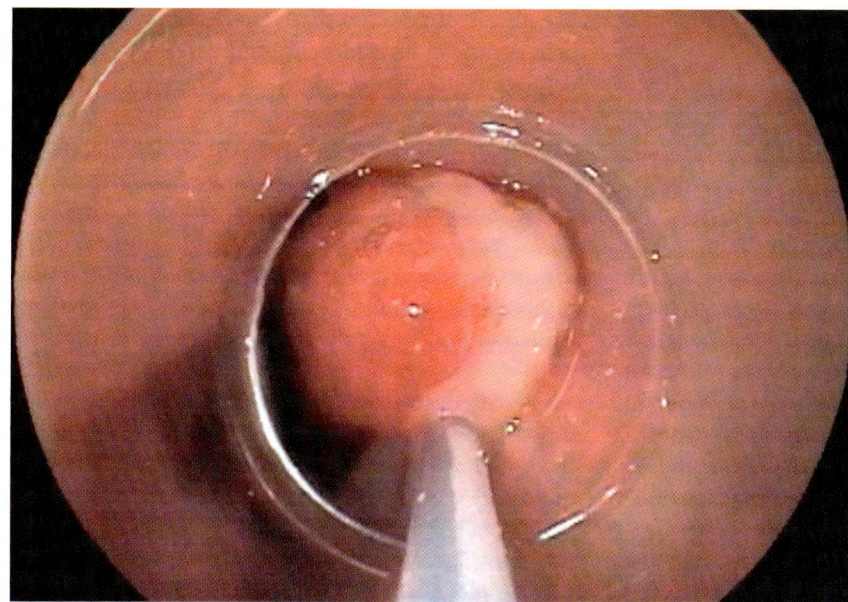

Figure 6
Cap mucosectomy of early
Barrett's carcinoma

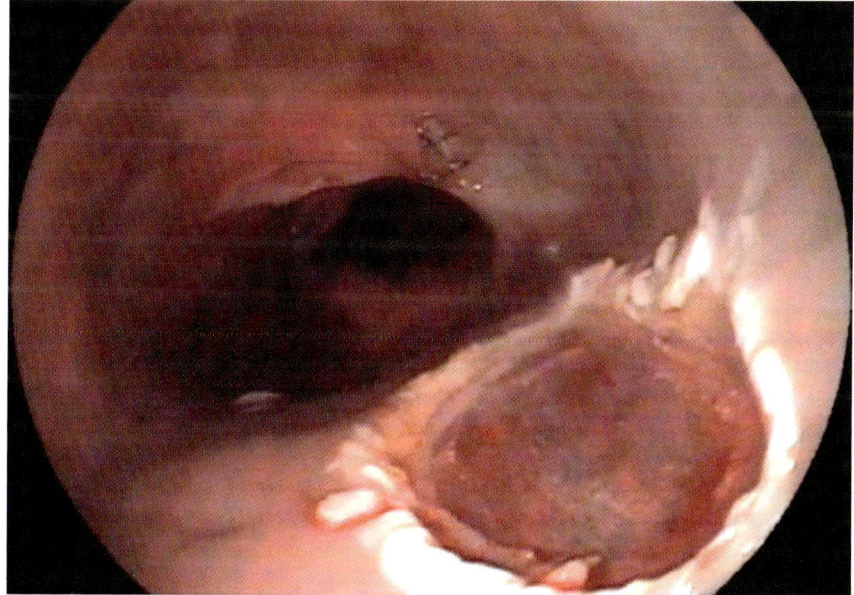

Figure 7
After cap mucosectomy

spite these results, APC thermodestruction represents a reserve method for local endoscopic treatment of dysplasias or carcinomas in Barrett's esophagus. The efficacy and safety of EMR and PDT have been confirmed in numerous studies, and they should therefore be preferred to thermal procedures.

Local endoscopic therapy should currently only be carried out at centers with expertise in the methods, i.e. with a high frequency of treatments and if possible with availability of all the treatment procedures. This is the only way of ensuring that if local treatment fails in these patients, surgical therapy can still be carried out early enough. In addition, this is the only way of obtaining results which, if positive, might lead in the medium term to a change in the treatment strategy for HGIN and early carcinomas in Barrett's mucosa.

Endoprostheses

In palliative situations in patients with tumor-related dysphagia, implantation of an endoprosthesis is usually associated with long-term symptomatic improvement. The method of choice here is self-expanding metal endoprostheses, which in contrast to plastic endoprostheses can be introduced in a compressed state using thin application systems (18–32 Fr) and then released step by step. This removes the need for extensive bougienage prior to implantation. After the stents have expanded, they reach a diameter of 18–20 mm, so that – in contrast to plastic endoprostheses – ingestion of even solid food is possible when they are used. Complications such as tumor ingrowth and overgrowth, and pocket formation on the upper margin of the stent, have been reduced by further development of metal endoprostheses (e.g. with silicon or polyurethane stent coverings). The dislocation rate can only be reduced through experience on the part of the endoscopist, with correct establishment of the indications and selection of a suitable stent.

Stent types that can be recommended include the Ultraflex (Boston Scientific, Cambridge, MA, USA) and the Gianturco-Z stent (Wilson-Cook, Winston-Salem, NC, USA). These stents both have a good configuration and are easy to use. The Ultraflex is attractive as it is highly flexible, and it is therefore above all suitable for bending stenotic courses. With its extremely high expansile strength, the Gianturco-Z stent has advantages for use in rigid stenoses.

The main disadvantage of metal stents is their high cost, at ca. € 1000–1500. For this reason, the indication has to be established relative to patient's life expectancy (with the exception of patients with esophagorespiratory fistulas).

Radiotherapy

The indication for radiotherapy is an advanced, inoperable tumor or a clearly increased surgical risk due to the patient's poor general condition, or concomitant diseases reducing operability. Radiotherapy can achieve effective reduction of the tumor volume in more than two-thirds of cases, so that a marked improvement in symptoms can be achieved. Tumor reduction only becomes effective about 4 weeks after irradiation; endoscopic procedures therefore have to be used temporarily to ensure esophageal passage. A percutaneous endoscopic gastrostomy (PEG) should be established in all cases before radiotherapy.

Radiotherapy can only achieve a definitive cure in individual cases. The criteria for potentially curative radiotherapy are T-3, N0–1, M0 tumors. The patients should not be over 70 years of age and should have a Karnofsky index >60%.

Percutaneous irradiation is carried out with a focal dose of 60 Gy, and intracavitary irradiation with afterloading technique (3 × 5 Gy) follows after a two-week pause.

Preoperative radiotherapy is usually carried out in combination with chemotherapy. In Barrett's carcinoma, preoperative radiotherapy appears to be associated with a survival advantage, but a general recommendation for adjuvant chemoradiotherapy cannot currently be made, and it should only be carried out in the context of clinical studies.

Postoperative radiotherapy can be carried out after R1 or R2 resections. No advantage has so far been confirmed with R0 resections.

Chemotherapy

Esophageal adenocarcinomas are moderately sensitive to chemotherapy. In comparison with monotherapy, high remission rates can be achieved with polychemotherapy. When the tumor spread is only local, the response rate is 30–60%, and with metastatic disease it is 20–40%. However, these effects are only of limited duration, and there is no evidence of a positive effect on the survival time. The most effective individual agents are cisplatin, mitomycin, paclitaxel, 5-fluorouracil and vinorelbine.

Chemoradiotherapy

The background for the combination of chemotherapy and radiotherapy is the synergistic effect of the chemotherapeutic agent as a radiosensitizer.

Neoadjuvant chemotherapy is used in primarily resectable tumors, as well as for down-staging purposes in locally advanced inoperable tumors. An established protocol is the combination of 5-fluorouracil/cisplatin and radiotherapy with a focal dose of 40 Gy [10]. Tumor reduction can be achieved in 30–50% of cases. Particularly in the case of locally advanced tumors, neoadjuvant chemoradiotherapy appears to lead to an improvement in the survival time. However, general recommendations regarding chemoradiotherapy are not currently possible, and these treatment methods should therefore only be used in the context of clinical studies.

Side effects of chemoradiotherapy, in addition to myelotoxicity in 20–40% of patients, include ulcerations, strictures, esophagitis, and esophagotracheal fistulas. At the start of radiotherapy, temporary tumor edema can cause a deterioration in dysphagia. A PEG should be established on principle before this procedure, so that enteral nutrition can be ensured if dysphagia deteriorates.

Prognosis

The prognosis in patients with Barrett's adenocarcinoma is decisively affected by the tumor stage at the initial diagnosis.

According to published data, patients with tumor restricted to the mucosa have a very good long-term prognosis after local endoscopic therapy. In a group of 115 patients (mean age 64, follow-up period 3 years), the actuarial 5-year survival rate was around 80%. This corresponds to the survival rate in the average population of the same age.

More advanced carcinomas require surgical treatment. If no lymph nodes are affected, the 5-year survival rate, depending on the local tumor stage, ranges from 44% (T3) to 80% (T1–2). When fewer than five lymph nodes are affected, it is ca. 37%, but it falls as low as 7% if more than five lymph nodes are involved. In patients in whom curative resection is not possible, the 5-year survival rate is 0%. The mean survival time in stage 4 tumors is 6–10 months.

Screening, Surveillance, Prevention

Depending on the histological findings, patients with Barrett's esophagus should receive endoscopic check-up examinations at regular intervals to ensure that any carcinoma that develops can be recognized and treated at an early stage [3].

Future Perspectives

The treatment strategy for HGIN and mucosal Barrett's carcinomas will change in the future. In these cases, local endoscopic therapy will replace radical esophageal resection as the therapeutic gold standard. In more advanced carcinomas, the surgical methods are still the treatment of choice. The value of neoadjuvant chemoradiotherapy requires further evaluation in controlled clinical studies.

Additional issues that need to be settled in the future are the value of long-term proton-pump inhibitor treatment and prophylactic ablation of Barrett's mucosa for the purposes of carcinoma prevention. The value of cyclooxygenase-2 inhibitors in carcinoma prevention is also not yet clear and requires further investigation.

Important further developments such as optical coherence tomography can also be expected in the field of endoscopic diagnosis, and these may make early recognition and localization of neoplasias in Barrett's esophagus easier.

References

1. Pech O, Gossner L, May A, Ell C. Management of Barrett's oesophagus, dysplasia and early adenocarcinoma. Best Pract Clin Res Gastroenterol 2001; 15: 267–84.
2. Lagergren J, Bergstrom R, Lindgren A, Nyren O. Symptomatic gastroesophageal reflux as a risk factor for esophageal adenocarcinoma. N Engl J Med 1999; 340: 825–31.
3. Sampliner RE. Practice guidelines on the diagnosis, surveillance, and therapy of Barrett's esophagus. The Practice Parameters Committee of the American College of Gastroenterology. Am J Gastroenterol 1998; 93: 1028–32.
4. Jankowski JA, Wright NA, Meltzer SJ, Triadafilopoulos G, Geboes K, Casson AG, Kerr D, Young LS. Molecular evolution of the metaplasia–dysplasia–adenocarcinoma sequence in the esophagus. Am J Pathol 1999; 154: 965–73.
5. Collard JM. Exclusive radical surgery for esophageal adenocarcinoma. Cancer 2001; 91: 1098–1104.
6. Stein HJ, Feith M, Mueller J, Werner M, Siewert JR. Limited resection for early adenocarcinoma in Barrett's esophagus. Ann Surg 2000; 232: 733–42.
7. Hölscher AH, Bollschweiler E, Schneider PM, Siewert JR. Early adenocarcinoma in Barrett's esophagus. Br J Surg 1997; 84: 1470–3.
8. Ell C, May A, Gossner L, Pech O, Guenter E, Mayer G, Henrich R, Vieth M, Mueller H, Seitz G, Stolte M. Endoscopic mucosal resection of early cancer and high-grade dysplasia in Barrett's esophagus. Gastroenterology 2000; 118: 670–7.
9. Gossner L, Stolte M, Sroka R, Rick K, May A, Hahn EG, Ell C. Photodynamic ablation of high grade dysplasia and early cancer in Barrett's esophagus by means of aminolevulinic acid. Gastroenterology 1998; 114: 448–55.
10. Walsh TN, Noonan N, Hollywood D, Kelly A, Keeling N, Hennessy TP. A comparison of multimodal therapy and surgery for esophageal adenocarcinoma. N Engl J Med 1996; 335: 462–7.

3 Other Tumors of the Esophagus

R. LAMBERT, J.Y. SCOAZEC

Summary

The burden of esophageal tumors is shared almost completely between two types of epithelial tumors that have been developed from the squamous Malpighian epithelium or from the metaplastic glandular mucosa in the distal esophagus.

Other tumors represent a very small fraction, just a few per cent, of the burden. Owing to their heterogeneity, they are present in different sections of the WHO classification of tumors (ICD-O). Non-epithelial mesenchymal tumors constitute a major group. Epithelial tumors are represented by the endocrine neoplasia, including the carcinoid and also the small cell esophageal cancer, which is classified in the group of carcinomas and has similar characteristics to the small cell cancer in the lung. Digestive lymphomas may be localized in the esophagus and are classified in a specific group. Finally, secondary tumors issuing from regional or distant primary tumors may offer a variety of tumor types.

Mesenchymal Tumors of the Esophagus

Definition

Mesenchymal tumors are less frequent in the esophagus than in the stomach. A few years ago, the 2 major groups of mesenchymal tumors were the leiomyoma corresponding to a smooth muscle tumor, eventually malignant (leiomyosarcoma), and the Schwannoma, a tumor of nervous origin which is benign. Histochemistry markers have shown that the protein CD 34 is a common marker for these tumors, while an overlap of muscular or nervous markers occurs between the two groups. Those tumors positive for CD 34 and having neither muscular, nor nervous markers were called gastrointestinal stromal tumors (GIST); this name was progressively adopted for all tumors of the group without considering the role of the specific muscle or nervous markers. More recently the c-KIT protein (tyrosine-kinase receptor) was shown to be the most specific marker of stromal or GIST tumors and they are now clearly separated from the pure Schwannoma and the pure leiomyoma, negative for the c-KIT marker and positive for their specific markers [1].

Epidemiology

Leiomyoma is the most common mesenchymal tumor in the esophagus [1]. It occurs in males at twice the frequency for females, the mean age distribution is 30–35 years. Most leiomyomas are benign. The malignant forms (leiomyosarcoma) with differentiated smooth muscle cells are rare, 4% of all smooth muscle and stromal tumors. They occur in older adults (60 to 80 years) and have a dismal prognosis. The leiomyosarcoma represents only 0.2% of malignant esophageal tumors in the Surveillance Epidemiology and End Results (SEER) registry during the period 1973–87. Multiple leiomyomas occur in leiomyomatosis where worm-like intramural benign tumors will extend down to the upper portion of the stomach. Esophageal leiomyomatosis can be associated with the Alport syndrome, an inherited nephropathy due to mutations in the COL4A5 gene, encoding the alpha5 chain of type IV collagen, a major component of the glomerular basement membrane.

The Schwannoma is exceedingly rare in the esophagus; it is not associated with neurofibromatosis types I and II and occurs in older adults than the leiomyoma. Most cases are benign, malignancy is exceedingly rare [2].

GISTs account for 2.2% of malignant gastric tumors but are much rarer in the esophagus. They occur either in males or in females in their sixth or eighth decade.

Gastrointestinal autonomic nerve tumors or GANT, previously classified as plexosarcomas, are extremely rare in the esophagus.

Granular cell tumors, found in the head and neck region, especially in the tongue, are rare in the esophagus. They are small (usually less than 1 cm) and well circumscribed lesions with a subepithelial location. In the Dutch registry [3], 52 cases of solitary esophageal lesions were collected in 6 years; they were localized in the distal esophagus in 75% of cases.

The Kaposi sarcoma is characterized by a dense vascular tumoral architecture.

Etiology

The histogenesis of GIST has been revisited with respect to the c-KIT marker, which is also expressed by the normal interstitial cells of Cajal. These are the pacemaker cells of the digestive wall controlling the peristaltic activity of smooth muscle. GISTs may therefore originate from the Cajal cells and have also been called gastrointestinal interstitial pacemaker cell tumors. GISTs coexpress c-KIT and CD 34 and one may consider that the Cajal cell could be a common precursor of mesenchymal tumors.

The granular cell tumor or Abrikosoff tumor is of neurogenic origin. Most cases are benign and malignancy occurs in 2 to 4%. Granular cell tumors are positive for the S 100 protein marker.

The Kaposi sarcoma occurs in patients with immunodeficiency from HIV and is positive for human herpes virus 8 by PCR.

Symptoms

Many tumors have a small diameter and are asymptomatic. This is the situation for most granular cell tumors and with many leiomyomas. They are incidentally detected when endoscopy has been carried out for another indication. Large non-obstructive tumors protruding into the mediastinum may also be asymptomatic and are detected incidentally during a chest X-ray or a CT scan. For large tumors protruding into the esophageal lumen, dysphagia is the usual complaint.

Diagnostics

Synopsis

Standard imaging techniques adopted for esophageal tumors are:
▶ endoscopic exploration
▶ endosonographic (EUS) exploration
▶ spiral computed tomography.

Assessment of histology:
▶ uncertain evaluation of malignancy in small samples.

Endoscopy is the standard detection procedure for mesenchymal esophageal tumors. Most lesions (leiomyomas, Schwannomas or GISTs) are located in the distal esophagus. The submucosal intramural lesions produce a swelling of the unaltered mucosa. On rare occasions, an ulcer is present. The size of most tumors varies between 2 and 3 cm. Tumors smaller than 3 cm are presumed to be benign. The granular cell tumor is also localized in the distal esophagus; this small and well-circumscribed lesion is grossly yellow, and firm on palpation, less than 5 mm in diameter in 50%, and over 1 cm in 20% of cases. The Kaposi sarcoma in the esophagus is characterized by multiple purpuric vascular lesions up to 1 cm in diameter.

Endoscopic tissue sampling is reliable for the diagnosis of mesenchymal neoplasia, but the prediction of malignancy is often uncertain when based on biopsy forceps or a needle aspiration biopsy.

Endoscopic ultrasound (EUS) is now required to determine the size and position of the tumor in the esophageal wall [4, 5], and is helpful for endoscopic treatment [6, 7]. The EUS analysis of stromal tumors is based on the following criteria: diameter, presence of a deep ulcer, hyper- or hypo-echogenic heterogeneity, presence of liquid, irregular or regular external limits, extraluminal extension.

Irregular external limits, presence of liquid and metastatic lymph nodes suggest malignancy. A small size (less than 3 cm), regular limits and homogeneity of the echoic structure suggest a benign tumor. The granular cell has a hypo-echoic solid pattern, placed in the inner layers of the esophageal wall and reaching the sub-epithelial layer.

The CT scan is useful complement to assess any extension in the mediastinum and explore the presence of liver metastases.

Histologic Classification and Molecular Genetics

Synopsis

Histochemical characteristics of esophageal tumors

▸ Leiomyomas are positive for desmin and actin and negative for CD 34 and CD 117 (KIT)
▸ Schwannomas are positive for S 100 and negative for desmin, actin and c-KIT
▸ GISTs are positive for CD 34 and c-KIT and negative for desmin
▸ GANTs are positive for S 100, vimentine and neurone-enolase and negative for keratin
▸ Granular cell tumors are positive for S 100 and negative for CD 34, desmin and c-KIT
▸ Kaposi sarcomas are positive for PAS, CD 34 and CD 31.

Leiomyoma is a spindle cell tumor with moderate cellularity and a low mitotic activity (Fig. 1). The tumor is positive for desmin and actin and negative for CD34 and CD 117 (KIT). Esophageal leiomyomas do not show *c-KIT*

gene mutations as is usual in GISTs, nor a loss in chromosome 11. Leiomyosarcoma, a malignant tumor with differentiated smooth muscle cells, has the same characteristics: desmin and actin positive and c-KIT negative. The exceedingly rare rhabdomyosarcoma, is characterized by skeletal muscle differentiation (cross-striation).

Schwannoma is a benign tumor with a spindle cell pattern and is positive for S 100 protein and negative for desmin, actin and c-KIT.

GISTs in esophagus, as in the stomach, have a spindle cell pattern (Fig. 2). Some tumors are rich in collagen and pauci-cellular with an epitheloid pattern. GISTs are positive for c-KIT and CD 34 with a *c-kit* mutation on exon 11; they are usually negative for desmin. Both benign and malignant GISTs show loss in chromosomes 14 and 22. GISTs are often malignant, with liver metastases. The assessment of malignancy is based on the size of the lesion and mitotic counts. Tumors less than 5 cm are usually benign.

The GANT of esophagus is exceedingly rare, showing a spindle cell pattern with moderate nuclear pleiomorphism. It stains for vimentin, neurone-specific-enolase, and S 100 protein and is negative for cytokeratin. Neurosecretory granules are present on ultra-structural studies.

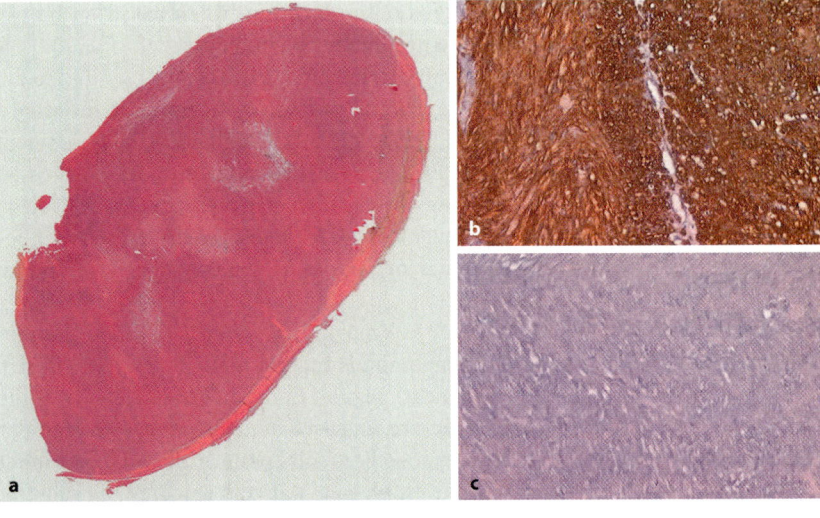

Figure 1a–c
Leiomyoma. The characteristic nodular appearance of the tumor is well visible at low magnification (**a**); spindle-shaped tumor cells, without atypia, strongly expressed smooth muscle actin (**b**) and lack c-kit (CD117) expression (**c**). (**a** HE, ×20; **b** and **c** immunoperoxidase staining, ×180)

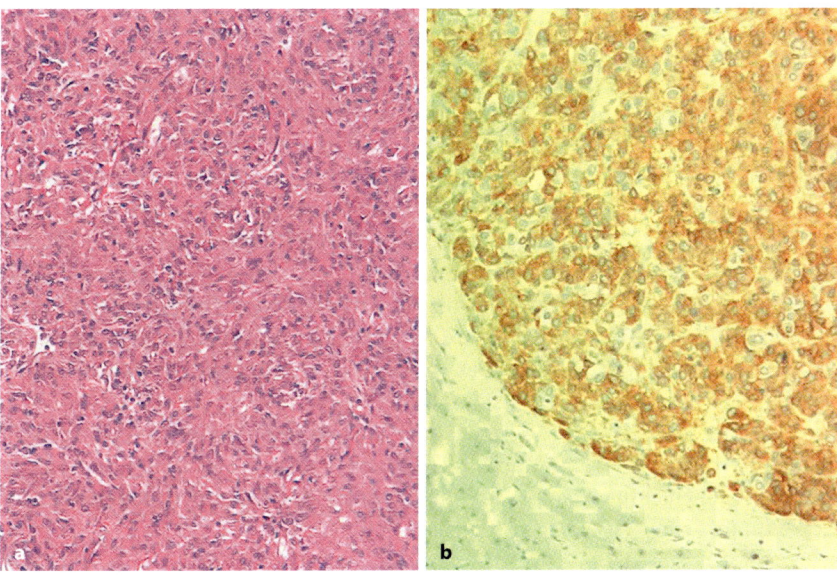

Figure 2a,b
Gastro-intestinal stromal tumor.
Spindle shaped tumor cells, presenting with a fascicular architecture (**a**), strongly express c-kit
(CD117) (**b**). (**a** HE, ×150; **b** immunoperoxidase staining, ×180)

The granular cell tumor or Abrikosoff tumor is constituted of sheets of oval to polygonal cells with abundant granular basophilic cytoplasm, lysosomes filled
with lamellar PAS-positive constituents. Granular cell
tumors are positive for the S 100 protein and negative for
desmin, CD 34 and KIT (Fig. 3).

The Kaposi sarcoma is composed of spindle cells
with vascular slit formation and scattered granules positive for PAS, CD 31 and CD 34 (Tab. 1).

Staging

Table 1
WHO histological classification of esophageal tumors

Epithelial tumors	
Non epithelial tumors	
Leiomyoma	8890/0
Schwannoma	9560/0
Lipoma	8850/0
Granular cell tumor	9580/0
Gastrointestinal stromal tumor	8936/1
– benign	8936/0
– uncertain malignancy	8936/1
– malignant	8936/3
Leiomyosarcoma	8890/3
Rhabdomyosarcoma	8900/3
Kaposi sarcoma	9140/3
Secondary tumors	

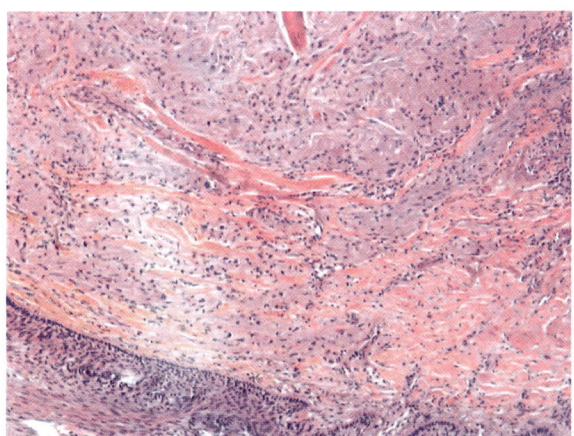

Figure 3
Granular cell tumor. Low power magnification of a submucosal
granular cell tumor; tumor cells are characterized by their large size,
abundant granular cytoplasm and small, centrally located nucleus;
the lesion is not encapsulated. (HE, ×60)

Note: TNM classification for staging applies only to carcinomas,
and is not presented. Morphology codes of the ICD-0. Behavior is
coded 0 for benign, 1 for unspecified or uncertain, 2 for in situ
carcinoma, 3 for malignant tumors.

Treatment

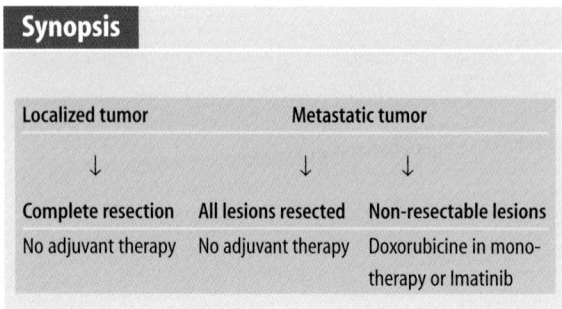

Localized tumor		Metastatic tumor	
↓		↓	↓
Complete resection	All lesions resected	Non-resectable lesions	
No adjuvant therapy	No adjuvant therapy	Doxorubicine in mono-therapy or Imatinib	

Surgery

The curative treatment of esophageal mesenchymal tumors requires complete removal. Large tumors entering into the mediastinum are treated by thoracic surgery in operable patients, aiming at a complete resection. Smaller tumors may be treated by a simple tumorectomy either through conventional or celioscopic thoracic surgery. In the presence of metastases, resection of metastases as well as the primary tumor is recommended. If the resection of the tumoral tissue is complete, no adjuvant chemotherapy is proposed.

Endoscopy

The endoscopic resection of small tumors not protruding into the mediastinum is possible [6, 7, 8]. Two techniques are used, as shown in a series of 62 cases. When the tumor is less than 2 cm a conventional polypectomy (snare resection) is used. Larger polypoid tumors and non-polypoid tumors require surgery or endoscopic resection based upon incisional enucleation, using a electrocautery snare and a coagulation electrode. This method has been adopted in about 40% of situations in a rather large series (62 cases) of tumors submitted to endoscopic treatment [8]. With granular cells tumors, the curative endoscopic treatment (excisional biopsy or snare resection) is the elective procedure, when treatment is preferred to surveillance.

In non-operable patients with large symptomatic tumors and dysphagia, endoscopic procedures may prove helpful in palliation; this includes luminal dilation or stenting.

Chemotherapy and Radiotherapy

Chemotherapy is used when a total resection is not possible, and adjuvant chemotherapy following a complete tumor resection is not recommended. Until recently, the most effective agent was doxorubicin (60 mg/m²) every 3 weeks. The polychemotherapy protocols (isofosfamide, deticene, vincristine (VCR), adriamycin) proved highly toxic with not much benefit. Great hope has arisen with the development of a polyvalent tyrosine-kinase inhibitor "Imatinib" or Gleevec [9] which proves highly efficient when there is over-expression of c-KIT in the tumor (CD 117).

There is no room for radiotherapy in the standard protocol of treatment. Palliative and antalgic radiotherapy is eventually proposed in painful situations.

Prognosis and Follow-Up

The prognosis of the tumor depends on its morphology and size. Malignancy (leiomyosarcoma or GIST) is suggested when the lesion is multinodular and protrudes into the mediastinum. A benign neoplastic lesion (leiomyoma, Schwannoma, GIST, granular cell tumor) is suggested when the lesion is small and spherical. Often, malignancy of larger tumors is uncertain after analysis of the tissue sample. The assessment of malignancy is dependent on the mitotic count, size, depth of invasion and presence or absence of metastases. Overall, the prognosis for esophageal stromal tumors is better than that of other stromal digestive tumors. In a larg multianalysis conducted in the Armed Forces Institute of Pathology [10] for the period 1954–97, the 5-year survival was estimated at 73% and the 10-year survival at 63%.

After endoscopic treatment, a coupled endoscopic and EUS surveillance of the esophagus is required for at least 5 years.

When a submucosal tumor has been left in place and untreated, coupled endoscopic and EUS surveillance is required; surgery is then recommended if the diameter of the tumor increases during the follow-up. This occurs when a small, morphologically benign, submucosal tumor is detected in the esophagus. A large majority of leiomyomas, the most common tumor with a size in the 2 to 3 cm range, are benign. The granular cell tumor is a very specific lesion because of its characteristic endoscopic pattern and exceedingly rare malignant potential. Such tumors have proved either stable or even regressive during follow-up.

Future Perspectives

Improvement in the management of mesenchymal esophageal tumors is based upon the endoscopic detection of small lesions and improved EUS staging. There is a trend towards enlarged indications of endoscopic resection for small tumors and much hope on the new protocols based upon tyrosine kinase inhibition, for the treatment of advanced disease.

Endocrine Tumors of the Esophagus

Definition

According to the ICD – Oncology classification of the WHO, the endocrine tumors of the esophagus are classified among epithelial tumors and include three distinct types: well differentiated endocrine neoplasms called *carcinoids*, poorly differentiated endocrine carcinomas called *small cell carcinomas* and mixed endocrine and exocrine carcinomas [11].

Epidemiology and Etiology

Carcinoids are very rare in the esophagus [12]. They represent no more than 0.05% of all gastrointestinal carcinoids, according to a large multicentric analysis on more than 8000 cases [13]. Similarly, carcinoids represent no more than 0.02% of all esophageal malignant tumors. The disease is seen in males more than in females, aged over 50 years.

Small cell carcinomas occur in the sixth or seventh decade of life and are more common in males. This tumor is more frequent than the carcinoid in the esophagus. Small cell carcinomas account for 0.5–5% of all esophageal tumors.

About 200 cases are found in the literature in 2001 [14].

The mixed endocrine-exocrine (squamous cell) cancers are also seen in males, rather than in females.

Etiology and Pathogenesis

All these tumors occur more frequently in males than in females. Most carcinoids occur as sporadic, without relation with the multgiple endocrine neoplasia (MEN) 1 and 2 syndromes. Patients with small cell carcinoma are usually heavy smokers. An anecdotal association between small cell carcinoma and a Barrett esophagus has been reported.

Symptoms and Clinical Signs

Most of these endocrine tumors are detected at an advanced stage, in the presence of dysphagia with severe weight loss, some patients complain of chest pain as the major symptom. Liver metastases may be present. A variety of biological abnormalities may be detected in patients with small cell carcinoma, involving the antidiuretic hormone, increased secretion of calcitonin, adrenocroticotrophic hormone (ACTH), secretin and parathyroid hormone-related protein. Clinical syndromes with hypercalcemia or with watery diarrhea may be present. Diarrhea suggests that extensive liver metastases are present. The watery diarrhea with hypokaliemia and achlorhydria syndrome with production of an ectopic vasoactive intestinal peptide (VIP) peptide hormone has been reported in mixed tumors with exocrine squamous cell carcinoma and endocrine carcinoma.

Diagnostics

Synopsis

▸ Standard imaging techniques adopted for esophageal endocrine tumors
▸ endoscopic exploration
▸ EUS exploration
▸ spiral computed tomography
▸ Biological parameters
▸ kaliemia, calcemia
▸ peptide hormones assays.

Most endocrine tumors in the esophagus are detected at an advanced stage, and therefore in patients complaining of dysphagia; endoscopy is often the first diagnostic procedure. All reported carcinoids were of large dimensions (4 to 7 cm) and completely infiltrated the esophageal wall. At endoscopy, the pattern is that of a large submucosal tumor covered by an intact mucosa, often localized in the distal esophagus. The small cell carcinomas appear as fungating and ulcerated masses of large size, invading the esophageal lumen and the mediastinum as well. The diameter of the tumoral mass may be over 10 cm. Tissue sampling is easier with fungating and ulcerated tumors and the diagnosis of endocrine tumor with trabecular acinar structure is easy. Specific immunostaining is required in complement. Tissue sampling in submucosal tumors is more difficult, requiring a partial excisional resection.

EUS, which is extremely useful in the assessment of small submucosal tumors and of their extension in the digestive wall, is less useful in presence of a very large tumor. EUS is still recommended to assess the amplitude of the submucosal extension at the periphery of the tumor and confirm whether there is invasion of the mediastinum.

Spiral computed tomography is required as a complement in the assessment of thoracic extension and of liver metastases.

Histologic Classification and Molecular Genetics

Synopsis

▶ Carcinoid: positive for Grimelius and neuron-specific enolase
▶ Small cell carcinoma: positive for neuron-specific enolase, synaptophysin, chromogranin, leu7
▶ Peptide hormones may be detected in both types of tumors.

Carcinoid or well-differentiated endocrine tumors in the esophagus are aggressive tumors organized in solid nests of cells with a high mitotic rate, staining positive for Grimelius and neuron-specific enolase. Membrane bound secretory granules are shown on electron microscopy. Most cases reported are advanced tumors with a large size, 4 to 7 cm, a transmural extension and frequent distant metastases.

Small cell carcinoma is similar to the small cell carcinoma in the lung with regard to histology and immunohistochemistry (Fig. 4). It is constituted of small cells with dark nuclei. In mixed types, there may be foci of squamous carcinoma/adenocarcinoma, associated with the trabecular acinar endocrine component. Immunohistochemical stains are positive for neuron specific eno-

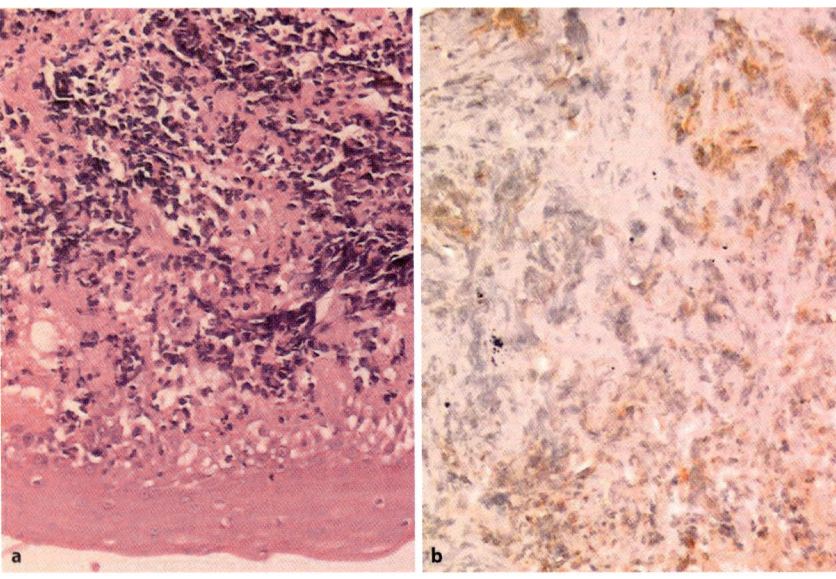

Figure 4a,b
Small cell carcinoma. Small, dark stained tumor cells are visible in the lamina propria of the esophagus; they present alterations due to crushing artifacts, frequent in biopsy samples (a). The diagnosis of small cell carcinoma is confirmed by the immunohistochemical demonstration of synaptophysin expression (b). (a HE, ×250; b immunoperoxidase staining, ×280)

lase, synaptophysin, chromogranin, and leu7. Telomerase activation is frequent in small cell carcinoma [15]. This suggests a potential application for anti-telomerase treatment. It is suggested that small cell carcinoma originates in the esophagus from a pluripotent cell in the squamous epithelium or in the ducts of esophageal glands.

Staging

See Table 2.

Treatment

Synopsis

Localized small tumor	Large and advanced tumor	
↓	↓	↓
Complete resection + adjuvant therapy	Without liver metastases: removal in some cases + multidrug therapy	With liver metastases: no operation, multidrug therapy + Imatinib?

Surgery

Surgical resection as a primary treatment of esophageal endocrine tumors, often gives disappointing results, because the disease is already generalized when it is detected. In a recent series of patients with a small cell carcinoma, surgery was adopted in 46% of cases. Very few cases have a long survival after surgery because liver metastases are frequent, even if the primary tumor had only a submucosal extension. In conclusion, surgical resection is not recommended if the tumor is very large or if liver metastases are present.

Endoscopy

There is no room for endoscopic procedures in the curative treatment of endocrine esophageal tumors. Endoscopic procedures (tumor destruction, dilatation, stenting) may play a role in palliation in inoperable patients. In a recent series of patients with a small cell carcinoma palliation or no treatment was adopted in 35% of cases.

Table 2

WHO histological classification of esophageal tumors

Epithelial tumors	
Carcinoma	
– Small cell Carcinoma	8041/3
– Carcinoid tumor	8240/3
Non epithelial tumors	
Secondary tumors	

Note: TNM classification for staging applies only to carcinomas, and is not presented. Morphology codes of the ICD-0. Behavior is coded 0 for benign, 1 for unspecified or uncertain, 2 for in situ carcinoma, 3 for malignant tumors.

Chemotherapy, Radiotherapy

Multidrug chemotherapy [16] sometimes offers a temporary remission. Esophageal endocrine tumors are poor responders to protocols based on adriamycin and streptozotocin, which remain a standard of care for endocrine pancreatic tumors. Poorly differentiated tumors and malignant esophageal carcinoids are treated with Cisplatinum and etoposide. As complementary treatments, somatostatin analogues (Octreotide) or α-interferon have been used. The tyrosine-kinase inhibitor Imatinib (Gleevec) is providing a recent hope for improved prognosis. Chemoembolisation can be complementary in the treatment of liver metastases. Radiotherapy can be used in palliation.

Prognosis and Follow-Up

The prognosis of small cell carcinoma is not significantly different from that of advanced squamous cell cancer or adenocarcinoma. This is a systemic disease requiring a multimodal treatment with chemotherapy. The median survival with chemotherapy is 16 months (only 2 months without chemotherapy). The overall survival is around 3 months.

Screening, Surveillance, Prevention

There is no specific argument to be developed for the prevention of such rare tumors, when the most specific etiologic factor is smoking. The surveillance intervals are determined according to which multidrug protocol has been adopted.

Future Perspectives

Progress is expected from the increased efficacy and decreased toxicity of multidrug protocols and eventually from the contribution of the tyrosine-kinase inhibitors or anti-telomerase agents. Human telomerase is a unique reverse transcriptase that is expressed in small cell carcinoma. The enzyme is responsible for telomere protection and supports the proliferative immortality of cancer cells. Thus, it has been proposed that the specific inhibition of telomerase activity in tumors might have beneficial therapeutic effects, resulting in apoptotic cell death or growth arrest. A number of oligonucleotides are presently being tested as telomerase inhibitors, without yet having a clinical application.

Lymphoma of the Esophagus

Definition

Primary lymphoma of the esophagus is defined as an extranodal lymphoma arising in the esophagus with the main bulk of the disease in the esophagus [17]. Most cases are low-grade B cell mucosa-associated lymphoid tissue (MALT) or large B cell types [18]. Primary esophageal T cell lymphoma is exceedingly rare [19]. Primary esophageal Hodgkin is also exceedingly rare.

Epidemiology

The esophagus is the least frequent site for primary lymphoma in the digestive tract, accounting for less than 1% of lymphoma patients. Patients are frequently of the male sex and over 50 years old.

   More frequently, the esophageal lymphoma is secondary to propagation from any type and site of lymphoma. The most frequent propagation is from mediastinal lymph nodes or from a primary gastric lymphoma.

Etiology and Pathogenesis

Immunostimulation associated with infectious agents in the digestive mucosae is considered as a pre-lymphoma condition. Infection by Helicobacter pylori plays a major role in the development of a lymphoma in the MALT of the stomach. The association with Helicobacter pylori infection does not play a role in the esophagus. Specific etiological factors and esophageal infections have not yet been identified for esophageal lymphoma. An increased risk of lymphoma occurs in patients with immunodeficiency such as seen in HIV and after transplantation. A lymphoma has developed in association with a long-term immunosuppression (azathioprine) in hepatitis C viral infection.

Symptoms and Clinical Signs

The esophageal lesion may be detected in a patient with an advanced primary lymphoma and complaining of dysphagia. The lymphoma can also be detected incidentally during upper gastrointestinal endoscopy in an asymptomatic patient or in a patient with suspicion of gastric MALT lymphoma.

Diagnostics

Endoscopy is the usual procedure of detection; superficial lesions show either as edematous and swollen areas or as multiple erythematous areas in the mucosa of the distal esophagus. Large tumors are obstructive. The diagnosis is established after tissue sampling with multiple biopsies and immunological phenotyping.

   Other procedures are helpful for the staging of the esophageal lymphoma in one of the four groups of the Ann Arbor classification. They include EUS to assess the extension of the lymphoma in the esophageal wall, spiral computerized tomography to explore the thorax and the abdomen and the assessment of immunodeficiency.

Histologic Classification and Molecular Genetics

The low grade, B cell MALT lymphoma has morphological and cytological features common to all digestive localizations of MALT. The proliferation is made of small lymphoid cells and contains centrocyte-like cells (CCL) or lymphoplasmocytic cells. The characteristic feature is the presence of lymphoepithelial lesions (Fig. 5). Immunohistologic studies show that CCL cells express pan B cell markers (CD 20 and CD 79 a), the bcl-2 protein and often the CD 43; they are negative for CD 5 and CD 10.

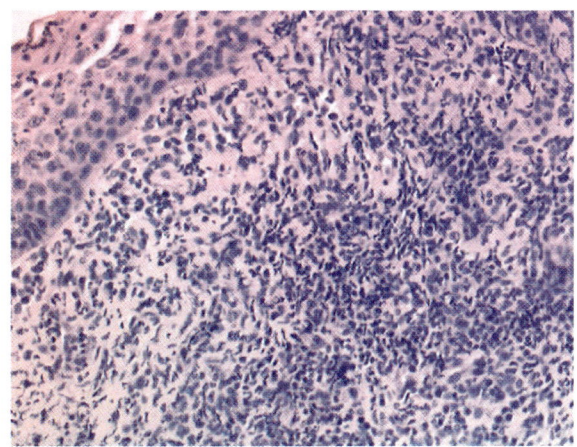

Figure 5
MALT. In this biopsy sample, a dense lymphoid infiltrate, formed by a majority of small lymphoid cells,covered by the malpighian epithelium, is visible in the lamina propria. (Mayer's hematoxylin, ×220)

cell rescue, improves with the adjuvant involved-field radiotherapy (IFRT). A risk-adapted therapy using the International Prognostic Index is essential for the treatment of aggressive non- Hodgkin lymphoma.

For a localized aggressive non-Hodgkin lymphoma, three courses of CHOP (cyclophosphamid/ doxorubicin/ vincristin/ predisone, CHOP protocol) are prescribed and followed by involved field radiation therapy (IFRT).

For an advanced stage aggressive non-Hodgkin lymphoma, 8 courses of CHOP are prescribed.

For the low-risk group of MALT lymphoma, eradication of Helicobacter pylori does not plays a significant role in the esophagus. There is no standard therapy for advanced stage MALT lymphoma.

Large B cell lymphomas are treated with a multiple drug course combining cyclophosphamide, doxorubicin, VCR, 6-mercaptopurine and prednisone and eventually radiation.

The high grade, large B cell type is morphologically similar to diffuse large B cell lymphomas arising in lymph nodes. There is complete destruction of the mucosa by large cells with vesicular nuclei, and the volume of the tumor is larger than that of the MALT lymphoma. They express pan B cell markers (CD 19, CD 20, CD 79a).

The primary T cell lymphoma is exceedingly rare, with densely packed small sized cells or with large cells. Immunohistologic studies show that they may express CD 3, CD4, CD8, CD 5, CD 7 and CD 5.

Staging

See Tables 3 and 4.

Treatment

Surgery has a limited place in the treatment of esophageal lymphoma. Resection of large tumors with a submucosal pattern at endoscopy has been reported and the lymphoma was confirmed only by the study of the specimen. The standard treatment of esophageal lymphoma is tailored to the stage and relies on chemotherapy combined with radiotherapy. The outcome for patients undergoing high-dose chemotherapy and autologous stem

Table 3
WHO histological classification of esophageal tumors

Epithelial tumors	
Non epithelial tumors	
Malignant lymphomas	
– B MALT type	9699/3
– B large cell	9680/3
– T cell lymphoma	9702/3
Secondary tumors	

Table 4
Ann Arbor Stage Classification of Lymphomas

Stage I	Localized extralymphatic organ involved or single lymph node involved.
Stage II	Localized extralymphatic organ involved + lymph nodes same side of diaphragmm or two or more lymph nodes involved same side of diaphragm.
Stage III	Localized extralymphatic organ involved + lymph nodes involved both sides of diaphragm.
Stage IV	Localized extralymphatic organ involved + distant lymph node involved or multifocal extralymphatic organs involved.

Note: the Ann Arbor stage classification of Hodgkin disease is now also adopted for Non-Hodgkin lymphoma.

Prognosis and Follow-Up

The prognosis of a primary esophageal lymphoma depends on the classification of the lesion after immunotyping and on its degree of diffusion. Secondary and metastatic esophageal lymphomas have the prognosis of a disseminated disease.

Future Perspectives

Improvements in the management of lymphoma are expected as a result of the typing of the tumors with multiple gene probes using micro-array technology. Promising results are expected with new anti-lymphoma drugs such as rituximab or purine analogs (cladribine and fludarabine).

Secondary Tumors of the Esophagus

Definition

These tumors originate from the esophagus, but are discontinuous with the primary lesion, which is located elsewhere in a distant organ, in a vicinal region (cardia) or even in the esophagus itself [20].

Epidemiology

Metastatic spread in the esophagus is uncommon in most countries, but reported to be more frequent in Japan.

Etiology and Pathogenesis

The metastatic spread from a distant tumor, occurs through a hematogenous propagation [21]. Any primary location – thyroid, breast, kidney, prostate, ovary – is a potential source of metastasis in the esophagus.

The metastases from vicinal tumors result from a lymphatic spread. This characterizes the intramural metastases occurring at some distance from a primary esophageal squamous cell cancer in about 11 to 16% of cases of advanced cancer [22]. Lymphatic spread in the esophagus from an adenocarcinoma of the cardia is also frequent [23]. The intramural metastases in the distal esophagus are discontinuous with the primary tumor.

They should be distinguished from the retrograde progression of the tumor in the submucosa of the distal esophagus; here the invasion is in continuity with the bulk of the primary tumor.

Symptoms and Clinical Signs

Esophageal symptoms occurring in patients with clinical signs of an advanced cancer at a distant site will suggest metastatic involvement at this level. Dysphagia is the most common symptom; hematemesis is less frequent. As a rule, the clinical characters of dysphagia suggest the presence of an obstructive lesion. When there is no tight obstruction, dysphagia may have the features of achalasia, when there is a perivisceral neoplastic infiltration around the distal esophagus [24].

If the primary tumor is in the esophagus or at the cardia, there is no specific clinical expression of the lymphatic metastatic spread, which is detected during endoscopy, EUS exploration or in the operative specimen.

Diagnostics

Endoscopy is the first procedure in the exploration of the esophagus in patients with dysphagia. The metastatic involvement of the esophagus may be mistaken for a primary esophageal tumor when there is an obstructive and fungating tumor. The etiology of the tumor will be corrected by the biopsies. This situation occurs when the primary tumor is distant. In other patients, a tight esophageal stricture is seen and is covered by the unaltered mucosa. Malignancy is suggested by the asymmetry of the luminal channel and the reduced mobility of the lesion. This situation occurs especially in the delayed metastatic peri-esophageal progression of breast cancer [25, 26].

Finally when a primary tumor in the esophagus or at the cardia is the cause of dysphagia, metastatic lymphatic spread is suspected when small ulcerated areas are seen at distance from the primary tumor .The detection of eventual lymphatic metastases surrounding a primary esophageal squamous cell cancer, or in the segment proximal to an adenocarcinoma of the cardia, is helped by chromoscopy with spraying of a iodine solution (Lugol, 1.5%) which stains the normal Malpighian epithelium dark brown.

Table 5
WHO histological classification of esophageal tumors

Epithelial tumors	
Non epithelial tumors	
Secondary tumors	code of the primary tumor

EUS is extremely helpful in appreciating the extension of the tumor in the esophageal wall and in the mediastinum. In complement, spiral computerized tomography is required for the detection of other distant metastases in the thorax or in the abdomen.

Histologic Classification and Molecular Genetics

The histology of the metastatic tumor in the esophagus is confirmed by forceps biopsy during endoscopy and is similar to that of the primary cancer.

Staging

See Table 5.

Treatment

The dysphagia provoked by a fungating tumoral mass in the esophagus, or by a extrinsic neoplastic stricture requires palliation. Endoscopic procedures are preferred to surgical palliation; they include laser photodestruction, bougiennage or stenting.

Lymphatic spread with intramural esophageal metastases, detected in patients with esophageal squamous cell cancer or adenocarcinoma at the cardia, has an impact on the extent of the segment resected during surgery. When such metastases are detected, shifting the proximal pole of the resection in the upper esophagus is recommended, even when the primary tumor is an adenocarcinoma at the cardia.

Prognosis and Follow-Up

The overall prognosis of secondary tumors in the esophagus is poor. Long-term survival is not expected, but the nature of the primary tumor has some influence on the global prognosis.

Melanoma of the Esophagus

Epidemiology

Gastrointestinal metastases of a cutaneous melanoma, often localized at the lower extremities, occur in nearly 5% of cases. Most melanomas in the esophagus are secondary metastatic tumors [20, 27]. Primary melanoma of the esophagus [28, 29] is very rare; about 200 cases have been published [28] and they are assumed to represent only 0.1 to 0.2% of all esophageal tumors. Primary or secondary, the tumor has an aggressive behavior and a dismal prognosis.

Symptoms and Clinical Signs

Dysphagia is always present, because the growth of the melanoma is expansive rather than infiltrative and the tumor bulk is polypoid and obstructive.

Diagnostics and Staging

Endoscopy is the first procedure in the exploration of the esophagus. The obstructive tumor is often dark in color, but achromic melanoma occurs in 25%, the tumor is then of a pink color. The extension of the tumor is further staged by EUS and spiral computerized tomography. When the parietal implantation of the polypoid tumor is superficial (mucosa or submucosa), the prognosis is still dismal.

Histologic Classification and Molecular Genetics

The melanoma is usually confirmed by forceps biopsies. The histology is identical to that of a cutaneous melanoma.

Staging

Table 6
WHO histological classification of esophageal tumors

Epithelial tumors	
Non epithelial tumors	
Malignant melanoma	8720/3
Secondary tumors	

Treatment

The response of esophageal melanoma to any form of treatment is poor. When the patient is operable, surgery is the preferred solution. However, even when the tumor is limited to the mucosa, cure is hazardous, only 1 patient out of 5 submitted to esophagectomy being alive at 7 months [28].

Most tumors are considered as inoperable and systemic chemotherapy is not effective; it is based on dacarbazine, numustine hydrochloride and VCR. Further progress is expected from immunotherapy, however the benefit of interferon alpha is not convincing.

There is no room for endoscopic procedures with a curative objective; in inoperable patients with dysphagia, palliation is recommended and stenting has been attempted.

Prognosis and Follow-Up

The overall prognosis is poor, with a 30% survival at one year. Most patients die with generalized metastases.

Future Perspectives

Further progress is expected in systemic chemotherapy, and there is a promising approach in the potential efficacy of anti-sense therapy. It is hoped to reduce the expression of Bcl-x(L) (a member of the anti-apoptotic Bcl-2 family) by anti-sense oligonucleotides.

References

1. Miettinen M, Blay JY, Sobin LH. (2000) Mesenchymal tumours of the oesophagus. In Hamilton SR and Aaltonen LA. (eds) .Pathology & Genetics. Tumours of the digestive system. International Agency for the Research on Cancer, Lyon, pp 28–29
2. Murase K, Hino A, Ozeki Y, Karagiri Y, Onitsduka A, Sugie S. (2001) Malignant Schwannoma of the esophagus with lymph node metastasis: literature review of Schwannoma of the esophagus. J Gastroenterol. 36, 772–777
3. Voskuil JH, van Dijk MM, Wagenaar SS, van Vliet AC, Timmer R, van Hess PA. (2001) Occurrence of esophageal granular cell tumors in the Netherlands between 1988 and 1994. Dig Dis Sciences. 46, 1610–1614
4. Palazzo L, Landi B, Cellier C, Cuillerier E, Roseau G, Barbier JP. (2000) Endosonographic features predictive of benign and malignant gastrointestinal stromal cell tumours. Gut 46, 88–92
5. Palazzo L, Landi B, Cellier C, Roseau G, Chaussade S, Couturier B, Barbier J. (1997) Endosonographic features of esophageal granular cell tumors. Endoscopy 29, 850–853
6. Waxman I, Saitoh Y, Raju GS, Watari J, Yokota K, Reeves AL, Kohgo Y. (2002) High frequency probe EUS-assisted endoscopic mucosal resection: a therapeutic strategy for submucosal tumors of the GI tract .Gastrointest Endosc. 55, 44–49
7. Sun S, Wang S, Sun S. (2002) Use of endoscopic ultrasound-guided injection in endoscopic resection of solid submucosal tumors.Endoscopy, 34, 82–85
8. Hyun JH, Jeen YT, Chun HJ, Lee HS, Lee SQW, Song CW, Choi JH, Um SH, Kim CD, Ryu SH (1997) Endoscopic resection of submucosal tumor of the esophagus: results in 62 patients. Endoscopy 29, 165–170
9. Joensuu H. (2002) Treatment of inoperable gastrointestinal stromal tumor (GIST) with Imatinib (Glivec, Gleevec). Med Klin. 97, Suppl 1: 28–30
10. Emory TS, Sobin LH, Lukes L, Lee DH, O'Leary TJ. (1999) Prognosis of gastrointestinal smooth-muscle (stromal) tumors: dependence on anatomic site. Am J Surg Pathol. 23, 82–87
11. Capella G, Solcia E, Sobin LH, Arnold R. (2000) Endocrine tumours of the oesophagus .In Hamilton SR and Aaltonen LA (eds) .Pathology & Genetics . Tumours of the digestive system International Agency for the Research on Cancer, Lyon, pp 26–27
12. Soga J (1998) Esophageal endocrinomas, an extremely rare tumor: a statistical comparative evaluation of 28 ordinary carcinoids, and 72 atypical variants. J Exp Clin Cancer Res. 17, 47–57
13. Modlin IM, Sandor A. (1997) An analysis of 8305 cases of carcinoid tumors. Cancer, 79, 813–829
14. Law SY, Fok M, Lam KY, Loke SL, MaLT, Wong J. (1994) Small cell carcinoma of the esophagus. Cancer 73, 2994–2899
15. Chow V, Law S, Lam KY, Luk JM, Wong J. (2001) Telomerase activity in small cell esophageal carcinoma. Dis. Esophagus 14, 139–142
16. Oberg K (2001) Chemotherapy and biotherapy in the treatment of neuroendocrine tumours. Ann. Oncol. 12 (Suppl 2), S11–S114
17. Wotherspoon A. Chott A, Gascoyne RD, Muller Hermelink HK (2000) Lymphoma of the oesophagus. In Hamilton SR and Aaltonen LA (eds) Pathology & Genetics . Tumours of the digestive system.International Agency for the Research on Cancer, Lyon, p 27
18. Oguzkurt L, karabulut N, Cakmacki E, Besim A (1997) Primary non Hodgkin lymphoma of the esophagus. Abdom Imaging 22, 8–20
19. Fujizawa S, Motomura S, Fujimaki K, Tanabe J, Tomita N, Hara M, Mohri H (1999) Primary esophageal T cell lymphoma. Leuk. Lymphoma 33, 199–202
20. Ilyes G, Kadar A, Carr NJ (2000) Secondary tumours and melanoma of the oesophagus. In Hamilton SR and Aaltonen LA (eds) Pathology & Genetics. Tumours of the digestive system. International Agency for the Research on Cancer, Lyon, p 30
21. Shimchuck EJ, Low DE (2001) Direct esophageal metastasis from a distant primary tumor is a submucosal process: a review of 6 cases. Dis. Esophagus 14, 247–250
22. Kuwano H (1998) Peculiar histopathologic features of esophageal cancer Surg. Today 28, 573–575.
23. Hirota T, Nishimaki T, Susuki T, Komukai S, Kuwabara A, Aizawa K, Hatakeyama K (1998) Esophageal intramural metastasis from an adenocarcinoma of the gastric cardia : report of a case. Surg. Today 28, 1160–1162
24. Manela FD, Quigley EM, Paustian FF, Taylor RJ (1991) Achalasia of the esophagus in association with renal cell carcinoma. Am. J. Gastroenterol. 86, 1812–1816
25. Wu CM, Hruban RH, Fishman EK (1998) Breast carcinoma metastatic to the esophagus. CT findings with pathologic correlation. Clin. Imaging 22, 343–345
26. Varanasi RV, Saltzman JR, Krims P, Crimaldi A, Colby J (1995) Breast carcinoma metastatic to the esophagus: clinicopathological and management features of four cases and literature review. Am J Gastroenterol. 90, 1495–1499
27. Panagiotou I, Brountzos EN, Bafaloukos D, Stoupis C, Brestas P, Kelekis DA (2002) Malignant melanoma metastatic to the gastrointestinal tract. Melanoma Res. 12, 169–173
28. Gollub MJ, Provda JC (1999) Primary melanoma of the esophagus: radiologic and clinical findings in 6 patients. Radiology 213, 97–100
29. Archer HA, Owen WJ Primary malignant melanoma of the esophagus. Dis. Esophagus, 2000, 13, 320–323

Stomach

II

4 Gastric Cancer

A.T.R. AXON, M.F. DIXON, H.M. SUE-LING

Summary

Gastric cancer is the second commonest cause of death from malignancy in the world. It arises usually in a stomach that has been chronically inflamed over many years leading to a pan-gastritis, gastric atrophy, hypochlorhydria and intestinal metaplasia. Risk factors include a high salt, low vegetable and fruit diet, duodenogastric reflux and *Helicobacter pylori* infection. These, in conjunction with other environmental factors and a genetic predisposition, lead to the development of cancer mainly in middle aged and elderly people. Histologically carcinomas are classified as "intestinal" or "diffuse"; both however are strongly associated with infection with *Helicobacter pylori*. The classical triad of symptoms; abdominal pain, anorexia and weight loss is usually associated with advanced cancer which carries a poor prognosis. Early gastric cancer may be identified by screening programmes, active investigation of minor dyspeptic symptoms or those typically associated with peptic ulcer. If the lesion has not invaded the muscularis propria the prognosis is good. Early cancer if limited in extent can be treated by endoscopic mucosal resection (EMR), however most cases of cancer are treated by partial or total gastrectomy with or without adjuvant chemotherapy. Screening for gastric cancer is not available, or practicable in most countries. A more logical method to reduce mortality might involve screening for *Helicobacter* infection in young adults and treatment of affected individuals with antibiotic therapy. Prospective studies have not been carried out, but it is likely that this approach would allow effective primary prevention of this disease.

Epidemiology

The incidence of gastric cancer varies widely both between and within countries. There is a notably high incidence in Japan, China, Colombia and Finland, but even in these countries, as elsewhere in the world, the incidence of carcinoma of the stomach is declining. Despite this fall, gastric cancer is still the second most frequent fatal malignancy (after lung cancer) in the world, with an estimated three-quarters of a million new cases diagnosed annually [1]. In several countries gastric cancer remains the most common form of malignant disease. Migrant studies indicate strong environmental influences; for example, when Japanese move to Hawaii or California the incidence of gastric cancer in that group falls, and after only one generation approximates to that of the local population. While formerly a high salt diet, low vitamin intake, and ingestion of smoked and pickled foods were incriminated, it is now appreciated that the major causative environmental factor is *H. pylori* infection (Fig. 1).

Evidence for this comes from several sources. Although there are some notable exceptions (e.g. the African enigma), the prevalence of *H. pylori* infection

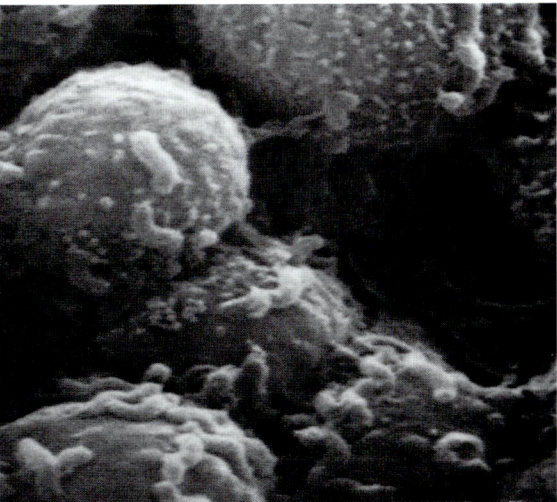

Figure 1
Scanning electron microscope photographs showing Heliobacter colonizing the gastric mucosa

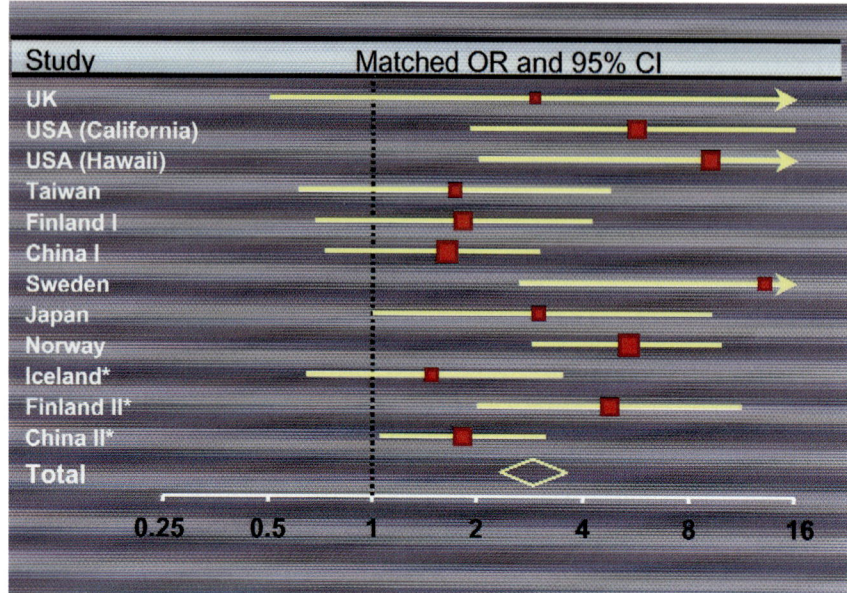

Figure 2
Meta-analysis of nested serological case control studies showing past infection with Heliobacter to be an important risk factor in non-cardia gastric cancer [3]. (Reproduced with the kind permission of author and editor)

runs parallel to the incidence of gastric cancer in the same populations [2]. Sero-epidemiological studies have shown that patients with evidence of prior *H. pylori* infection have a higher risk of gastric cancer than uninfected controls [3], and a meta-analysis of serological case-control studies has confirmed past infection as an important risk factor (Fig. 2).

Epidemiological studies under-estimate the risk of *Helicobacter* as a cause of cancer because as the stomach becomes atrophic, the load of infection within it declines and eventually the organism disappears altogether and serology becomes negative. One study from Japan has shown the odds ratio for infected patients to be very much higher in young patients and those with early cancer (Table 1) [4].

In Japan it has been reported that each year gastric cancer develops in 300,000 (0.5%) of the 60 million people who are infected with *H. pylori* [5], or, put another way, gastric cancer will develop in 5% of infected individuals over a 10 year period. The strength of the epidemiological link is such that the International Agency for Research into Cancer has declared *H. pylori* a Class 1 carcinogen [6].

Etiology and Pathogenesis

For many years a sequence of events, starting with chronic gastritis (Fig. 3) and passing through atrophy and intestinal metaplasia (Fig. 4) to intra-epithelial neoplasia (dysplasia) (Fig. 5), has been acknowledged as the precursor to cancer of the stomach [7].

Given that *H. pylori* has now been accepted as the major cause of chronic gastritis, it is logical to implicate this infection in the causation of gastric cancer. However, given the high prevalence of infection and the compara-

Table 1
Relationship between gastric cancer and Hp serology in patients aged <40 years. (Taken from Kikuchi et al. [4])

Subjects	Odds ratio	(95% CL)
All patients	13.3	(5.3–35.6)
Men	6.8	(2.4–18.8)
Women	32.8	(6.2–330.4)
Early gastric carcinoma patients	20.8	(3.8–220.4)
Advanced gastric carcinoma patients	10.8	(3.7–34.8)
Intestinal type gastric carcinoma	18.0	(1.9–1744.6)
Diffuse type gastric carcinoma	12.8	(4.7–36.8)
Proximal carcinoma	11.3	(2.6–68.8)
Distal carcinoma	14.8	(4.8–53.9)

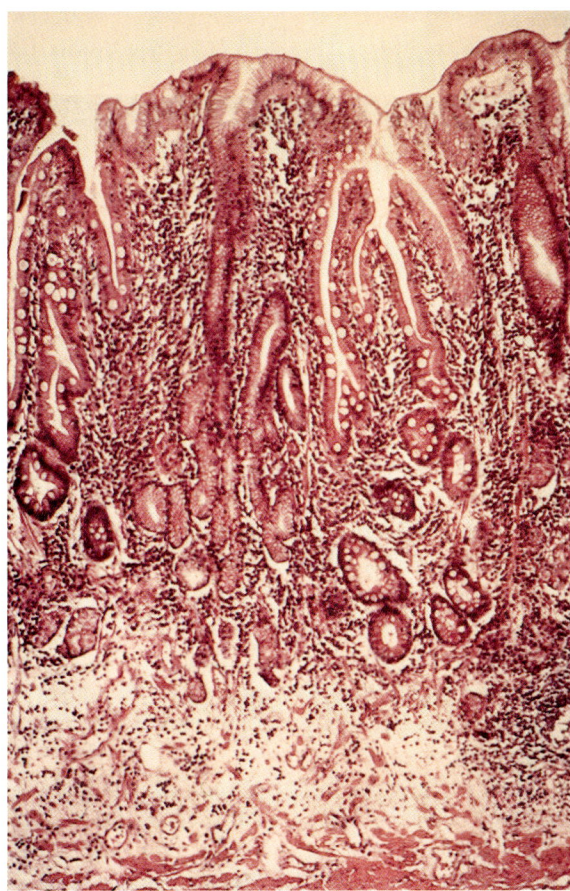

Figure 3
Antral mucosa showing chronic inflammation (*H. pylori* positive), glandular atrophy and intestinal metaplasia

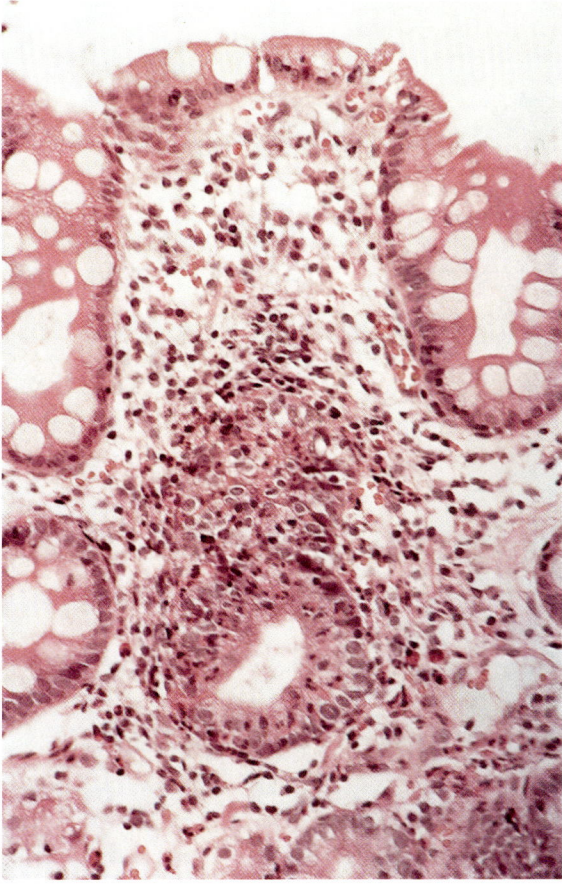

Figure 4
Gastric mucosa showing intestinal metaplasia. Active chronic inflammation is concentrated around residual normal foveolar epithelium where *H. pylori* are found

tive infrequency of gastric cancer it is unlikely that the organism or its products are direct-acting mutagens. On the other hand, there are a number of indirect mechanisms which could link *H. pylori* infection to gastric cancer.

Long-term infection leads to corpus atrophy and a gradual decline in acid secretion. Hypochlorhydria allows other (enteric) bacteria to proliferate in the gastric juice; these bacteria are capable of reducing nitrate ions to nitrite and can catalyze nitrosation of amines and amides present in the diet to give rise to potentially carcinogenic N-nitroso compounds [8]. *H. pylori* possesses an inducible alcohol dehydrogenase which is capable of producing acetaldehyde from alcohol substrates. Acetaldehyde is a highly reactive product which damages epithelial cells and is genotoxic, but its role *in vivo* is in dispute.

A more likely source of genomic DNA damage in *H. pylori* gastritis is attack by reactive oxygen species [9] including superoxide and hydroxyl radicals, monochloramines and nitric oxide produced by activated polymorphs and macrophages. Interestingly, nitrosation and oxidative damage is minimized by anti-oxidant vitamins, among which ascorbic acid is the most important, and diets rich in fresh fruit and vegetables have long been recognized as protective against gastric cancer. As-

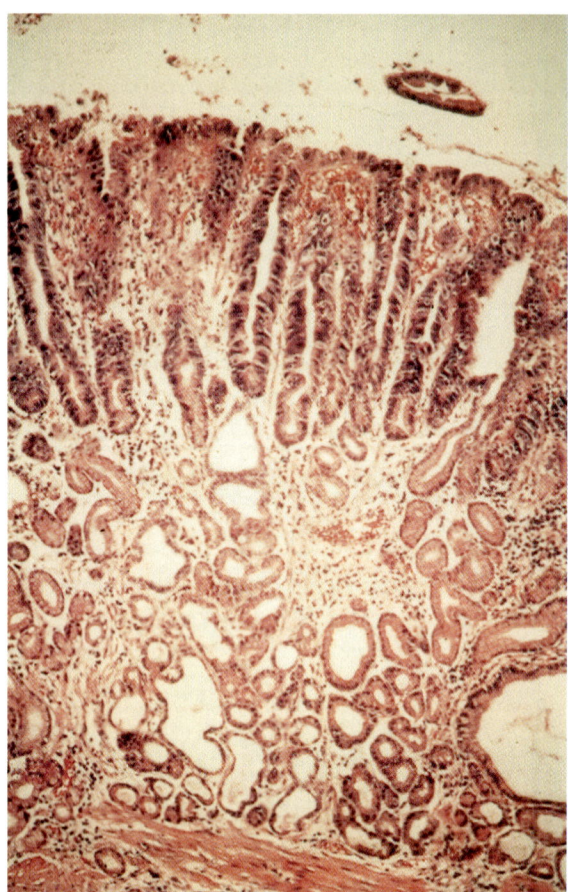

Figure 5
High grade dysplasia arising in the antral-corpus transitional zone affected by atrophy and pyloric metaplasia

Table 2
8 year prospective study of 1526 patients. (Taken from Uemura et al. [5])

Diagnosis	No	Cancer [%]
Hp+ve	1246	*36 (2.9)
Hp-ve	280	0 (0)
NUD	445	21 (4.7)
GU	297	10 (3.4)
Hyperplastic polyps	229	5 (2.2)
DU	275	0 (0)

*$p<0.001$.

cause, DNA repair is compromised and the probability of a mutation escaping repair and being transmitted to daughter cells is increased. In this way mitogenesis promotes mutagenesis.

Further evidence in favor of *Helicobacter* being an important contributory factor in the development of gastric cancer comes from experimental work using the Mongolian gerbil which develops a gastritis similar to that in humans and which can progress also to gastric cancer [12].

More recent work in Japan from Uemera and colleagues has shown that in a prospective study comparing the outcome of patients treated for *Helicobacter pylori* infection those who have received effective eradication therapy were protected (Table 2) [5].

Cancer of the Gastric Cardia

Cancer arising from the cardia of the stomach (Fig. 6) appears to have a completely different epidemiology and pathogenesis from non-cardia (or distal) gastric cancer.

It is much less common than distal cancer, but is increasing in incidence in developed countries just as distal cancer is declining.

Cardia cancer is believed to arise from the specialized cardia mucosa, a non-acid secreting columnar tissue that extends from the squamo-columnar junction of the esophagus for a short distance into the upper stomach. Unlike cancer of the distal stomach there is no evidence that *Helicobacter* plays a role in its pathogenesis [3]. Nevertheless, taking account of the small area of mucosa from which these tumors arise, it is apparent that, in the West at any rate, some important change has taken

corbic acid secretion into gastric juice is severely compromised in *H. pylori* gastritis and gradually returns after eradication of infection [10].

Perhaps the most important factor underlying the relationship between *H. pylori* and gastric cancer is a promotional effect through high cell turnover [11]. The production of cytotoxins and ammonia by the organism, and indirect epithelial damage brought about by cytokines and polymorph products, induce increased cell turnover. These effects may be exacerbated by increased gastrin-induced cell proliferation both as a consequence of hypergastrinemia and autocrine stimulation, and by a high salt diet. In hyperplastic states, from whatever place in the environment which has made this mucosa vulnerable to malignant change. Cardia cancer may arise from intestinal metaplasia of the cardia mucosa. However, this is common (5.3%–23% of dyspeptic patients). The presence of acidic glycoproteins and goblet cells together is indicative of intestinal metaplasia. Four histological types of cancer have been described, papillary (Fig. 7), tubular, mucinous and signet-ring adenocarcinoma (Fig. 8).

Signet-ring cancer is much less common in the proximal stomach than distally and proximal stomach cancer is generally not accompanied by atrophic gastric [13].

It is often difficult to distinguish cancer of the cardia from that of the lower esophagus. This latter disease which is also increasing in developed countries has been attributed to the increased prevalence of Barrett's esophagus, a condition where in some individuals reflux esophagitis leads to a change in the nature of the lower esophageal epithelium from its normal squamous phenotype to one of specialized intestinal metaplasia (usually type II or III). Figure 9 demonstrates the difficulty in distinguishing between the two.

The two photographs were taken at the same endoscopic examination, one showing the lesion in the esophagus, the other in the stomach. In this instance no Barrett's mucosa could be seen within the distal esophagus. Problems with identifying the site of origin of these lesions cause confusion in studies of the epidemiology and pathogenesis of the two tumors.

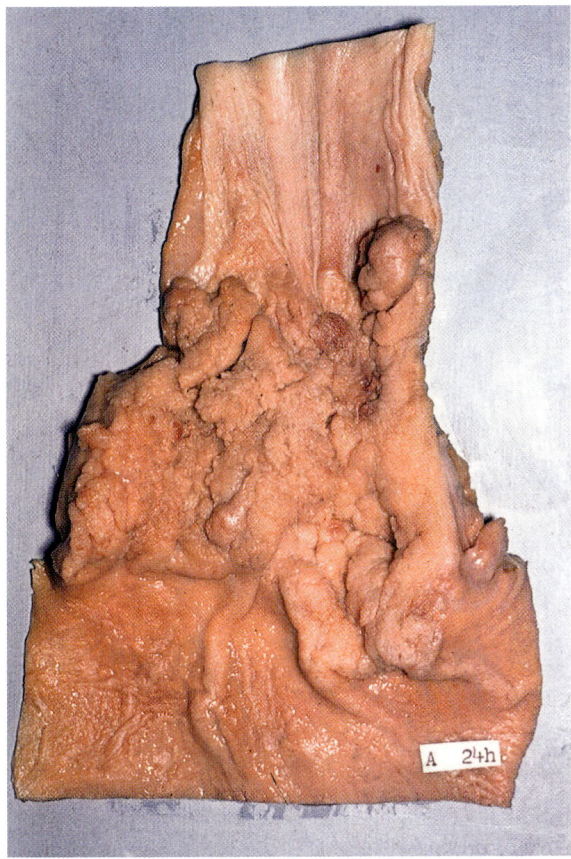

Figure 6
Large ulcerated and fungating carcinoma at the gastric cardia

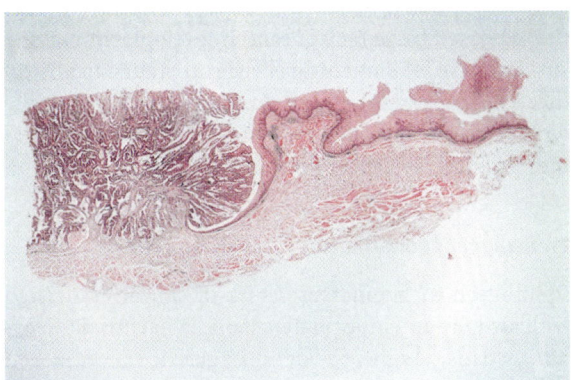

Figure 7
Papillary adenocarcinoma arising at the cardia abutting onto the squamous junction

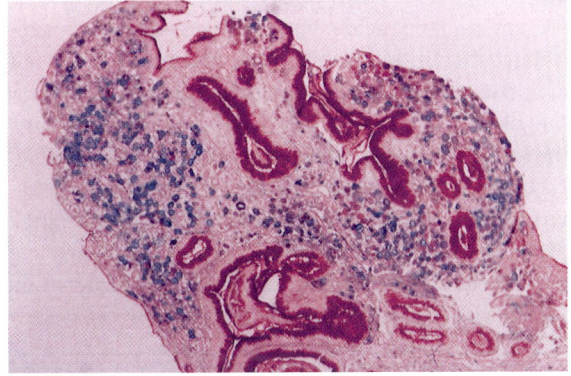

Figure 8
Biopsy of cardia mucosa stained by alcian blue/PAS to show neutral (*magenta*) and acidic (*blue*) mucins. The lamina propria of the mucosal is widely infiltrated by signet-ring cell adenocarcinoma

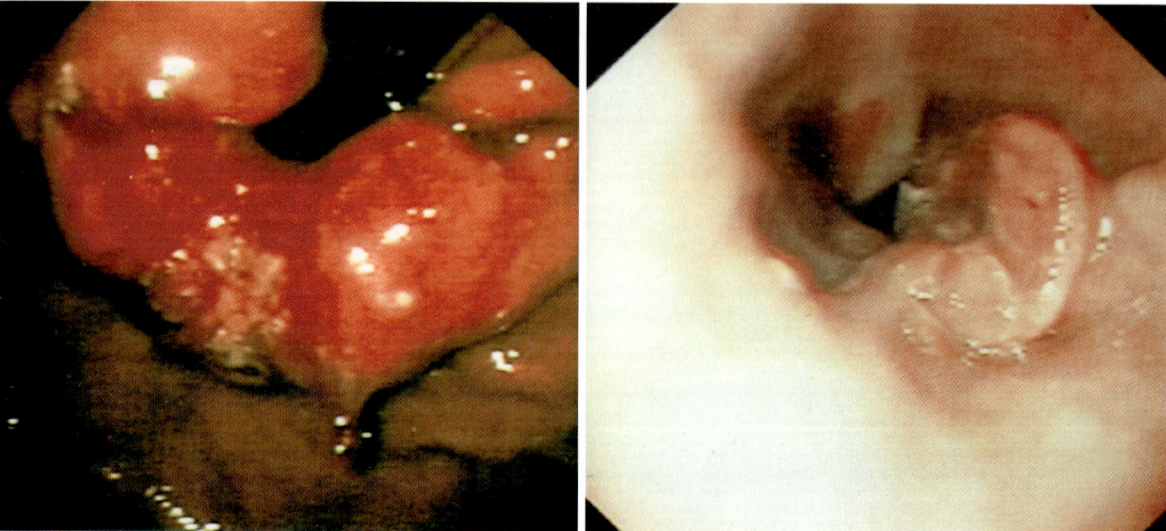

Figure 9
Endoscopic photographs taken at the same examination showing cancer at the cardio-oesophageal junction present both in the oesophagus and in the stomach, no Barrett's mucosa was macroscopically apparent

Work from McColl's group in Glasgow has shown that a micro-environment exists in close vicinity to the gastro-esophageal junction. Following a meal, gastric acid in the distal stomach is buffered and the pH rises, however, the gastric juice in the vicinity of the cardia remains at a low pH. It seems that relatively little mixing takes place, possibly due to a fatty layer that floats on the top of the gastric contents [14]. Further work by this group has shown that not only is the post-prandial micro-environment acidic but, following ingestion of nitrate-containing food, nitric oxide concentrations in this area rise to high levels. The underlying mechanism is that dietary nitrate is absorbed and re-excreted through the saliva. Much of it is then metabolized by oral bacteria to nitrite. When nitrite reaches the acidic micro-environment it is rapidly converted to nitric oxide in the presence of ascorbic acid. Nitric oxide is a mutagen and McColl has suggested that this may be the explanation for the rise in cardia cancer resulting from the hugely increased nitrate content of food over the past 50 years [15] as a result of intensive farming.

Role of Gastrointestinal Reflux

While *Helicobacter* infection is the single most important etiological factor, it is not the only identifiable contributor to gastric carcinogenesis. Well before the *H. pylori* era, reflux of bile and other pancreatico-duodenal contents were known to be an important risk factor for the development of gastric cancer. Breakdown products of bile are known to be carcinogenic [16] and the increased frequency of cancer development in post-surgical gastric remnants has been attributed to bile reflux [17]. Interestingly, bile reflux may act synergistically with *H. pylori* infection to increase cell turnover and thereby increase cancer risk [18].

Premalignant Conditions

In addition to the increased risk of cancer associated with atrophy and intestinal metaplasia in chronic *H. pylori* gastritis, a higher incidence of gastric cancer is seen in patients with pernicious anemia and following partial gastrectomy for benign ulcer disease. Patients with pernicious anemia exhibit a threefold increase in the risk of gastric cancer over the general population, while post-gastrectomy patients develop an excess risk about 15–20 years after surgery. A common denominator in all such patients is the presence of hypochlorhydria or achlorhydria as a result of glandular atrophy and/or alkaline and bile reflux. Thus it is likely that the development of most "environmental" gastric cancers can be explained in terms of longstanding mucosal injury giving rise to a continuing hyperproliferative state, combined with low acid secretion and luminal conditions conducive to genotoxin formation. Hyperproliferation also underlies the increased cancer risk in Menetrier's disease.

While intestinal metaplasia (IM) is commonly present in stomachs which harbor malignancy, its role in the histogenesis of gastric cancer is in doubt. For instance, IM could be a general response of the mucosa to injury without being directly linked to cancer development. There have been many attempts to relate certain subtypes of IM to cancer risk. While the link appears to be strongest for Type III (incomplete, sulphomucin positive) IM, it is not sufficiently close for IM typing to be of value in clinical management or surveillance. It seems likely that the other subtypes are epiphenomena with regard to cancer development.

There are patients with gastric cancer who have neither a recognized premalignant condition nor chronic gastritis and hypochlorhydria. Genetic factors are likely to be involved, but little is known of these beyond a link with blood group A and the appearance of frequent gastric cancers in certain families often at a young age. It is likely that such individuals have inherited defects in DNA repair genes as, for instance, in HNPCC kindreds.

Symptoms and Clinical Signs

Advanced Gastric Cancer

The symptoms of advanced gastric cancer are well known. They include anorexia and weight loss, non-specific upper abdominal pain and nausea. If the lesion is sited at the cardia, dysphagia may be the presenting symptom. In those with pyloric cancer, the symptoms of pyloric obstruction may be present, these include vomiting of food ingested many hours before, foul eructations and upper abdominal discomfort. Sometimes the clinical picture is more typical of that found in gastric ulcer, with epigastric pain precipitated by eating and sometimes relieved by vomiting, hematemesis and melena are other presentations in this group. Sometimes the disease presents insidiously with the symptoms of iron deficiency anemia, tiredness, fatigue, lethargy, pallor, angular stomatitis and glossitis. Occasionally patients present with an abdominal mass which they have noticed or symptoms relating to metastases such as enlargement of Virchow's node, jaundice from infiltration of the liver or back pain if the lesion penetrates posteriorly.

The physical signs of advanced cancer include those relating to the symptoms already outlined. Abdominally the primary lesion may be palpable or the liver may be enlarged, hard and irregular from metastases. Left sided supra-clavicular lymph nodes may be palpable. In patients with outlet obstruction, a succussion splash may be elicited more than four hours after ingestion of food. Ascites may be present from peritoneal seeding. There may be muscular wasting, pallor and koilonychia.

In the majority of patients who present with the above symptoms the carcinoma will already be at an advanced stage. However, of those presenting with symptoms more typical of gastric ulcer, a significant subset will be found to have early gastric cancer, or at any rate no distant metastases or penetration into adjacent organs.

Early Gastric Cancer (EGC)

The concept of early EGC has been promoted by the pioneering work of Japanese radiologists and endoscopists [19]. EGC is defined as a lesion limited to the mucosa or submucosa, ie. it has not penetrated the muscularis propria. Patients with these lesions have a five year survival of over 90% following surgery [20]. The identification of EGC is therefore extremely important. As indicated above the symptoms of EGC may be those of simple gastric ulcer but in the majority of cases the lesion is pre-symptomatic and often diagnosed in Japan as a result of radiological or endoscopic screening of asymptomatic patients, or the early investigation of patients with mild dyspepsia. In general, patients with EGC have a longer history than those with advanced cancer and it is possible that many of these have been identified as a result

Table 3
Symptom distribution in early gastric cancer (per cent of patients with specified symptom). (Reproduced from Everett and Axon [20], with kind permission of the author and editor)

Reference	Cases [n]	Epigastric Pain/dyspepsia	Anorexia	Weight loss	Gastrointestinal Bleeding	Anaemia	Nausea/ Vomiting	None
Pinto et al. 1994	142	91.2	–	42.3	–	–	40.1	–
Belcastro et al. 1998	19	84.2	5.3	5.3	–	5.3	–	5.3
Gozzetti et al. 1997	49	82.6	–	–	–	–	–	–
Houghton et al. 1985	35	74	23	63	37	14	26	–
Ballantyne et al. 1987	20	75	–	–	15	15	25	–
Sue-Ling et al. 1992	46	73	18	24	11	–	49	9
Eckardt et al. 1990	51	70	12	25	8	–	11	–
Craanen et al. 1991	28	67.8	–	10.7	25	–	17.9	–
Oleagoita et al. 1986	142	75.3	–	–	5	–	6.4	4.2
Moreaux et al. 1993	101	84.2	–	3.9	6	1	–	5.9
Carter et al. 1984	5	80	–	40	–	–	20	–
Farley et al. 1992	48	62.5	39.6	39.6	25	–	39.6	–
Lawrence et al. 1991	60	–	–	21.7	21.6	–	–	–
Chia et al. 1988	52	67.3	–	–	19	11.5	23.1	–

of the widespread use of endoscopy in patients with functional dyspepsia, that is to say the symptoms for which the endoscopy has been performed may not have been generated by the cancer itself. Table 3 indicates the symptom distribution of early gastric cancer and it can be seen that those complaining of weight loss and anorexia were in the minority, most complained of epigastric pain.

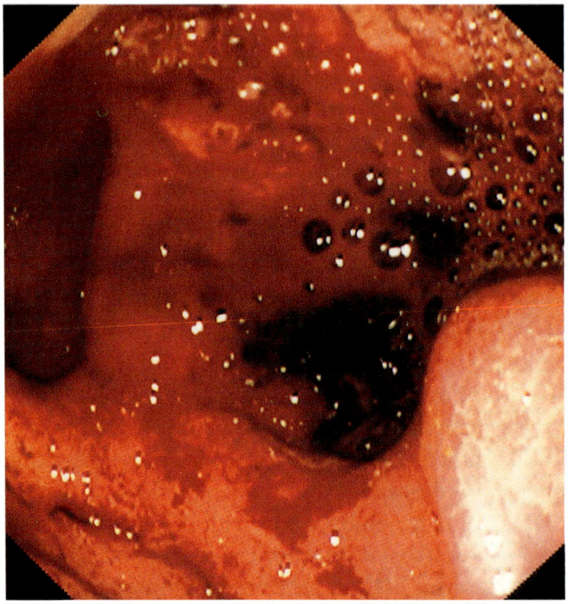

Figure 10
Endoscopic image of advanced gastric cancer

Diagnostics

The diagnosis of gastric cancer today is made by upper digestive endoscopy. The appearances in most cases of cancer diagnosed in the West are typical and unmistakable (Fig. 10) however, in some cases it may be difficult to distinguish benign from malignant peptic ulceration endoscopically.

It is extremely important to do this however because early ulcerative cancer carries a good prognosis. Figure 11 [21] outlines the differences in appearance between malignant and benign ulceration.

Of even greater difficulty however is the identification of early gastric cancer that is neither ulcerated nor protruberant. Japanese endoscopists have drawn attention to "a gastritis- like" lesion, a condition rarely identified in the West. Yoshida [22] has divided them into four appearances. Those with an erythematous (reddish appearance), those with a discoloured (pale) appear-

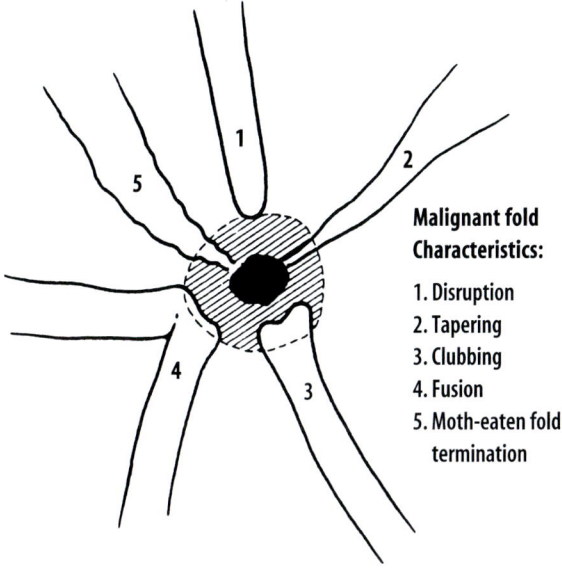

Figure 11
Gastric fold characteristics in proximity to an ulcer that suggest malignancy. (Reproduced from Mellinger and Ponsky [21], with kind permission of Kluwer Academic Publishers and the authors)

Malignant fold Characteristics:

1. Disruption
2. Tapering
3. Clubbing
4. Fusion
5. Moth-eaten fold termination

The Japanese have classified early gastric cancer into three types, I, II and III, type II being subdivided into a, b and c. In principle type I is protruding, type II is flat, type III excavated (ulcerated). Type IIa is where the lesion is flat in the sense of being rather like a plateau but is raised above the level of the mucosa. Type IIb (rather rare) is where the lesion is completely flat and type IIc (probably the most common form of early gastric cancer) where the lesion is depressed below the level of the surrounding mucosa. A diagram of the classification is shown in Fig. 14 [21].

A not uncommon combination is a type IIc + III where the lesion is essentially flat at the edge and slightly depressed but excavated (ulcerated) in the center.

The diagnosis of early gastric cancer is difficult and lesions are frequently missed in the West. The reason why the Japanese have had such success in identifying early cancer is because of the care they take with each individual endoscopy and because their system of quality control includes many photographs which are reviewed and followed up. The Japanese endoscopist insists on a clean stomach without bubbles, so patients are often given a drink of Infacol before the examination. They spend longer inspecting the stomach for asymptomatic lesions, paying attention in turn to the antrum, the body, the corpus and the cardia region. They ensure that the stomach is adequately inflated and if they are in any

ance, others with roughened mucosa and those with an abnormal vascular appearance. Examples of these are shown in Figs. 12 and 13.

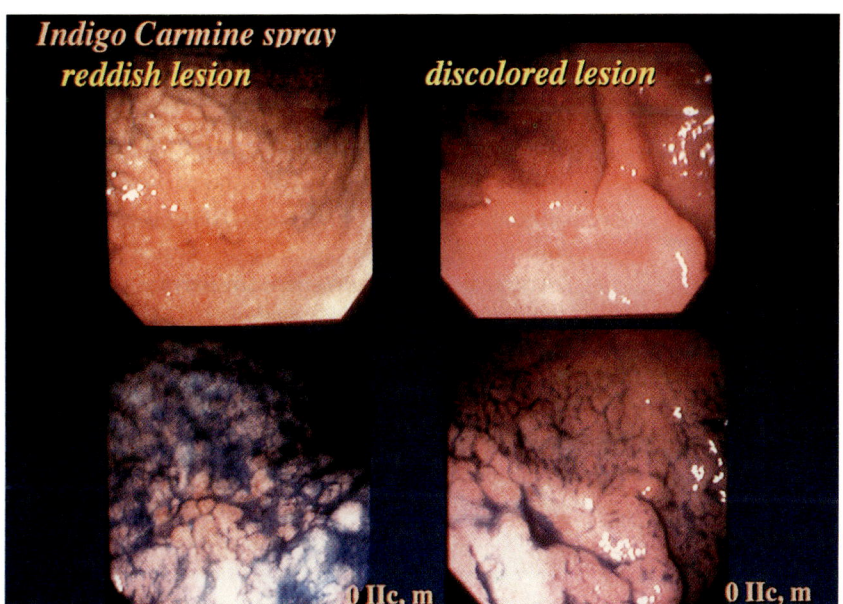

Figure 12
Gastritis-like early cancer showing erythematous and discoloured lesions. (Reproduced with kind permission of Dr Hitoshi Kondo, The Centre for Digestive Diseases, Tonan Hospital, Japan)

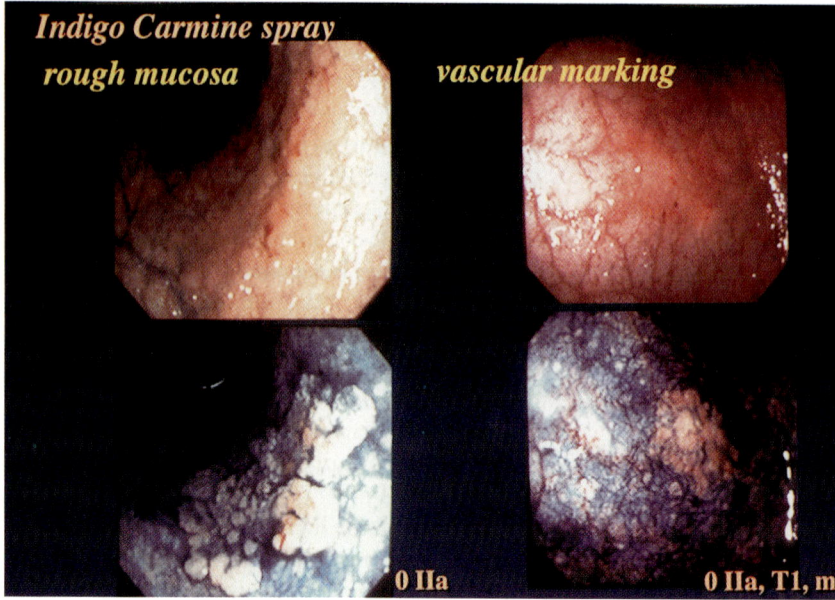

Figure 13
Gastritis-like early gastric cancer showing roughened type lesion and a lesion associated with abnormality of the vascular appearance. (Reproduced with kind permission of Dr Hitoshi Kondo, The Centre for Digestive Diseases, Tonan Hospital, Japan)

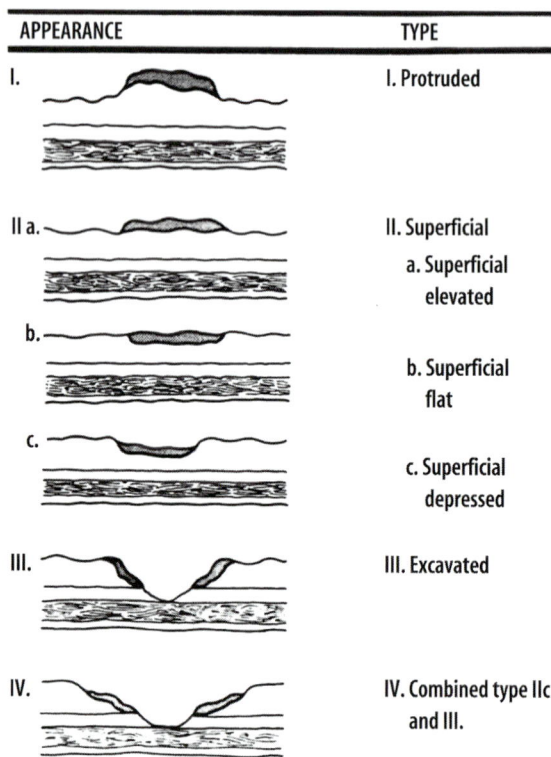

Figure 14
Sakita classification of early gastric cancer. (From Mellinger and Ponsky [21], with kind permission of Kluwer Academic Publishers)

doubt they spray the lining with dilute indigo carmine which enhances the contours and displays differences between normal and abnormal mucosa (Fig. 15a,b).

In the West early cancers are usually diagnosed only in patients with the ulcerative (type III) early cancer and this used to be the case in Japan. The adoption of Japanese methods into Western endoscopy should improve the identification of these important early lesions.

Biopsy Findings

Lesions of high-grade intra-epithelial neoplasia may be endoscopically visible as slightly elevated plaques or shallow depressions. Histologically, *in-situ* neoplasia is distinguished from intra-mucosal carcinoma according to whether or not invasion of the lamina propria has occurred. However invasion can only be excluded by examination of multiple sections from the entire area of involvement. Likewise a biopsy diagnosis of intra-mucosal carcinoma must be considered an interim one, as confirmation of the maximal depth of invasion will only be revealed in a resection specimen. Thus further management of high grade neoplasia should be based on the findings at endoscopy and by imaging; circumscribed lesions confined to the mucosa can be treated by EMR or local surgical resection, more advanced lesions will require gastrectomy.

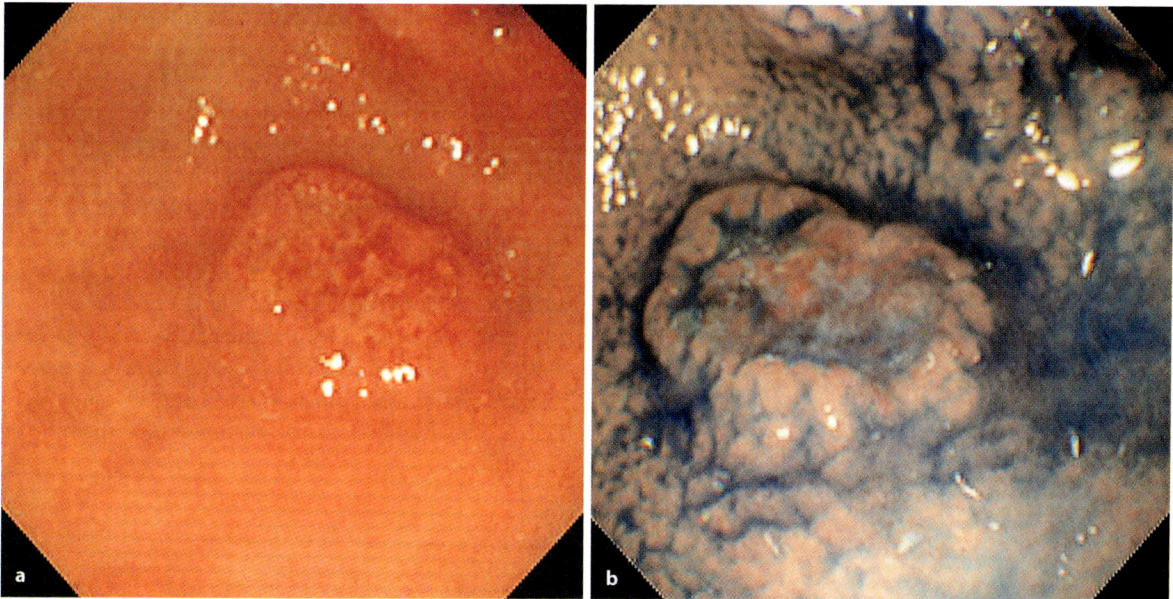

Figure 15
a An early gastric cancer before and **b** after dye spray, immediately prior to endomucosal resection (EMR). (Illustrations courtesy of Dr. B. Rembacken, Locum Consultant Gastroenterologist, Leeds General Infirmary)

With increasing size, the elevated lesions develop into *polypoid* and later into *fungating* carcinomas, while depressed carcinomas frequently progress to an excavated *ulcerated* appearance mimicking that seen in chronic peptic ulcer.

Histological Classification and Molecular Genetics

Carcinomas of the stomach are almost exclusively *adenocarcinomas* derived from either native or metaplastic mucus-secreting epithelial cells. Cancers which are not adenocarcinomas are thus distinctly uncommon. Neuroendocrine tumors are to be distinguished from adenocarcinomas showing some degree of neuroendocrine differentiation, and from mixed carcinoid tumor and adenocarcinoma ("collision" type). Adeno-squamous carcinoma is an uncommon variant, while pure squamous carcinomas are exceedingly rare. Other rare variants include hepatoid, parietal-cell, embryonal and chorio-carcinomas.

While there are several approaches to categorizing and grading gastric cancers only the Lauren classification into "intestinal" or "diffuse" types is widely employed in Western countries.

Intestinal type carcinomas (Fig. 16) show tubular or glandular formations lined by mucus-secreting cells with plentiful cytoplasm; they are more likely to have an expansive growth pattern.

Diffuse carcinomas (Fig. 17) consist of chains of single, non-cohesive cells infiltrating the wall with a poorly demarcated invasive margin.

Mucus secretion is generally less apparent, and usually takes the form of intra-cytoplasmic vacuoles which may compress the nucleus to form so-called "signet ring" cells.

An alternative division into "expansive" and "infiltrative" gastric cancers (Ming) has proved to be prognostic in multivariate analyses after stage has been taken into account. Expansive tumors are associated with longer survival than infiltrative forms [23]. The nature of the invasive margin is also of importance in EGC. However in EGC, in contrast to the claimed effect in advanced

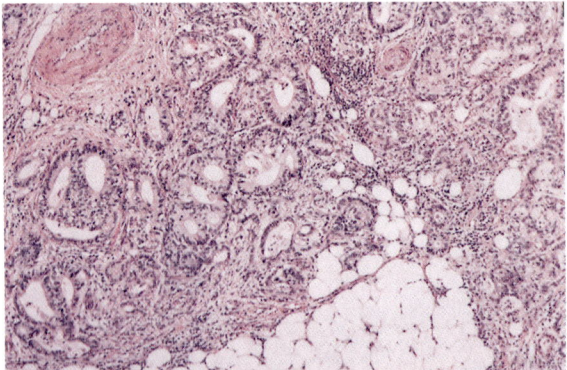

Figure 16
Intestinal-type gastric adenocarcinoma that has invaded through the main muscle coat to involve sub-peritoneal fat

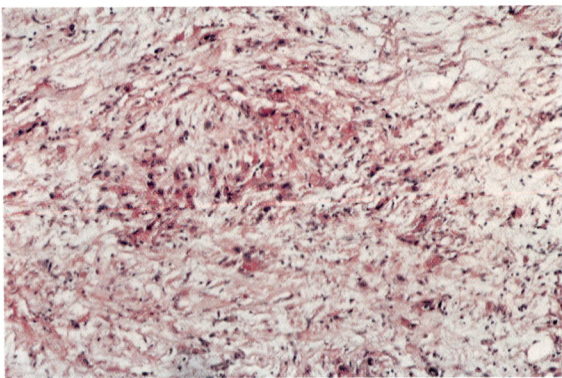

Figure 17
Widely invasive diffuse-type adenocarcinoma infiltrating the gastric wall (Alcian Blue-PAS stain for mucins)

cases, expansive tumors have a worse prognosis than infiltrative lesions. Nevertheless this has to be put in the context of the generally favorable outlook in EGC and the rarity of "aggressive" subtypes.

With regard to conventional tumor grade, a simple two-tier division into *poor,* and combined *good* or *moderate* differentiation (based on the predominant appearance) is considered sufficient. This dichotomous separation is more in keeping with the Japanese practice of distinguishing "poor" or "undifferentiated" and "well" or "differentiated" gastric cancers. Japanese pathologists have achieved further refinement by distinguishing

"gastric", "intestinal" and "mixed" phenotypes based on immunostaining for mucin gene products and brush border antigens [24]. These phenotypes have a bearing on clinical behavior, with tumors of "gastric" phenotype having a more aggressive course and a higher incidence of lymph node metastases. Interestingly, small "early" carcinomas are more frequently "differentiated" and have an intestinal phenotype, whereas larger tumors exhibit an increased frequency of undifferentiated, non-cohesive growth and a gastric phenotype. In keeping with these observations, it is generally acknowledged that poorly (and un-) differentiated gastric carcinomas have usually spread more extensively and are more likely to have disseminated via the peritoneum at the time of diagnosis than well-differentiated tumors.

Genetic and Epigenetic Abnormalities

Several molecular genetic changes have been demonstrated in gastric cancer involving loss of tumor suppressor genes, over-expression of oncogenes, and abnormalities in DNA repair genes, cell-cycle regulators and cell adhesion molecules.

In all cell lineages, telomere maintenance by activation of telomerase results in cellular immortalization. In this regard, increased activity of telomerase has been found in most gastric cancers irrespective of stage or histological type [25]. Mutations and deletions of tumor suppressor genes, notably p53, K-*ras* and the APC gene, and over-expression of oncogenes such as c-*myc* and c-*erb*B-2, have been demonstrated most frequently in well-differentiated or intestinal carcinomas [26]. Other abnormalities are more closely associated with poorly differentiated or diffuse carcinomas; for example, inactivation of cadherins and amplification of the K-*sam* and c-*met* genes. Abnormalities in cell cycle regulation are indicated by the amplification of cyclin E found in 15–20% of gastric cancers [27].

Genetic instability is an important general feature of carcinogenesis particularly in its early phase. While high frequency microsatellite instability is observed in only 4% of gastric cancers, low frequency instability (MSI-L) is found in about 30%, including early gastric cancers [26]. MSI-L is also found in some cases of intestinal metaplasia and in a proportion of adenomas, suggesting that in these instances there is a greater risk of malignant transformation [28].

In addition to these genetic abnormalities, epigenetic alterations are also of importance. DNA hypermethylation is known to be accompanied by allelic loss at the same locus and may account for inactivation of tumor suppressor genes following methylation of the gene promoter region. Hypermethylation of CpG islands (sites of enriched cytosine-guanine dinucleotides) in genes involved in DNA repair (*hMLH1, MGMT* and *p16$^{MTS1/INK4A}$*) is found in 20–30% of gastric cancers [29]. Reduced *hMLH1* expression resulting from CpG island hypermethylation is also found in intestinal metaplasia, suggesting that this is an early event in carcinogenesis. However, a more important general factor in gastric carcinogenesis may be the presence of genetic polymorphisms which determine the host inflammatory response to *H. pylori* and, in consequence, the extent of mucosal damage, atrophy and acid production. For instance, inherited variations in the genes controlling interleukin-1β production have been shown to be associated with a higher risk of gastric cancer [30]. Other polymorphisms in genes controlling anti-oxidant enzymes (e.g. glutathione S-transferase) could also play a part [31].

In conclusion, host genetic factors may dictate both the severity of the inflammatory response to *H. pylori* and the ability to counteract cellular injury by reactive oxygen species. In a few individuals, inherited abnormalities in DNA repair genes predispose to cancer development. In a far greater number, acquired epigenetic changes mediated by hypermethylation lead to defective repair and genomic instability. An accumulation of mutations in tumour suppressor genes, oncogene activation and disturbances of cell regulation ultimately leads to the malignant phenotype. The pattern of genes involved differs between intestinal and diffuse type cancers indicating that despite their common origin on a background of *H. pylori* gastritis there are (at least) two distinct routes of carcinogenesis.

Staging

Clinical Staging

Despite advances in radiological techniques, a careful history and physical examination is still a vital part of the early assessment of patients with gastric cancer. Detection of widespread metastatic disease by simple examination may avoid subjecting a patient to needless and expensive further investigations. Patients with malignant cachexia who have an abdominal mass in the epigastrium, Virchow's nodes in the neck, hepatomegaly, ascites and so on may only require a simple needle biopsy under ultrasound control or aspiration of fluid for cytology to confirm the presence of metastatic disease. If such gross physical signs are not present, then the next line of investigation is usually a computed tomography (CT) scan.

Whilst conventional CT imaging and the more up to date, third-generation spiral CT have been used widely in staging gastric cancer, the results have been disappointing [32]. Detection of disseminated disease such as liver secondaries and gross intraperitoneal involvement can be readily identified by CT scanning, but accurate assessment of the depth of penetration through the gastric wall (T stage) or nodal involvement (N stage) have proven more elusive. Whilst the presence of enlarged lymph nodes may indicate malignant disease, it is virtually impossible to differentiate metastatic disease from benign lymph node hyperplasia. It is also well known that normal sized lymph nodes can contain cancerous deposits. Small peritoneal metastases, which are not uncommon in gastric cancer, are also usually beyond the resolution of the CT scanner. Direct invasion into adjacent organs such as the liver, pancreas and transverse colon can also prove difficult to determine using this mode of imaging.

A more accurate assessment of the T and N stage of gastric cancer is obtained using endoscopic ultrasound scan (EUS) [33]. Unlike CT scan, EUS can distinguish five layers within the gastric wall which appear as a series of alternating bright and dark bands (Fig. 18a,b).

Invasion of any of these layers by the tumor can be more accurately assessed by EUS than CT scan. Whilst lymph node metastases can only be determined by the size of the nodes on the CT scan, EUS provides additional useful information such as the shape of the lymph nodes, their echogenicity and echotexture and whether they have a well-defined or demarcated border. Such additional information makes EUS much more sensitive at detecting lymph node metastases than CT scan. Interventional EUS, with for example biopsy of lymph nodes, is another additional useful role for EUS for the staging of patients with gastric cancer.

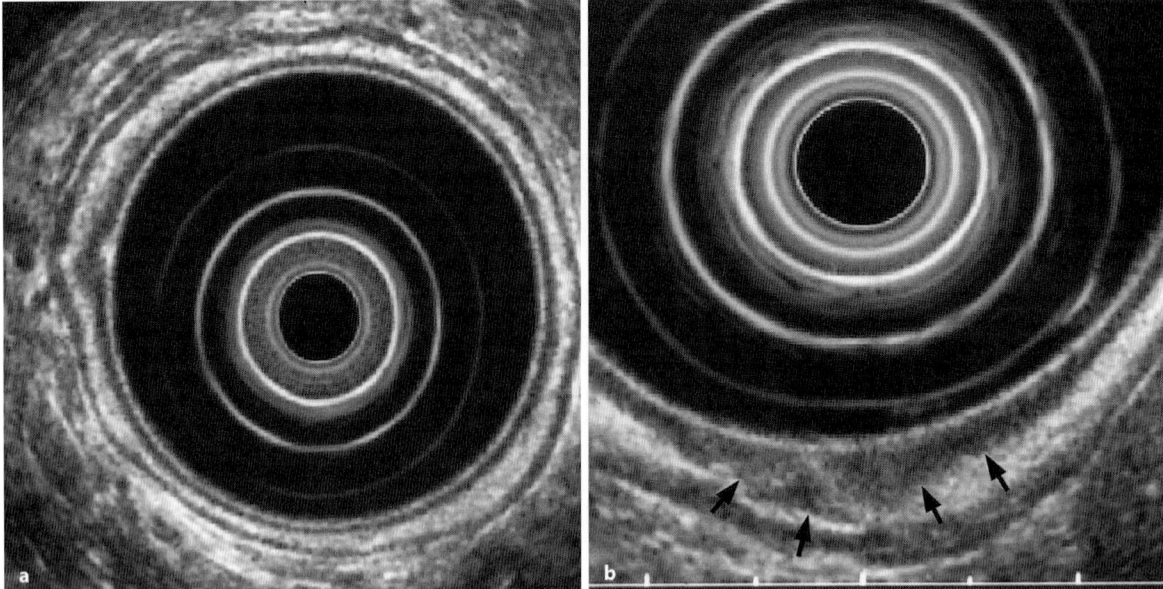

Figure 18a,b
In **a**, the 5 layers of the normal gastric wall, as seen on EUS, appear as a series of alternating *bright and dark bands*: mucosa (*bright*, innermost layer), mucularis mucosa (*dark*), submucosa (*bright*), muscularis propria (*dark*) and serosa (*bright*). Note the presence of an early gastric cancer which has invaded submucosa (*arrowed*) in **b**. (Illustrations courtesy of Dr. K. Harris, Consultant Radiologist, Leeds General Infirmary)

Staging laparascopy is frequently used in patients with advanced gastric malignancy as it provides additional information to EUS and CT. Laparoscopy can detect the presence of peritoneal seedlings, small hepatic metastases, distant lymph node involvement and presence or absence of direct invasion of adjacent organs such as the pancreas. These findings are important in determining whether a patient may have advanced and incurable disease and help to avoid needless laparotomies that were not uncommon in the past. Laparoscopy is also a useful tool in clinical trials of adjuvant chemotherapy, as it can exclude patients who would not benefit from such treatment.

Pathological Staging

Gastric cancers are classified as either "early" or "advanced" on the basis of direct spread through the stomach wall. A carcinoma that is either limited to the mucosa or extending no deeper than submucosa regardless of its lateral extent is early gastric cancer (stage T1). Within this stage, it is of value to distinguish between carcinomas restricted to the mucosa and those with submucosal invasion as the latter are associated with an increased risk of lymph node metastasis. Indeed further precision can be achieved by assessing whether superficial, mid- or deep submucosa (Sm1-Sm3) is involved [34].

A carcinoma that extends beyond the submucosa is by definition "advanced". Tumor extending into the muscularis propria or subserosa *but not penetrating through the peritoneal surface* is T2; tumor which penetrates through the peritoneal surface without invading contiguous structures is T3; and tumor which penetrates through the peritoneal aspect and involves adjacent structures is T4. "Adjacent structures" include transverse colon, spleen, liver, pancreas, abdominal wall, adrenal gland, kidney, small intestine and retroperitoneum.

Lymph node spread is initially to the perigastric nodes along the lesser and greater curvatures and the nodes along the left gastric, common hepatic, hepatoduodenal, splenic and coeliac arteries. The updated UICC TNM classification (1997) is used to assign tumors to No = no regional node involvement, N1 = involvement in 1–6 regional nodes, N2 = involvement of 7 to 15 regional lymph nodes, and N3 = involvement of more than 15 regional lymph nodes. Involvement of more remote intra-abdominal lymph nodes such as retro-pancreatic, mesenteric and para-aortic groups, is considered to be distant metastasis (M1). Involvement of the liver or the presence of peritoneal seedlings is also M1.

Treatment

Synopsis

The management of patients with gastric cancer is very much dependent on the stage of disease at presentation as well as the fitness and the wishes of the patient. Early cancers confined to the mucosa or submucosa (T1) can be treated endoscopically (endomucosal resection) or by laparoscopic or conventional surgical resection. The results of treatment of early gastric cancer are often excellent, with 5 year survival in excess of 90%. Patients with more advanced disease with invasion through the muscularis propia (T2) or serosa (T3) often have significant lymph node involvement and consequently a much worse prognosis. Treatment of such patients may often involve multi-modality treatment in addition to surgical resection, including chemotherapy, immunochemotherapy or chemoradiotherapy. Ideally, patients with advanced gastric cancer should therefore be discussed at a multi-disciplinary team meeting, with involvement of surgeons, oncologists, pathologists, radiologists and palliative care specialists. Not infrequently, patients with advanced gastric cancer are often also elderly and treatment in such cases needs to be carefully tailored to the individual patient.

Endoscopic Treatment

EMR of early gastric cancers was pioneered in Japan and is used to treat up to 40% of early gastric cancers in some Japanese centers. Tumors confined to the mucosa that are less than 3 cm in size, histologically well-differentiated, or moderately well-differentiated and macroscopically type I (protruded) or type II (flat) lesions without ulceration are deemed suitable for EMR [22]. These types of tumors are common in Japan due to their mass-screening program, but unfortunately are rarely found in the West. The technique of EMR involves careful mapping of the tumor using indigo carmine dye spray, submucosal infiltration with saline to lift the tumor off the gastric wall and removal using a diathermy snare (Fig. 19a–c).

The specimen is then carefully pinned out and examined histologically for evidence of completeness of resection and submucosal invasion. If the resected specimen shows evidence of incomplete resection, submucosal infiltration or involvement of blood vessels, then a more conventional surgical resection is recommended. Complications of this procedure, such as excessive bleeding and perforation of the gastric wall are not uncommon, though thankfully these problems can be resolved by endoscopic clipping or suturing. Endomucosal resections should be performed by skilled endoscopists in specialist centers with appropriate surgical backup so as to minimize morbidity and mortality from this procedure.

Surgery

Surgical resection remains the mainstay of treatment of gastric cancer either for cure or for palliation. The extent of gastric resection depends on the site of the tumor in the stomach. Tumors in the distal third or antrum of the stomach require a subtotal gastrectomy, whereas tumors of the middle or proximal stomach, a total gastrectomy is necessary. Reconstruction is best achieved by a Roux-en-Y anastomosis to keep bile and pancreatic juice away from the gastric remnant or esophagus.

The extent of lymph node dissection in patients undergoing a "curative" resection has evoked much controversy. The Japanese have long favored a radical surgical approach, with dissection of N2 (distant perigastric, hepatic, splenic and left gastric), N3 (retro-pancreatic) or even N4 (para-aortic) nodes which correspond to a D2, D3 or D4 level of dissection. This surgical philosophy is based on extensive histopathological studies of the pattern of lymph node spread in patients with gastric cancer. In Japan, the standard operation is a D2 gastrectomy, though in some centers, a D3 or even a D4 resection is performed in patients with more advanced disease. The Japanese have reported very impressive results using this type of radical surgical approach [35], with operative mortality of 1–2% and improvement in survival

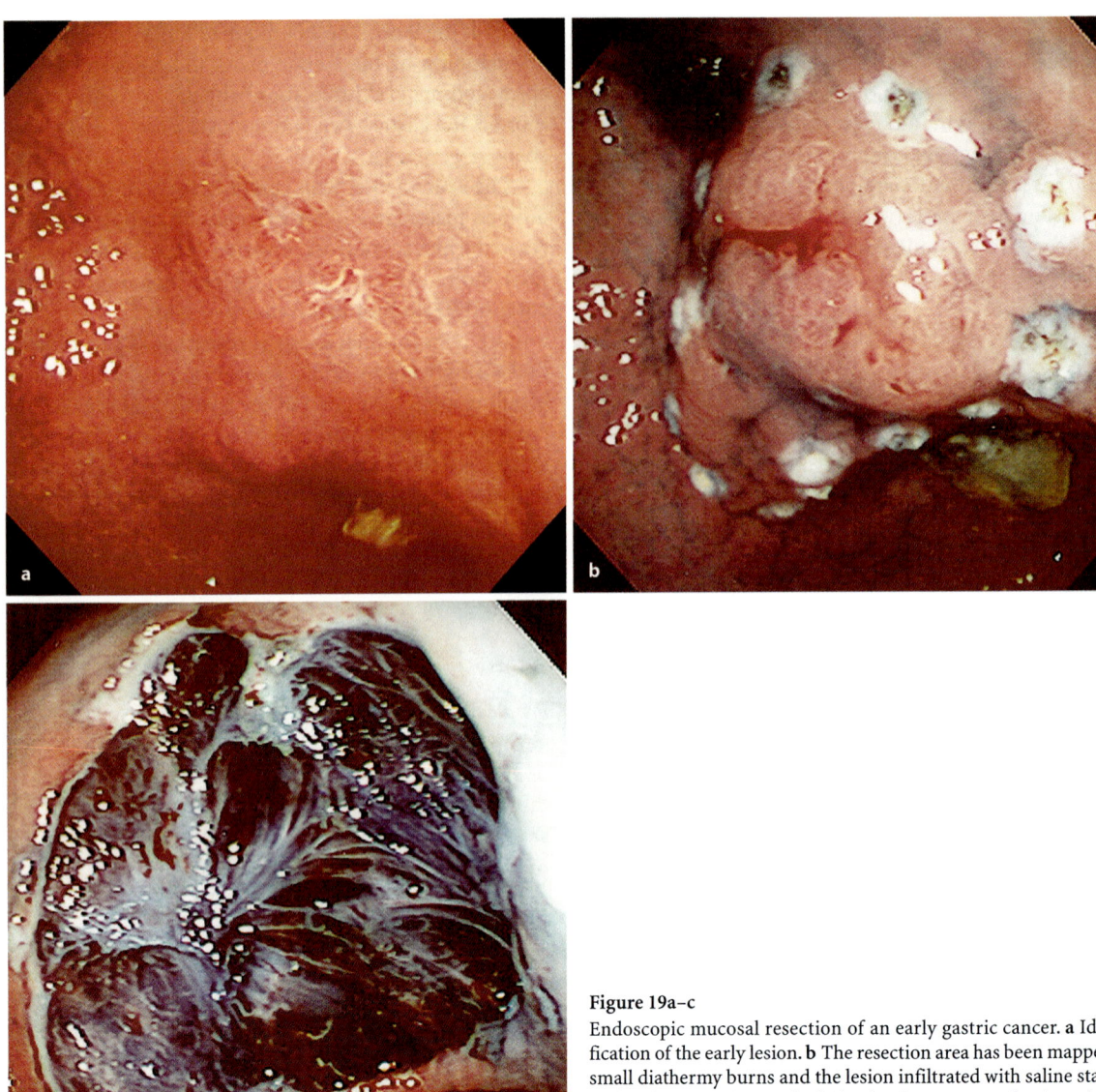

Figure 19a–c
Endoscopic mucosal resection of an early gastric cancer. **a** Identification of the early lesion. **b** The resection area has been mapped by small diathermy burns and the lesion infiltrated with saline stained with indigo-carmine. **c** The lesion has been removed using wire diathermy and the base (*stained*) with indigo-carmine is visible. It can be seen that the margin of the excision follows the mapping on the previous photograph

particularly in patients with node-positive and serosa-positive disease, though these results have been criticized as the studies have all been retrospective.

Attempts to reproduce similar results in the West have met with mixed fortunes. Two recently concluded prospective randomized studies in Europe have shown that operative mortality was much higher (10% to 13%) after a radical D2 resection and there was little evidence of survival benefit from this more radical surgical approach [36]. Much of the increased morbidity and mortality in these two randomized studies appeared to have been related to the resection of the spleen and pancreas in patients having a radical D2 total gastrectomy and there were also some criticism of these studies because of the lack of experience of the surgeons carrying out this type of radical surgical resection. Much more encouraging results have been reported from several specialist centers in Europe who have adopted the Japanese radical surgical approach, with operative mortality a more acceptable 3%–5% and improvement in survival more closely resembling the Japanese experience [37]. Whilst controversy still remains regarding the most appropriate type of curative resection for gastric cancer, it would seem reasonable from the results published that radical surgical resection for gastric cancer in the West should perhaps be confined to specialist centers.

Patients with advanced disease in whom "curative" surgery is not possible need palliation of symptoms such as pain, vomiting, bleeding and gastric outlet obstruction. Palliation is often best achieved in these circumstances by simple gastric resection: subtotal gastrectomy for obstructing tumors of distal stomach and total gastrectomy for more proximal cancers. If a resection is not feasible because of the extensive nature of the tumor or the patient not fit enough to withstand a major resection, then bypass gastroenterostomy or a Devine exclusion bypass procedure may be necessary to relieve obstruction.

The complication rate after palliative surgical procedures is often very high, largely because the patients have a heavy tumor burden as well as being very frail and nutritionally depleted. Some of these patients may also only have a few months to live because of the advanced nature of the tumor and therefore the potential benefits of a palliative surgical procedure must be carefully weighed up against the downside of surgical intervention in the individual patient. This is particularly so in patients who may have quite advanced disease but no symptoms of obstruction of the stomach. In this latter group, an attractive alternative would be the use of palliative chemotherapy which in some cases can produce a dramatic improvement in patients' quality of live as well as duration of life [38]. There is a limited role for the use of endoscopic stents in patients with gastric outlet obstruction who are deemed not suitable for surgery. However, unlike its role in esophageal cancer, the success rate of stents in gastric cancer is often disappointing because of the extensive nature of the tumors in the stomach.

A new and exciting development is the use of laparoscopic surgery in the treatment of gastric cancer. With the advancement of laparoscopic techniques, it is now feasible to carry out not only local excisions of tumors but also partial gastrectomies with limited D1 lymph node dissection and bypass procedures. Tumors suitable for such procedures would include early gastric cancers confined to the mucosa as well as stromal tumors that do not have lymph node metastases. The advantages of laparoscopic over conventional surgery include less post-operative discomfort and a quicker return to normal activity as well as perhaps a better quality of life. However, careful selection of the patient for this type of procedure is required. For example, early gastric cancers through to the submucosa have a 20% incidence of lymph node involvement and some of these lymph nodes may be more distant N2 disease which would make such tumors unsuitable for limited laparoscopic resection. The risk in such cases would be to convert disease which is eminently curable by conventional surgery into incurable disease. These procedures also need to be carried out by skilled laparoscopic surgeons familiar with the techniques of conventional gastric surgery.

Chemotherapy

Whilst gastric cancer in its early stages is eminently curable by radical surgery alone, there is a high risk of recurrence and long-term failure in patients with more advanced disease, particularly those with serosal involvement or lymph node involvement. The need to improve the outcome in the latter group of patients has led to exhaustive studies of chemotherapy as adjuvant treatment to surgery in the last three decades. There have been some exciting developments during this time but sadly, to date, there is no convincing evidence that adjuvant chemotherapy can significantly improve survival in patients who have undergone "curative" resection for locally advanced disease, unlike the more established role of chemotherapy in the palliation of patients with advanced and metastatic disease.

Gastric cancer is relatively sensitive to chemotherapy, with response rates of 10%–20% using single agents such as 5-fluoro-uracil (5FU) or mitomycin C. Response rates are greater when these agents are used in combination, such as ECF (epirubicin, cisplatinum and 5FU) which produces a 50% response rate [39] but such combinations also lead to greater toxicity. There have been numerous randomized trials of various chemotherapeutic agents given intravenously after surgery, with only a few showing a positive outcome. Meta-analysis of these trials published in 1993 and again in 1999 has shown only a small survival benefit of doubtful significance [40], though there may be subsets of patients such as those with lymph node involvement who may benefit from adjuvant chemotherapy. Part of the difficulty in interpreting the results of these studies lies in the lack of uniformity of the trials to date. Patients entered into these trials have variable stage of disease, with, for example, the inclusion of patients with T1 tumors or stage I disease who are unlikely to derive any benefit from adjuvant chemotherapy. Another criticism has been the lack of standardization of the surgery performed particularly in Western countries, which means that the residual tumor burden would be variable even after apparent "curative" resection. The timing and duration of chemotherapy has also been somewhat haphazard, with trials in Japan starting chemotherapy immediately after surgery whereas in the West, chemotherapy is often delayed for a least four to eight weeks to allow the patient to recover from their operation. These confounding variables have hampered the interpretation of the results of adjuvant chemotherapy after surgical resection and, given the toxicity of these drugs, systemic adjuvant chemotherapy cannot at present be recommended except within the context of clinical trials.

Several other promising avenues of treatment using chemotherapy in the adjuvant setting are under investigation. One such approach is the use of chemotherapy intraperitoneally, which seems logical as recurrence after surgery for advanced disease usually occurs loco-regionally or intraperitoneally. Another advantage of this approach is that higher concentrations of the drugs can be delivered intraperitoneally and systemic side effects are uncommon as very little of the drugs enter the systemic circulation. Studies in Japan using mitomycin C bound to carbon particles given intraperitoneally at the end of operation have held out much promise with significant improvement in survival of patients with serosal positive disease [41]. However, attempts to reproduce these results in a Western setting have failed due to the high rate of post-operative complications. Whilst intraperitoneal chemotherapy still holds much promise, its role in the adjuvant setting is yet to be proven.

Another approach that has been investigated is the use of chemotherapy given systemically before operation (neo-adjuvant). The advantages of such an approach are that systemic micro metastases are treated relatively early during the course of the disease and the primary tumor can be downstaged which would increase the proportion of patients likely to undergo "curative" resection. There are several ongoing phase III trials, including the MRC ST02 (MAGIC) trial, the results of which are eagerly awaited. Future trials of adjuvant chemotherapy are likely to evaluate newer cytotoxic agents such as irinotecan, docetaxel, paclitaxel and TS-1 either singularly or in combination. These new agents have shown significantly higher response rates in the treatment of patients with advanced gastric cancer and therefore hold out much promise.

Patients with advanced and metastatic disease often require palliation of symptoms such as pain and vomiting, loss of appetite and malignant cachexia. Several studies have shown that chemotherapy can effectively palliate symptoms of advanced, metastatic disease and in some cases lead to a dramatic improvement in both the quality of life as well as the duration of life of such patients. This is particularly so in patients with advanced disease who do not have symptoms of gastric outlet obstruction, where palliation by surgical resection of bypass procedure may still be necessary.

Chemoimmunotherapy

It has been recognized for some time that the immune system is depressed in patients with advanced cancer and this observation has also been seen in patients after surgery. This has led scientists to develop drugs to reverse the immunosuppression caused by cancer and surgery by stimulating the body's own natural immune defence mechanisms. In gastric cancer, a number of immunostimulants have been investigated, including levamisole, BCG, OK432 (Picabanil) and PSK (Krestin). Of these agents, perhaps the most widely studies is PSK which is a protein polysaccharide extracted from the fungus *Coriolus versicolour*. PSK has been shown to induce the interleukins IL1, IL6 and IL8 as well as tumor necrosis factor. On its own, PSK does not appear to lead to any improvement in the outcome of patients with gastric cancer. However, when given in combination with chemotherapy after "curative" resection for locally advanced gastric cancer, PSK has been shown in several randomized studies to improve outcome compared with chemotherapy alone [42]. Whether this effect is due to a reversal of the immunosupression caused by surgery and chemotherapy or due to direct effect of the immunostimulant on cancer cells is not clear. Most of the trials of chemoimmunotherapy have been carried out in Japan and Korea and, to date, there are very few similar studies in the West.

Chemoradiotherapy

Radiotherapy has, until recently, not had a role to play in the treatment of gastric cancer, apart from relieving symptoms such as bone pain caused by metastatic disease. However, a recent study from the United States using combined chemotherapy and radiotherapy after surgical resection for gastric cancer has generated a great deal of interest. In an Intergroup 116 trial, patients were randomized to either surgery alone (control group) or surgery plus 5FU and leucovorin with radiotherapy (45 Gy). There was an improvement in both the disease-free survival and overall survival in patients who received chemoradiotherapy compared to the surgery alone group [43]. Whilst these results are encouraging, the surgery performed in a significant proportion of patients was rather limited and only 10% of patients had radical D2 resection. It therefore begs the question as to whether the chemoradiotherapy may have made up for less than adequate surgery and this treatment therefore needs to be investigated further in patients who undergo radical D2 resection.

Prognosis

The importance of accurate pathological data in determining prognosis is self- evident. Patients with confirmed early gastric cancer undergoing complete removal have a 5-year survival in excess of 90%. The prognosis of advanced cases rests to some extent on the precise stage but is largely dependent on whether or not surgery has been truly "potentially curative". Thus involvement of the resection margins by carcinoma carries a dire prognosis, as does the presence of covert hepatic or distant lymph node metastases.

The two most important factors that determine outcome after potentially curative resection are lymph node involvement (N stage) and depth of penetration of the tumor through the gastric wall (T stage). Five-year survival for patients with node-negative gastric cancer is 80%, whereas it is a grim 35% or less for patients with node-positive disease. The number of involved lymph nodes also has a bearing on prognosis. Five-year survival of patients with N1 disease (<6 nodes involved) is 60%, N2 disease (7–16 nodes involved) 25% and N3 disease (>16 nodes involved) a mere 5%. Likewise, depth of penetration of the tumor through the gastric wall has a major bearing on prognosis. Five-year survival of patients with T1 tumors is over 90%, T2 tumors 65%, T3 30% and T4 10% [44].

Follow-Up

After surgical resection, patients should ideally be followed up in a specialist gastric clinic, with ample support from dieticians and oncologists. Recurrence after surgery for gastric cancer usually occurs within the first two to three years and careful evaluation of the patients during this period of time is vital to spot early signs of recurrent disease. Patients should perhaps be seen every three months for the first two to three years and six-monthly thereafter. If there is any clinical suspicion of recurrent disease, then a CT scan with or without an endoscopy is necessary to determine the site and extent of recurrence.

Patients also need continued psychological support and counseling as well as good dietary advice to ensure an adequate intake of calories. They should be encouraged to eat smaller, frequent meals, particularly in the first few months after gastric resection and to supplement their diet with multivitamins and iron as well as B12 injections every 3–6 months. Quality of life is often impaired in the first few months after surgery, but gradually improves with time and patients should be reassured of this.

Screening, Surveillance, Prevention

Gastric cancer is responsible for more deaths worldwide than any other malignant tumor apart from the lung. Furthermore throughout most of the world the prognosis is appallingly bad, five year survival rates being less than 10%. It follows that only screening or prevention will have a major impact on the disease. *Helicobacter pylori* infection is the environmental factor that contributes most to the development of non-cardia gastric cancer (numerically the most important type of gastric cancer worldwide). Epidemiological data over the last century has shown a gradual but continued decline in infection rates throughout the developed world with a concomitant reduction in the incidence and mortality of gastric cancer. The mode of transmission of this infectious disease is unknown. It is contracted primarily in childhood and it is associated particularly with the socially disadvantaged. As the mechanism of transmission is unknown primary prevention (other than trying to improve the standard of living of the world's population) is not feasible.

Fortunately it is relatively easy and comparatively inexpensive to screen populations for *Helicobacter pylori*. Furthermore effective treatments are available to eradicate the infection (Fig. 20).

No prospective studies have been performed to test the hypothesis that *Helicobacter* eradication will prevent cancer and until this is done, governments, health providers and indeed physicians are unlikely to support a campaign of "test and treat" in the general population, even though on circumstantial grounds this is likely to be effective. The advantage of this approach is not only that eradication of *Helicobacter* will prevent gastric cancer but that it would also protect against peptic ulcer and help a small proportion of patients with uninvestigated dyspepsia. A prospective study has shown that testing and treating of patients infected with the organism actually saves money over a ten year period, at the end of that time the lives saved by preventing cancer would cost nothing [45].

Alternative methods of preventing cancer have also been suggested. Diets rich in fruit and vegetables protect, but it is not easy to change the dietary habits of populations. Prospective studies have been undertaken to see whether supplementation with micro-nutrients such as vitamin C, selenium and retinoids are effective but to date none of these studies have demonstrated significant benefit.

Prevention of cardia cancer is a more difficult area. In developed countries the incidence of this type of cancer is increasing *pari passu* with the rise in adenocarcinoma of the esophagus (which is believed to be secondary to Barrett's esophagus). As indicated earlier, it may be that a reduction in the use of nitrogenous fertilizers may be desirable. More research is required in this area.

A number of medical conditions are associated with an increased risk of gastric cancer. These include pernicious anemia, previous operation for a peptic ulcer and the presence of gastritis with type III intestinal metaplasia. At present there is no prospective data to suggest that surveillance of these groups is effective or desirable. Patients who have hypogammaglobulinemia in addition to pernicious anemia are at considerably higher risk and it is sensible to endoscope these patients periodically.

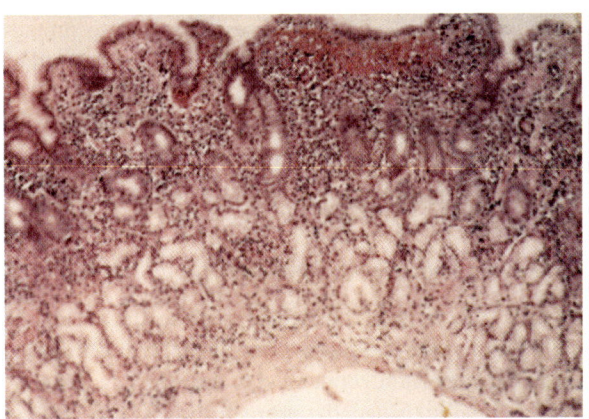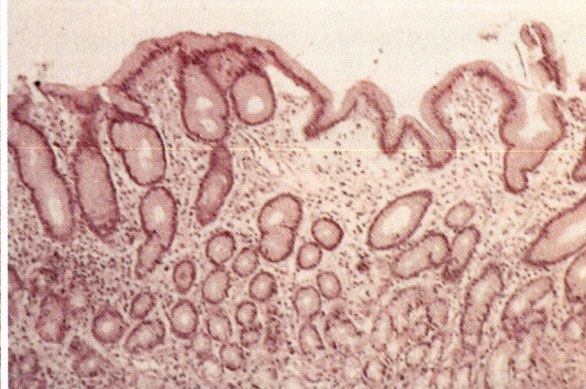

Figure 20

H and E sections from a stomach before and one month after treatment for *Helicobacter pylori*. Note the decline in the acute inflammatory cell infiltrate and the improvement in the morphology of the superficial epithelium

It may also be desirable to survey those in whom pernicious anemia arises at an early age. There are a number of rare familial syndromes associated with gastric cancer that also require surveillance.

Future Perspectives

Although the prevalence of *Helicobacter pylori* is falling rapidly in the developed world the number of people dying from gastric cancer is set to increase. The reason for this is that the condition is a disease of the elderly and within increasing longevity and demographic changes throughout the world increasing numbers of individuals will be at risk. Non-cardia cancer should continue however to decline in the West and with the passage of time will die out. Whether this will be associated with an increase in patients with cardia cancer remains to be seen.

If the developing world follows the same pattern as occurred in developed countries during the 19th and 20th centuries the incidence of gastric cancer and peptic ulcer will rise initially, as the average age of the population increases and further industrialization occurs. It should then decline in parallel with the fall in numbers of people infected with *Helicobacter*. Unlike the developed world however where the cause of the disease was unknown we now have the advantage of knowing the major environmental risk and within the foreseeable future public health measures to speed the elimination of *Helicobacter pylori* may be introduced.

References

1. Murray CJL, Lopez AD (1997). Alternative projections of mortality and disability by cause 1990–2020 – global burden of disease study. Lancet 349: 1498–1504
2. The Eurogast Study Group (1993). An international association between *Helicobacter pylori* infection and gastric cancer. Lancet 341: 1359–1362
3. Helicobacter and Cancer Collaborative Group (2001). Gastric cancer and *Helicobacter pylori*: a combined analysis of 12 case control studies nested within prospective cohorts. Gut 49: 347–353
4. Kikuchi S, Wada O, Nakajima T, Nishi T, Kobayashi O, Konishi T, Inaba Y (1995). Serum anti-*Helicobacter pylori* antibody and gastric carcinoma among young adults. Research Group on Prevention of Gastric Carcinoma among Young Adults. Cancer 75: 2789–2793
5. Uemura N, Okamoto S, Yamamoto S, Matsumura N, Yamaguchi S, Yamakido M, Taniyama K, Sasaki N, Schlemper RJ (2001). *Helicobacter pylori* infection and the development of gastric cancer. N Engl J Med 345: 784–789
6. International Agency for Research on Cancer (1994). Schistosomes, liver flukes and *Helicobacter pylori*. Monograph 61. Lyon, France: IARC: 177–240
7. Sipponen P, Kekki M, Haapakoski J, Ihamaki T, Siurala M (1985). Gastric cancer risk in chronic atrophic gastritis: statistical calculations of cross-sectional data. Int J Cancer 35: 173–177
8. Correa P, Haenszel W, Cuello C, Tannenbaum S, Archer M (1975). A model for gastric cancer epidemiology. Lancet ii: 58–60
9. Drake IM, Mapstone NP, Schorah CJ, White KLM, Chalmers DM, Dixon MF, Axon ATR (1998). Reactive oxygen species activity and lipid peroxidation in *Helicobacter pylori* associated gastritis: relation to gastric mucosal ascorbic acid concentrations and effect of H pylori eradication. Gut 42: 768–771
10. Sobala GM, Schorah CJ, Shires S, Lynch DAF, Gallacher B, Dixon MF, Axon ATR (1993). Effect of eradication of *Helicobacter pylori* on gastric juice ascorbic acid concentrations. Gut 34: 1038–1041
11. Lynch DAF, Mapstone NP, Clarke AMT, Sobala GM, Jackson P, Morrison L, Dixon MF, Quirke P, Axon ATR (1995). Cell proliferation in *Helicobacter pylori* associated gastritis and the effect of eradication therapy. Gut 36: 346–350
12. Watanabe T, Tada M, Nagai H, Sakaki S, Nakao M (1998). *Helicobacter pylori* infection induces gastric cancer in Mongolian gerbils. Gastroenterology 115: 642–648
13. Wang HH, Antonioli DA, Goldman H (1986). Comparative features of esophageal and gastric adenocarcinomas: recent changes in type and frequency. Human Pathology 17: 482–487
14. Fletcher J, Wirz A, Young J, Vallance R, McColl KEL (2001). Unbuffered highly acidic gastric juice exists at the gastroesophageal junction after a meal. Gastroenterology 121: 775–783
15. Iijima K, Henry E, Moriya A, Wirz A, Kelman AW, McColl KEL (2002). Dietary nitrate generates potentially mutagenic concentrations of nitric oxide at the gastroesophageal junction. Gastroenterology 122: 1248–1257
16. Busby WF, Shuker DEG, Charnley G, Newberne PM, Tannenbaum SR, Wogan GN (1985). Carcinogenicity in rats of the nitrosated bile acid conjugates N-nitrosoglycocholic acid and N-nitrosotaurocholic acid. Cancer Res 45:1367–1371
17. Miwa K, Hattori T, Miyazaki I. (1995) Duodenogastric reflux and foregut carcinogenesis. Cancer 75: 1426–32
18. Lynch, D.A.F., Mapstone, N.P., Clarke, A.M.T., Jackson, P., Dixon, M.F., Quirke, P., Axon, A.T.R. (1995) Cell proliferation in the gastric corpus in *Helicobacter pylori* associated gastritis and after gastric resection. Gut 36: 351–353.
19. Murakami T (1971). Pathomorphological diagnosis. Definition and gross classification of early gastric cancer. Gann Monogr Cancer Res 11: 53–55
20. Everett SM, Axon ATR (1997). Early gastric cancer in Europe. Gut 41: 142–150
21. Mellinger JD, Ponsky JL (1991). Endoscopy in gastric malignancy. In: Sugarbaker P (ed) Management of gastric cancer. Kluwer Academic Publishers, Boston, volume 55: p 51–68
22. Yoshida S (1998). Endoscopic diagnosis and treatment of early cancer in the alimentary tract. Digestion 59: 502–508
23. Ribiero MM, Sarmento JA, Simoes S, Bastos J (1981). Prognostic significance of Lauren and Ming classifications and other pathologic parameters in gastric carcinoma. Cancer 47; 780–784
24. Tajima Y, Shimoda T, Nakanishi Y, Yokoyama N, Tanaka T, Shimizu K, Saito T, Kawamura M, Kusano M, Kumagai K (2001). Gastric and intestinal phenotypic marker expression in gastric carcinomas and its prognostic significance: immunohistochemical analysis of 136 lesions. Oncology 61:212–20
25. Kim NW, Piatyszek MA, Prowse KR, Harley CB, West MD, Ho PL (1994). Specific association of human telomerase activity with immortal cells and cancer. Science 266; 2011–2015
26. Yokozaki H, Yasui W, Tahara E (2001). Genetic and epigenetic changes in stomach cancer. Int Rev Cytol 204; 49–95
27. Yasui W, Oue N, Kuniyasu H, Ito R, Tahara E, Yokozaki H (2001). Molecular diagnosis of gastric cancer: present and future. Gastric Cancer 4: 113–121

28. Hamamoto T, Yokozaki H, Senba S, Yasui W, Yunotani S, Miyazaki K, Tahara E (1997). Altered micro-satellites in incomplete-type intestinal metaplasia adjacent to primary gastric cancers. J Clin Pathol 50; 841–846

29. Kanai Y, Ushijima S, Kondo Y, Nakanishi Y, Hirohashi S (2001). DNA methyltransferase expression and DNA methylation of CPG islands and peri-centromeric satellite regions in human colorectal and stomach cancers. Int J Cancer 91; 205–212

30. El-Omar E, Carrington M, Chow WH, McColl KE, Bream JH, Young HA, Herrera J, Lissowska J, Yuan CC, Rothman N, Lanyon G, Martin M, Fraumeni JF Jr, Rabkin CS (2000). Interleukin-1 polymorphisms associated with increased risk of gastric cancer. Nature 404: 398–402

31. Rebbeck TR (1997). Molecular epidemiology of the human glutathione S-transferase genotypes GSTM1 and GSTT1 in cancer susceptibility. Cancer Epid Biomarkers & Prevention 6; 733–743

32. Sussman SK, Halvorsen RA, Illescas FF, et al (1988). Gastric adenocarcinoma: CT versus surgical staging. Radiology 167: 335–340

33. Dittler HJ, Siewert JR (1993). Role of endosonography in gastric carcinoma. Endoscopy 25: 162–166

34. Gotoda T. Sasako M. Ono H. Katai H. Sano T. Shimoda T (2001) Evaluation of the necessity for gastrectomy with lymph node dissection for patients with submucosal invasive gastric cancer. Brit J Surg 88; 444–449

35. Maruyama K, Okabayashi K, Kinoshita T (1987). Progress in gastric cancer surgery in Japan and its limits of radicality. World J Surg 11: 418–425

36. Cuschieri A, Weeden S, Fielding J, et al (1999). Patient survival after D1 and D2 resections for gastric cancer: long term results of the MRC randomized surgical trial. Br J Cancer 78: 1522–1530

37. Sue-Ling HM, Johnston D, Axon ATR, et al (1993). Gastric cancer: a curable disease in Britain. Br Med J 307: 591–596

38. Seymour MT, Dent JT, Papmichael D, et al (1999). Epirubicin, cisplatin and oral UFT with leucovorin (ECU): a phase I-II study in patients with advanced upper gastrointestinal tract cancer. Ann Oncol 10: 1329–33

39. Webb A, Cunningham D, Scarffe H, et all (1997). Randomized trial comparing epirubicin, cisplatin and fluorouracil versus fluorouracil, doxorubicin, and methotrexate in advanced esophagogastric cancer. J Clin Oncol 15: 261–267

40. Earle CC, Maroun JA (1999). Adjuvant chemotherapy after curative resection for gastric cancer in non-Asian patients: revisiting a meta-analysis of randomised trials. Eur J Cancer 35: 1059–1064

41. Hagiwara A, Takahashi T, Kojima O, et al (1992). Prophylaxis with carbonabsorbed mitomycin against peritoneal recurrence of gastric cancer. Lancet 339: 629–631

42. Kim JP (1987). The concept of immunochemosurgery in gastric cancer. World J Surg 11: 4650–472

43. Macdonald JS, Smalley S, Benedetti J, et al (2000). Postoperative combined radiation and chemotherapy improves disease-free survival (DFS) and overall survival (OS) in resected adenocarcinoma of the stomach and GE junction. Results of Intergroup Study INT-0116 (SWOG 9008). Proc Am Soc Clin Oncol 19: A1

44. Maruyama K, Gunven P, Okabayashi K, et al (1989). Lymph node metastases of gastric cancer. General pattern in 1931 patients. Ann Surg 210: 596–602

45. Mason J, Axon ATR, Forman D, Duffett S, Drummond M, Crocombe W, Feltbower R, Mason S, Brown J, Moayyedi P (on behalf of the Leeds HELP Study Group) (2002). The cost-effectiveness of population Helicobacter pylori screening and treatment: a Markov model using economic data from a randomized controlled trial. Aliment Pharm Ther 16: 559– 568.

5 Lymphoma of the Stomach

B.A. DRAGOSICS

Summary

Lymphomas of the stomach mostly arise from the mucosa-associated lymphoid tissue (MALT) and represent the largest subgroup of all extranodal lymphomas. They have become a focus of interest in recent years due to their unique *Helicobacter pylori* (*H. pylori*) associated etiopathogenesis resulting in complete remission (CR) of MALT-type lymphoma in early stage in up to 80%, following cure of infection by antibiotic therapy only. Gold standard diagnostic procedures include gastroduodenal endoscopy, tissue biopsy for histological workup and gastric endosonography (EUS).

The outcome for patients with gastric lymphomas (GLs) is substantially more favorable than that with gastric cancer. As opposed to gastric cancer, lymphoma cells are highly sensitive towards chemotherapy (CTX) as well as irradiation (RTX) thus providing the option of a non-invasive, multimodal therapeutic approach pushing aside surgery from the first-line position. To date, both RTX and CTX have given excellent results in treating indolent as well as aggressive lymphomas, equalizing results from surgical therapy and exceeding them with respect to quality of patient life. Stage at diagnosis and the histology of the lymphoma are the most important factors predicting prognosis, which is reflected by 5-year overall survival rates between 90 and 100% for stage EI, but 50–80% for stage EII according to the Ann Arbor system and between 90% for indolent and 60% for aggressive lymphoma, respectively.

Lifelong follow up of patients in CR is recommended, because of relapses later than 10 years in other MALT locations, due to the homing properties of tumor cells and a slight increase in secondary malignancies.

In the future, gastric MALT-type lymphoma may set an example for evolving molecular and cytogenetic factors into major markers predicting prognosis and selecting the mode of treatment.

Epidemiology

Primary non-Hodgkin's lymphomas of the stomach represent a group of clinicopathological entities deriving from B-lymphocytes and their precursor cells and account for about 4–8% of all malignancies of this organ. They are defined as extranodal lymphomas originating from the gastric mucosa, confined to the stomach and its associated lymph nodes without dissemination to other organs or bone marrow at diagnosis and constitute about 70% of the large extranodal group of primary gastrointestinal lymphomas.

Although occurring worldwide, incidence data of primary gastric lymphomas (GLs) are scarce and show considerable geographic variability. According to cancer registry data from 14 European countries, the incidence rate has been calculated to be as low as 0.21 per 100 000 inhabitants per year [1] showing an annual increase of 3 to 5%. However, incidence in the USA has recently been estimated as between 1:30000 and 1:80000 in the *H. pylori* infected population and in northeastern Italy an incidence of 13.2 per 100000 per year has been reported from a population with excessively high *H. pylori* prevalence. In Vienna, Austria, the number of cases diagnosed as GL in the past five years was twice the number for the previous 5-year period, thus reflecting the increasing awareness of this diagnosis among clinicians and pathologists. In addition to the acknowledged epidemiological role of *H. pylori*, yet unknown environmental, genetic or dietary factors may also play a role in oncogenesis.

Overall, primary GL is mainly a disease of middle age (mean 62 years) with an age peak in the eighth decade and a slight male predominance (1.4:1). In contrast, secondary involvement of the stomach in the course of nodal lymphoma of any type occurs at any age and in either sex. It has been prospectively evaluated in 27% of non-Hodgkin's lymphoma and may be found in up to 65% at autopsy, eventually causing fatal complications like bleeding or perforation.

Etiology and Pathogenesis

In 1983 two events revolutionized the understanding of both the etiology and the pathogenesis of primary GLs: first, the discovery of *H. pylori* and its pathogenic effect on the gastric mucosa by Warren and Marshall and second, the formulation of the concept of MALT by Isaacson and Wright as a distinct entity of structure and function. Since that time, *H. pylori* infection has been identified as primarily inducing the acquisition of MALT in the gastric mucosa, which is normally devoid of lymphoid tissue, through ongoing antigenic stimulation and, furthermore, to promoting the development of GL in particular cases.

To date, many epidemiologic, biologic and molecular genetic studies provide sufficient evidence for the causal role of *H. pylori* in the oncogenesis of marginal zone B-cell lymphoma, the "classical" indolent lymphoma of MALT-type. Reports of sustained CR of such lymphomas after cure of bacterial infection by antibiotic therapy only, further strongly support the causal relationship between *H. pylori*-associated gastritis and malignant transformation of the gastric MALT. However, the gap between the high prevalence of *H. pylori* infection worldwide, amounting to about 40% in European countries, and the low incidence of GLs is poorly understood and may implicate an immunologic cross-talk between "host" and "germ" as of significant importance for determining outcome in the individual case.

For recognizing pathogenesis and biology of GLs the understanding of the MALT concept is crucial [2]. This concept ingeniously combines anatomical structure and specific receptor-mediated lymphocyte traffic. While the term MALT designates every association of lymphatic tissue and mucosa in the body, it is usually applied to the lymphatic system along the intestinal mucosa (which indeed is the largest "lymphatic organ") named gut associated lymphoid tissue. It is composed of different lymphoid compartments acting in concert in order to protect mucosal tissue, which is directly in contact with antigens from the external environment. The most prominent structures and the most relevant to lymphoma genesis are the Peyer's patches, which consist of a central follicle surrounded by a prominent marginal zone of B-lymphocytes, which occasionally give rise to the "classical" lymphoma of MALT-type. Following antigen stimulation, MALT B-cells leave the mucosa, enter the circulation *via* the thoracic duct and "home" back to the gut mucosa. This exquisite homing property of B-cells is thought to be operative through a receptor on the cell surface collaborating with its ligand expressed on the endothelium of mucosal venules. Such a "homing" mechanism may explain both features of indolent MALT-type lymphoma, the tendency to remain localized for long periods and the pattern of dissemination to other sites along the MALT system elsewhere in the body, respectively. However, the etiopathogenesis of primary gastric, aggressive, diffuse large B-cell lymphoma (DLBCL) is still unknown, not even an association with *H. pylori* has yet been assessed.

Symptoms and Clinical Signs

The presenting symptoms of primary GLs are generally non-specific dyspepsia (70%) accompanied by loss of appetite and weight or symptoms suggestive of peptic ulcer disease (50%) sometimes masked by complications such as anemia or overt gastrointestinal bleeding (10%). The presence of an abdominal mass is a rare finding. The duration of symptoms before diagnosis has been reported to be from a few days to 36 months (mean 5 months) [3]. Clinically indolent MALT-type GL presents mostly in the sixth decade, mean age 57 years, while aggressive DLBCLs come to diagnosis at a mean age of around 66 years, suggesting a period of about one decade for transformation from indolent to "secondary aggressive" GL.

Symptoms of gastric lymphoproliferative disorders in the course of primary or acquired immunodeficiency syndromes or concomitant to immunosuppressive therapy (e.g., post-transplant) are dominated by those of underlying disease and may occur at any age. Symptoms of GLs secondary to nodal non-Hodgkin's lymphoma are usually non-specific, but may cause hemorrhage or perforation in end-stage disease.

Diagnostics

Synopsis

Imaging Procedures for Detection of GL and Assessing Histological Diagnosis – Golden Standard

1. Gastroduodenal endoscopy with multiple (8–12) biopsies from every visible lesion for assessment of histological diagnosis
2. Assessment of *H. pylori* status
3. Endosonographic ultrasound of the upper gastrointestinal tract for evaluation of localized lymphoma extension
4. Transabdominal ultrasound for assessment of intraabdominal lymphoma spread

Imaging techniques for the diagnosis of GL include double contrast radiography of the stomach, gastroduodenal endoscopy, transabdominal as well as gastric endoscopic ultrasound (EUS) and computerized tomography (CT). Radiography is expected to reveal pathologic structures in about 90% of cases, compelling subsequent endoscopy for further characterization of the lesion. The definite diagnosis, however, is made by gastroduodenal endoscopy and is histologically classified by multiple biopsy specimens. The endoscopic features may range from non-specific macroscopic gastritis or thickened folds to infiltrative (15%), polypoid (35%) or ulcerative (69%) lesions, as reported recently in a large prospective series [4]. Macroscopically tumors grow unifocally in 89% of cases and are localized in the corpus (79%) or antrum (64%) ventriculi predominantly, rarely in the fundus (15%), and are >5 cm in diameter in up to 80%. Multiple biopsies (8–12) from the lesion are generally acquired to adequately assess histological diagnosis and to either exclude or identify focal high-grade transformation of low-grade, indolent disease. In addition, gastric mapping (i.e. taking probes from different anatomical parts of the stomach) is recommended to document multifocal microscopic disease. Moreover, evidence for *H. pylori* or, in very rare cases, of *H. heilmannii* infection should come from evaluation of histologic specimens, which sometimes require Warthin Starry stain. Rapid urease testing or microbial cultivating of native biopsy tissue are further options for assessing *H. pylori* status. However, a note of caution has to be sounded as to the procedure of histological diagnosing of lymphoma by endoscopic biopsy specimens in general. Data comparing histological diagnosis from preoperative biopsies with that from resection specimens report a mismatch of 27%, missing aggressive foci in 13% of cases [4].

Gastric EUS allows an evaluation of both depth of infiltration into the gastric wall and locoregional lymphoma extension, especially with respect to serosal penetration and involvement of perigastric lymph nodes. Fortunately, EUS imaging is increasingly available at gastrointestinal centers and is highly recommended, especially for initial, pretreatment staging of GL [5]. Nevertheless, the reliability of EUS evaluation to date is still under debate. The accuracies of assessing depth of tumor infiltration and lymph node involvement were 76% and 74% respectively, as compared to the surgical specimens. Over- and under-staging of depth each occurred in 12% of cases and over-staging of perigastric lymph node involvement in 23%.

Transabdominal ultrasound and CT scan of the abdomen as well as crista biopsy for investigating bone marrow histology are the techniques used for lymphoma staging. Among the laboratory tests an abnormal smear of peripheral blood cells, elevated serum lactate dehydrogenase activity or an increase in beta2-microglobulin are of importance in the diagnosis of GL, indicating generalized disease. Search for serological *H. pylori* antibody, ^{13}C urea breath test or *H. pylori* antigen testing of Stool probes are complementary methods of assessing *H. pylori* association with GL (Figs. 1–4).

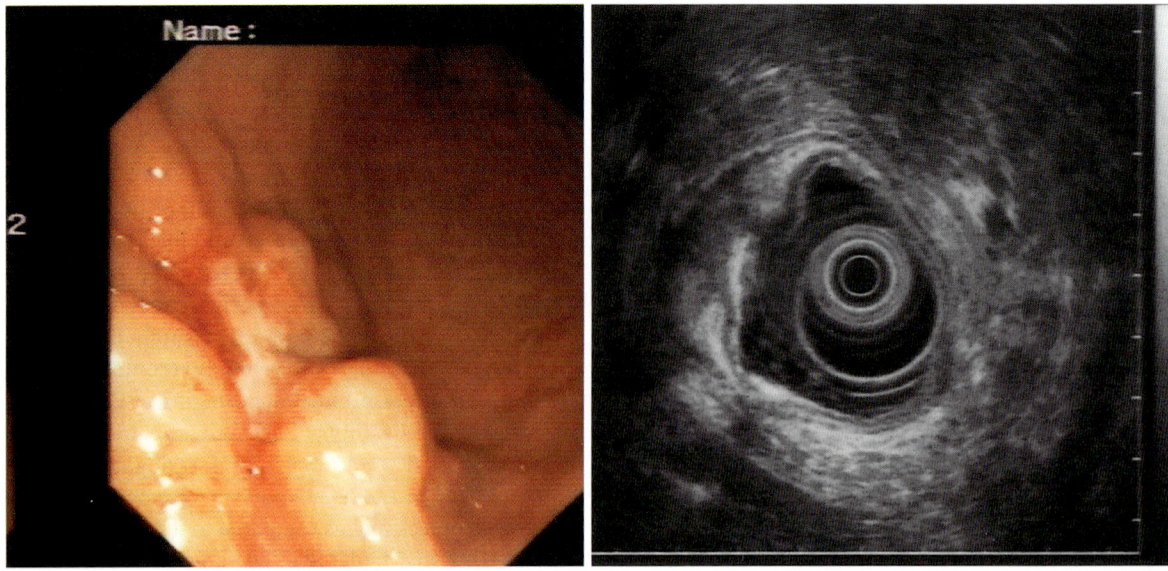

Antrum ventriculi proximal   Antrum ventriculi (US) proximal

Figure 1
Primary gastric lymphoma of diffuse large B-cells (DLBCL). *Left*: Endoscopic feature of ulcerated tumorous infiltration in the proximal antrum ventriculi; *right*: Gastric endoscopic ultrasound imaging of the lesion demasking infiltration of mucosal, submucosal as well as muscularis propria layers of the gastric wall. No evidence of serosal involvement or of perigastric lymph node infiltration. (By courtesy of Andreas Püspök, Vienna)

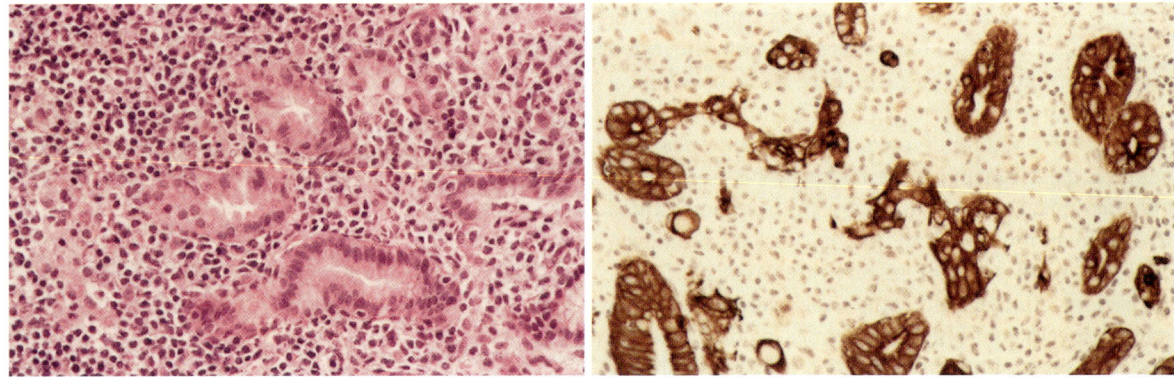

Figure 2
Gastric marginal zone B-cell lymphoma of MALT-type. Left: Partial destruction of gastric foveolar epithelium by centrocyte-like cell (HE stain); *right:* Visualization of infiltration and partial destruction of gastric gland epithelium by immunohistochemistry for cytokeratin (LU5 antibody, *brown stain*). (By courtesy of Andreas Chott, Vienna)

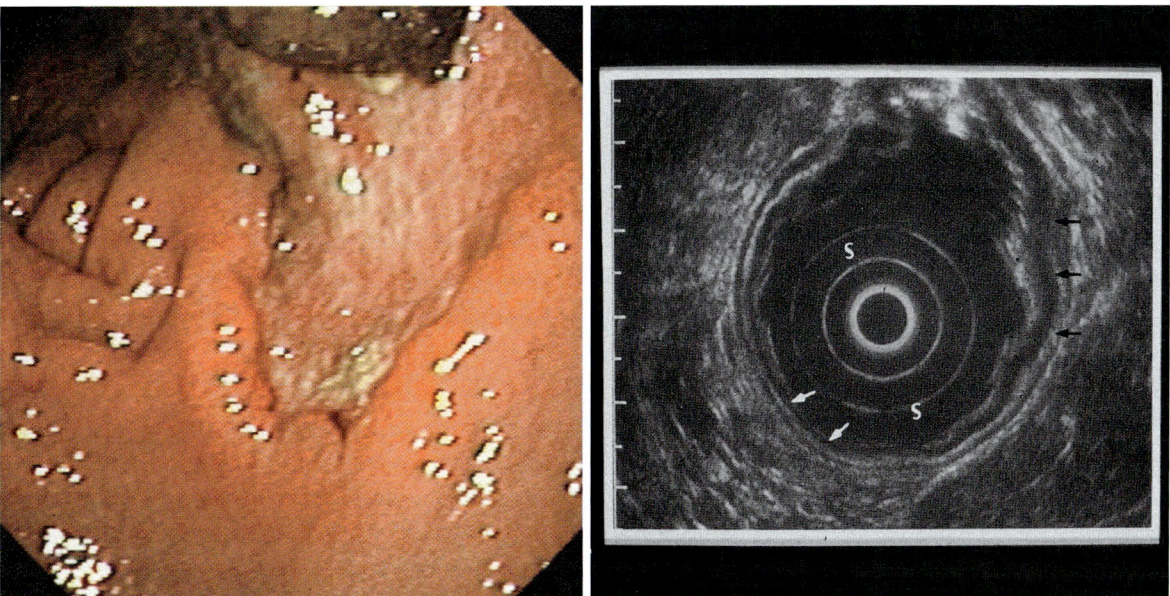

Figure 3
Left: "Classical" MALT-type lymphoma in the gastric antrum with mixed protruding and depressed endoscopic appearance; *right*: Endoscopic ultrasound revealing tumorous infiltration of mucosal and submucosal layers of the gastric wall (black arrows), no infiltration of perigastric lymphnodes

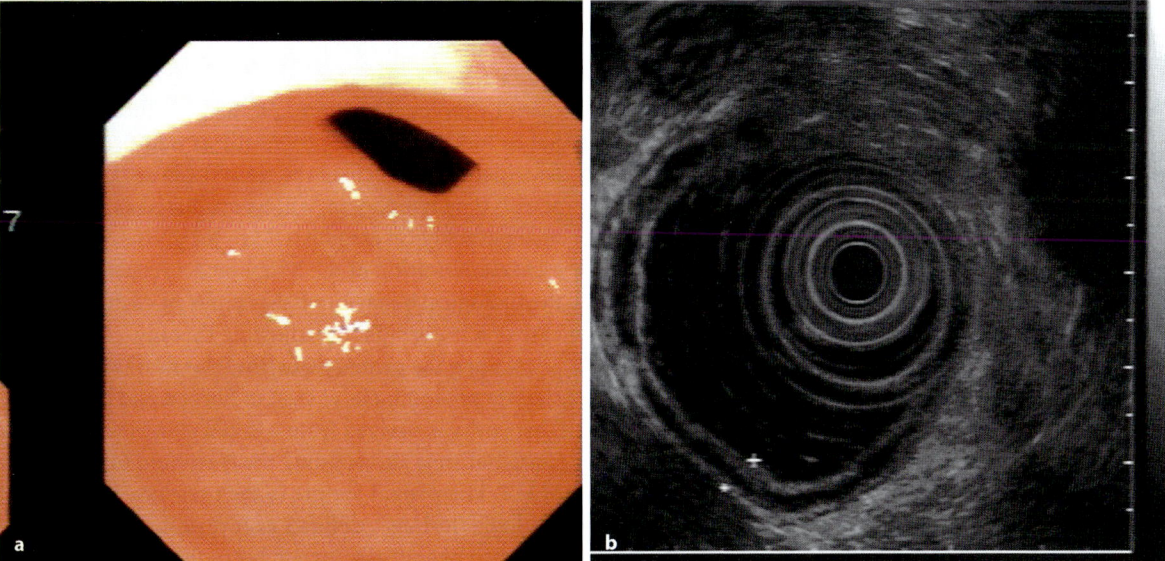

Figure 4
Left: Thickened fold in the prepyloric antrum, histologically confirmed marginal zone lymphoma, so-called "classical" MALT type lymphoma; *right*: Endoscopic ultrasound reflects a diffuse thickening of the mucosal layer of the gastric wall marked with two *white crosses*; so called "early" lymphoma. (Courtesy of Andreas Püspök, Vienna)

Histological Classification and Molecular Genetics

Synopsis

Spectrum of Lymphoma Entities Occuring in the Stomach and Duodenum According to the WHO Classification [6]

	Stomach (n)*	Intestine [n]
Primary		
B-Cell Lymphomas		
Extranodal marginal zone	75	10
B-cell lymphoma of MALT-type		
Follicular lymphoma	0	23
Mantle cell lymphoma		
(lymphomatouse polyposis)	1	48
Diffuse large B-cell lymphoma		
(+/– MALT-type component)	77 (10)	26
Burkitt lymphoma	6	8
Immunodeficiency associated		
lymphomas	0	7
T-Cell Lymphomas		
Intestinal T-cell lymphoma,		
enteropathy associated	1	29
Secondary		
Extragastrointestinal lymphoma		
of MALT-type		
Primary nodal lymphoma and B-CLL		

* Data from the Viennese Lymphoma Registry (1997–2001) provided by Andreas Chott, University of Vienna, Department of Clinical Pathology, illustrating the prevalence and distribution of gastrointestinal lymphomas in the population of Austria, Europe.

Immunohistochemistry of Gastrointestinal B-cell Proliferations

	CD20	Cyclin D1	CD5	CD10	bcl2	Ki-67(%)
MALT-L.	+	–	–	–	+	5–20
Follikular L.	+	–	–	+	+	15–50
MZL	+	+	+	–	+	15–50
DLBCL	+	–	–	–/+	+/–	>50
Burkitt L.	+	–	–	+	–	100

MZL mantle cell lymphoma, *DLBCL* diffuse large B-cell lymphoma

Lymphoma Entities and Characteristic Genetic Aberrations

Gastric MALT-type	t(11;18) (q21;q21)	30–40%
	Trisomy 3	60%
Follicular lymphoma	t(14;18) (q32;q21)	70–95%
Mantle cell lymphoma	t(11;14) (q13;q23)	>90%
Diffuse large B-cell lymphoma	Trisomy 12, alteration of p53, p16, c-myc	
Burkitt lymphoma	c-myc rearrangement	100%
	t(8;14) (q24;q32)	

The REAL (Revised European American Lymphoma) Classification established in 1994 terminated the confusion of nomenclatures applied for lymphomas in the previous decades. The recently proposed WHO Classification of lymphoid neoplasia [6] represents an update of the REAL Classification and comprehensively defines all non-Hodgkin's lymphomas, including those occurring in the gastrointestinal tract, as distinct entities. Accordingly, the gold standard of histological diagnosis of lymphomas of the stomach and the duodenum relies on the combination of morphology and immunohistochemistry of tumor cells. To reach this goal, the clinician has to provide sufficient tumor tissue for histopathological analysis, usually collected endoscopically by forceps biopsy. If, nevertheless, diagnostic problems arise, they can usually be managed by a rebiopsy or, in individual cases by molecular studies. In the near future, additional factors relevant for prognostic as well as therapeutic considerations, such as the t(11;18) (q21;q21) in gastric MALT-type lymphoma, will be evaluated as part of the histopathological diagnosis. As to prognosis, the histological classification of the lymphoma adequately reflects the biological behavior of the tumor in each individual case and is essential for adjusting therapy.

Among the primary GLs, the "classical" MALT-types slightly predominate, at least in Europe and in the USA. This entity is derived from a B-cell clone located in the marginal zone surrounding the lymphoid follicle of the MALT. The pivotal feature is the presence of "lymphoepithelial lesions", defined as invasion and partial destruction of epithelial structures of the gastric glands by aggregates of tumor cells with centrocyte-like morphology. The course of these GLs is indolent. They have been shown to regress completely after *H. pylori* eradication in up to 80% of cases when confined to mucosa and submucosa and not exhibiting the translocation of t(11;18), in particular (Fig. 5).

DLBCL of the stomach and the duodenum is almost equal in incidence with MALT-type lymphoma and may in part evolve from marginal zone B-cell lymphoma secondarily [7]. Mostly, however, DLBCL may develop primarily *de novo* from a clone of large B-cells with characteristic immunophenotype and a proliferation index as indicated by a Ki-67 stain of >50%. Knowledge of molecular genetics is still scarce, but t(11;18) is lacking. As opposed to MALT-type lymphoma, the clinical course is aggressive and the therapeutical approach differs markedly.

In conclusion, the precise histological classifying of lymphoma as apart from clinical staging is mandatory for selecting an adequate therapeutic strategy.

Staging

Synopsis

Initial staging of GL is necessary first, for discriminating primary from secondary GL and, second, for selecting the mode of therapy. In the case of indolent "classical" MALT-type lymphoma, the spectrum of therapeutic options ranges from antibiotic therapy in *H. pylori*- (or *H. heilmanii*) associated "early lymphoma" (stage EI1 Ann Arbor) to RTX or CTX in non-responders as well as in the case of more advanced disease (stage >EI2 Ann Arbor). Surprisingly, a recent report (8) did not find any difference in estimated 5-and 10-year overall survival rates (86% and 80%, respectively) between localized and disseminated MALT-type disease. This entity has been shown to present multifocally along the MALT, spreading to the tonsils, to lacrimal or salivary glands, to thyroid, lung or small or large bowel. Gastric DLBCL, however, is more likely to grow aggressively focally, causing complications or to generalize.

Staging systems in use are given above: the Ann Arbor System has been applied for staging GLs most widely in the past 30 years, whereas the TNM system may more adequately document depth of infiltration as assessed by EUS. Currently, a new staging system adjusted to the specific features of gastrointestinal lymphomas is in preparation by the European Gastrointestinal Study Group.

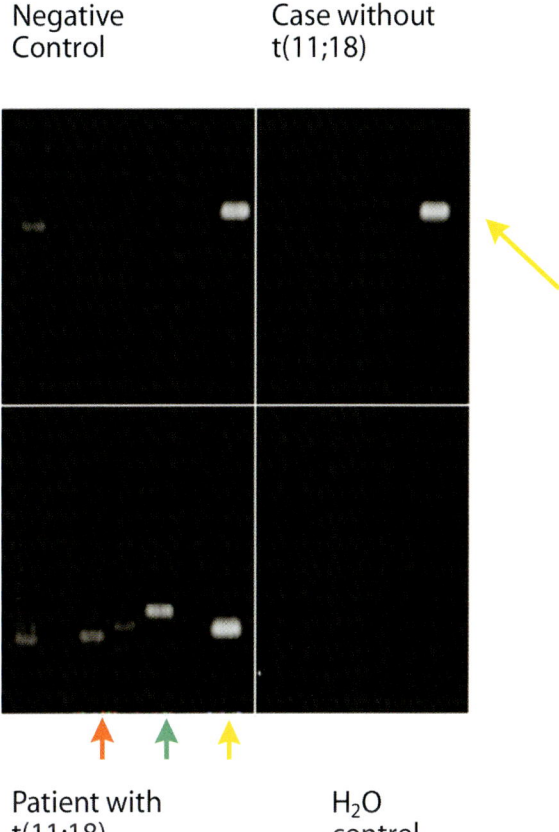

Figure 5

RT-PCR for the detection of the t(11;18) from paraffin tissue of gastric MALT-type lymphoma. The *red arrow* depicts the fusion transcript generated by breakpoints at 1446 bp and 814 bp of the *API2* and the *MALT1* gene, respectively. Another band (*green arrow*) is produced by primers annealing outside of this product. The *yellow arrow* points at the band produced by the actin control amplification. (Courtesy of Andreas Chott, Vienna)

Treatment

Synopsis

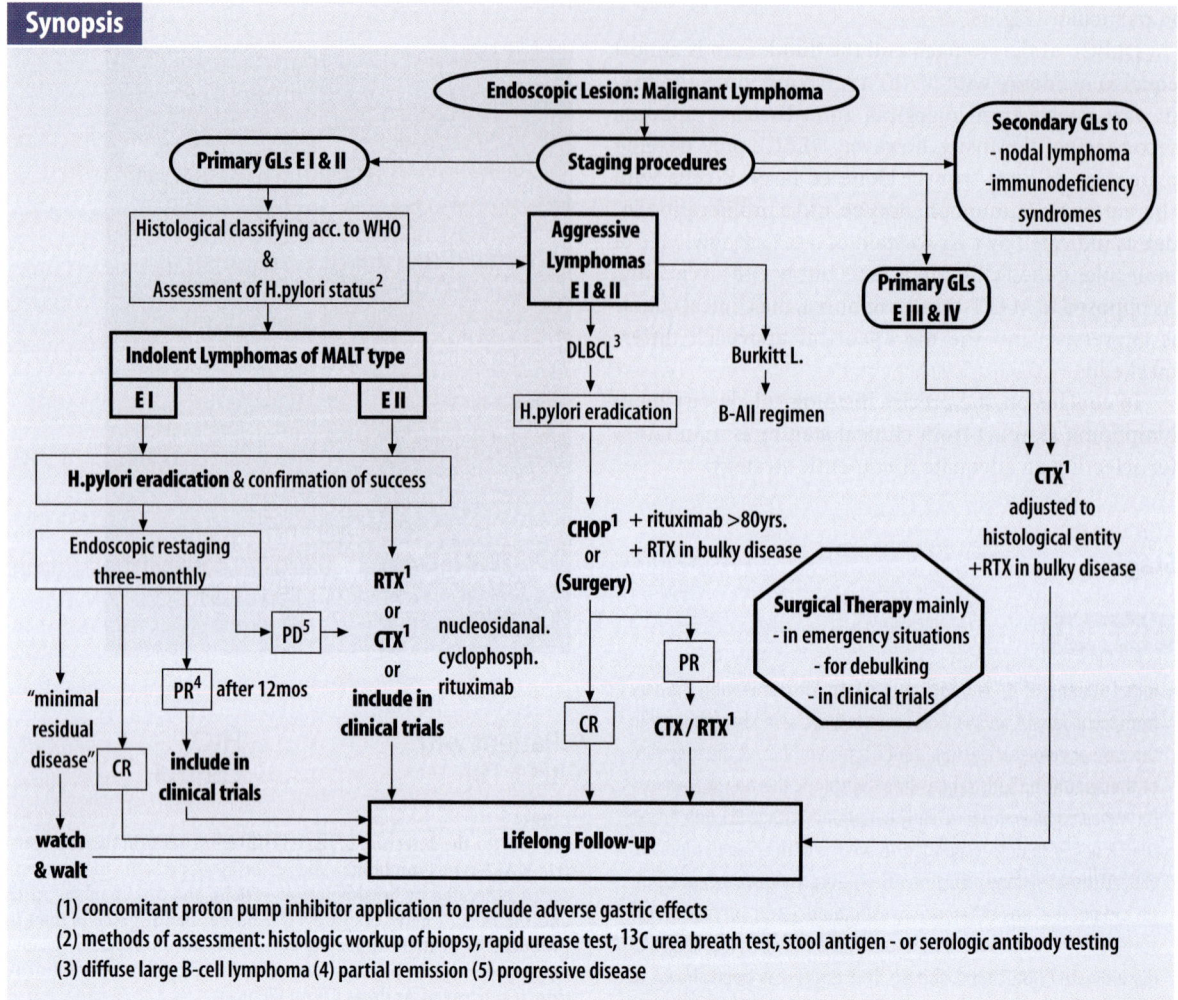

(1) concomitant proton pump inhibitor application to preclude adverse gastric effects
(2) methods of assessment: histologic workup of biopsy, rapid urease test, ^{13}C urea breath test, stool antigen - or serologic antibody testing
(3) diffuse large B-cell lymphoma (4) partial remission (5) progressive disease

While surgery has been the most commonly applied therapy in the past for primary GLs, there is a clear trend in favor of organ-conserving strategies, since retrospective analyses have shown equal efficacy with probably lower morbidity as compared to gastrectomy. Especially the risk of bleeding and perforation with conservative management has been diminished in the last decade by concomitant therapy with proton pump inhibitors (PPI), effectively preventing production of acid gastric juice, an important co-factor of such complications. As evidence from prospective studies on successful management of GLs with non-invasive treatment modalities is increasing recently, surgical therapy should mostly be restricted to rescuing emergency situations, replacing its previous position as "first-line therapy".

Assessment of both histological classification and stage is mandatory for adequately adjusting therapy in the individual case. Attention has to be paid to *H. pylori*-associated "early" MALT-type lymphoma (stage EI1 Ann Arbor) to avoid over-treatment.

Surgery

Resection of GLs has been shown to result in CR of disease in about 87% of cases in several retrospective studies. However, surgical therapy was combined with postoperative CTX or RTX or both in >50% of cases, impairing the evaluation of the surgical part of the treatment. Results of large prospective studies indicate similar rates of CR after either resection combined with stage-adjusted CTX and/or RTX or non-surgical multi-modal therapy [4]. Two to 5% of patients undergoing total gastrectomy may die postoperatively, up to 20% may suffer from post-gastrectomy syndromes with up to 5% remaining symptomatic lifelong. Moreover, relapses involving a distant site many years after local therapy of the initial localization have been repeatedly reported, suggesting systemic therapeutic approaches.

With respect to surgical therapy, the assessment of lymphoma histology and stage is essential (Fig. 6). *H. pylori*-associated MALT-type lymphoma in stage EI and the subgroup of locally advanced DLBCL have been shown to benefit substantially from non-invasive therapy [4]. In conclusion, with constantly improving efficacy and tolerability of stomach-conserving methods, surgery is pushed aside from the first-line treatment position, focusing on particular cases as well as on emergency situations in future.

Endoscopy

Gastroduodenal endoscopy is applied therapeutically only in order to stop bleeding, occurring spontaneously or in the course of CTX or RTX. Laparoscopic approach for staging procedures such as lymph node sampling or imaging of abdominal tumor extension is under investigation.

Radiotherapy

GL appears highly sensitive towards irradiation as has been repeatedly reported from the Netherlands Cancer Center since 1970. Without respect to lymphoma histology, the overall 5-year survival rate amounts to 71% for RTX alone, not significantly different from the 82% after resection plus RTX. Recent data from Princess Margret Hospital, Canada, report excellent 5-year overall survival rates of 96%, with 76% disease-free in stages EI and II of

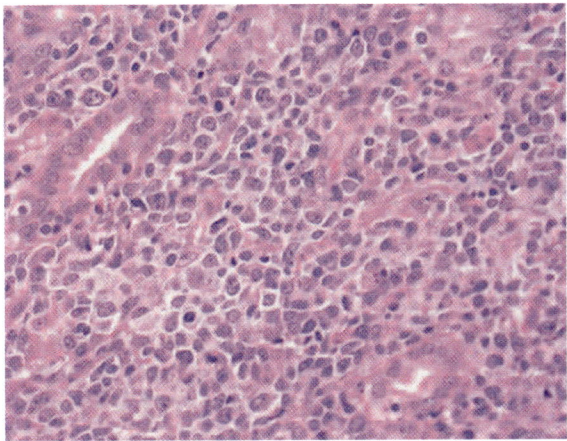

Figure 6
Histology of diffuse large B-cell lymphoma of the stomach. Sheets of atypical large cells are spreading between gastric glands. (Courtesy of Andreas Chott, Vienna)

MALT-type lymphoma, following moderate-dose (30 Gy, range 17.5 to 35 Gy) RTX. Prospective results from the Memorial Kettering Cancer Center for a similar cohort indicate up to a 100% event-free survival rate after follow-ups of median 27 months. In addition, RTX has earned merits as an adjunct to surgical therapy from the very beginning in particular cases. In conclusion, moderate-dose RTX may be considered as one of the preferred treatment modalities for localized MALT-type lymphoma to date. RTX is recommended for patients not responding with CR to antibiotic *H. pylori* therapy after 12 months or for those presenting with > stage EI disease.

Chemotherapy

CTX as sole management of localized GLs has only been applied reluctantly, especially in Europe, because of side-effects like bleeding or perforation, but concomitant PPI therapy has accumulated confidence in preventing such complications. For indolent GLs, the administration of nucleoside analogs is theoretically compelling. Both, fludarabine and 2-chlorodesoxyadenosine (2CdA) have been shown to be associated with a pronounced T-cell depletory activity, suggesting an interesting additional mechanism of controlling the role of *H. pylori*-specific T-cells in gastric, MALT-type lymphoma. To date only pilot series with 2CdA treatment have been published, giving impressive response rates; mature results with prolonged follow-up are needed.

Evidence for successful CTX of gastric DLBCL, either secondarily transforming from MALT-type or primary arising in the stomach, is accumulating rapidly in recent years. A prospective study from the Viennese Lymphoma Study Group including 37 patients with localized DLBCL achieved CR in 86% sustained for a median of 39 months, after a maximum of only three cycles of CHOP, an anthracyclin based treatment regimen, containing cyclophosphamide, doxorubicin, vincristine and oral prednisolone. An additional *H. pylori* eradication therapy is recommended.

Thus, the data of CTX for localized GL available are promising but scarce and should be further evaluated in trials comparing different organ conserving strategies. The rare cases of gastric Burkitt lymphoma are known to run an extremely aggressive course frequently involving the central nervous system and need more aggressive therapy according to the B-ALL regimen.

Radiochemotherapy

These combined modalities are warranted in cases not responding to monotherapy, they are mostly applied in consecutive mode or, in particular, in cases of relapse.

Immunotherapy

At present, the efficacy of the monoclonal CD-20 antibody rituximab has been tested only in a small series. Though theoretically interesting, this therapy only works in the presence of small tumor mass, or combined with CTX such as CHOP. In addition, the substance is very expensive.

Antibiotic Therapy

This mode of therapy is of relevance for localized GLs of MALT-type and, probably also for transformed DLBCLs in very early stage. As has been shown above, *H. pylori* is a key factor in the development of GL in generating T-cells necessary for maintenance of the malignant B-cell clone in its early stages. In fact, more than 90% of MALT-type lymphomas are associated with *H. pylori* infection of the gastric mucosa. In addition, GLs associ-

ated with H. heilmannii infection have been shown to behave almost identically to *H. pylori*-associated GL in clinical as well as therapeutical respects.

Since the early nineties of the twentieth century, more than 650 patients worldwide have been treated for gastric MALT-type lymphoma with antibiotics, experiencing CR of disease in up to 80% of cases [9]. The treatment regimen of first choice, according to the Maastricht consensus 2000 of the European Helicobacter Pylori Study Group, is a combination of PPI twice daily with two antibiotics, preferably clarithromycin 500 mg and amoxicillin 1 g twice daily for a minimum of 7 days. The most predictive factors for response are lymphoma restriction to stages EI1 (78%) and EI2, with stepwise decreasing response rates from submucosa (43%) to serosa (20 to 25%) as well as indolent histology. However, the bias of over- or under-staging by clinical procedures like EUS amounts to about 23%. It is even higher with CT scan and has to be considered when evaluating the response. Other factors predictive for positive treatment response are high expression of CD86 on B-lymphoma cells and the absence of t(11;18), respectively [5, 9].

CR after successful antibiotic eradication of *H. pylori* should be defined on the basis of endoscopic appearance and of histological diagnosis as gold standard. CR of lymphoma may most likely occur between 3 and 12 months (mean 6 months) after *H. pylori* eradication and should be confirmed by endoscopic and histologic reassessment twice in an interval of 3 months. Monoclonality of small B-cell aggregates, however, is reported to persist in about 50% of cases after a median follow-up period of 33 months and is designated as "minimal residual disease" [9]. As the meaning of this finding is not yet clear, endoscopy including a mapping procedure is advisable within 12 to 24 months after diagnosis of CR, in order to detect recurrent disease.

Refined methods of further investigating the molecular genetics of GLs in general, are currently being investigated to provide more insight into the biologic behavior of this disease.

Prognosis and Follow-Up

Lymphomas of the stomach, in general, run a substantially better course than gastric cancer, their epithelial counterpart. While stage at clinical presentation is of major influence on prognosis in both instances, the high sensitivity of lymphoma cells towards CTX as well as RTX favors the success of such treatment. In consequence, overall 5-year survival rates of *H. pylori*-associated gastric MALT-type lymphoma in stage EI range between 90 and 100%, including cases responding to antibiotic therapy of infection only, which previously have been designated as "pseudolymphomas". Indolent GLs in stages EII experience a 5-year overall survival expectancy of about 80% without respect to mode of therapy applied. Even for GLs with aggressive histology in stage EI, 5-year survival rates ranging between 86 and 100% are reported [10] after either multimodal therapy or mono-CTX. However, for aggressive GLs in more advanced stages or with macroscopic tumor residues after gastrectomy or without reaching CR after multimodal therapy, 5-year survival drops to around 50%.

Follow-up of patients in CR is indicated at intervals of 12 to 24 months – especially of MALT-type lymphoma with "minimal residual disease" after antibiotic therapy – to detect recurrence of disease. In general, restaging procedures at intervals of 2 to 3 years are advisable lifelong, as late relapses on other MALT-sites have been reported. In addition, a slight increase of secondary malignancies has been observed in GL patients, encouraging regular follow-up.

Screening and Prevention

Patients with autoimmune disease such as Hashimoto thyroiditis or Sjögren's syndrome are at 70-fold risk for developing lymphomas in the respective glands and moreover may develop asymptomatic gastric MALT-type lymphoma. Gastrointestinal tract screening of these patients and of patients with MALT-type lymphomas at any other location is recommended.

Worldwide, there are ongoing trials investigating the effect of *H. pylori* eradication on prevention of gastric cancer, which calculate a diminishing of this condition by about 60%. As this association in the case of lymphoma is even higher than in that of cancer, results will be of relevance for lymphoma prevention as well.

Future Perspectives

With respect to the increase in stomach conserving therapy, there is a need for improving clinical procedures in order to minimize failures in staging as well as in classifying the histological entity. With this purpose, the use of high frequent miniechoendoscopes and EUS-guided biopsy will probably contribute to diagnostic accuracy.

Large-scale studies comparing different non-surgical treatment modalities in well-defined settings are needed for further validation of preliminary results.

Ongoing investigations are focusing on refined molecular methods to predict responsiveness of GLs to *H. pylori* eradication and upcoming therapeutic modalities such as application of monoclonal antibodies.

References

1. Gurney KA, Cartwright RA, Gilman EA (1999) Descriptive epidemiology of gastrointestinal non-Hodgkin's lymphoma in a population-based registry. Brit J Cancer 79:1929–1934
2. Isaacson PG (1995) Primary gastric lymphoma. Brit J Biomed Science 52:291–296
3. Radaszkiewicz Th, Dragosics B, Bauer P (1992) Gastrointestinal Malignant Lymphomas of the Mucosa-Associated Lymphoid Tissue: Factors Relevant to Prognosis. Gastroenterology 102:1628–1638
4. Fischbach W, Dragosics B, Kolve-Goebeler ME, et al. (2000) Primary gastric B-cell lymphoma: results of a multicenter study. Gastroenterology 119:1191–1202
5. Ruskone-Fourmestraux A, Lavergne A, Aegerter Ph (2001) Predictive factors for regression of gastric MALT lymphoma after anti-Helicobacter pylori treatment. Gut 48:297–303
6. Jaffe E, Harris N, Diebold J, Müller-Hermelink H (1999) World Health Organization classification of neoplastic diseases of the hematopoietic and lymphoid tissues: A progress report. Am J Clin Pathol 111(Suppl1) S8–S12
7. De Jong D, Boot H, Van Heerde P, Hart GAM, Taal BG (1997) Histological Grading in Gastric Lymphoma: Pretreatment Criteria and Clinical Relevance. Gastroenterology 112:1466–147
8. Thieblemont C, Berger F, Dumontet C, Moullet I, Bouafia F, Felmann P, Salles G, Coiffier B (2000) Mucosa-associated lymphoid tissue lymphoma is a disseminated disease in one third of 158 patients analyzed. Blood 95(3): 802–806
9. Morgner A, Miehlke S, Fischbach W, Schmitt W, Müller-Hermelink HK (2001) Complete remission of primary high-grade B-cell gastric lymphoma after cure of Helicobacter pylori infection. J Clin Oncol 19: 2041–8
10. Ruskone-Fourmestraux A, Aegerter Ph, Delmer A, et al. (1993) Primary digestive tract lymphoma: a prospective multicentric study of 91 patients. Gastroenterology 105:1662–1671

6 Gastric Tumors Other than Adenocarcinoma and Lymphoma

N.C.T. VAN GRIEKEN, G.A. MEIJER, E.J. KUIPERS

Summary

In the previous chapters, gastric adenocarcinomas and lymphomas have been discussed. In addition to these two main tumor types, a variety of other gastric tumors are classified by the WHO according to their origin. These lesions are described in this chapter (Table 1).

Most tumorous lesions of the stomach are of epithelial origin. Among them, adenocarcinomas are the dominating tumor type. However, a variety of other epithelial and non-epithelial tumors can occur in the stomach, ranging from benign polyps with little tendency for malignant degeneration, such as fundic gland polyps, to malignant tumors such as carcinoids. In between, we find lesions with the potential for malignant degeneration like adenomas and (some) hyperplastic polyps. The aim of this chapter is to review epidemiological, pathogenetic, histological and clinical data for these less frequent epithelial and mesenchymal tumors of the stomach.

Epithelial Tumors

Fundic Gland Polyps

Epidemiology

Fundic gland polyps (FGPs) are the most common gastric polyps and occur predominantly in the fundus and corpus. Within Western populations, FGPs are found in 0.8–1.9% of the subjects undergoing upper gastrointestinal endoscopy. FGPs occur in a sporadic form, as well as in a syndromic form associated with familial adenomatosis polyposis (FGP-FAP). The sporadic form most often affects women, while the syndromic polyps have no sex preference. FGPs mostly arise between 40 and 70 yrs, although syndromic FGPs occur at a younger age.

Table 1

Epithelial tumors	Mesenchymal tumors
Fundic gland polyps	GIST
Hyperplastic polyps	GANT
Adenomas	Schwannoma
Neuroendocrine tumors	Leimyoma/leiomyosarcoma
Others (Peutz-Jeghers, juvenile polyposis, Cowden, Cronkite-Canada)	Others (Granular cell tumor, Glomus tumor, Kaposi sarcoma, Lipoma)

Etiology, Pathogenesis and Molecular Genetics

The etiology of sporadic FGPs is still unclear. Because of the female predominance, a role for female hormones has been suggested for sporadic FGPs. The development of FGPs has, however, in particular, been associated with the use of proton-pump inhibitors (PPIs), profound acid-suppressive drugs. It has been suggested that PPI-induced parietal cell protrusions lead to fundic gland cysts (FGCs) and finally FGP, but more indirect mechanisms have also been proposed, such as hypergastrinemia-related hyperproliferation of the glandular epithelium. In contrast to this hypothesis, a large retrospective study of 2251 cases and 28,096 controls observed a similar FGP prevalence among PPI users and controls. The contrast between this study and previous smaller reports has not yet been fully elucidated. It may be that the former clinical experience, originating from smaller series, was biased and presumptive. It may however also be that there is an association between PPI use and FGP development, in which case the low prevalence of registered PPI use among the FGP patients in the German study has to be explained otherwise. The study seemed to have been based on the retrospective use of a central pathology database. Unfortunately, such pathology databases are often insufficient with respect to clinical data. For the present time, the hypothesis of an association between PPIs and FGPs needs further evaluation. Both the German study and others reported that FGPs in particular occur in *H. pylori*-negatives [1].

Fundic gland polyps have for long been regarded as non-neoplastic lesions, but recently, FGPs harboring dysplastic areas or adenocarcinoma have been described. In addition, the association of FGPs with FAP suggested a role for the APC gene in FGP development. Indeed, a high frequency of somatic mutations in the APC gene were found in FGP-FAP, while in sporadic FGP, activating mutations of the β-catenin gene have been found in 91% of cases (52 out of 57). This is strong evidence that disruption of the Wnt signaling pathway is the central molecular biological mechanism in the pathogenesis of FGP. At the same time one should realize that in the vast majority of FGP, this does not lead to dysplasia and subsequent progression towards cancer.

Symptoms, Clinical Signs, and Diagnosis

Like most gastric polyps, fundic gland polyps do not cause specific clinical symptoms. They are often small (2–5 mm), although they may gradually increase in size to reach a diameter up to 2–3 cm. In most cases, they appear as multiple, sessile, whitish pink polyps, often with a partially translucent surface (Fig. 1a). They are particularly located in the fundus and corpus mucosa of the stomach, the region with parietal cells. Histological evaluation confirms the diagnosis.

Histological Classification

Sporadic and syndromic fundic gland polyps share the same histology. Microscopically, fundic gland polyps show a (partial) distortion of the normal acid secreting gastric mucosa with dilated, cystic glands (Figs. 1b and c). The glandular epithelium is lined with flattened parietal cells. These changes are frequently associated with parietal cell hyperplasia. In this case, the parietal cells tend to have an abundant cytoplasm that protrudes into the glandular lumen at the apex of the cells. The chief cells, which are also still present, have a normal aspect and the surrounding mucosa is normal.

Treatment, Prognosis and Follow-Up

FGP do not require specific treatment. After confirmation of the histological diagnosis by sampling of standard biopsy specimens from a representative number of polyps, an expectative approach is sufficient. Although the occurrence of adenocarcinoma in sporadic FGP has been reported in a number of case reports, the incidence is most likely very low. In the few large series of FGP that have been studied, no cancer or dysplasia has been reported. Therefore, the cancer risk in patients with sporadic FGP is probably too low to warrant any specific treatment or follow up. There is no need to withdraw PPI treatment, although the FGPs may increase in number and size during ongoing treatment. In FAP patients, endoscopic surveillance may be necessary for early detection of malignancies, despite the absence of histologically neoplastic signs.

Hyperplastic Polyps

Epidemiology

Valid data on the prevalence of hyperplastic polyps of the stomach in the general population are scarce. Studies from reference centres have reported that they comprise approximately 30% of all gastric polyps while in other series they make up 90% of all gastric polyps. As with sporadic fundic gland polyps, they are more frequently found in women than in men, usually occurring in subjects older than 60 years of age. They are equally distributed throughout different parts of the stomach [2], in which respect they differ from fundic gland polyps.

Etiology, Pathogenesis and Molecular Genetics

Hyperplastic polyps virtually never occur in normal gastric mucosa, but always against a background of chronic gastritis. They are thought to result from regeneration after mucosal damage, e.g. due to *H. pylori* gastritis. Eradication of *H. pylori* has been reported to be associated with regression of hyperplastic gastric polyps. In this respect, hyperplastic polyps are regenerative lesions to a certain extent, resembling inflammatory polyps of

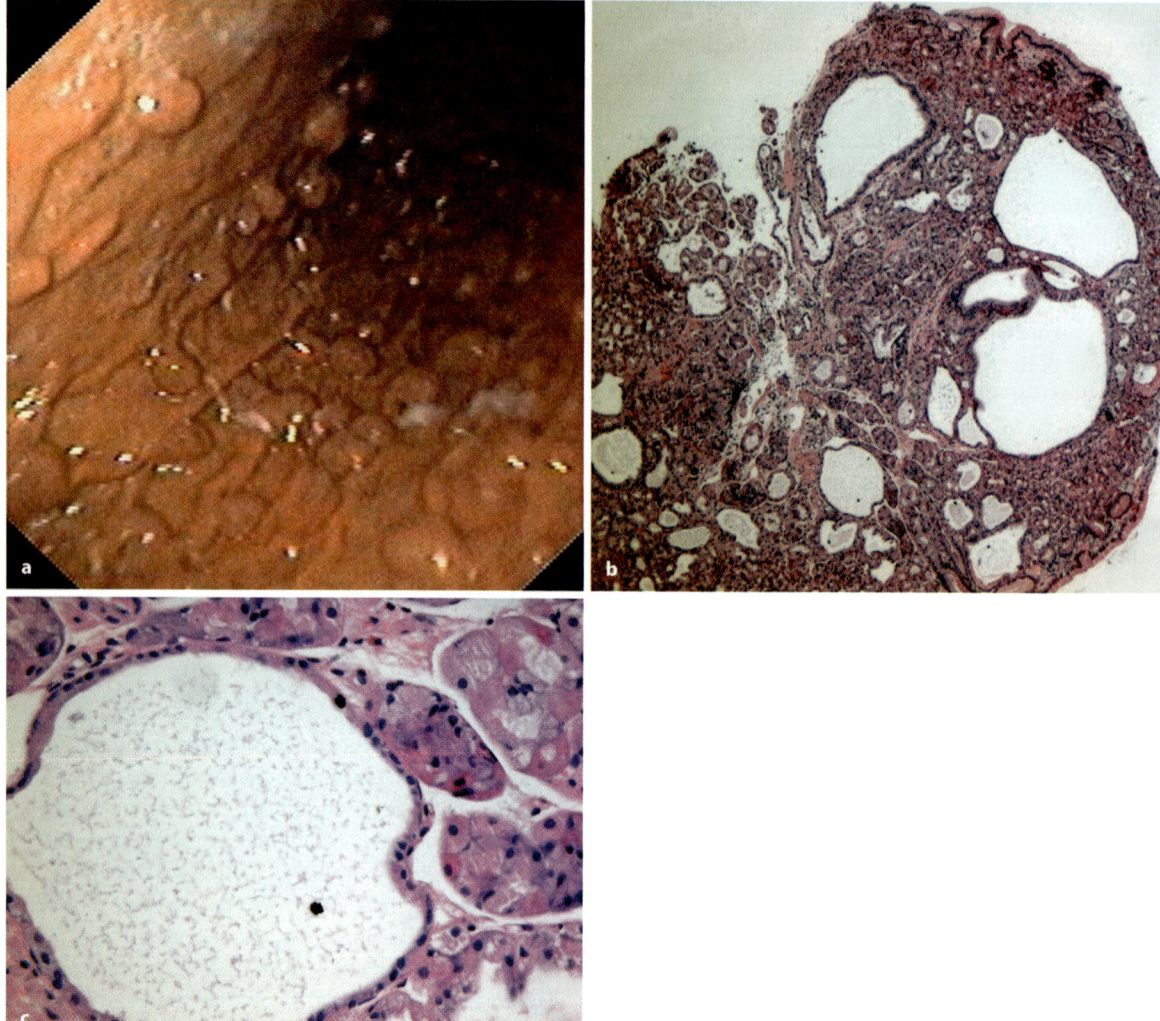

Figure 1a–c
Fundic gland polyps mostly present as small (2–5 mm), multiple, sessile, whitish pink polyps, often with a partially translucent surface. They are particularly located in the fundus and corpus mucosa of the stomach, the region with parietal cells (**a**). Microscopically, fundic gland polyps show a (partial) distortion of the normal acid secreting gastric mucosa with dilated, cystic glands lined with flattened parietal cells (**b** and **c**)

the large bowel rather than hyperplastic polyps of the large intestine. Whether hyperplastic polyps develop via foveolar hyperplasia as a precursor is not clear. Familial occurrence of hyperplastic polyps, suggesting a genetic factor, has been reported, and was found to be associated with gastric cancer. Although in principle hyperplastic polyps are non-neoplastic, dysplastic changes in hyperplastic polyps can occur. These probably reflect neoplastic changes in a background of chronic inflammation and regeneration rather than a neoplastic origin of the hyperplastic polyp itself.

Symptoms, Clinical Signs, and Diagnosis

Like most gastric polyps, hyperplastic polyps do not cause specific clinical symptoms.

They mostly are incidental findings during gastroscopy. Endoscopic ultrasonography (EUS) is required for the evaluation of gastric submucosal polypoid lesions.

Histological Classification

Most hyperplastic polyps arise against a background of chronic gastritis and microscopically they show irregular elongation of gastric pits, often accompanied by cystic dilatation of glands which are of the antral type (Fig. 2). The foveolar epithelium can become serrated and is often hyperplastic with basal nuclei and prominent intracytoplasmic mucin, which may resemble goblet cells. The lamina propria shows edema with infiltration of inflammatory cells and presence of smooth muscle cells and small blood vessels. There is a resemblance to granulation tissue, which reflects the regenerative character of the lesion. At the surface, erosions may occur with further inflammatory response including polymorphic neutrophils. Regenerative epithelium in these areas may yield an impression of atypia. Rarely, true dysplasia does occur in hyperplastic polyps and even adenocarcinoma arising in gastric hyperplastic polyps has been described. Indeed, chromosomal aberrations can be found in such lesions.

Treatment, Prognosis and Follow-Up

Although there is consensus that all gastric adenomatous polyps should be removed, as should gastric hyperplastic polyps that are symptomatic and/or bear dysplastic foci on forceps biopsy, controversy still exists over the management of asymptomatic gastric hyperplastic polyps that do not show any dysplastic focus on forceps biopsies. *H. pylori* eradication should be considered, even though there is no evidence as to what extent patients with hyperplastic polyps benefit from such a strategy.

Gastric Adenomas

Epidemiology

The term adenoma is used for pre-malignant neoplastic lesions of the gastric mucosa with a circumscript, often polypoid nature, as in the large intestine. As such, they are a precursor of gastric cancer of the intestinal type.

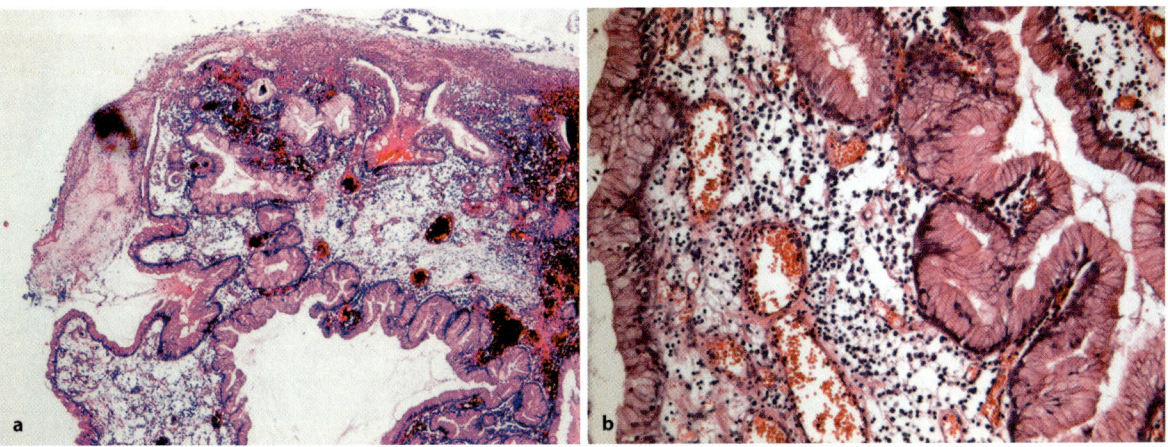

Figure 2a,b
Hyperplastic polyps of the stomach microscopically show irregular elongation of gastric pits, often accompanied by cystic dilatation of antral type glands (**a**). The foveolar epithelium can become serrated and is often hyperplastic with basal nuclei and prominent intracytoplasmic mucin, which may resemble goblet cells. The lamina propria shows edema with infiltration of inflammatory cells and presence of smooth muscle cells and small blood vessels. At the surface, erosions with a further inflammatory response including polymorphic neutrophils are present (**b**)

However, most gastric cancers of the intestinal type arise from flat dysplastic lesions, simply referred to as dysplasia. Adenomas comprise only 9% of all gastric polyps, show an equal sex distribution and occur mainly in subjects over 60 years of age. Gastric adenomas are more common in patients with FAP.

Etiology and Pathogenesis

Adenomas by nature are neoplastic lesions, i.e. proliferations with a clonal origin caused by (epi)genetic changes. The etiology of gastric adenomas is not yet fully understood. Some are associated with chronic atrophic gastritis, which in its turn is caused by *H. pylori*-infection. The common gastric adenomas, i.e. adenomas of the intestinal type, arise from intestinal metaplastic gastric mucosa. In sporadic gastric adenomas, several types of genetic changes have been found, including chromosomal aberrations (including loss of 17p) and microsatellite instability, but the underlying sequence of genetic changes is far from understood, other than the recognition that the sequence differs from the genetic changes that are known to induce the colorectal adenoma to carcinoma sequence. In FAP-associated adenomas in contrast, a very high prevalence of APC mutations has been found.

Symptoms, Clinical Signs, and Diagnosis

Like most gastric polyps, adenomas do not cause specific clinical symptoms.

Most adenomas are incidental findings during gastroscopy. EUS is of relevance for further evaluation of gastric submucosal polypoid lesions.

Histological Classification and Molecular Genetics

Despite differences in genetic aberrations, the histology (and the histological classification) of the common type of gastric adenomas is comparable to those of the large intestine. Architecturally these intestinal types of adenomas can show a spectrum from pure tubular adenomas, through tubulovillous adenomas to pure villous adenomas. Japanese classifications rather stress the difference between papillary and flat adenomas. Adenomas by definition are dysplastic lesions, and dysplasia is graded on a two or three grade scale by assessing changes such as nuclear size, shape, polymorphism, stratification, hyperchromasy and chromatin structure, together with mitotic rate, complexity of glands and mucin depletion (Fig. 3). The risk of finding carcinoma in a given adenoma correlates with size and grade of dysplasia. In particular, adenomas which are larger than two centimeters carry a more than 50% risk for the presence of cancer.

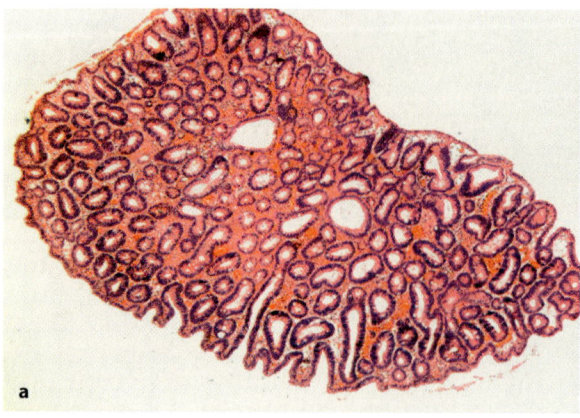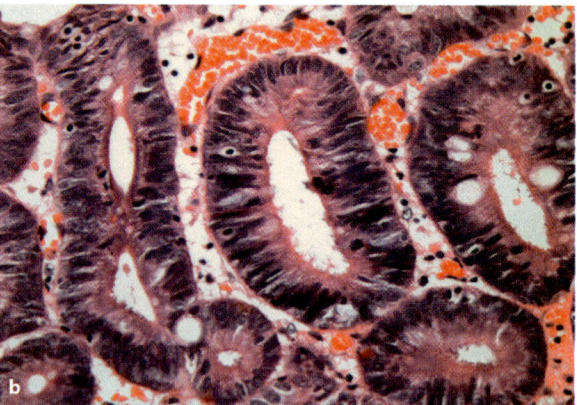

Figure 3a,b
Gastric adenomas histologicaly resemble those of the large intestine. This adenoma has a tubular architecture (**a**), and the epithelial cells have enlarged, elongated to polymorphic and hyperchromatic nuclei, which lie crowded and stratified in the epithelium (**b**). Furthermore, there is an increased mitotic rate and mucin depletion. This lesion would classify as low-grade dysplasia in a two-grade system and as moderate dysplasia in a three grade system

Treatment, Prognosis and Follow-Up

Since gastric adenomas are premalignant neoplastic lesions, they should all be completely removed. Literature on post-polypectomy surveillance in patients with gastric adenomas is not as comprehensive by far as that for post polypectomy surveillance of colorectal adenomas.

Neurendocrine Tumors of the Stomach (see also chapter 15)

Introduction

Neuroendocrine tumors occur throughout the body in different organ systems, in particular in the pulmonary and gastrointestinal tract. Unfortunately, terminology of neuroendocrine tumors is confusing, because of inconsistencies over time, between different organ systems, and even within organ systems. The terms carcinoid, microcarcinoid, enterochromafin-like (ECL)-cell hyperplasia, endocrine tumor, neuroendocrine tumor, small cell carcinoma. and others have been used to describe entities that are part of a spectrum of neoplastic changes in cells with neuroendocrine differentiation such as the ECL cells of the fundus and the G-cells of the antrum. In addition, these lesions are classified in different ways:

1. By etiology:
   ▸ Type I; associated with autoimmune atrophic gastritis (A-CAG)
   ▸ Type II; associated with multiple endocrine neoplasia type 1 (MEN1) or Zollinger-Ellison syndrome (ZES)
   ▸ Type III; sporadic neuroendocrine tumors, not associated with other clinical disorders.
2. By clinical behaviour
   ▸ Benign:
   Nonfunctioning, well differentiated, <1 cm, limited to mucosa/submucosa, no angioinvasion
   ▸ Benign or low-grade malignant:
   Nonfunctioning, well differentiated, 1 cm < X <2 cm, limited to mucosa/submucosa, no angioinvasion or <2 cm with angioinvasion
   ▸ Low grade malignant:
   Nonfunctioning, well differentiated, >2 cm, or extending beyond the submucosa
   Functioning, well differentiated tumor of any size and extension
   ▸ High grade malignant:
   Functioning or non-functioning, poorly differentiated intermediate or small cell carcinoma.
3. By histologic appearance
   ▸ ECL-cell hyperplasia
   ▸ Micro carcinoids
   ▸ Carcinoids
   ▸ Small cell carcinoma

The fact that these classifications are not mutually exclusive adds to the confusion with respect to this topic. As a basic biological concept, one should keep in mind that gastric epithelial cells with neuroendocrine differentiation (i.e. ECL cells or G-cells) belong to the normal cell population of the gastric mucosa. Due to inherited (e.g. MEN1 syndrome) and/or environmental factors (e.g. hypergastrinemia), these cells can show hyperplasia as a result of a disturbed balance between cell proliferation and apoptosis. By further accumulation of (epi)genetic changes neoplastic clones arise with a clinical behavior that may range from indolent to highly aggressive (as is the case with small cell carcinoma of the stomach). In this respect, understanding of these general biological principles makes more sense than semantic debates on classifications.

Epidemiology

The exact incidence of carcinoid tumors of the stomach is unknown, but the stomach is not an uncommon site for the development of gastrointestinal carcinoids. In fact, recent observations indicate that gastric neuroendocrine tumors may account for up to 40% of the neuroendocrine tumors arising in the gastrointestinal tract. Most gastric carcinoids are non-functioning, well differentiated lesions arising in the fundus or corpus mucosa. Type I carcinoids account for 74% of cases and show a female predominance. Type II represents about 6% of cases with an equal sex distribution, while Type III carcinoids comprise about 14% of cases and predominantly occur in males in their 6th decade. Small cell carcinoma has been reported to account for 6% of neuroendocrine tumors with a predominance in males in their 7th decade. Gastrin cell tumors comprise only 1% of gastric neuroendocrine tumors, occurring in patients over fifty years of age.

Etiology and Pathogenesis

Gastrin can act as a growth factor for ECL cells through the CCK-B/gastrin receptor. As a consequence, hypergastrinaemia leads to hyperplasia of ECL-cells as a first step. This phenomenon may explain the observed development of ECL-cell hyperplasia during long-term profound acid-suppressive maintenance treatment for gastro-esophageal reflux disease. However, development of ECL-cell hyperplasia in these patients was, in particular, observed in association with atrophic gastritis. This observation led to the hypothesis that the suggestion of hyperplasia in these cases might also result from the disappearance of specialized cells, instead of a true increase of ECL-cells. Once hyperplasia is present, additional (epi)genetic changes are required for tumor progression, and several other growth factors like TGFalfa and bFGF are thought to play a role. In addition, *H.pylori* may play a synergistic role. In Type II lesions, the MEN1 tumor suppressor gene on chromosome 11q13 may be involved. However, knowledge of the molecular pathogenesis of these tumors is still incomplete. Progression of hyperplasia towards dysplasia has never been observed to our knowledge in patients on long-term PPI therapy.

Symptoms, Clinical Signs, and Diagnosis

Most gastric neuroendocrine tumors are non-functioning and symptoms from carcinoid syndrome are rare. Type I carcinoids are frequently multiple, smaller than 1 cm and detected in the clinical setting of A-CAG. In the case of Type II carcinoids, symptoms of ZES prevail. Type III carcinoids present as a solid mass with symptoms resembling those of gastric adenocarcinoma, including hemorrhage, obstruction and metastases. Patients with malignant metastasizing tumors may present with clinical symptoms related to hormone hyper production such as flushing, diarrhea, wheezing and right heart disease, which is predominantly associated with the serotonin- and tachykinins-producing carcinoids. These tumors, however, occur mainly in the midgut rather than in the stomach.

Diagnosis of gastric neuroendocrine tumors depends on endoscopy and histopathological evaluation. EUS and radiologic evaluation are of help for staging of the disease.

Histological Classification and Molecular Genetics

Histologically, well-differentiated neuroendocrine (carcinoid) tumors appear at the bottom of the mucosa in small clusters or ribbons of regular cells with rounded nuclei with a diffuse chromatin pattern. The cells have moderately abundant cytoplasm which stains strongly with neuroendocrine markers like chromogranin a (Fig. 4).

Poorly differentiated tumors show a typical small cell phenotype with large atypical nuclei with homogenous chromatin, scant cytoplasm and frequent mitotic and apoptotic figures. Vascular and perineural invasion is virtually always present. Immunohistichemical neuroendocrine markers show a markedly decreased staining in poorly differentiated tumors as compared to the well differentiated neuroendocrine markers. Large cell neuroendocrine tumors in the stomach are very rare.

Treatment

In cases with fewer than five small lesions (most Type I lesions) endoscopic resection is the therapy of choice. In Type II lesions, the therapeutic approach depends on the presence of associated pancreatic and/or duodenal lesions. Most Type III lesions require surgery.

Prognosis and Follow-Up

Lymph node metastases are found in 5% of Type I lesions, 30% of type II lesions and 71% of type III lesions. Distant metastases are found in 2.5% of Type I lesions, 10% of type II lesions and 69% of type III lesions. Tumor related death is exceptional in Type I lesions while in case of Type II and Type III lesions about 10% and 27% of patients die of their disease, respectively. Higher histological grade, larger size (≥3 cm), and mitotic index ≥9/10HPF are indicators of poor prognosis. Patients with poorly differentiated neuroendocrine tumors (small cell cancers) often already have metastatatic disease at the time of diagnosis, a condition associated with a very poor short term prognosis.

Other Polyposis Syndromes

Rare colorectal tumor syndromes include Peutz Jeghers, juvenile polyposis, Cowden's syndrome, Croncite Canada, and New colorectal cancer syndromes.

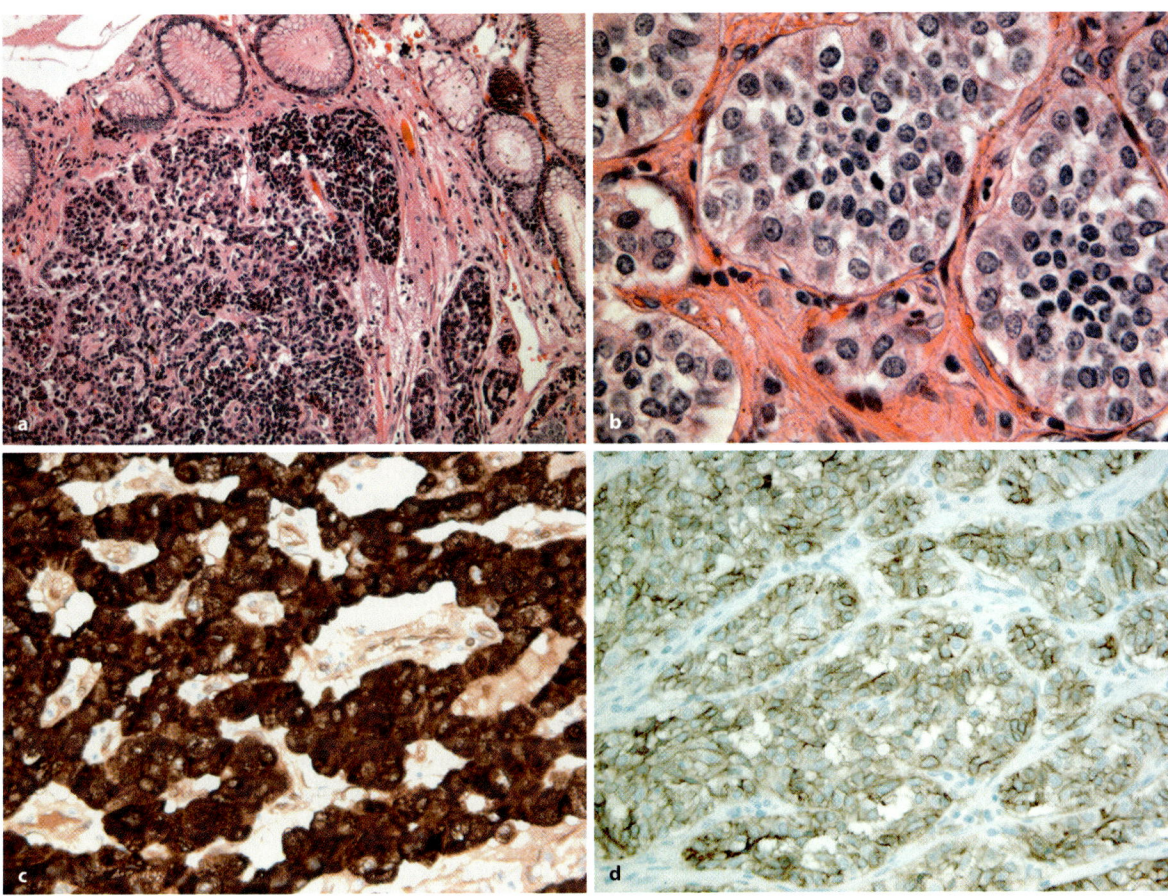

Figure 4a–d
Gastric carcinoid tumor appearing at the bottom of the mucosa (**a**) in small clusters or ribbons of regular cells with rounded nuclei with a diffuse chromatin pattern (**b**). The cells have moderately abundant cytoplasm, which stains strongly with neuroendocrine markers like chromogranin A (**c**) and CD56 (**d**).

Peutz Jeghers Syndrome

This is an autosomal, dominantly inherited condition characterized by hamartomatous gastrointestinal polyps and cutaneous pigmentation. It is about one tenth as common as FAP. STK11 on chromosome 19 has recently been identified as the Peutz Jeghers gene. The polyps in Peutz Jeghers syndrome show a characteristic arborizing framework of smooth muscle with an overlying normal mucosa. The risk of gastrointestinal cancer in this condition is 2–13%, but extra-intestinal malignancies (breast, cervix, pancreas and ovary) are also common, with a cancer risk of up to 48% [3].

Juvenile Polyps

Juvenile polyps are benign, non-neoplastic tumors, particularly with an overgrowth of the lamina propria in which cystically dilated glands are often found, hence the name retention polyp. The polyps occur most commonly in the colon and can give rise to rectal bleeding or anal prolapse of a polyp, but they may occur throughout the gastrointestinal tract. "Isolated juvenile polyposis" refers to the presence of a single or a few polyps. This occurs in 1–2% of all children. This condition is not hereditary. Juvenile polyposis refers to an entity with multiple polyps (more than 10, but usually 50–200). It may be familial with an autosomal dominant inheritance pattern. Germ line mutations of the SMAD4 gene on chromosome 18 are involved in some of the juvenile polyposis cases. Dysplastic change in juvenile polyps has been reported and the cancer risk in inherited juvenile polyposis, which has been estimated to be approximately 50%, includes gastric cancer.

Cowden's Syndrome

This rare syndrome is synonymous with multiple hamartoma syndrome characterized by mucocutanous abnormalities, breast cancer and gastrointestinal polyps that include hamartomatous polyps and hyperplastic polyps. The PTEN tumor suppressor gene on 10q23.3 is responsible for the Cowden and the related Bannayan-Zonana syndrome.

Cronkite-Canada Syndrome

Cronkite-Canada syndrome is a rare, nonhereditary syndrome with multiple hamartomatous polyps of both the large intestine and the upper digestive tract, hyperpigmentation of the skin, alopecia and atrophy of the nails, usually occurring in the middle-aged and elderly. Polyps show an overgrowth of lamina propria covered with essentially normal epithelium. The glands may be dilated. Some polyps are morphologically indistinguishable from juvenile polyps. Dysplastic changes in polyps have been described.

Mesenchymal Tumors of the Stomach

Like many other organs, the stomach may be not only the origin of epithelial tumors and lymphomas, but also of a wide range of mesenchymal tumors. About 1–3% of all gastric malignant tumors belong to this category. Many of these tumors are rare, and a detailed discussion of these entities would go beyond the scope of this chapter. For information on these lesions, the reader is referred to specialized literature [4]. This second part of the chapter will, in particular, focus on the most frequent, and clinically most relevant, mesenchymal tumor found in the stomach, i.e. the gastrointestinal stromal tumor (GIST), and on a partially overlapping entity, the gastrointestinal autonomic nerve tumor (GANT).

GIST (Gastrointestinal Stomach Tumor)

Introduction

A decade ago, classification of mesenchymal tumors almost completely depended on histological examination of standard hematoxylin eosin staining, to some extent supplemented with electron microscopy. Based on this, spindle cell tumors in the stomach were frequently classified as leiomyo-tumors, or to a lesser extent as schwannomas. Rapid development and application of broad panels of antibodies for immunohistochemistry have resulted in reappraisal of classification systems and designation of new entities in many areas of soft tissue pathology. Upon the finding that most of the so-called leiomyo-tumors of the gastrointestinal tract did not show any smooth muscle differentiation (i. e. absence of a clear expression of desmin and actin), or nervous differentiation (S100 or NSE expression), the neutral term GIST was proposed. Today, the nomination GIST is used for soft tissue tumors of the gastrointestinal tract that show cKIT (CD117) expression by immunohistochemistry. The vast majority of gastric soft tissue tumors fall in this category. As a consequence, older literature referring to gastric leiomyo-tumors mostly dealt with GISTs.

Epidemiology

The incidence of GISTs is estimated to be 10–20 per million inhabitants per annum, with a peak incidence between 55–65 years. In some series, a male predominance has been found. Gastrointestinal stromal tumors arise predominantly in the stomach (60–70%) and the small intestine (20–30%), while the esophagus, colon and rectum are less frequently affected. In the case of tumors with extensive intra-abdominal spread at the time of presentation, it may be impossible to determine the actual site of origin.

Etiology and Pathogenesis

The etiology of GIST is still unresolved. Activating mutations in the gene encoding KIT form the main pathogenetic mechanism, and familial occurrence due to a germline mutation in this gene has been described. The c-kit proto-oncogene has been mapped to 4q11–21 and encodes a type II tyrosine kinase growth factor receptor. In addition, loss of chromosomes 1p, 14q and 22q has

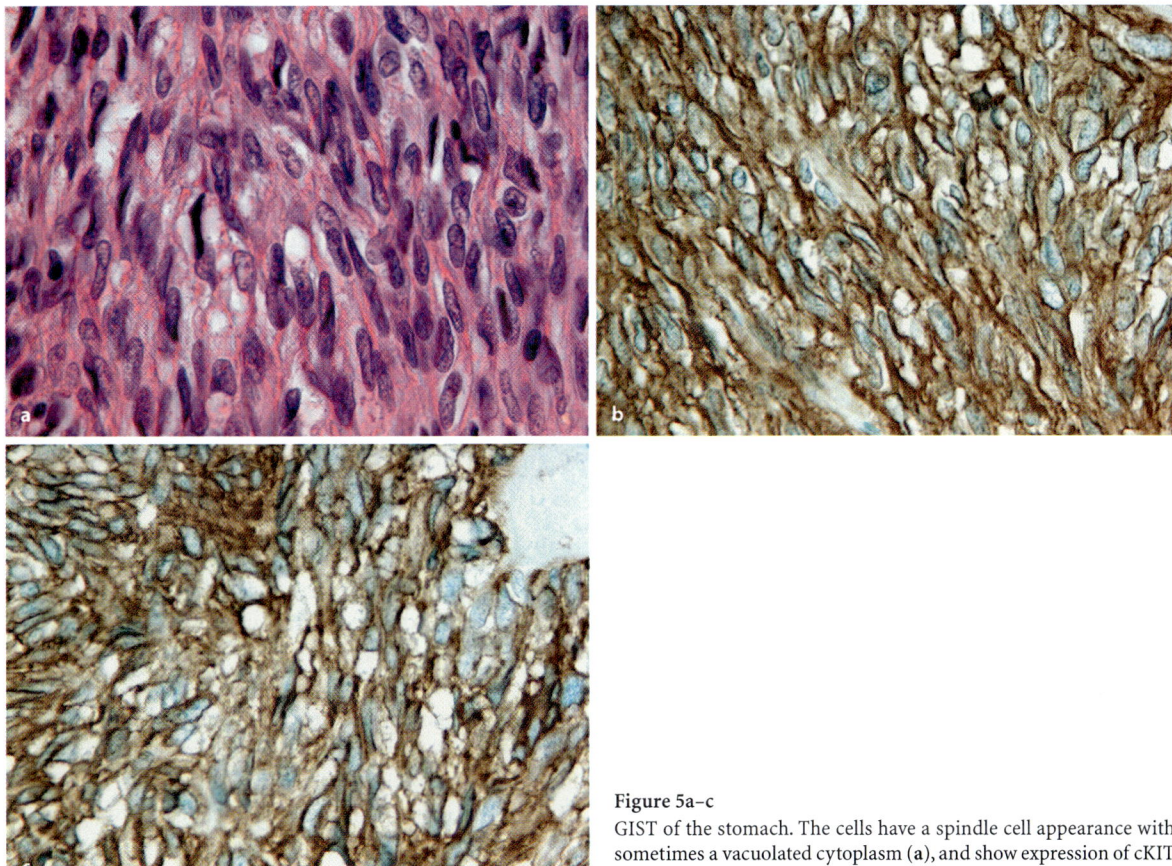

Figure 5a–c
GIST of the stomach. The cells have a spindle cell appearance with sometimes a vacuolated cytoplasm (**a**), and show expression of cKIT (**b**) and CD34 (**c**)

been reported, while additional chromosomal gains and high level amplifications of chromosomes 3q, 8q, 5p and Xp occur. GISTs share KIT expression with the interstitial cells of Cajal, which show autonomic nerve differentiation and serve as pacemaker cells of the gastro-intestinal tract. Whether Cajal cells are the cells of origin of GISTs, or whether both share a common ancestor, is yet unclear.

Symptoms, Clinical Signs, and Diagnosis

Symptoms of GIST are those of a gastric tumor, and thus usually rather unspecific, and include nausea, vomiting, abdominal pain, anemia and melena. Diagnosis of GIST depends on endoscopy and histopathological evaluation. EUS and radiologic evaluation are of help for staging of the disease.

Histological Classification and Molecular Genetics

Most GISTs show a cellular spindle cell appearance, while variations include less cellular, more collagen-rich variants, epitheloid variants and GISTs with prominent cytoplasmic vacuolisation (Fig. 5). In addition to KIT expression, a typical membrane staining for CD34 is seen in 60–70% of cases while, alternatively, 30–40% of cases may show some form of positivity for alpha-smooth muscle actin. Positivity for desmin and S100 is rare (about 5% of cases).

Tumor size and mitotic activity correlate with malignancy, which has been estimated to occur in 30% of cases. Small GISTs (i.e. <5 cm) usually behave benignly, as do tumors with a mitotic rate of <5 per 50 high power fields. These characteristics, however, do not exclude subsequent metastasis. Tumors with >5 mitoses per 50 high power fields are regarded as malignant, while tumors with >50 mitoses per 50 high power fields are called high-grade malignant.

Treatment

Surgery is the therapy of choice for GIST tumors. Metastatic and inoperable disease may respond to chemotherapy with Imatinib (Gleevec, Novaitis, Basel, Switzerland), a KIT tyrosine kinase activity inhibitor [5]. Imatinib induced a sustained objective response in more than half of patients with advanced tumors.

Prognosis and Follow-Up

As mentioned above, high mitotic activity and tumor size are predictors of poor prognosis, which presents as intra-abdominal tumor spread as multiple nodules and liver metastasis. Additional prognostic factors include DNA aneuploidy, presence of tumor necrosis and a high proportion of Ki67 (a proliferation marker) positive cells. In addition, site of origin plays a role. GISTs from the stomach of a given size and mitotic rate seem to behave less aggressively than their counterparts from the small intestine.

GANT (Gastrointestinal Autonomic Nerve Tumor)

A mesenchymal tumor exists with histological similarities to GIST, but with neurosecretory type granules. This lesion therefore is named GANT. A subset of these tumors, formerly called plexosarcomas, has been reported to be KIT positive, indicating that the entities GIST and GANT (at least partially) overlap. The fact that the diagnosis of GANT requires electron microscopy, which is not available everywhere, might cause these lesions to be classified as standard GISTs.

Leiomyoma/-sarcoma

According to recent classifications, leiomyomas and leiomyosarcomas are clearly positive for desmin and smooth muscle actin, whilst being negative for CD34 and CD117 (KIT). Tumors fulfilling these criteria are very rare in the stomach, although they do occur in the esophagus and large intestine. Most tumors formerly assigned to this category turned out to be gastrointestinal stromal tumors. As a consequence, data on true leiomyomas and

leiomyosarcomas of the stomach are rare, and the reader is referred to specialized literature on soft tissue tumors [4].

Schwannoma

Schwannomas are rare in the gastrointestinal tract, but when they occur it is most frequently in the stomach, with a peak incidence in the 6th decade. There is no relation with neurofibromatosis types I or II. Histologically schwannomas resemble GISTs, but they show a different immunohistochemical profile: KIT (–), actin (-), desmin (-), and S100 (+). There may also be admixed lymphocytes. Mitoses may be present, but this is an irrelevant finding since schwannomas are benign lesions.

Other Mesenchymal Tumors

Other mesenchymal tumors reported in the stomach at a very low incidence include glomus tumors, granular cell tumors, lipoma and Kaposi sarcoma. The reader is referred to specialized literature on soft tissue tumors [4].

In conclusion, the stomach may harbor a large variety of epithelial and mesenchymal tumors, ranging from benign lesions with very little potential for malignant degeneration, to aggressive malignancies giving rise to early metastases and poor prognosis. These lesions are usually diagnosed by endoscopy, either by chance as a coincidental finding, or because of symptoms such as pain, weight loss, or bleeding. For submucosal lesions, EUS may contribute to the diagnostic workup, but is needed in all cases for a definite diagnosis.

References

1. Vieth M, Stolte M. Fundic gland polyps are not induced by proton pump inhibitor therapy. Am J Clin Pathol 2001; 116: 716–20
2. Oberhuber G, Stolte M. Gastric polyps: an update of their pathology and biological significance. Virchows Arch 2000; 437: 581–90
3. Wirtzfeld DA, Petrelli NJ, Rodriguez-Bigas MA. Hamartomatous polyposis syndromes: molecular genetics, neoplastic risk, and surveillance recommendations. Ann Surg Oncol 2001; 8: 319–27
4. Weiss SW, Goldblum JR. Ensinger and Weiss's Soft tissue tumors 4th ed., Mosby Inc, St. Louis, 2001
5. Heinrich MC, Blanke CD, Druker BJ, Corless CL. Inhibition of KIT tyrosine kinase activity: a novel molecular approach to the treatment of KIT-positive malignancies. J Clin Oncol 2002; 20:1692–703
6. Hamilton SR, Aaltonen LA (Eds.): World Health Organization Classification of Tumors. Pathology and genetics of tumors of the digestive system. IARC Press: Lyon 2000
7. Miettinen M, Lasota J. Gastrointestinal stromal tumors – definition, clinical, histological, immunohistochemical, and molecular genetic features and differential diagnosis. Virchows Arch 2001, 438:1–12

Small Intestine

III

7 Neoplasms of the Small Intestine

K. GEBOES, C. DE WOLF-PEETERS

Summary

Despite its anatomical location between the stomach and the colon, two regions with high cancer risk, malignancies rarely occur in the small bowel. Careful follow-up is mainly indicated for patients with medical conditions carrying an increased risk for small bowel malignancy, in particular for patients with celiac disease, Crohn's disease, inherited disorders such as familial adenomatous polyposis (FAP) and immunodeficiency. Four main histological subtypes of small bowel cancer can be distinguished: adenocarcinoma, carcinoid, malignant lymphoma and malignant gastro-intestinal stromal tumors (GIST). The incidence of these tumors is increasing, especially for the first three types and various medical conditions are now recognized to be associated with an increased cancer risk. The clinical presentation and symptoms of small bowel tumors are non-specific and therefore the diagnosis is made late in the course of the disease. Small bowel tumors are often in an advanced stage at diagnosis and the overall 5-year survival rate is rather poor (approximately 50%). Except for lymphoma where the treatment of choice is chemotherapy, treatment is essentially surgical. The role of adjuvant or palliative chemotherapy for adenocarcinoma, carcinoid and malignant GIST is unclear. Recently good results have been obtained with the introduction of new therapeutic modalities.

Epidemiology

The small intestine constitutes 75% of the total length of the gastrointestinal (GI) tract and over 90% of its mucosal surface. Yet small bowel tumors are rare, although approximately two-thirds are malignant. Malignant small bowel tumors constitute less than 5% of GI malignancies. Four major different histological types of malignant small bowel tumors can be distinguished (Table 1).

Adenocarcinoma is the most common type. As in the large bowel, most adenocarcinomas arise from pre-existing adenomas that occur sporadically or in the context of familial adenomatous polyposis (FAP), hereditary non-polyposis colorectal cancer (HNPCC) or variant syndromes. Adenomas are found most commonly in the duodenum. In a prospective study of 100 patients with FAP (mean age 34 yrs; range 13–73 yrs; 48 male), upper gastrointestinal endoscopy revealed adenomatous polyps in the duodenum in 33. The incidence of adenomas is higher in older patients. Adenocarcinomas of the small intestine represent less than 2% of all malignant tumors of the GI tract (Table 2). The age-adjusted incidence in the USA (period 1988–1992) is 1.2 per 100,000 per year (esophagus 3.9; stomach 7.7; colon/rectum 47.7).

Table 1
Malignant tumors of the small intestine: relative frequency

	Overall	Duodenum	Jejunum	Ileum
Adenocarcinoma	32–47%	38.5%	41.8%	19.7%
Endocrine tumours	19–35%	9.3%	6.7%	83.8%
Lymphoma	17–20%	3.5%	39.5%	57.0%
Malignant GIST	11–14%	17.3%	40.0%	42.7%
Miscellaneous	0.5%			

Table 2
Estimated new cancer cases (USA 1997)

All sites	1,382,400
All digestive	225,900
Esophagus	12,500
Stomach	22,400
Small intestine	4,900
Colon	94,100
Rectum	37,100

A slight increase has been noted over the years. In general, the incidence is higher in developed Western countries. Within the USA the incidence is higher in blacks and males have higher incidence rates than females. The age of the patients ranges from 30 to 80 with a peak in the seventh decade.

Endocrine tumors of the small intestine include carcinoid tumors (well differentiated), small cell carcinomas (poorly differentiated) and malignant large cell neuro-endocrine carcinomas. Carcinoid tumors are derived from the diffuse endocrine system. They can therefore be ubiquitous, but most originate from the jejuno-ileum, appendix, rectum and bronchus. About 74% of all carcinoid tumors occur in the GI tract. In the GI tract, most carcinoid tumors occur in the small bowel (29% of total) with the highest frequency in the ileum. The age-adjusted incidence rate of malignant carcinoid tumors of the small intestine rose from 0.2 to 0.3 per 100,000 population per year from 1973 to 1982. A significant percentage of these tumors remain asymptomatic. In most series, the tumors are distributed about equally between males and females. Patients range in age from the third to the tenth decade with a peak in the sixth and seventh decades.

Table 3
Primary intestinal lymphomas

B celql	T cell
Low-grade MALToma	Enteropathy-associated lymphoma (EATL)
High-grade MALToma	Other
Immunoproliferative small intestinal disease (IPSID, α chain disease)	
Lymphomatous polyposis (Mantle cell zone lymphoma)	
Burkitt's-like	
Immunodeficiency-associated lympho-proliferative disease:	
– AIDS-associated	
– post-transplant lymphoproliferative disorder (PTLD)	
Other:	
– follicular lymphoma	
– lymphocytic lymphoma	

In general, lymphoma incidence rates rose especially in the 1980s, reflecting the spread of the acquired immunodeficiency syndrome (AIDS) and the introduction of immunosuppressive therapies. Lymphomatous infiltrates in the GI tract are frequently found as part of a disseminated disease. Primary gastrointestinal lymphoma defined as an extra-nodal lymphoma arising in the GI tract with bulk of the lesion in this site, is a rare disorder. These lymphomas represent 5 to 10% of all NH lymphomas. Despite the fact that the small intestine is the part of the gut where the mucosa associated lymphoid tissue (MALT) is preferentially localized as Peyer's patches, less than 25% of the GI lymphomas affect the small intestine. In comparison with gastric lymphomas, they affect a younger age group and may present as multifocal disease. Different types of lymphomas can be identified in the small intestine (Table 3). Almost 65% of these lymphomas correspond to diffuse large B cell lymphomas, with in addition 20% of Burkitt's lymphoma, which localizes in the ileocecal region. MALT type lymphomas as well as other small B cell lymphomas e.g. mantle cell lymphoma and follicular lymphoma are extremely rare. Nevertheless, within the group of multifocal intestinal lymphomas they represent almost half of the cases. A variant of MALT lymphoma known as immunoproliferative small intestinal disease (IPSID) is common in the Middle East and South Africa. This disease affects young patients, usually with severe malabsorption. All other primary intestinal lymphomas (almost 25%) are of T cell origin, mostly corresponding to Enteropathy-associated T-cell lymphoma (EATL). The increase in relative risk in celiac disease is approximately 40% although the exact prevalence is unknown.

The majority of the small intestinal mesenchymal tumors are gastrointestinal stromal tumors (GISTs). They are defined as KIT (CD117, stem cell factor receptor)-positive mesenchymal neoplasms. They are the most common mesenchymal tumors of the GI tract. The small intestine is the second most common location (20–25%) after the stomach (60–70%). The incidence rate is approximately 0.2 per 100,000 per year. Males are affected somewhat more than females. The peak incidence is in the sixth to eighth decades and somewhat lower than for carcinomas. Forty to fifty per cent of the small intestinal GISTs are malignant. Genuine leiomyosarcomas are less common [1, 2].

Primary small intestinal malignant tumors have to be differentiated from secondary tumors, originating from an extra-intestinal malignancy or discontinuous with a primary tumor elsewhere in the GI tract. Metastatic spread to the small intestine is more frequent than to any other site of the GI tract and secondary carcinomas of the small bowel are as common as primary carcinomas at this site. Melanoma, lung, breast, colon and kidney are the most frequent primary sites.

Etiology

Little is known regarding the etiology of small bowel neoplasms. The reasons for the relatively rare occurrence of malignancies are not known but it has been suggested that the small intestine may have protective mechanisms. These could include the rapid transit time limiting the exposure to carcinogens, alkalinity, the high level of benzopyrene hydroxylase, an enzyme that may detoxify potential carcinogens, the low bacterial population and greater concentrations of IgA.

Important risk factors for small bowel cancer include associated diseases such as Crohn's disease and inherited syndromes such as FAP. Patients with HNPCC, and the Peutz-Jeghers syndrome, celiac disease, cystic fibrosis and other types of cancer are at less risk. Other medical conditions carrying a risk are cholecystectomy, peptic ulcer disease and radiation. Behavioral risk factors include dietary fat and protein intake, cigarette smoking and alcohol consumption (Table 4).

Apart from the genetic susceptibility for endocrine tumors of the duodenum in Neurofibromatosis type I and MEN-1 (multiple endocrine neoplasia) syndrome, there is little knowledge about etiological factors involved in the pathogenesis of carcinoids or endocrine tumors.

Helicobacter pylori infection resulting in a T cell induced B cell proliferation against autoantigens, Epstein-Barr virus infection, immune deficiency resulting from HIV infection or immune suppressive therapy (in transplant recipients) and celiac disease are risk factors for GI lymphomas. Patient with chronic idiopathic inflammatory bowel disease probably do not have an increased

Table 4
Risk factors for small bowel cancer [1] and lymphoma

Lymphoma	Adenocarcinoma	
Risk factor	Risk factor	Strength of association for carcinoma only
Crohn's disease	Crohn's disease	++++*
Malabsorptive conditions	Adenomas & FAP	+++
Celiac disease	Celiac disease	+++
Autoimmune disorders	Cholecystectomy	+
Congenital immune disorders	Peptic ulcer disease	+
Previous organ transplant	Other intestinal cancers	+++
Chronic immunosuppressive therapy	Other cancers	?
AIDS	Alcohol use	?
Previously treated peripheral lymphoma	Dietary intake of animal fat	+
	Dietary intake of animal protein	+
	Dietary intake of sugar	+
	Tobacco use	+
	Radiation	+
	Socioeconomic status	?

*+ means positive association (numbers of signs refers to strength of association).

Table 5

Clinical symptoms in 66 patients with small bowel malignancies [3]

Symptoms	% of patients
Abdominal pain	43.8
Weight-loss more than 5 kg	25
Palpable tumour	21.9
Ileus, obstipation, acute abdomen	21.9
Colics	18.8
Nausea/vomiting	17.2
Iron deficiency anaemia	14.1
Melena	12.5
General weakness	12.5
Loss of appetite	10.9
Diarrhoea	6.25
Aszites	4.7
Jaundice	1.6
Hydronephrosis	1.6

risk of lymphoma as compared with the general population. A modest increased risk with immunosuppressive therapy cannot be completely ruled out, but has not yet been observed with, for instance, azathioprine or 6-mercaptopurine.

Malignant GISTs are associated with mutations in the KIT protein. This is a transmembrane growth factor receptor for stem cell factor (SCF). It belongs to the family of receptor tyrosine kinases and is involved in the signal transduction pathway that ultimately carries the proliferation signal to the nucleus [1, 3].

Symptoms and Clinical Signs

Many sporadic adenomas of the small bowel are asymptomatic and discovered incidentally. They may produce low-grade bleeding, vague abdominal pain or nausea. Approximately 75% of all malignant small intestinal tumors are symptomatic. The symptoms may be nonspecific and vague, especially early in the clinical presentation. The consequence of this is that small bowel malignancies are frequently diagnosed late in their course. The mean time to diagnosis in most series ranges from 6 to 26 months. The most common symptoms

are abdominal pain (30–85%) and weight loss (30–70%) (Table 5). Pain is variable in character, occurring as epigastric burning, cramps or dull aches. Nausea and vomiting is found in 17 to 54%. Obstruction develops in 15 to 35%. It may be intermittent and partial as for benign tumors. Intussusception is most frequently the result of a benign tumor.

Most small intestinal carcinoids do not cause specific symptoms. In the duodenum, the most frequently encountered carcinoid tumors are the small gastrinomas, which cause 13% of the cases of Zollinger-Ellison syndrome, and the larger, histologically unique, psammomatous somatostatinomas. The latter may cause no endocrine symptoms but they may be associated with MEN and von Recklinghausen's syndrome. Carcinoids in the ileum can cause fibrosis of the mesentery resulting in kinking of the small bowel, intestinal obstruction or intussusception and vascular involvement causing gut infarction. The most common clinical presentation for carcinoids is periodic abdominal pain and intermittent crises of obstruction. Ileal carcinoids must not be confused with Crohn's disease.

Intestinal lymphomas predominantly affect male patients. The reported median age varies from one study to the other but is considerably younger than for gastric lymphoma. Lymphomas do not usually present with specific symptoms. Pain is the main diagnostic symptom in most of the cases, followed by loss of appetite and weight loss. Constipation and ileus do occur as signs of intestinal occlusion. Bleeding may be found but is mainly present when the lymphoma affects the stomach or the ileocecal area. Perforation occurs infrequently. EATL is a well-known complication of celiac disease. Most patients (25–65%) will have a previous history of gluten enteropathy and the disease must be suspected in any of these patients, usually in their fifties, who deteriorates for no apparent reason. Development of fever and skin rash are not uncommon. However, in approximately 20% of the cases, the associated celiac disease is clinically occult.

Hemorrhage occurs to varying degrees, being more common with GISTs, less frequent with adenocarcinomas and distinctly rare with carcinoids. Perforation develops in about 10% of patients with small bowel malignancy, usually with lymphoma and sarcomas. Patients with GISTs may also present with a palpable abdominal mass at physical examination [4, 5].

Diagnostics

Synopsis

Standard imaging techniques

▸ Upper gastrointestinal barium study – enteroclysis
▸ Endoscopy including upper GI endoscopy, colonoscopy with ileoscopy and if possible total enteroscopy
▸ Transabdominal ultrasound
▸ Computed tomography

Most small intestinal neoplasms can be visualized by radiological techniques using contrast material (i.e., a barium swallow with small bowel follow-through or a small bowel "enema" (enteroclysis) or by endoscopic examination. The sensitivity of upper GI barium examination for small bowel malignancies varies between 53 and 83%. Radiology is especially useful for duodenal tumors. Double-contrast duodenography is superior to single-contrast barium study. Enteroclysis with radiological imaging and computed tomography scan (CT) currently represent the technique of choice for visualization of the small bowel tumors distal to the duodenum with a sensitivity of approximately 90%. The two methods can be complementary. With enteroclysis, adenocarcinoma appears as a filling defect, thickening of the folds with wall rigidity, slowed motility, eccentric passage of the contrast medium or a clear stenosis. On CT scan it may appear as an annular lesion, a discrete nodular mass or an ulcerative lesion. The diagnosis of a small intestinal carcinoid cannot usually be made with certainty on the basis of a barium examination because the condition can mimic lesions similar to those produced by other diseases. The results of CT are variable but in general 60–73% of symptomatic patients can be diagnosed accurately. Serological determination of chromogranin can be useful for the confirmation of the diagnosis. MRI scans can be useful for the detection of mesenteric involvement by carcinoids. CT is in general also useful in detecting extraluminal tumors and mesenteric metastases. It may be particularly helpful with carcinoid tumors, which often have small primaries and with GISTs. In the case of small intestinal lymphoma, it can provide supplemental information useful in the typing and staging. Malignant lymphomas have a variety of different macroscopic (radiographic and endoscopic) manifestations. MALT lymphomas can occur at any level of the intestine. They usually present as single ulcerating or polypoid lesions. In most cases of IPSID, a diffuse thickening of the jejunum with enlarged mesenteric lymph nodes is noted. Mantle cell zone lymphoma presents with numerous polyps. The larger polyps tend to concentrate in the terminal ileum. The lesions of enteropathy-associated lymphoma arise in the jejunum. The lymphoma is commonly multifocal and causes multiple ulcers, strictures or tumor nodules. Bone marrow aspiration and biopsy, as well as lumbar puncture should be performed for staging the lymphoma.

Abdominal ultrasonography and scintigraphy can be useful but the tumor detection rate of these techniques is limited in retrospective series, although ultrasonography can be especially useful for the detection of malignant GISTs. The tumors detected by endoscopy are usually located in the duodenum, upper jejunum and ileum. Endoscopy is particularly useful for the assessment of the severity of duodenal adenomas in FAP. Intraoperative endoscopy can be very useful. Total enteroscopy may in the future improve diagnostic accuracy. In a combined series of 413 patients examined for iron deficiency anemia of undetermined origin, 9 malignant tumors of the small intestine (5–10% of all lesions) were detected. Mucosal biopsies are useful for adenocarcinomas and lymphomas. However, in the case of EATL, the neoplastic population may be small and difficult to differentiate from the reactive intra epithelial T cells. In these cases, molecular analysis is mandatory. Endoscopic biopsies are usually inadequate for the identification of submucosal GISTs and carcinoids [6].

Histological Classification and Molecular Genetics

Synopsis

▸ Approximately two-thirds of small bowel tumors are malignant.
▸ More than 95% of these are adenocarcinomas, carcinoids, lymphomas or malignant GISTs.
▸ The histology of the tumors correlates with the anatomic subsite in which they arise.

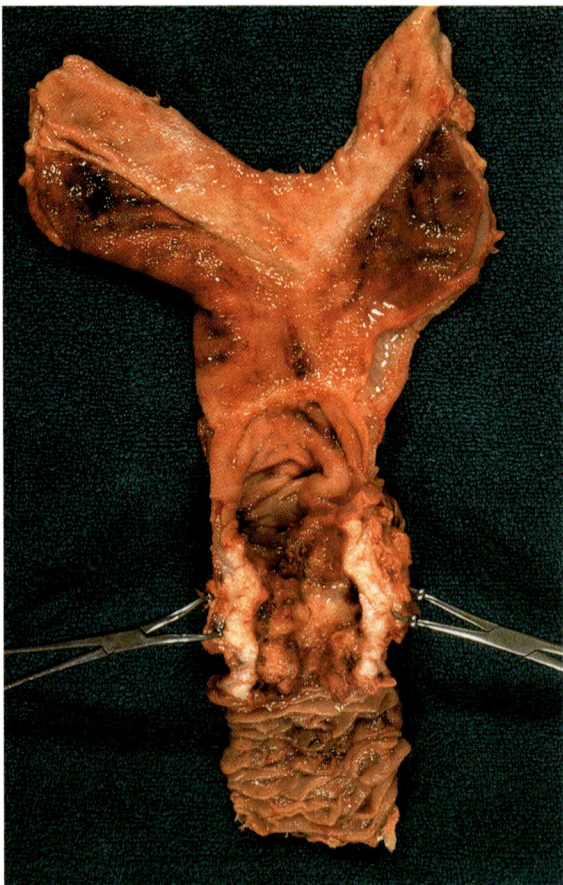

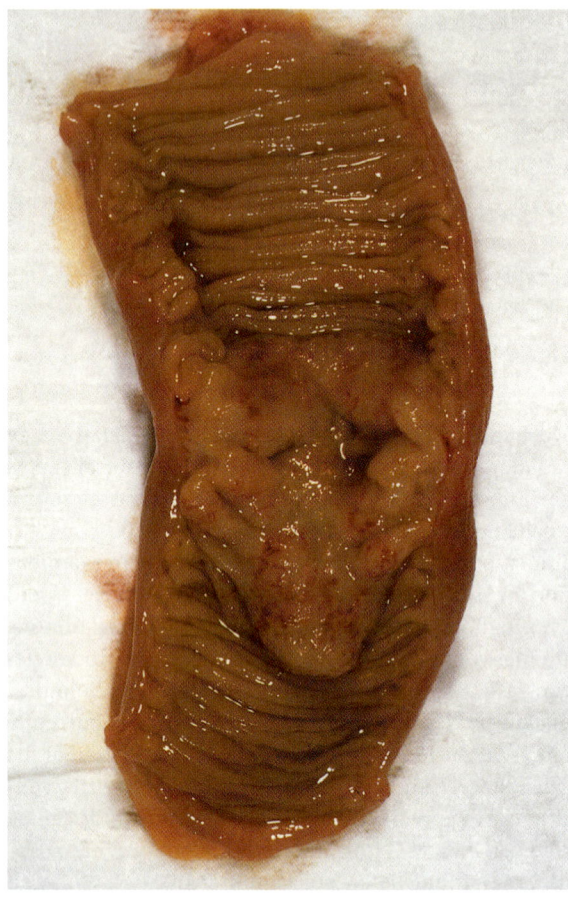

Figure 1
The site at the highest risk for adenocarcinoma of the small intestine is the duodenum. Duodenal carcinomas tend to be polypoid but can be annular and constrictive as in this case

Figure 2
Most small intestinal adenocarcinomas present as an annular lesions

Duodenal adenomas occur mainly in the second part of the duodenum but may involve also the first and third parts.

The site at the highest risk for adenocarcinoma of the small intestine is also the duodenum (Fig. 1). The location of the adenocarcinomas is however influenced by the precancerous conditions from which they arise. Seventy five per cent of the carcinomas associated with Crohn's disease, for instance, occur in the ileum. These carcinomas develop from dysplastic epithelium. Adenocarcinomas of the proximal small intestine tend to be polypoid or fungating, possibly related to their origin in adenoma, whereas those of the distal segments are often ulcerated and infiltrating. However, in about 80% of the cases the cancer is annular and constrictive (Fig. 2). The histology of the premalignant lesions (adenoma and dysplasia or intraepithelial neoplasia) and of the malignant lesions is essentially the same as that of similar lesions in the large bowel. Duodenal adenomas may be tubular or predominantly villous in character. Villous adenomas are composed of a thin fibrovascular core and crowded high columnar epithelium. Paneth cells can be present scattered all along the crypts, singly or in small clusters. Brunner's glands may be present in the endoscopic biopsies of these lesions and can appear prominent and associated with mild cystic dilatation. In

FAP patients, the grade of dysplasia of the duodenal adenomas tends to be worse in older patients. Adenocarcinomas are composed of tubular glandular and villous structures. Most neoplastic cells are columnar, with varying degrees of microvillar development. Mucous cells and argyrophilic cells are commonly present. Paneth cells may be present, occasionally in large numbers. Most adenocarcinomas are well to moderately differentiated and frequently mucin production can be demonstrated with appropriate staining methods. Mucinous adenocarcinomas (a tumor with a substantial amount of mucin – more than 50%) are seen, but signet-ring cell carcinoma is rare. A morphologic adenoma-carcinoma sequence has been described in the small intestine similar to the well-described sequence in the colon. At the molecular level, several abnormalities in the expression of cell-cycle related proteins have been detected in both small bowel adenomas and adenocarcinomas. These include a decrease in the expression of the p27 protein in 20% of the tumors and an increase in cyclin D, cyclin E, p21 and the p16 and p53 proteins. Increased expression of p53 is associated with tumor progression. It is over-expressed in 45% of the adenomas and 65% of the adenocarcinomas [7]. Like large bowel cancers, small bowel adenocarcinomas have been found to have K-ras mutations (14–54%). One report found no 5q loss, while another found the frequency to be 60%. Fifteen to forty-five per cent of small bowel cancers have high levels of microsatellite instability and mutations in the TGF beta-RII gene have been identified. Mutations in the mutation cluster region (MCR) of the APC gene are however unusual. This suggests that adenocarcinoma of the small intestine may follow a different genetic pathway to colorectal cancer.

The small intestine is rich in lymphatics. Lymphatic permeation is common in the primary lesion. The majority of small intestinal carcinomas are already deeply invasive at the time of diagnosis. Early carcinoma is rarely diagnosed except as a focal lesion in an adenoma. Many of the small intestinal adenocarcinomas have already also metastasized to regional lymph nodes, liver, or the peritoneal surface by the time of diagnosis. Carcinomas of the duodenum metastasize to the posterior pancreaticoduodenal lymph nodes, those of the jejunum and ileum to the mesenteric nodes, and those of the terminal ileum to the ileocolic and posterior cecal nodes.

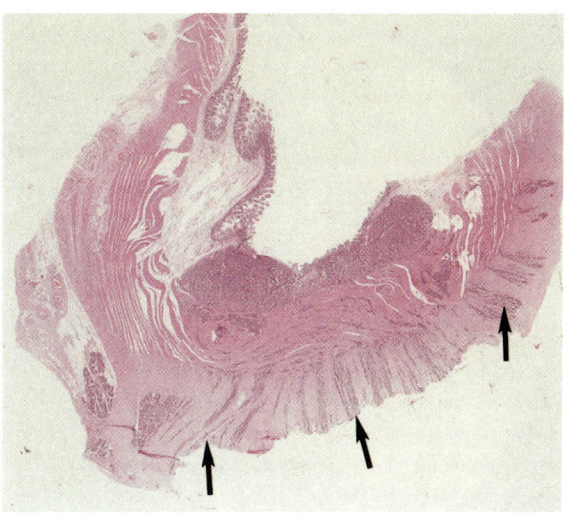

Figure 3
Extensive involvement of the mesentery is not uncommon with endocrine tumours of the distal small intestine (*arrows*)

Endocrine tumors exhibit site-related differences. In the duodenum and upper jejunum, they usually form small (<2 cm in diameter), gray, polypoid lesions within the submucosa with an intact overlying or focally ulcerated mucosa. Some tumors may appear as larger, infiltrative lesions. The tumors are multiple in about 13% of the cases. Jejuno-ileal endocrine tumors are multiple (2 to 100 lesions) in about 25–30% of cases. The size of the tumor is less than 1 cm in 13% and 2 cm or more in 47% of cases. They usually appear also as deep mucosal-submucosal nodules with apparently intact or slightly eroded surfaces, but deep infiltration of the muscular wall and peritoneum is frequent (Fig. 3). Extensive involvement of the mesentery produces angulation, kinking of the bowel, obstruction of the lumen or infarction of the involved loop. In the stomach, ECL-cell hyperplasia has been identified histologically as a precursor lesion, but for the small bowel, little is known about the incipient stages. Duodenal endocrine tumors include gastrin cell tumors, somatostatin cell tumors, EC-cell tumors (serotonin-producing carcinoid) and gangliocytic paraganglioma. Gastrin tumors are formed by uniform cells with scanty cytoplasm, arranged in broad trabeculae and show predominant immuno-reactivity for gastrin (other peptides include insulin, cholecystokinin and pancreatic polypeptide (PP). Somatostatin cell

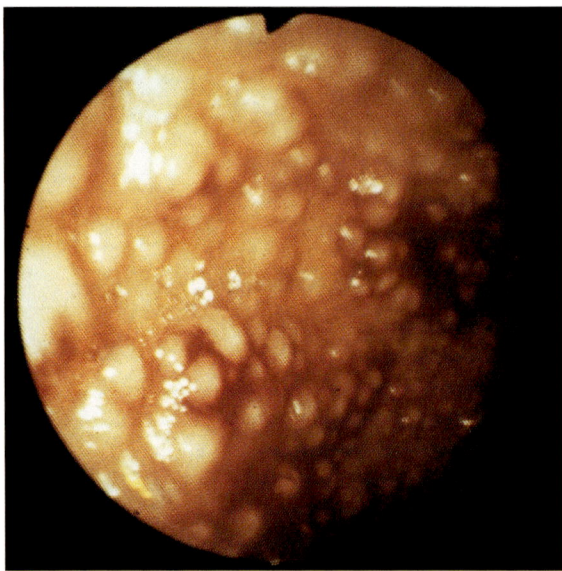

Figure 4
Mantle cell lymphoma of the small intestine usually presents as multiple lymphomatous polyposis. The polyps are of variable size and usually covered by a smooth surface

tumors exhibit a mixed pattern with a predominant tubulo-glandular component. Concentrically laminated psammoma bodies are detected mostly within glandular spaces. The tumor is characteristically composed of solid, somewhat rounded nests of closely packed cells, often with peripheral palisading. Rosette-type and gland-like structures can be present. Tumor cells are monomorphous round to polygonal cells. They show indistinct cell membranes, abundant granular cytoplasm enclosing centrally placed small round nuclei with stippled chromatin, inconspicuous nucleoli, and sharply defined nuclear membrane. Mitoses and cellular pleiomorphism are rare. There is often an intense desmoplastic stromal reaction. In such areas, tumor cells may be oriented into cords or files. The identification of the tumor can be accomplished using different histochemical methods. Most tumor cells are intensely argyrophilic and reactive with chromogranin antibodies. Several growth factors and related receptors such as insulin-like growth factor (IGF-1), platelet-derived growth factor (PDGF), transforming growth factor (TGF) β and α have been localized in tumor cells. PDGF and TGF β are involved in the stromal reaction. Other markers than

have been identified include substance P and neural cell adhesion molecule (NCAM). Deep infiltration of the muscular wall and peritoneum is a frequent finding. Metastases are usually confined to the regional lymph nodes and liver. They may be larger than the primary tumor. Few data are available on molecular studies. The p53 protein seems not involved in the pathogenesis of these tumors. Point mutations of K-ras at codon 12 are also absent. Clonality study of multifocal ileal carcinoids by X-chromosome inactivation analysis suggests that multiple carcinoids are generated by metastasis of a primary tumor.

Primary intestinal lymphomas can be subtyped into B cell and T cell malignancies, according to the recently published WHO classification which is based on the REAL classification.

Most B cell lymphomas correspond to "diffuse large B cell lymphoma", a heterogenous group of B cell lymphomas, not yet subdivided into well characterized clinico-pathological entities. These lymphomas are composed of centroblast-like large B cells, of immunoblast-like B cells or of a mixture of both. Evaluating the proliferation fraction of the tumor cells using a marker, e.g. Ki67 or MIB1, may provide some additional information on the biological behaviour of the neoplasm. Burkitt's lymphoma cannot always be differentiated from other large B cell lymphomas. This particular diagnosis should be considered in young patients with an ileocecal localization. The diagnosis can be confirmed by the identification of a cMYC rearrangement resulting from t(8;14) associated with this particular lymphoma.

More rarely the intestinal B cell lymphoma is composed of small B cells. In such a case differential diagnosis between MALT type lymphoma, mantle cell lymphoma and follicular lymphoma is mandatory. The latter is recognized by its nodular growth mimicking the B follicle, and its cellular composition comprising a mixture of centrocytes and centroblasts. Most follicular lymphomas are associated with t(14;18), resulting in BCL2 gene rearrangement. The resulting gene overexpression and aberrant bcl2 protein production can be identified by immune histochemistry or by molecular techniques. Mantle cell lymphoma as a primary GI lymphoma is the lymphoma *par excellence* to present as a lymphomatous polyposis (Fig. 4). The tumor is composed of a rather monotonous proliferation of small irregular lymphocytes (centrocyte-like) with or without a nodular growth pattern and with or without preservation of some residual reactive germinal centers. The neoplastic B cells of this lymphoma express in addition to several B cell markers, CD5 a pan T cell marker. Moreover and as a result of t(11;14) found in more than 60% of mantle cell lymphomas, a nuclear over-expression of cyclin D1 can be demonstrated by immunohistochemistry. Finally, MALT type lymphoma, mostly found in the stomach, may rarely affect the small intestine. This lymphoma is characterized by its growth pattern, surrounding residual B follicles with preserved reactive germinal center and lymphocytic corona, thereby mimicking the marginal zone of Peyer's patches. Most MALT-type lymphomas of the GI tract are associated with Helicobacter pylori infection and almost half of them are associated with t(11;18). At present, no antibodies are available to identify the presence of an aberrant protein expression resulting from this genetic abnormality but molecular techniques can be used to identify the fusion gene. However an aberrant nuclear expression of bcl10 protein is found in all cases documented by t(11;18). Occasionally MALT-type lymphoma cells demonstrate a prominent plasma cell differentiation resulting in a very high immunoglobulin production recognized previously as Mediterranean alpha heavy chain disease or indicated as immuno-proliferative intestinal disease.

Peripheral T cell lymphomas not infrequently affect the intestine. Most of the cases are found in patients with celiac disease and correspond to the clinico-pathological entity indicated as EATL. These lymphomas are considered to be related to the intra-epithelial cytotoxic T cells. The cytotoxic character of the neoplastic cells is easily demonstrated by immunohistochemistry. The lymphoma is composed of small, medium sized or large cells. Angiotropism of the neoplastic cells may be a prominent feature resulting in ischemic necrotic lesions. Only rarely the T cell lymphoma can be recognized as an anaplastic CD30-positive large cell lymphoma.

Stromal tumors occur throughout the small bowel. They are situated within the submucosa, the muscularis propria or both layers (Fig. 5). GISTs of the small bowel are different from those that occur in the stomach. They tend to be more aggressive, although they may be smaller. They are usually highly cellular and composed of uniform small spindle cells. They may show an organoid vascular pattern and often contain extracellular collagen globules (skeinoid fibers). They show a positive staining with antibodies directed against CD117 while the expression of CD34 is less common than for similar tumors in the stomach (33% positive cases in the jejunum and 87% in the stomach). GISTs show c-kit mutations in exon 11. Alterations have also been described in exons 9 and 13 which encode portions of the extracellular and kinase domains respectively. Comparative genomic hybridization shows common losses in chromosome 14 and 22. Various chromosomal deletions, including deletions of 1p and 9p, coincide with malignant progression. Gains and high-level amplifications at 5p, 8q, 17q and 20q are also significantly more frequent in malignant and metastatic GISTs. Gut autonomic nerve tumors (GANT) are essentially a subtype of GIST. Genuine leiomyosarcomas are composed of well-differentiated smooth muscle cells with cigar-shaped nuclei and well-differentiated cytoplasm. They are negative for KIT and CD34 (the hematopoietic progenitor cell antigen) and positive for smooth muscle actin (SMA) and usually for desmin. Angiosarcomas are recognized by an anastomosing proliferation of atypical endothelial cells, usually reacting positively with antibodies against CD31.

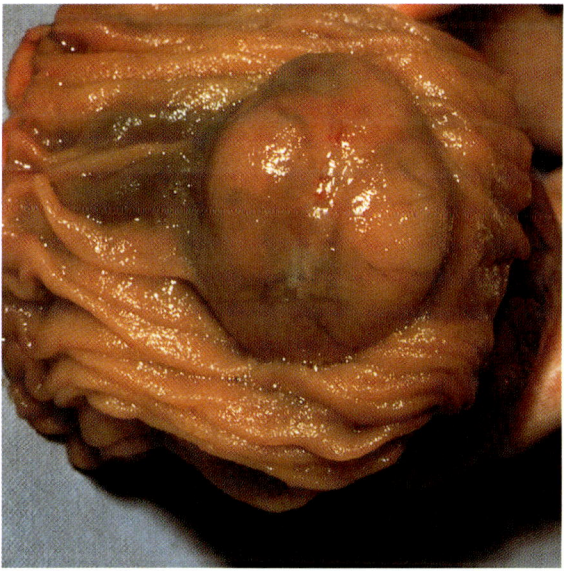

Figure 5
Stromal tumours are localized in the submucosa, the muscularis mucosae or both layers. Therefore they often present as submucosal tumours, with or without ulceration at the top. Endoscopic biopsies are usually inadequate for precise histologic diagnosis

Staging

TNM classification of small intestinal cancers

T	Primary tumor
TX	primary tumor cannot be assessed
T0	no evidence of primary tumor
Tis	Carcinoma in situ (intraepithelial neoplasia)
T1	lamina propria, submucosa
T2	Muscularis propria
T3	Subserosa, non-peritonealized perimuscular tissues (mesentery, retroperitoneum) with extension 2 cm or less
T4	visceral peritoneum, other organs/structures (including mesentery, retroperitoneum) >2 cm, and the abdominal wall by way of the serosa; for the duodenum only, includes invasion of the pancreas
N	Regional lymph nodes
N1	regional

Stage groupings	T	N	M
Stage 0	Tis	N0	M0
Stage I	T1	N0	M0
	T2	N0	M0
Stage II	T3	N0	M0
	T4	N0	M0
Stage III	any T	N1	M0
Stage IV	any T	any N	M1

Histologic grade

Grade X	cannot be assessed
Grade 1	well differentiated (>95% of tumor forms glands)
Grade 2	moderately differentiated (50 to 95% of tumor forms glands)
Grade 3	poorly differentiated (5 to 49% of tumor forms glands)
Grade 4	undifferentiated (<5% of tumor forms glands)

Absence of presence of esidual tumor following non-surgical therapy

RX	cannot be assessed
R0	no residual tumor
R1	microscopic residual tumor
R2	macroscopic residual tumor

Preoperative staging techniques include primarily transabdominal ultrasound, endoscopic ultrasound and spiral computerized tomography.

A special endoscopic staging system has been designed for duodenal polyps in patients with FAP. The lesions are subdivided according to the polyp number, size and histological type. Polyp number: 1–4 polyps = 1 point; 5–20 polyps = 2 points, >20 polyps = 3 points; Polyp size: 1–4 mm = 1 point; 5–10 mm = 2 points; >10 mm = 3 points; histological type: tubular/hyperplastic/inflammation = 1 point; tubulovillous = 2; villous = 3; dysplasia (mild = 1, moderate = 2, severe = 3). An overall score of 0 points is stage 0. Stage I corresponds to a score of 1–4. Stage II means a score of 5–6. Stage III corresponds to a score of 7–8 and stage IV is a score of 9–12.

The TNM classification essentially applies to the carcinomas [8]. For carcinoids, a close relationship was found between the size of the primary tumor and the incidence of metastases: when lesions measured less than 1 cm in diameter, 1 to 2 cm, and 2 cm or more, metastases were found in 2%, 50%, and 80% respectively. The depth of invasion into the intestinal wall is also significant in this respect.

The Musshoff modification of the Ann Arbor system is generally used for the staging of primary gastrointestinal lymphomas. In this system, stage I indicates that the lesion is confined to the wall of the intestine. Stage II(1 E) indicates involvement of contiguous lymph nodes and stages II(2 E) and III refer to involvement of lymph nodes at a distance.

Once a diagnosis of GIST is made in a tumor with no known metastases, two prognostic factors, tumor size and mitotic index, provide the most useful histologic indication of the future biologic behavior. Mitotic index is measured by counting the number of mitotic figures in 50 high-powered fields. Features of malignancy are a tumor larger than 5 cm and mitotic counts of more than 2/10 or 5/50, evidence of gross invasion, necrosis, increased proliferation as assessed with antibodies directed against the proliferation marker Ki67 (more than 7 to 20% positive cells), DNA aneuploidy and the presence of a c-kit mutation (exon 11). A positive immunohistochemical staining with antibodies directed against c-kit might indicate that the tumor will react with adjuvant chemotherapy.

Treatment

Synopsis

▸ Surgery is the treatment of choice for adenocarcinoma, carcinoid and malignant GIST.
▸ Adjuvant chemotherapy can be effective for metastasized carcinoid and GIST.
▸ Chemotherapy (with radiotherapy and surgery) is the treatment of choice for lymphoma.

Surgery

Surgical resection is the treatment of choice for adenocarcinomas, carcinoids and GISTS. For adenocarcinomas, the reported resectability rate is, on average, 72% for carcinomas of the duodenum, 76% for those of the jejunum, and 82% for those of the ileum. The decision for surgery depends on the results of preoperative staging and the existence of concomitant diseases. Sometimes, if the tumor was not directly detected preoperatively, exploratory laparotomy may be indicated. The infrequency of the lesion has precluded much comparative surgical analysis but total removal of the malignancy with contiguous excision of surrounding zones of anticipated spread is accepted as being the most rational approach. Depending on the location of the tumor, this can be achieved by resection of a jejunal or ileal segment with a wedge of the mesentery to include regional lymph nodes, a small bowel resection extended by transversum resection or appendectomy, right hemicolectomy, ileocecal resection, pancreaticoduodenectomy or a Whipple procedure. Bypass surgery can be considered as palliative treatment [8].

Aggressive and radical surgery is also the treatment of choice for carcinoids although a less aggressive approach may be employed for small tumors (<1 cm). The abdomen should be thoroughly explored for multicentric lesions. Lesions of the terminal ileum may best be treated by right hemicolectomy. Small duodenal tumors can be excised locally.

For primary lymphoma of the small intestine, surgery can be considered for diagnostic purpose, and for complications such as a perforation. There is no general agreement for surgery as primary treatment except in rare cases when the disease is limited as may be the case in low-grade MALT lymphoma. If the mass is resectable, *en bloc* removal of the involved bowel and the attached mesentery, with clear margins, can be potentially curative. Metallic clips should be placed at the margins to guide radiotherapy simulation if needed. The operative mortality is between 5 and 8%. The presence of multifocal disease can reduce the chance for a curative resection. Some authors propose surgery for tumor reduction. Usually however a combination of chemotherapy, radiation and surgery has to be considered, depending upon the type and the grade of the lymphoma and the staging. In advanced cases, surgery should not be considered. Surgery has also probably no role in the treatment of Burkitt lymphoma.

For malignant GISTs complete resection is feasible in approximately 70% of the cases.

Chemotherapy

The role of adjuvant or palliative chemotherapy for adenocarcinomas of the small intestine remains unclear. In older series, chemotherapy with 5-fluorouracil (5FU) appears to be of little benefit. The new drugs such as camptothecins, which can extend life expectancy and may achieve a significant benefit in metastatic disease patients with colorectal cancer, may be useful for small intestinal cancer, because of the epidemiologic and other similarities between small and large intestinal cancers.

For carcinoids, chemotherapy should be considered only if metastases are present. Monotherapy with Streptozotocine, 5FU, adriamycin and DTIC is of some benefit but the duration of the response is limited (3 to 10 months). Combination therapy shows better results. The introduction of somatostatin analogues in the treatment of patients with carcinoids has modified positively the natural history of many patients with metastatic disease. The drugs are effective in controlling symptoms and in stabilizing tumor progression and survival seems substantially prolonged. The role of interferon alpha is not yet clear. Intra-arterial chemotherapy through the hepatic artery using adriamycin and lipiodol (chemo-embolization) has been used successfully for the treatment of liver metastases.

Chemotherapy (with or without radiotherapy) is the treatment of choice for lymphoma. For low-grade lymphoma, extended-field radiotherapy with total abdominal irradiation can be considered for patients in stage IE and IIE. An additional boost can be given in case of residual tumor after resection. In addition, for patients with stage IIE disease chemotherapy (for instance COP which is a combination cyclophosphamide, vincristine and prednisone) can be given in cycles before radiotherapy. For patients in stages IIIE and IVE remission induction is strived for by chemotherapy alone. For high-grade B-cell lymphoma or T-cell lymphoma, protocols identical as those proposed for similar lymphomas elsewhere should be considered. These include cycles of CHOP (cyclophosphamide, doxorubicin, vincristine and prednisone) followed by radiotherapy [9]. Complications of chemotherapy include bleeding and perforation. For mantle cell zone lymphoma, chemotherapy associated with total body radiation and bone marrow transplantation should be considered, especially when the disease is disseminated or in cases where clinical response is incomplete. Remission has been achieved in the early stages of IPSID with broad-spectrum antibiotics. The lesions of post-transplantation lymphoproliferative disorders may regress following reduction or discontinuation of immunosuppressive therapy. However, in some cases the lesions progress despite aggressive chemotherapy.

Classic chemotherapy and radiotherapy are ineffective for malignant GISTs. However, recently drugs targeting the tyrosine kinase activity of c-kit have been introduced with promising results. *In vitro* studies have shown inhibition of kit activity. Early clinical trial data with Imatinib (Gleevec) are very encouraging, even for patients with metastatic disease. Side effects of Imatinib treatment have been mostly mild dyspepsia and diarrhea. Long-term follow up does not exist however. The appropriate treatment for patients with the diagnosis of high-risk (i.e. malignant) GIST, but without metastases is not yet clear.

Radiotherapy

Radiotherapy has no particular role in the treatment of adenocarcinoma, carcinoid or malignant GISTs. Radiation therapy alone has been used for small intestinal lymphoma, especially stages IE and IIE. It can be associated with a high incidence of tumor necrosis and bleeding. Radiotherapy (with or without surgery) can be considered in cases of low-grade MALT lymphoma and, in association with chemotherapy, in high-grade MALT lymphoma and mantle cell zone lymphoma.

Prognosis and Follow-Up

The overall 5-year disease-specific survival for adenocarcinomas is low, with an average of 24% (15 to 51%) and the mortality rate is 0.3 per 100,000 population. For patients undergoing "curative" resection, 5-year survival varies between 32 and 54%. Survival may be lower for cancer of the ileum because of late detection. Survival rates appear to decrease with advancing stage and lymph node involvement.

Reported 5-year survival rates for carcinoids range from 60 to 100% and the 10-year survival rate is approximately 43%. When only invasive tumors are considered, the 5-year survival is low (40%) and decreases with increasing incidence of distant metastases and lymph node involvement. In patients with no liver metastases, the 5- and 10-year survival rates were 72% and 60% respectively as opposed to 35% and 15% for patients with liver metastases.

For lymphomas, the prognosis is highly variable, depending on the type and grade of the lesion. The clinical behavior of intestinal MALT lymphoma is not as favorable as that of gastric lymphoma. Five-year survival rates of 44%–75% and 25%–37% are reported for low- and high-grade lymphoma respectively. Histological grade, stage and resectability are all significant factors. IPSID runs a prolonged course, often over many years and rarely spreads out of the abdomen, until the terminal stage following transformation into high-grade. Restaging after completion of treatment includes diagnostic endoscopy with biopsies of the primarily involved site, if possible, endoscopic ultrasound, abdominal and pelvic CT, chest X-ray and blood analysis. Lymphomatous polyposis disseminates widely early in its course and involvement of liver, spleen, bone marrow and lymph nodes soon follows identification of the polyps or may be present at the time of diagnosis. The prognosis of post-transplantation lymphoproliferative disorders is generally good. The prognosis of T-cell lymphoma is worse than for B-cell lymphoma. Current therapy for EATL is unsatisfactory and survival rates are very low: 1-year survival is 31% and 5-year survival is 11%.

The 5-year survival for patients with malignant GISTs averages 50% [9]. GISTs arising in the small intestine show malignant behavior at lower levels of mitotic counts than do GISTs in the stomach. For adenocarcinoma there is no well-established post-operative follow-up scheme. For lymphoma, regular (every 6–12 months) follow-up based on clinical examination, hematological screening and radiology is indicated.

Screening, Surveillance, Prevention

There are only very few data available except for patients with FAP and related syndromes. There is good evidence for the existence of the adenoma – carcinoma sequence in the duodenum of patients with FAP. An estimated incidence of 2–4% for developing periampullary carcinoma has been reported. Endoscopic surveillance using the above mentioned staging system or gross appearance and histological assessment suggests that most patients undergo little change over a period of 40 months to 7 years. Based on these data it has been suggested that upper gastrointestinal endoscopy every 3 years is safe. Surveillance (from the age of 30 yrs on) may lead to a moderate increase in life expectancy by seven months. Treatment with Sulindac, a non-steroidal anti-inflammatory drug seems to have little or no benefit for the control of periampullary adenomas in FAP.

Adequate treatment of celiac disease and strict follow-up of the patients is indicated in order to prevent malignant complications. The overall risk for lymphoma is clearly reduced in patients following a correct diet [10].

Future Perspectives

Early diagnosis and better treatment are two major challenges for those dealing with small bowel malignancy. Virtual endoscopy or better techniques for total enteroscopy are therefore needed. The role of capsule endoscopy in diagnosing small bowel neoplasms awaits further evaluation. In addition, a better understanding of the molecular mechanisms involved in the development of the tumor might lead to better therapy.

References

1. Neugut AI, Jacobson JS, Suh S, Mukherjee R, Arber N. (1998) The epidemiology of cancer of the small bowel. Cancer Epidemiol, Biomarkers Prev 7: 243–251
2. Spigelman AD, Williams CB, Talbot IC, Domizio P, Phillips RKS. (1989) Upper gastrointestinal cancer in patients with familial adenomatous polyposis. Lancet II: 783–785
3. Ojha A, Zacherl J, Scheuba C, Jakesz R, Wenzl E. (2000) Primary small bowel malignancies. Single-center results of three decades. J Clin Gastroenterol 30: 289–293
4. North JH, Pack MS. (2000) Malignant tumors of the small intestine: a review of 144 cases. Am Surg 66: 46–51
5. Angeletti S, Annibale B, Marignani M, Corleto VD, Fave GD. (1999) Natural history of intestinal carcinoids. Ital J Gastroenterol Hepatol 31: S108–110
6. Bouhnik Y, Bitoun A (1997) L'entéroscopie: technique, indications, résultats. In: Colombel JF, Dupas JL (eds) Pathologie du Grêle – Progrès en hépato-gastroentérologie, Nouvelle série 2, Doin, Paris, p 107–118
7. Arber N, Hibshoosh H, Yasui W, Neugut AI, Hibshoosh A, Yao Y, Sgambato A, Yamamoto H, Shapira I, Rosenman D, Fabian I, Weinstein IB, Tahara E, Holt P (1999) Abnormalities in the expression of cell cycle-related proteins in tumors of the small bowel. Cancer Epidemiol, Biomarkers Prev 8: 1101–1105
8. Contant CME, Damhuis RAM, Van Geel AN, Van Eijck CHJ, Wiggers T (1997) Prognostic value of the TNM classification for small bowel cancer. Hepato-gastroenterology 44: 430–434
9. Koch P, del Valle F, Berdel WE et al. (2001) Primary Gastrointestinal non-Hodgkin's lymphoma: I. Anatomic and histologic distribution, clinical features, and survival data of 371 patients registered in the German multicenter study GIT NHL 01/92 J Clin Oncol 19: 3861–3873
10. Holmes GKT, Prior P, Lane MR et al (1989) Malignancy in celiac disease – effect of a gluten-free diet. Gut 30: 333–338

Colon and Rectum

IV

8 Colorectal Cancer

R.S. BRESALIER, S.B. HO

Summary

Cancer of the colon and rectum (colorectal cancer) is a major cause of cancer-associated morbidity and mortality world-wide. It has been suggested that carcinogens introduced into the bowel act in concert with other luminal factors (e.g., bile acid and other tumor promoters) to affect epithelial cells in the colonic mucosa. Carcinogenesis is, however, a multistage process. Cells must be genetically primed (through either hereditary disposition or genotoxic events), must be induced to proliferate and must pass through a series of stages *en route* to immortalization and uncontrolled growth. Specific molecular changes related to enhanced cancer stage and metastatic potential have been identified. The diagnosis of colorectal neoplasms relies on screening strategies in patients without symptoms. These include the use of fecal occult blood testing with or without screening flexible sigmoidoscopy, radiological procedures or screening colonoscopy. Patients with symptoms of iron deficiency anemia, rectal bleeding or changes in bowel habits should be evaluated by colonoscopic examination. Treatment of colorectal cancer is by excision, either by colonoscopy for early lesions or by surgical means. Patients with evidence of extension of rectal cancer into the bowel wall or lymph nodes are treated with adjuvant chemo- and radiation therapies. Patients with colon cancer and regional lymph node metastases are treated with adjuvant chemotherapy. Chemotherapy of advanced disease has evolved, but is still often palliative. Rapidly evolving knowledge of the pathogenesis of colorectal cancer, especially in high-risk groups, is leading to the development of new tools for identifying which persons will benefit most from cancer surveillance and from adjuvant therapy following potentially curative surgery.

Epidemiology

Cancer of the colon and rectum represents a major cause of cancer-associated morbidity and mortality in North America, Europe, and regions with similar lifestyles. The fourth most common newly diagnosed cancer overall in the United States (behind breast, prostate, and lung cancer), colorectal cancer represents 11% of new cancer cases in men and 12% in women. In 2002, there were an estimated 148,000 new cases in the United States and 57,000 related deaths (a rate second only to that of lung cancer). The incidence rates for colorectal cancer in men and women are similar in the United States, but there appears to be a slight male predominance world-wide. Approximately 6% of the American population will eventually develop invasive colon or rectal cancer, and an individual's lifetime risk of dying from colorectal cancer has been estimated to be 2.5%. Globally, it is the fourth most common cancer in males and third most common in females, with mortality paralleling incidence. Countries where colorectal cancer mortality was low before 1950 (e.g. Japan) have reported substantial increases.

Etiology and Pathogenesis

Interregional differences in the incidence of colorectal cancer, including differences among populations who live in geographic proximity but with different life-styles, strongly suggest that environment plays a role in the development of this disease. Migrant studies and rapid changes in incidence in countries assimilating Western practices support this concept. Population studies and preclinical animal studies have attempted to delineate the effects of various fats and proteins, carbohydrates, vegetable and fiber components, and micronutrients on the genesis of cancer of the large bowel. Colon cancer rates are high in populations whose total fat intake is high and are lower in those who consume less fat. Case-control and cohort studies have also suggested that the incidence and mortality rates from colon cancer, and in some cases rectal cancer, are positively correlated with dietary fat, but these findings are less convincing than data based on descriptive epidemiology studies. A prospective study, which assessed the relationship between meat, fat, and fiber intake among 88,751 women aged 34 to 59 years, demonstrated that the intake of animal fat was significantly correlated with the risk of colon cancer after adjustment for energy intake. Other recent cohort and case-control studies, however, failed to provide clear-cut evidence for the association between dietary fat and colorectal cancer observed in earlier studies. The intakes of red meat and saturated fat appear to correlate more strongly with the incidence and recurrence of colorectal cancers and adenomas than total fat intake. An inverse relationship has been reported between physical activity and risk for colorectal cancer in men. Obesity is associated with elevated risk of colorectal cancer.

Animal studies lend additional support for the role of dietary fat in the development of colon cancer. These studies involve the injection of carcinogens such as 1,2-dimethylhydrazine or azoxymethane into rodents fed various diets. Animals fed a variety of polyunsaturated and saturated fats develop greater numbers of carcinogen-induced colonic adenocarcinomas than those on low-fat diets. It has been proposed that dietary fat enhances cholesterol and bile acid synthesis by the liver, increasing amounts of these sterols in the colon. Colon bacteria convert these compounds to secondary bile acids, cholesterol metabolites, and other potentially toxic metabolic compounds. Little is known about how lipid and sterol metabolites promote tumors, but both bile acids and free fatty acids have been shown to damage the colonic mucosa and increase the proliferative activity of the epithelium. Bacterial enzymes such as 7-alpha-dehydroxylase (which converts cholic to deoxycholic acid), beta-glucuronidase, nitroreductase, and azoreductase may be induced by a high-fat diet and could also convert compounds ingested in the diet to active carcinogens. Bile acids may also induce the release of arachidonic acid and its conversion to prostaglandins, which can increase the proliferation of colonic epithelial cells.

Dietary fiber is plant material that resists digestion by the upper gastrointestinal tract and is composed of a heterogeneous mix of carbohydrates (cellulose, hemicellulose, pectin) and noncarbohydrates (e.g., lignin). Although the protective role of fiber is not completely clear (owing to the lack of definition of fiber components in many studies) the majority of both observational epidemiological and case-control studies support the protective effect of fiber-rich diets with regard to colonic neoplasia. These studies however, do not define the relationship between fiber-rich food and the importance of nonfiber vegetable components, nutrients and micronutrients in fruits and vegetables. This may explain the inability of recent randomized controlled trials to demonstrate an effect of dietary fiber intake on adenoma recurrence in the colon.

The possibility that specific genotoxic carcinogens may play a role in the genesis of colorectal cancer was raised when it was noted that the stools of certain persons exhibited mutagenic activity for bacteria *in vitro*. Mutagenic activity is frequently present in the feces of populations at high risk for large bowel cancer and is low or absent in low-risk populations.

Epidemiological, clinical and laboratory evidence suggest that calcium and vitamin D intake may protect against carcinogenesis in the colon. The potential chemopreventive activity of these compounds was originally suggested by epidemiological studies reporting an inverse relationship between intakes of vitamin D and calcium and colorectal cancer. A recent study demonstrated that dietary calcium supplementation in the form of low-fat dietary foods may affect a variety of "intermediate biomarkers" thought to be associated with tumor progression in the colon. A recent prospective double-blind placebo controlled trial demonstrated that supplemental calcium (3000 mg of calcium carbonate per day, equivalent to 1200 mg elemental calcium) reduced the number of recurrent adenomas after index polypectomy to a modest degree (19% reduction in adenoma recurrence and 24% reduction in the number of adenomas over 3 years). Calcium increases fecal excretion of phosphate and bile acids, and modifies the composition of bile. Some, but not all, studies have demonstrated that calcium supplementation reduces the rate and pattern of proliferation in the colorectal mucosa. Calcium may also affect a variety of cellular processes after activation of calcium-sensing receptors in intestinal epithelial cells and downstream effects mediated in part by protein kinase C. The effects of calcium may be most pronounced in tumors demonstrating K-ras mutations (see below). Vitamin D_3 metabolites and analogs play a role in the regulation of proliferation differentiation and apoptosis (programmed cell death) in addition to their role in mineral homeostasis. The vitamin D receptor, a member of the steroid hormone nuclear receptors, is found in normal and malignant colonocytes. Vitamin D metabolites produce genomic effects involving the vitamin D receptor and other transcription factors, as well as rapid effects that do not involve gene transcription or protein synthesis.

Clinical case-control and cohort studies have shown a 40%–50% reduction in colorectal cancer-related mortality in individuals taking aspirin and other nonsteroidal anti-inflammatory drugs (NSAIDs) on a regular basis compared with those not taking these agents (see below). The mechanism for cancer protection may relate to altered synthesis of arachidonic acid metabolites (eicosanoids) that include prostaglandins, thromboxanes, leukotrienes, and hydroxyeicosatetraenoic acids. These compounds modulate a number of signal transduction pathways that may affect cellular adhesion, growth, and differentiation. Cyclooxygenase (COX or prostaglandin-endoperoxide synthase) oxidizes arachidonic acid to prostaglandin G_2, reduces prostaglandin G_2 to prostaglandin H_2 and is the key enzyme responsible for production of prostaglandins and other eicosanoids. The COX-2 isoform is induced by cytokines, mitogens, and growth factors, and its level has been shown to be elevated in both murine and human colorectal cancers. Expression of COX-2 is markedly increased in 85% to 95% of colorectal cancers, and in preclinical animal models of colonic tumorigenesis. COX-2 inhibition leads to prevention of cancer development during both the initiation and promotion/progression stages of carcinogenesis. Genetic or pharmacological knockout of COX-2 results in suppression of intestinal polyposis in animal models of familial adenomatous polyposis (FAP), where dose-dependent reductions in polyp number and size, alterations in polyp morphology and accompanying reductions in proliferation, membrane-bound vascular endothelial growth factor and angiogenesis have been demonstrated. Over-expression of COX-2 decreases apoptosis, while COX-2 inhibition leads to an increase in apoptosis. Another mechanism by which COX-2 may influence tumorigenesis in the colon involves its role in signal transduction pathways. The nuclear hormone receptor peroxisome-proliferator-activated receptor δ (PPARδ) activates genes involved in cell growth differentiation and apoptosis after exposure to a variety of lig-

ands, including eicosanoids dependent upon COX-2 for synthesis. COX-2 inhibition also leads to alterations in cellular adhesion to extracellular matrix proteins, inhibition of angiogenesis, and reduction in carcinogen activation. Aspirin and non-selective NSAIDS (e.g. sulindac) may have COX-2 dependent and independent effects on inhibiting neoplasia in the colon. Human clinical trials in patients with FAP have shown significant reductions in adenoma number in patients treated with the NSAID sulindac and the COX-2 inhibitor celecoxib, leading to approval of the latter by the U.S. Food and Drug Administration as an adjunct to usual care in this group. Prospective clinical trials of NSAIDS and specific COX-2 inhibitors for prevention of adenoma recurrence in patients with sporadic adenomas are in progress. Data from a large randomized prospective trial using aspirin in this group will soon be reported, and demonstrate a significant chemopreventive effect of low-dose aspirin on adenomas in the large bowel. There is growing evidence that NSAIDS including COX-2 inhibitors may be effective chemopreventive agents for adenomas and cancer occurrence in the colon, either alone or in combination with other agents. Assessment of their full potential awaits additional trials designed to further elucidate their mechanisms of action and to confirm their efficacy in both average and high-risk groups.

Observational studies continue to find the risk of colorectal cancer to be lower among populations with high intakes of some vitamins and micronutrients. Studies suggest protective effects associated with intake of dietary folate, selenium, and organosulfur compounds. The suggestion from population studies that foods rich in the antioxidants carotene (vitamin A) and vitamin C may have protective effects against colonic neoplasia has not been confirmed by prospective trials.

The strength of evidence for potential chemopreventive agents in preventing colorectal neoplasia is summarized in Table 1.

Symptoms and Clinical Signs

Adenocarcinomas of the colon and rectum grow slowly and may be present for years before symptoms appear. Individuals with asymptomatic disease often have occult blood loss from their tumors, and the bleeding rate increases with tumor size and degree of ulceration.

Table 1
Chemopreventive agents and colorectal neoplasia

| Strenght of Evidence | Weak | | | | Randomized Human Trials | Strong |
Agent	Animal Studies	Case Control	Cohort Studies	Mucosal Proliferation	Polyposis Patients	Sporadic Adenoma
		Observational Studies				
Aspirin/NSAIDS	↑	↑	↑		↑	↑
COX-2 inhibitors*	↑				↑	?
Vitamins A, C, E	↑	↑	↑	↑	→	→
Calcium	↑	↑	↑	→		↑
Fiber	↑	↑	↑	↑	→	↓
Selenium	↑	↑	→			
Fish Oil		↑			↑	
Organosulfur	↑					

*Cyclooxygenase-2. ↑ Most studies positive; ↓ most studies negative; → studies equivocal; ? studies ongoing.

Symptoms depend to some extent on the site of the primary tumor. Cancers of the proximal colon usually grow larger before they produce symptoms than those of the left colon and rectum. Constitutional symptoms (fatigue, shortness of breath, angina) secondary to microcytic hypochromic anemia are often the principal manner of presentation of right colon tumors. Less often, blood from right colon cancers is admixed with stool and appears as "maroon stool" (Fig. 1).

More advanced tumors may produce vague abdominal discomfort or present as palpable masses. Obstruction is uncommon because of the large diameters of the cecum and ascending colon, although cecal cancers may block the ileocecal valve and cause distal small bowel obstruction.

The left colon has a narrower lumen than the proximal colon, and cancers of the descending and sigmoid colon often involve the bowel circumferentially and cause obstructive symptoms (Fig. 2). Patients may present with colicky abdominal pain, and changes in bowel habits. Constipation may alternate with increased frequency of defecation, as small amounts of retained stool move beyond the obstructing lesion. Hematochezia is present more often with distal lesions than with proximal ones, and bright red blood which coats the stool surface is common with cancers of the distal colon and rectum. Rectal cancers also cause obstruction and changes in bowel habits, including constipation, diarrhea, and tenesmus. Rectal cancers may invade locally to involve the bladder, vaginal wall, or surrounding nerves, resulting in perineal or sacral pain, but this is a late occurrence.

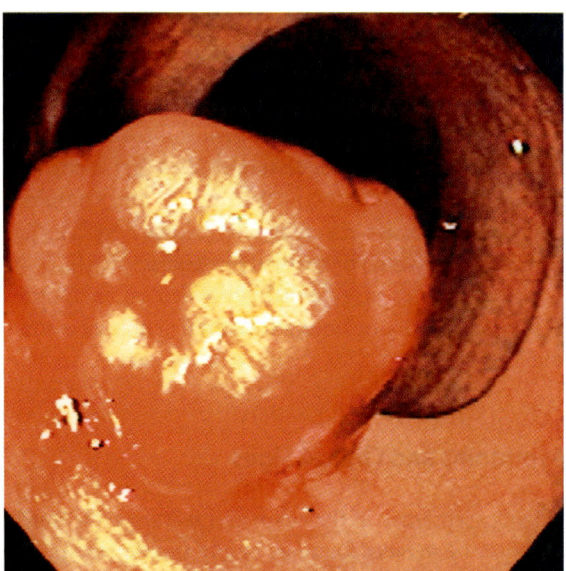

Figure 1
Bleeding polypoid cancer of the colon at colonoscopy. Chronic blood loss may lead to microcytic anemia and constitutional symptoms such as fatigue, shortness of breath or angina.

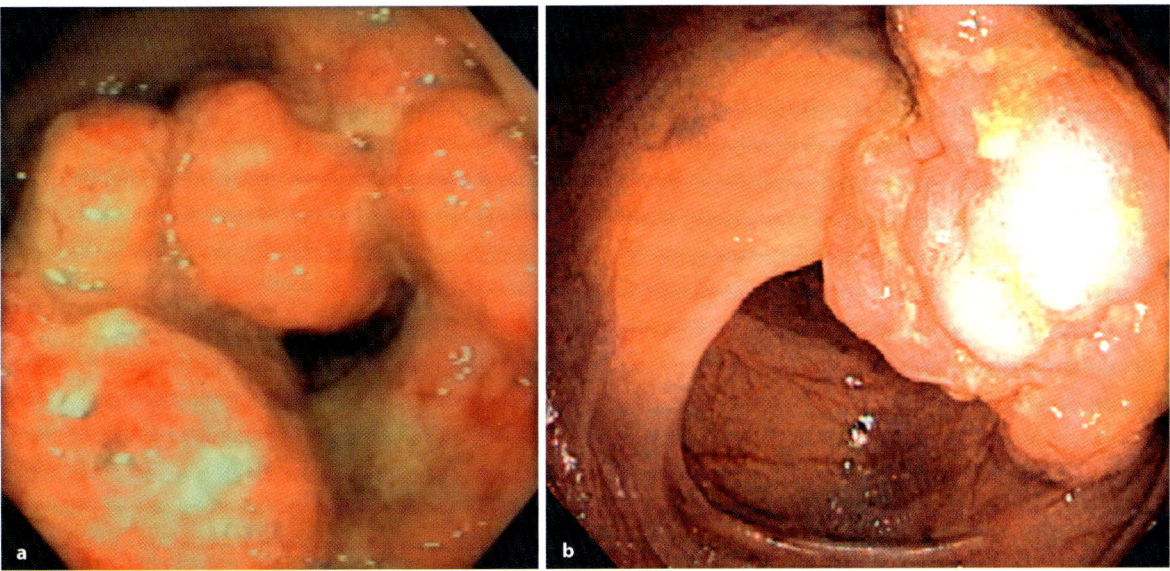

Figure 2a,b
Carcinomas of the colon seen at colonoscopy. a Obstructing carcinoma with circumferential involvement of the bowel wall. **b** Polypoid carcinoma

Diagnosis of colorectal cancer in asymptomatic individuals may be associated with an improved prognosis, while patients presenting with bowel obstruction or perforation have a diminished prognosis.

Diagnostics

Synopsis

Colorectal cancers can be diagnosed by endoscopy or radiological procedures. When there is an indication to examine the whole colon, colonoscopy is the procedure of choice due to its greater accuracy and ability to perform biopsies and polypectomies. Cohort and case-control studies indicate that endoscopic polypectomy reduces the subsequent incidence and mortality of colorectal cancer.

The use of various procedures to diagnose asymptomatic preneoplastic and early neoplastic colorectal lesions is discussed below (screening, surveillance, prevention) and in accompanying chapters.

When colorectal cancer is suspected because of clinical signs and symptoms or when screening suggests the possibility of a large bowel tumor, prompt endoscopic or radiographic diagnostic evaluation should be undertaken. Colonoscopy is more accurate than air-contrast barium enema, especially for detecting small lesions such as adenomas less than 1 cm, but up to half of even larger adenomas may be missed by barium enema. If colonoscopy is unavailable, technically difficult, or refused by the patient, an air-contrast barium enema should be performed following flexible sigmoidoscopy. Neoplasms in the rectum and sigmoid colon are sometimes difficult to diagnose radiologically, and proctosigmoidoscopy should be used as a complement to double-contrast enema imaging. Virtual colonoscopy involving the use of helical computed tomography (CT) to generate high-resolution three-dimensional reconstructed images of the colon has been predominantly utilized in the context of screening and is discussed below. CT is useful in detecting recurrence after resection of rectosigmoid tumors. The use of endorectal ultrasound and magnetic resonance imaging (MRI) has allowed accurate staging of rectal disease and facilitated preoperative therapy. CT or MRI are useful in detecting distant metastases. Intraoperative ultrasonography increases the ability to detect small and deep hepatic lesions that are not palpable during surgery. The role of positron emission scanning is also being evaluated. Determination of serum levels for the carcinoembryonic antigen (CEA) is insensitive for diagnosis, but confers prognostic information, and may be useful in indicating recurrent disease. Expression of other tumor-associated carbohydrate antigens such as sialyl Lewis X and the carbohydrate binding protein galectin-3 have been associated with the metastatic potential of tumor cells, and are being evaluated as potentially useful clinical tumor markers.

Histological Classification and Molecular Genetics

Synopsis

Carcinomas of the large bowel are predominantly adenocarcinomas, which form moderately to well-differentiated glands and secrete variable amounts of mucin. The depth of transmural tumor penetration and the extent of regional lymph node spread are the most important determinants of prognosis.

The development of advanced adenomas results from accumulated genetic damage in colonic epithelial cells. Alteration in the adenomatous polyposis coli (*APC*) tumor suppressor gene is an early step in adenoma formation, and has been shown to occur in dysplastic aberrant crypts. Subsequent genetic damage primarily occurs in the setting of chromosomal instability, characterized by aneuploidy and alterations of *SMAD2, SMAD4, DCC*, and *p53* genes. Approximately 10–15% of sporadic adenomas may develop in the setting of defective DNA mismatch repair, and are characterized by normal DNA content, microsatellite instability, and frequent mutations of TGFβRII.

Carcinomas of the large bowel are predominantly adenocarcinomas, which form moderately to well-differentiated glands (Fig. 3) and secrete variable amounts of mucins, high-molecular weight glycoproteins, which are the major secreted products of both normal and neoplastic glands of the colon. Poorly differentiated tumors, comprising approximately 20% of colorectal adenocarcinomas, demonstrate less prominent gland formation and mucin production and are associated with a worse prognosis than well-differentiated carcinomas. "Signet-ring" cells, in which a large vacuole of mucin displaces the nucleus to one side, are a feature of some tumors. In approximately 15% of tumors, large lakes of mucin con-

tain scattered collections of tumor cells (Fig. 3). These mucinous or colloid carcinomas are most frequent in patients with hereditary non-polyposis-related carcinomas, in the setting of ulcerative colitis, and in patients whose carcinomas occur at an early age. Scirrhous carcinomas are uncommon and are characterized by sparse gland formation, with marked desmoplasia and fibrous tissue surrounding glandular structures. Sometimes tumors demonstrate a mixed histological picture, with glands of varying degrees of differentiation. Cancers other than adenocarcinomas account for fewer than 5% of malignant tumors of the large bowel. Medullary carcinomas, often associated with high degrees of microsatellite instability (MSI), are characterized by uniform polygonal cells in nested, organoid or trabecular patterns. Small cell carcinoma is a malignant neuroendocrine tumor that resembles small cell carcinoma of the lung histologically and in biological behavior. Tumors arising at the anorectal junction include squamous cell carcinomas, cloacogenic or transitional cell carcinomas, and melanocarcinomas. Primary lymphomas and carcinoid tumors of the large bowel comprise fewer than 0.1% of all large bowel neoplasms.

Colorectal cancers begin as intramucosal epithelial lesions, usually arising in adenomatous polyps or glands. As cancers grow they become invasive, penetrating the muscularis mucosae of the bowel and invading lymphatic and vascular channels to involve regional lymph nodes, adjacent structures and distant sites. Adenocarcinomas of the colon and rectum grow at varying rates, most often with long periods of silent growth before producing bowel symptoms. Patterns of spread depend on the anatomy of the individual bowel segment as well as its lymph and blood supplies.

Colon cancers invade transmurally to penetrate the bowel wall and involve regional lymphatics and then distant nodes. The liver is the most common site of hematogenous spread from colon tumors, and this spread occurs via the portal venous system. Pulmonary metastases from colon cancer result, in general, from hepatic metastases.

Cancers of the rectum advance locally by progressive penetration of the bowel wall. Extension of the primary tumor intramurally is most often limited, and lymphatic and hematogenous spreads are unusual before penetration of the muscularis mucosae. Exceptions appear to be

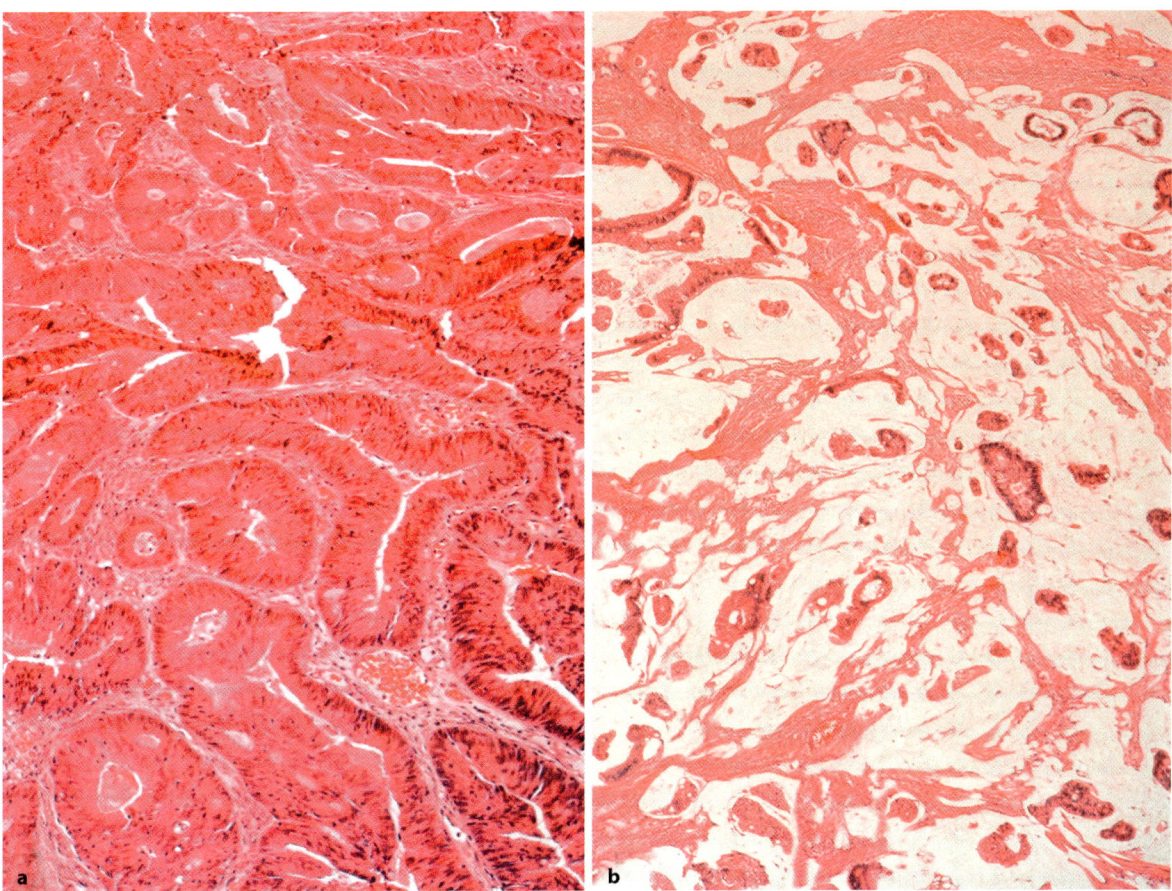

Figure 3a,b
Photomicrographs of **a** well differentiated adenocarcinoma of the colon, **b** mucinous colloid carcinoma of the colon

poorly differentiated tumors, which may metastasize lymphatically or hematogenously before penetrating the bowel. Rectal cancers tend to spread contiguously to progressively involve local structures. Tumors in the lower one third of the rectum may metastasize hematogenously to the liver via the superior hemorrhoidal vein and portal system or to the lungs by way of the middle hemorrhoidal vein and inferior vena cava. The blood of the upper and middle thirds of the rectum drain into the portal system, and tumors in these segments first spread hematogenously to the liver. Occasionally, lumbar and thoracic vertebral metastases may result from hematogenous spread via portal-vertebral communications (Batson's vertebral venous plexuses).

Colorectal carcinomas result from molecular alterations in normal colonic cells that result in dysregulated cell growth. Accumulation of multiple molecular defects drives the histological progression of early adenomas to late adenomas and then into cancers (Table 2, Fig. 4). Continued cell growth necessary for adenoma formation results from genetic alterations causing deregulated cell cycle checkpoints, loss of programmed cell death (apoptosis) and deregulated intracellular signaling pathways. These genetic alterations occur in two major classes of genes – proto-oncogenes and tumor suppressor genes. Activation of proto-oncogenes can occur by several mechanisms, including point mutations, gene amplification/rearrangement or loss of promoter methylation.

Table 2

Genes altered in sporadic colorectal cancer

Gene	Chromosome	Tumors with alterations [%]	Class	Function
K-ras	12	50	Proto-oncogene	Encodes guanine nucleotide-binding protein that regulates intracellular signaling
APC	5	70	Tumor suppressor	Regulation of β-catenin involved in activation of Wnt/TcF signaling (activates c-myc, cyclin D1)[+]; regulation of proliferation, apoptosis. Interaction with E-cadherin (? cell adhesion)
DCC	18	70	? Tumor suppressor	Netrin-1 receptor; caspase substrate in apoptosis; cell adhesion
SMAD 4 (DPC4, MADH 4)	18	?	Tumor suppressor	Nuclear transcription factor in TGF-β1 signaling; regulation of angiogenesis; regulator of WAF1 promoter; downstream mediator of SMAD2
p53	17	75	Tumor suppressor	Transcription factor; regulator of cell cycle progression after cellular stress, of apoptosis, of gene expression, and of DNA repair
hMSH2	2	*	DNA mismatch repair	Maintains fidelity of DNA replication
hMLH1	3	*	DNA mismatch repair	Maintains fidelity of DNA replication
hMSH6	2	*	DNA mismatch repair	Maintains fidelity of DNA replication
TGF-β1 RII	3	**	Tumor suppressor	Receptor for signaling in the TGF-β1 pathway; inhibitor of colonic epithelial proliferation, often mutated in tumors with MSI

*Approximately 15% of sporadic colorectal cancers demonstrate microsatellite instability associated with alterations in mismatch repair genes (principally hMSH2 and hMLH1 but also hMSH3, hMSH6, hPMS1 and hPMS2). ** Mutated in 73% to 90% of MSI colon cancers. Up to 55% of MSS colon cancer cell lines may demonstrate a TGF-β signaling blockage distal to TGF-β1 RII. [+]β-Catenin mutations (downstream of APC) are found in 16% to 25% of MSI (microsatellite instability) colon cancers, but not in microsatellite stable (MSS) cancers.

Tumor suppressor genes inhibit cell growth. In general, both alleles of a tumor suppressor gene must be disabled by mutation, gene loss, or deactivation by promoter methylation for the cell to be affected.

Loss or inactivation of the APC tumor suppressor gene at chromosome location 5q is an early step in the formation of sporadic adenomas. APC mutations have been shown to occur in dysplastic aberrant crypts, and are ultimately found in over 80% of sporadic colorectal cancers. APC functions in regulation of the Wnt signaling pathway (Fig. 5). Wnt ligands initiate a signaling cascade involving translocation of the protein β-catenin from the cytoplasm to the nucleus. APC interacts with at least 6 cytoplasmic proteins, including glycogen synthetase 3β and axin to down-regulate β-catenin through phosphorylation. Loss of APC function leads to lack of degradation of cytoplasmic β-catenin, allowing its translocation to the nucleus at higher levels. Nuclear β-catenin activates another protein Tcf-4, which in turn transcriptionally activates target genes such as C-myc,

Cyclin D, PPARδ, TCF-1 and other genes which are involved in cell cycle control, regulation of cell growth and prevention of apoptosis. The most common mechanism responsible for loss of APC-mediated regulation is through biallelic inactivating mutations of the APC gene. APC mutations most often result in a truncated protein that loses all but one or two of the seven catenin binding/degradation sites. As a result, the APC protein cannot down-regulate cytoplasmic β-catenin levels. In some cases dominant mutations of the β-catenin gene render β-catenin-Tcf-regulated transcription insensitive to the regulatory effects of wild-type APC. APC abnormalities may also lead to disruption of normal cell-cell adhesion by altered binding to the cell adhesion molecule E-cadherin. The dysplastic aberrant crypt is characterized by persistent replication of dysplastic cells near the crypt surface, coupled with loss of apoptosis, leading to infolding and branching patterns in the crypt. Activating mutations of the K-ras proto-oncogene also occur at an early stage in adenoma formation, and are documented

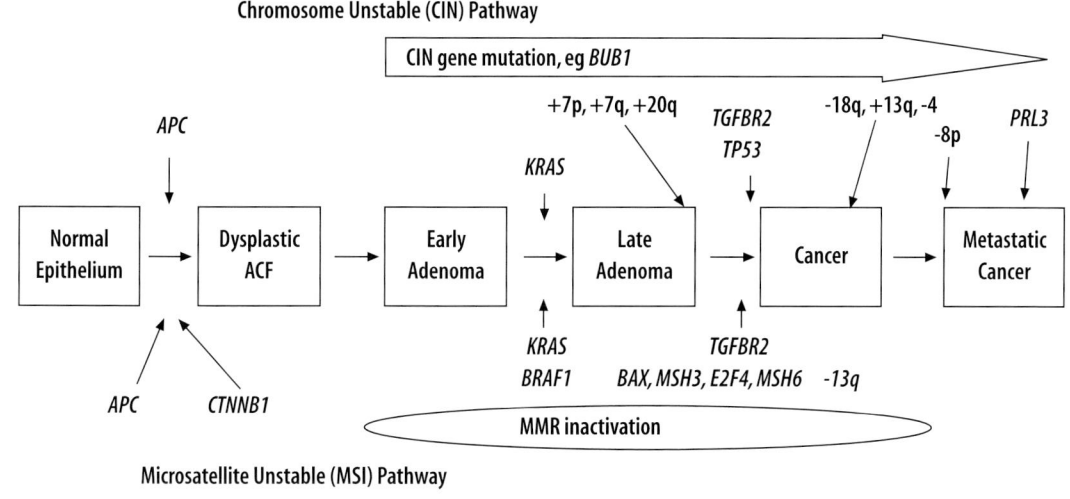

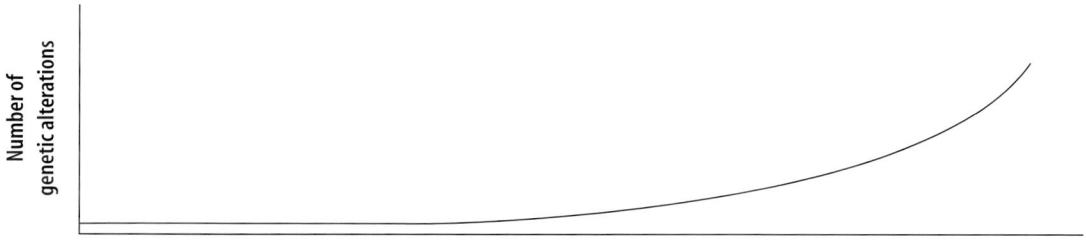

Figure 4

Model of colon cancer in which the progression from normal epithelium through the adenoma to carcinoma sequence is associated with an accumulation of genetic alterations, and genetic instability marked by chromosomal instability (CIN) or microsatellite instability (MSI). ACF, aberrant crypt focus; TGF, transforming growth factor. (Modified from Grady WM and Markowitz S (2000) Genomic instability and colorectal cancer. Curr Opin Gastroenterol; 16: 62–67)

in approximately half of colonic neoplasms. COX-2 levels are increased in the majority of adenomas and cancers, whereas levels of COX-1 remain unchanged. The potential mechanism by which increased COX-2 activity promotes adenoma progression has already been discussed.

Stepwise molecular alterations resulting in the progression of a small tubular adenoma to an advanced adenoma or cancer can occur via two types of pathways. Approximately 85% of sporadic adenomas and cancers are characterized by chromosomal instability (CIN). These cancers display marked losses or gains in large portions of chromosomes. Tumor cells with abnormal quantities of DNA are termed aneuploid. In sporadic adenomas and cancers, the most frequently reported chromosomal losses involve 5q, 18q, and 17p, whereas the most common gains involve 8q and 20q. Stepwise tumor progression is associated with loss of tumor suppressor gene activity located on chromosome 18q in more than 75% of cases. Genes located at the 18q locus include the "deleted in colon cancer" gene, and DPC4 a member of the SMAD gene family involved in the transforming growth factor β (TGFβ) signaling pathway. Deletions of 17p involve the p53 tumor suppressor gene, whose prod-

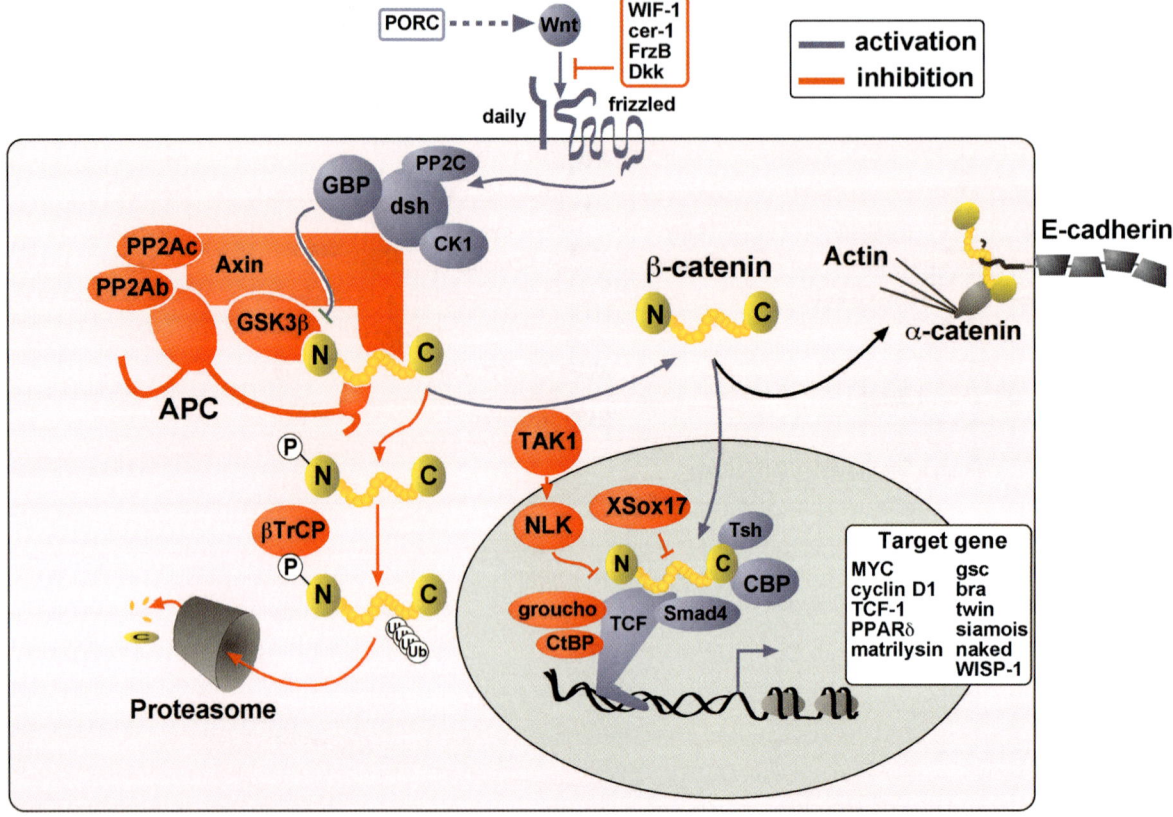

Figure 5
The Wnt signaling pathway. This pathway is important in activating several key genes involved in cell cycle control and regulation of cell growth. The product of the APC gene plays a key role in regulating this pathway, and abnormalities of APC are important events in colorectal tumorigenesis. (Reproduced from Hulsken J and Behrens J (2000) The Wnt signaling pathway. J Cell Science 113:35–45)

uct prevents damaged DNA from progressing from G1 to the S phase of the cell cycle. Loss of 17p is also associated with reduced apoptosis. Inactivation of p53 mediates the progression from adenoma to carcinoma. Distant metastases are also associated with high fractional allelic loss and deletions of 18q and 17 p. CIN is an early event in tumor formation that increases with tumor progression. The molecular basis for CIN is not clear, but may involve genes concerned with kinetochore structure and function, centrosome and microtubule formation and behavior, chromosome condensation, sister chromatid cohesion and cell cycle checkpoint control.

Inactivation of a component of the DNA mismatch repair system causes genomic instability by increasing the rate of polymerase-generated replication errors. This increases the error rate in DNA replication, particularly at microsatellite repeat sequences. Microsatellites is a term given to nucleotide repeat sequences (commonly An/Tn or CAn/GTn) that are distributed throughout the genome. Replication errors in dinucleotide repeats result in an increase in the numbers of these repeats in the tumor DNA, and is termed MSI. At least six genes have been identified that function in the human DNA repair system. Patients with hereditary non-polyposis colorectal cancer (HNPCC) have a germline mutation in a DNA mismatch repair gene, usually MSH2 or MLH1, resulting in cancers with microsatellite instability. Approximately 10–15% of sporadic colorectal cancers are also characterized by MSI. These cancers are diploid and do not have increased rates of chromosomal aberrations. Most patients with sporadic MSI cancers do not have mutations in the known DNA mismatch repair genes. In contrast, hypermethylation of the MLH1 promoter has been shown to occur in approximately 70% of these cancers, resulting in mismatch repair inactivation. The molecular alterations that occur in the microsatellite mutator phenotype pathway are different from those of the chromosomal instability pathway. The most frequently mutated gene in the microsatellite pathway is the TGF-β receptor type II tumor suppressor gene, which occurs at the adenoma-carcinoma transition. β-catenin mutations are found in 16–25% of cancers with the microsatellite mutator phenotype, but are not found in microsatellite-stable cancers. Mutations of; Bax and caspase 5 (proteins that regulate apoptosis), insulin growth factor 2 receptor, E2F (a transcription factor) and MSH3 and MSH6 DNA mismatch repair proteins have been described in adenomas and cancers with the microsatellite mutator phenotype, but the timing of these events remains to be mapped. Colorectal cancers with the microsatellite mutator phenotype are more common on the right side of the colon, may be more poorly differentiated and may have a mucinous or signet ring phenotype. Paradoxically, patients with these MSI tumors may have a better prognosis than others with colorectal cancer.

Staging

The American Joint Committee for Cancer Staging and End Results Reporting and the International Union Against Cancer introduced the tumor-node-metastases (TNM) classification for colorectal cancer in order to provide a uniform and orderly classification for colorectal cancers (Table 3). This system classifies the extent of the primary tumor (T), the status of regional lymph nodes (N) and the presence or absence of distant metastases (M). Cases are assigned the highest value of TNM that describes the extent of the disease and are grouped into five stages (0 through IV). This system is recommended by the College of American Pathologists and has become important in uniformly randomizing patients for therapeutic trials. The TNM classification is widely accepted internationally and should be considered the classification of choice for staging colorectal tumors. The Dukes' classification has been to a large extent supplanted by the TNM System, but is still commonly used.

On the basis of observations of what he believed to be an orderly progression of local-regional invasion by rectal cancer, Cuthbert Dukes proposed a classification in 1929, which has since been modified many times in

Table 3

Staging of colorectal cancer. American joint committee on cancer (TNM classification)

Stage 0	Carcinoma in situ intraepithelial or invasion of lamina propria*(Tis N0 M0)
Stage I	Tumor invades submucosa (T1 N0 M0) Dukes' A
	Tumor invades muscularis propria (T2 N0 M0)
Stage II	Tumor invades through the muscularis propria into subserosa or into nonperitonealized pericolic or perirectal tissues (T3 N0 M0) Dukes' B
	Tumor perforates the visceral peritoneum or directly invades other organs or structures and/or perforates visceral peritoneum** (T4 N0 M0)
Stage III	Any degree of bowel wall perforation with regional lymph node metastasis
	N1 Metastasis in 1 to 3 regional lymph nodes
	N2 Metastasis in 4 or more regional lymph nodes
	Any T N1 M0, Dukes' C
	Any T N2 M0
Stage IV	Any invasion of bowel wall with or without lympho node metastasis, but with evidence of distant metastasis.
	Any T Any N, M1

Dukes' B (corresponds to stage II) is a composite of better (T3, N0, M0) and worse (T4, N0, M0) prognostic groups, as is Dukes' C (corresponds to stage III) (Any T, N1, M0 and Any T, N2, M0).

Definitions: **NX** = regional lymph nodes cannot be assessed, **N0** = no regional lymph node metastasis, **MX** = distant metastasis cannot be assessed, **M0** = no distant metastasis, **M1** = distant metastasis.

*Tis includes cancer cells confined within the glandular basement membrane (intraepithelial) or lamina propria (intramucosal) with no extension through the muscularis mucosae into the submucosa. **Direct invasion in T4 includes invasion of other segments of the colorectum by way of serosa; for example, invasion of the sigmoid colon by a carcinoma of the cecum.

attempts to increase its prognostic value for cancers of both the rectum and the colon. The most commonly employed modification of Dukes' system is that of Astler and Coller. This classification uses the following designations: A, tumors limited to the mucosa; B1, tumors extending into, but not through, the muscularis propria; B2, tumors penetrating the bowel wall but without lymph node involvement; and C, tumors with regional lymph node involvement by tumor. Stage C tumors are further divided into primary tumors limited to the bowel wall (C1) and those that penetrate the wall (C2). In the system proposed by the Gastrointestinal Tumor Study Group, C1 lesions are those in which one to four regional lymph nodes contain tumor, and C2 lesions are those in which more than four lymph nodes contain tumor. Another modification by Turnbull and Associates adds a D category to account for distant metastases.

Treatment

Synopsis

Surgical resection is the treatment of choice for most colorectal cancers. Preoperative colonoscopy should be performed, if possible, to rule out synchronous lesions. Malignant sessile polyps can be managed by colonscopic polypectomy if the resected specimen has no prognostic features that may indicate an increased risk of nodal metastases. Liver metastases can be resected if there is no evidence of other metastatic disease. 5-fluorouracil (5-FU) plus leucovorin is the standard for adjuvant treatment of colorectal cancer with lymph node metastases. It is not clear whether patients with stage II, node-negative colon cancer should receive adjuvant chemotherapy, since the risk-benefit ratio has not been established. Patients with modified Dukes' B2 and C (stage II and III) rectal cancer following curative surgery should receive combined-modality adjuvant therapy.

Surgery

Surgical resection is the treatment of choice for most colorectal cancers. Despite evidence that five-year survival is 90% when colorectal cancer is diagnosed at an early stage, less than 70% of cancers are diagnosed when still localized. Preoperative colonoscopy should be performed, if possible, to rule out synchronous lesions and serum CEA should be measured to inform staging and

postoperative follow-up. CT or MRI are not indicated as a routine preoperative staging procedure, but can be useful for the evaluation of focal hepatic metastases if partial hepatectomy or regional hepatic artery infusion of chemotherapeutic agents is contemplated. CT is also useful for postoperative detection of pelvic recurrence in patients with rectosigmoid tumors. Transrectal ultrasonography and MRI are of value in the preoperative assessment of patients with rectal cancer.

The extent of resection for cure is determined by the location of the tumor, the blood supply and the distribution of regional l'ymph nodes. The resection should include a segment of colon at least 5 cm on either side of the tumor, although wider margins are often included because of obligatory ligation of the arterial blood supply. The resected specimen should be carefully examined for lymph nodes, and at least 10–12 nodes should be submitted for histological examination for metastatic cells. Extensive "super-radical" colonic and lymph node resection does not increase survival over that associated with segmental resection. The approach toward rectal cancers depends on location of the lesion. For lesions of the rectosigmoid and upper rectum, low anterior resection can be performed through an abdominal incision and primary anastomosis accomplished. Even for low rectal lesions, a sphincter-saving resection can be performed if a distal margin of at least 2 cm of normal bowel can be resected below the lesion – an aim now facilitated by end-to-end stapling devices. The inability to obtain an adequate distal margin, the presence of a large, bulky tumor deep within the pelvis, and extensive local spread of rectal cancer, dictate the need for abdominoperineal resection of the rectum.

The prognosis for patients with colorectal cancer who undergo potentially curative surgery is strongly correlated with the stage of the primary tumor at surgery. Despite resection of all macroscopic tumors, patients whose primary tumor has penetrated the serosa or who have regional lymph node metastases at the time of surgery have high recurrence rates. Microscopic and molecular pathologic features which may affect prognosis are listed in Table 4.

In a patient with colorectal cancer, the primary tumor should be resected, even in the presence of distant metastases, to prevent obstruction or bleeding. In patients with advanced disease and multiple medical problems, repeated palliative fulguration of rectal tu-

Table 4

Pathologic and molecular features that may affect prognosis in patients with colorectal cancer

Feature	Effect on prognosis
Surgical or pathologic stage	
Depth of bowel wall penetration	Increased penetration diminishes prognosis
Number of regional lymph nodes involved by tumor	1–4 nodes better than >4 nodes
Histologic findings	
Degree of differentiation	Well-differentiated better than poorly differentiated
Mucinous (colloid or signet-ring cell histologic findings)	Diminished prognosis
Scirrhous histologic findings	Diminished prognosis
Venous invasion	Diminished prognosis
Lymphatic invasion	Diminished prognosis
Perineural invasion	Diminished prognosis
Local inflammation and immunologic reaction	Improved prognosis
Tumor size	No effect in most studies
Tumor morphologic findings	Polypoid or exophytic better than ulcerating or infiltrating
Tumor DNA content	Increased DNA content (aneuploidy) diminishes prognosis
Molecular markers	
Deletions in chromosome 18q, (DCC, DPC4), 17p (p53), or 8p	Diminished prognosis
Mutation in BAX gene	Diminished prognosis
Microsatellite instability	Improved prognosis
Increased labeling index of p21$^{WAF/CIP1}$ protein	Improved prognosis

mors may be preferable to surgery. Newer modalities, such as laser photoablation, are being tested as alternative means of palliation in these patients. Polypoid carcinomas may be removed endoscopically by snare polypectomy techniques.

Synchronous metastases to the liver are evident at initial presentation in approximately 20% of patients with large bowel cancer, and 25% to 30% develop metachronous liver metastases. Seventy percent to 80% of hepatic metastases appear within two years after primary resection. The uniformly poor prognosis for patients with untreated hepatic metastases dictates an aggressive surgical approach in selected patients. Candidates for resection of hepatic lesions are those whose primary tumor has been resected with curative intent and in whom where is no evidence of extrahepatic disease. Surgical resection for isolated liver metastases results in a 5-year survival of 24% to 38% in selected patients, but only 10% to 15% of patients with liver metastases are appropriate surgical candidates. Staging laparoscopy and laparoscopic ultrasound may aid in ruling out inappropriate candidates. Patients with a large number of metastases (74) and bilobar metastases are at increased risk for post-surgical recurrence. Cryotherapy utilizes an ultrasonically guided probe to ablate malignant lesions intraoperatively, while maintaining preservation of surrounding tissue. Rapid freezing results in crystal formation and cellular damage and death.

Adjuvant Chemotherapy

Patients whose primary tumor has penetrated the serosa or who have regional lymph node metastases at the time of potentially curative surgery have high recurrence rates. Patients who undergo aggressive surgical resection of isolated hepatic metastases also have high tumor recurrence rates in the liver and elsewhere. The principal of adjuvant therapy is that survival can be improved by treatment of micrometastatic disease. Adjuvant therapy with the fluoropyrimidine 5-FU plus levamisole was evaluated in 1296 patients with resected colon cancer that was either locally invasive (Dukes' B2; stage II) or had regional lymph node involvement (Dukes' C; stage III). 5-FU plus levamisole reduced the risk of cancer recurrence by 42%, and the overall death rate by 33% relative to surgery alone in patients with stage III disease. The results in patients with stage II disease were equivocal.

Comparison of 5-FU/levamisole *versus* 5-FU/leucovorin in randomized clinical trials suggests a small advantage in disease-free and overall survival in favor of 5-FU plus leucovorin. Review of the combined data suggests that while 5-FU/levamisole given for one year is still considered an acceptable regimen, 5-FU/lecovorin given for 6 months after "curative" surgery is superior with regard to convenience and efficacy. 5-FU plus leucovorin should therefore be considered the new standard for adjuvant treatment of colorectal cancer. It is not clear whether patients with stage II, node-negative colon cancer should receive adjuvant chemotherapy, since the risk-benefit ratio has not been established. Anatomic or biologic features may, in the future, define subsets of patients with stage II colon cancer who will benefit from adjuvant therapy. One recent analysis suggested that retention of 18q alleles in microsatellite stable cancers, or mutations of the TGF-βRII gene in cancers with high levels of MSI confers a favorable outcome after adjuvant therapy with FU-based regimens in patients with stage III colon cancer. Regimens containing the oral 5-FU prodrug UFTC (uracil, 5-FU, tegafur), oxaliplatin and irinotecan (CPT-11) are currently under investigation for use in the adjuvant setting. The use of portal vein infusion of chemotherapeutic agents to treat hepatic micrometastases is also being evaluated.

Adjuvant therapy for rectal cancer should be considered separately from that for colon cancer, since patterns of failure are different. Local recurrence for stage II rectal cancer after primary resection approaches 25% to 30%, with a 50% or greater local recurrence rate in those with stage III tumors. Local recurrence is associated with significant morbidity, and patients with locally invasive rectal cancer are at high risk for systemic relapse. Studies during the past two decades have shown a significant decrease in local recurrence of rectal cancer in patients who receive moderate to high doses of preoperative and/or postoperative radiation (40 to 50 Gy), but with little impact on systemic recurrence and survival. Combined adjuvant radiation and chemotherapy has been used to address this potential for local and systemic recurrence. Prospective trials have strongly indicate that postsurgical combined-modality therapy decreases tumor relapse and improves survival over those with surgery alone or with full-dose postoperative radiation therapy. Based on these data, patients with resected rectal cancer with transmural extension (TNM stage II; Dukes' B2) or with positive lymph nodes (TNM stage III; Dukes' C) should be considered for such combined-modality therapy. Patients with rectal cancer should have preoperative staging including transrectal ultrasound, which has 90% to 95% accuracy in staging the extent of transmucal involvement, and 80% accuracy in detecting lymph node metastases. The relative benefits of pre-*versus* postoperative multimodality adjuvant therapy (radiation and chemotherapy) for rectal cancer are currently under investigation.

Chemotherapy for Advanced Disease

The approach to therapy of patients with advanced colorectal cancer has, for the most part, utilized regimens containing fluoropyrimidines (5-FU, 5-fluorodeoxyuridine). 5-FU interacts with thymidylate synthetase, inhibiting the methylation of deoxyuridylic to thymidylic acid, thereby inhibiting DNA synthesis. 5-FU has been administered intravenously in bolus doses or by continuous intravenous infusion. Oral formulations have been developed including UFT, an oral 5-FU prodrug composed of a 1:4 fixed molar ratio of tegafur and uracil. The combination of 5-FU and high-dose intravenous leucovorin (tetrahydrofolate) has become standard therapy. Studies suggest that continuous infusion 5-FU is associated with a higher response rate (22% versus 14%; $p=0.0002$ in a recent meta-analysis) and a small survival advantage as compared with bolus 5-FU regimens. Intensive-course 5-FU plus low-dose leucovorin may have a superior therapeutic index with less toxicity in comparison with weekly 5-FU plus high-dose leucovorin. CPT-11 inhibits topoisomerase I, a nuclear enzyme involved in the unwinding of DNA during replication. Weekly treatment with CPT-11 plus 5-FU and leucovorin may be superior to 5-FU and leucovorin with regard to progression free survival and overall survival in patients with metastatic colon cancer. CPT-11 has also been shown to be of efficacy in patients refractory to 5-FU.

Oxaliplatin is a third generation platinum analogue that induces DNA cross-linkage and apoptosis. Oxaliplatin also has demonstrated efficacy in 5-FU-refractory colon cancer, and has been used in combination with 5-FU and leucovorin. Other agents currently under investigation include topotecan and 9-aminocamptothecin, trimetrexate (an antifolate), tamudex (a thymidylate synthase inhibitor), and WFT (tegafur and uracil).

Selective infusion of chemotherapeutic agents into the hepatic arterial system may be employed to treat hepatic metastases. This method delivers more concentrated drug into the tumor capillary bed than do conventional means. The infusion catheter is usually implanted into the common hepatic artery via the gastroduodenal artery at the time of laparotomy. The development of implantable infusion pumps has led to increasing use of such therapy in major centers. Fluorinated pyrimidines, such as 5-FU and floxuridine (FUDR), have high hepatic extraction (80% to 95%), and it is felt that high concentrations of these drugs can be delivered with low systemic toxicity by direct hepatic arterial infusion. Continuous hepatic arterial infusion of FUDR to treat hepatic metastases from colorectal cancer in patients not previously treated may achieve response rates of 54% to 83%, but the influence on survival is unclear.

Radiation therapy is used preoperatively or postoperatively to decrease local recurrence in those with high-risk rectal and rectosigmoid cancers, or in a combined preoperative and postoperative "sandwich approach." It is also used to convert unresectable large tumors and those fixed to pelvic organs to resectable lesions. Radiation therapy may occasionally be useful for palliation of bleeding and pain due to advanced rectal disease.

Preoperative radiation reduces local recurrence in patients with rectal and rectosigmoid cancers, but there is no convincing evidence that it improves survival. Sphincter preservation is a major goal of preoperative therapy. When sphincter preservation is the goal, the use of preoperative therapy should be limited to those who are not technically able to undergo excision. Postoperative radiotherapy is generally restricted to patients at high risk for local recurrence of rectal cancer (penetration of the bowel wall, positive lymph nodes). Prospective series show a substantial reduction in local recurrence for those receiving postoperative radiotherapy, with an overall reduction in local-regional recurrence from 25% to 16% in one randomized trial. Distant metastases remain a problem, however, and it is not clear whether survival is altered substantially. Combined postoperative radiation and chemotherapy decreases

recurrence and increases survival in patients with rectal cancer, making this the treatment of choice for high-risk patients with transmural tumor extension or lymph node metastases extension or lymph node metastases.

Screening, Surveillance, Prevention

Screening

Screening involves large populations and is aimed at identifying asymptomatic individuals who are at risk for development of colorectal cancer. Surveillance relates to monitoring those with a personal history of disease (adenoma, colorectal cancer, inflammatory bowel disease).

Colorectal cancer represents a major health problem and localized lesions are curable by surgical resection. Furthermore, the prolonged natural history of colonic neoplasia affords time to detect and eliminate preneoplastic and early neoplastic lesions before they reach an advanced, incurable stage. Effective, easily administered and cost-effective screening tests are needed for screening large asymptomatic populations and to optimize compliance. Current evidence indicates that screening for colorectal cancer reduces related mortality. Current screening options include fecal occult blood testing (FOBT) annually, flexible sigmoidoscopy every five years, annual FOBT plus flexible sigmoidoscopy every five years (preferred to either alone), double contrast barium enema every five years, or colonoscopy every 10 years.

Screening and surveillance guidelines have been adopted by most medical and surgical societies, and most recently have been presented as option menus to offer a broad set of screening options and to enhance compliance (Table 5). Each of the choices has inherent characteristics related to accuracy, prevention, potential costs and risks. Recommendations for screening can be categorized according to personal risk (average, moderate, high). Moderate-and high-risk categories are further subdivided according to personal and family history of adenoma, carcinoma or predisposing disease. Compliance with screening recommendations has a major impact on the effectiveness and cost-effectiveness of screening programs.

FOBT has been proven to detect earlier lesions and to improve survival in large prospective randomized controlled trials of symptomatic average-risk populations. Results of 18-year cumulative follow-up from the Minnesota FOBT trial confirmed a 33% reduction in

Table 5

Guidelines for screening average risk individuals for colorectal cancer

Screening tool	USPSTF[a]	Multidisciplinary expert panel[b]	American cancer society[c]
FOBT	Recommended annually	Recommended annually	Recommended annually as an option
Flexible sigmoidoscopy	Recommended "periodicity unspecified"	Recommended every 5 years	Recommended every 5 years as an option
FOBT + flexible sigmoidoscopy	Recommended as an option	Recommend as an option	Annual FOBT plus flexible sigmoidoscopy every 5 years recommended as an option
Colonoscopy	Insufficient evidence	Recommended as an option every 10 years	Recommended as an option every 10 years
Double-contrast barium enema	Insufficient evidence	Recommended as an option every 5–10 years	Recommended as an option every 5 years

[a]U.S. Preventative Services Task Force 1995; [b]Endorsed by numerous medical and surgical societies (Gastroenterology 1997;112:594); [c]Updated guidelines 2001 (CA Cancer J Clin 2001;1:51) provides menu of options rather than recommending any specific option in order to increase compliance with screening. FOBT should use take home sample method. All positive tests should be followed up with colonoscopy.

cancer mortality in those screened annually with FOBT compared to controls, and a 21% reduction with biennial screening. European trials have also demonstrated 15% to 18% reductions in mortality with random or biennial screening (Table 6). These studies utilized chromogen-based tests, which depend upon the pseudoperoxidase activity of hemoglobin. More specific immunochemical tests are available, and have been extensively utilized in screening trials in Asia.

Case-control trials have suggested that screening sigmoidoscopy can result in a 70% to 80% reduction from cancers within reach of the sigmoidoscope, but most have studied patients undergoing rigid as opposed to flexible sigmoidoscopy. The overall impact of screening flexible sigmoidoscopy on lesion detection has been inferred from trials utilizing colonoscopy, using the distal portion of the examination as a surrogate for flexible sigmoidoscopy. These studies suggest that approximately 50% of individuals with advanced adenomas (larger than 1 cm in size, with vilious features, severe dysplasia or cancer) in the colon will not have lesions within range of the flexible sigmoidoscope. However, only 1.5% to 2.7% of patients with negative distal exams will have proximal advanced adenomas. The true impact of screening sigmoidoscopy on mortality awaits results of trials such as the National Cancer Institute sponsored Prostate, Lung, Colorectal, and Ovarian Cancer Screening Trial. It has been assumed that combining FOBT and flexible sigmoidoscopy is superior to either test alone, but definitive data is lacking.

Colonoscopy visualizes the entire colon and allows for biopsy of lesions and removal of adenomatous polyps at the time of examination. While the impact of screening colonoscopy on cancer-related mortality has not been assessed in randomized prospective trials, indirect evidence from the National Polyp Study strongly suggests a reduction in colorectal cancer mortality as the result of removing adenomas at colonoscopy. Recent analyses suggest that screening colonoscopy maybe a cost-effective option, since a positive FOBT or sigmoidoscopy will themselves generate a subsequent colonoscopic examination. Given the long "dwell time" of adenomas, colonoscopy may be performed at 10-year intervals, adding to the cost-effectiveness of the procedure. The cost-effectiveness of colonoscopy is also less susceptible to the impact of compliance than tests which must be performed at more frequent intervals. The sensitivity of colonoscopy for detecting colonic neoplasia has been estimated at 95%. The most frequent reason for the failure to detect cancer is the inability to reach the lesion in question. "Virtual" colonoscopy involves the use of helical CT to generate high-resolution, two-dimensional images of the abdomen and pelvis. Three-dimensional images of the colon are then generated. This examination may prove a rapid and safe method of providing full structural evolution of the entire colon. Initial trials have been promising, but the need for expensive, rapid, high-resolution CT scanners and high false-positive rates will have to be overcome.

Table 6

Controlled trials of fecal occult blood testing (FOBT) in screening asymptomatic persons for colorectal cancer

	Minnesota	Nottingham	Goteborg	Funen	New York
Study population	46,000 (50–80 yrs)	152,850 (50–74 yrs)	28,000 (60–64 yrs)	61,933 (45–74 yrs)	22,000 (≥40 yrs)
Study design	Random; annual vs. biennial vs. control	Random	Random	Random; biennial vs. control	Allocation by month-assigned
Rehydration of test cards[a]	Yes-most	No	Yes-most	No	No
Compliance	Annual 75%; biennial 78%	50%		56%	
Positivity rate	2.4% (nonhydrated) 9.8% (rehydrated)	1st screen: 2.1% 2nd screen: 1.2%	1st screen: 1.9% (nonhydrated); 5.8% (rehydrated) 2nd screen: 4.8% (prev. rehydrated); 8.0% (prev. non-hydrated)	1st screen: 1.0% 2nd screen: 0.8% 3rd screen: 0.9% 4th screen: 1.3% 5th screen: 1.8%	Regular attendees: 1.4% first time screen: 2.6%
Positive predictive value for colorectal cancer	2.2% (rehydrated) 5.6% (nonhydrated)	1st round: 9.9% 2nd round: 11.9%	1st round: 5.0% (nonhydrated) 2nd round: 4.2% (rehydrated)	1st round: 17.7% 2nd round: 8.4%	10.7%
Colorectal cancer (CRC) mortality[b]	**18-yr follow-up:** 33% reduction for annual group 21% reduction for biennial group **CRC mortality/1000:** Annual: 9.46% [7.75–11.17] Biennial: 11.19% [9.39–12.99] Control: 14.09% [12.01–16.17] **Mortality ratio:** Annual 0.67 [0.51–0.83] Biennial: 0.79 [0.62–0.97]	**7.8-yr follow-up:** 15% reduction in cumulative CRC mortality **Mortality ratio:** 0.85 [0.74–0.98]	Not yet available	**10-yr follow-up:** 18% reduction in CRC-related mortality in screened group **Mortality ratio:** 0.82 [0.68–0.99]	**10-yr follow-up:** 43% reduction in CRC mortality in screened group

[a]Hemoccult test cards were used – rehydrated or nonhydrated. [b]Reductions in mortality area relative risk reductions. Data in brackets represent 95% confidence intervals.

Air contrast barium enema is included as an option in most screening guidelines, but no study has directly addressed the effectiveness of this modality for colon cancer screening. Data from the National Polyp Study suggests that barium enema may be less sensitive than previously thought. Comparison of 862 paired barium enema and colonoscopic exams found that barium enema detected only 48% of adenomas greater than 1 cm and 39% of smaller adenomas.

Increasing knowledge regarding the molecular genesis of colorectal neoplasia has raised substantial interest in the use of molecular markers for colorectal cancer screening. Multi-targeted DNA-based assays have been developed to detect neoplasia-related alterations in DNA shed into stool by colorectal neoplasms. One recent study targeted a panel of DNA markers, and reported a sensitivity of 91% for detecting cancers and 82% for detecting adenomas greater than 1 cm, with a specificity of

93%. While exciting, these results need to be confirmed in large prospective screening trials before being applied to screening large populations.

Screening and surveillance of individuals with increased or high risk for development of colon cancer is discussed in accompanying chapters (sporadic adenomas, polyposis syndromes, HNPCC, inflammatory bowel disease).

Future Perspectives

Primary prevention of colorectal adenomas holds the promise of preventing colorectal cancer, and prospective trials of chemopreventive agents are underway to determine the efficacy of a variety of agents (e.g. aspirin, COX-2 inhibitors, calcium and vitamin D, HMG-CoA reductase inhibitors) in preventing the recurrence of sporadic adenomas in at-risk individuals. Current screening and treatment strategies for colorectal adenomas have the promise of reducing colorectal cancer mortality. The situation will continue to improve with new technologic advances and continued basic science research. New diagnostic techniques for screening average and high-risk populations continue to be developed. These include the use of radiological "virtual" colonscopy and the use of molecular markers in blood and stool. Technologic advances in fiber optic colonoscopes will increase the efficacy, safety and comfort of colonoscopic procedures and allow better detection of early preneoplastic lesions. Finally, increased understanding of the molecular pathways involved in adenoma formation and of predisposing genetic susceptibility genes will enable us to tailor specific interventions to populations at greatest risk.

References

1. Baron JA, Beach M, Mandel JS, vanStolk RU, Haile RW, Sandler RS, Rothstein R, Summers RW, Snover DC, Beck GJ, Bond JH, Greenberg ER. (1999) Calcium supplements for the prevention of colorectal adenomas. N Engl J Med 340:101–107.
2. Steinbach G, Lynch PM, Phillips RK, Wallace MH, Hawk E, Gordon GB, Wakabayashi N, Saunders B, Shen Y, Fujimura T, Su LK, Levin B. (2000). The effect of celecoxib, a cyclooxygenase-2 inhibitor, in familial adenomatous polyposis. N Engl J Med 342(26):1946–1952.
3. Grady WM, Markowitz, S. (2000). Genomic instability and colorectal cancer. Current Opinion in Gastroenterology 16:62–67.
4. Watanabe T, Wu TT, Catalano PJ, Ueki T, Satriano R, Haller DG, Benson AB 3rd, Hamilton SR. (2001). Molecular predictors of survival after adjuvant chemotherapy for colon cancer. N Engl J Med 344(16):1196–1206.
5. Imperiale TF, Wagner DR, Lin CY, Larkin GN, Rogge JD, Ransohoff DF. (2000). Risk of advanced proximal neoplasms in asymptomatic adults according to distal colorectal findings. N Engl J Med 343(3):169–174.
6. Burt R. (2000) Colon Cancer Screening. Gastroenterology 119:837–853.
7. Ahlquist DA, Skoletsky JE, Boynton KA, Harrington JJ, Mahoney DW, Pierceall WE, Thibodeau SN, Shuber AP. (2000). Colorectal cancer screening by detection of altered human DNA in stool: feasibility of a multitarget assay panel. Gastroenterology 119(5):1219–1227.
8. Sonnenberg A, Delco F, Inadomi JM. (2000).Cost-effectiveness of colonoscopy in screening for colorectal cancer. Ann Intern Med 133(8):573–584.
9. Winawer SJ, Stewart ET, Zauber AG, Bond JH, Ansel H, Waye JD, Hall D, Hamlin JA, Schapiro M, O'Brien MJ, Sternberg SS, Gottlieb LS. (2000). A comparison of colonoscopy and double-contrast barium enema for surveillance after polypectomy. National Polyp Study Work Group. N Engl J Med; 342(24):1766–1772.
10. Saltz LB, Cox JV, Blanke C, Rosen LS, Fehrenbacher L, Moore MJ, Maroun JA, Ackland SP, Locker PK, Pirotta N, Elfring GL, Miller LL (2000). Irinotecan plus fluorouracil and leucovorin for metastatic colorectal cancer. Irinotecan Study Group. N Engl J Med 343(13):905–914.

9 Sporadic Adenomas of the Large Intestine

S.B. Ho, J.H. Bond

Summary

Sporadic adenomas of the colon are extremely common in the general western population. The risk increases with age and is higher in men than women. The etiology of sporadic polyps is related to the individual's genetic background and exposure to environmental agents. Environmental factors that increase the risk of adenoma development include increased levels of dietary fat and decreased levels of specific vitamins and physical activity. Genetic events in colonic epithelium that set the stage for adenoma development include the early events of *APC* and *k-ras* gene mutations. The development of advanced adenomas results from accumulated genetic damage in cells within dysplastic or aberrant crypts. This primarily occurs in the setting of chromosomal instability, characterized by aneuploidy and alterations of *SMAD2*, *SMAD4*, *DCC*, and *p53* genes. A minority of sporadic adenomas develop as a result of inactivated DNA mismatch repair genes, and are characterized by normal (diploid) DNA content, microsatellite instability, and frequent mutations of TGFβRII. Sporadic adenomas are largely asymptomatic, but may occasionally present with rectal bleeding, anemia, or obstructive symptoms. Diagnosis and treatment of adenomas is primarily by colonoscopy. Screening for the presence of adenomas is accomplished by fecal occult blood testing and/or flexible sigmoidoscopies or colonoscopies. Once adenomas are removed current practice guidelines call for repeat surveillance colonoscopies at 3–5 year intervals. Calcium supplementation can reduce adenoma formation in patients with a previously resected adenoma, but the effect is modest. Primary prevention of colonic adenomas is best accomplished by diets low in fat and high in fiber, fruits, and vegetables; increased physical exercise; and avoidance of smoking, excessive alcohol, and obesity. Primary prevention by dietary supplements of vitamin E, vitamin C, selenium, or calcium; or the use of cyclooxygenase inhibitors (aspirin, sulindac) or selective cyclooxygenase (COX-2) inhibitors is currently under investigation and cannot be recommended for general use.

Epidemiology

Sporadic adenomas in the large intestine are common. They are detected by colonoscopy in 24–47% of asymptomatic persons over the age of 50 years in North America and Europe. The incidence of colorectal adenomas increases with age, and approximately 50% of patients 70 years and older may have an adenoma. The lifetime risk of developing colorectal cancer in patients with an adenoma is 1 in 20. Single small tubular adenomas are unlikely to develop into an invasive cancer, whereas the risk of malignant potential increases with the increasing adenoma size, villous histology, dysplasia, and age of the patient. The progression from an adenoma to invasive cancer takes from 4–11 years, depending on the degree of dysplasia.

Etiology and Pathogenesis

Adenomas develop from monoclonal derivatives of mutated colonic epithelial cells. Mutations result from the interactions of environmental factors such as diet and carcinogens and the underlying genetic susceptibility of an individual. Populations in high incidence countries tend to consume a diet high in animal meat and total fat and low in dietary fiber, fruits and vegetables. Excessive coloric intake leading to obesity is also a risk factor for adenoma development. Smoking, excessive alcohol intake, and a sedentary lifestyle also contribute to an increased risk.

A family history of colorectal cancer or adenomatous polyps identifies individuals who are at increased risk for sporadic adenomas and cancer. The specific genetic factors responsible for this predisposition are unknown. Specific genetic defects have been described for familial adenomatous polyposis and hereditary nonpolyposis colorectal cancer syndromes, but these account for only 1% and 6% of all colorectal cancers, respectively. Data from the National Polyp Study indicates that parents and siblings of patients with adenomas diagnosed at any age have a relative risk of colorectal cancer of 1.78 compared to spouse controls. The relative risk for siblings of patients in whom adenomas were diagnosed before the age of 60 was 2.59. The relative risk of siblings of patients with adenomas diagnosed at any age, who also had a parent with a history of colorectal cancer diagnosed at any age was 3.25.

Symptoms and Clinical Signs

Colorectal adenomas are largely asymptomatic. When symptoms occur, they are usually related to overt or occult rectal bleeding. Hematochezia usually occurs from adenomas in the descending colon, sigmoid, and rectum, whereas melena more commonly occurs from adenomas in the right colon. Occult bleeding is more common than overt bleeding, and can occur with both left and right-sided adenomas. Occult colon bleeding may go unrecognized until symptoms related to iron deficiency anemia develop. Rarely, large adenomas can present with symptoms suggestive of partial bowel obstruction.

Diagnostics

Synopsis

Colorectal adenomas can be diagnosed by endoscopy or barium enemas. When there is an indication to examine the whole colon, colonoscopy is the procedure of choice due to its greater accuracy and ability to perform biopsies and polypectomies. Cohort and case-control studies indicate that endoscopic polypectomy reduces the subsequent incidence and mortality of colorectal cancer.

Several studies have compared the accuracy of colonscopy to barium enemas for the detection of colorectal adenomas. Accuracy rates of 94% for colonoscopy and 67% for barium enemas were reported. The National Polyp Study found that barium enema studies missed 52% of polyps that were =1 cm in size. Studies of "tandem" colonscopy procedures in the same patient indicated an appreciable miss rate for small adenomas, but very few polyps =1 cm were missed by the initial colonoscopy. Colonscopy may be inadequate in 5–10% of patients when the instrument is not able to pass into the cecum, usually in those with extensive diverticulosis or previous pelvic surgery. Flexible sigmoidoscopy is used most commonly for screening average-risk asymptomatic patients.

Perforation from a diagnostic colonoscopy is rare, and has been reported in <0.1% of cases performed by experienced endoscopists. Perforation and clinically significant bleeding occur after colonoscopic polypectomy in approximately 0.2% and approximately 1%, respectively. Perforations resulting from colonoscopic polypectomy can occasionally be managed non-operatively, but if worsening signs of peritonitis occur an exploratory laparotomy is indicated. Perforations from diagnositic colonoscopy may represent a larger mucosal tear rather than a small perforation, and likely will require operative intervention. Major complications occur less frequently with barium enema (0.02%) and flexible sigmoidoscopy (0.01–0.04%).

Several case control studies have shown that endoscopic polypectomy reduces the subsequent incidence and mortality of colorectal cancer in the part of the colon examined by 50–79%. The National Polyp Study consisted of 1418 patients who had colonscopy and removal of at least one adenom a. After an average follow-up of 5.9 year, the incidence of colorectal cancer was 76–90% lower than expected compared to three reference groups.

A new radiologic method of imaging the large bowel, CT colonography or "virtual colonoscopy," combines rapid helical CT scanning of the abdomen with sophisticated computer hardware capable of rendering two- and three-dimensional views of the colon and rectum. Since its introduction in 1994, this promising new technique has undergone rapid refinement. Several published studies comparing the accuracy of virtual colonoscopy and standard colonoscopy show that this new method already is more accurate than double-contrast barium enema for detecting colorectal polyps of all sizes, and approaches the accuracy of standard colonoscopy for detecting large (>1 cm) polyps. Additional studies are underway to make this examination more acceptable to patients, shorten the time it takes for a radiologist to set-up and read the scans, and improve sensitivity and specificity for detecting colorectal neoplasia. Many predict that this method soon will become an effective screening option that will help increase public compliance for screening.

Histological Classification and Molecular Genetics

Synopsis

The risk of malignant transformation is increased in advanced adenomas, which are larger (=1 cm), contain appreciable villous histology or high grade dysplasia. The development of advanced adenomas results from accumulated genetic damage in colon epithelial cells. Alterations of the adenomatous polyposis coli (APC) tumor suppressor gene is an early step in adenoma formation, and have been shown to occur in dysplastic aberrant crypts. Subsequent genetic damage primarily occurs in the setting of chromosomal instability, characterized by aneuploidy and alterations of SMAD2, SMAD4, DCC, and p53 genes. Approximately 10–15% of sporadic adenomas may develop in the setting of defective DNA mismatch repair genes, and are characterized by normal DNA content, microsatellite instability, and frequent mutations of TGFbRII.

Adenomas are classified according to size and amount of villous histology. Adenomas are classified by the World Health Organization as tubular, tubulovillous, or villous, depending on the presence and volume of villous tissue (Fig. 1). Non-neoplastic polyps include hyperplastic polyps, hamartomas, lymphoid aggregates, juvenile polyps, and inflammatory polyps. Approximately 70% of polyps removed at colonoscopy are adenomas. Small (<1 cm) tubular adenomas are common and have a low risk of malignant potential. In contrast, larger (=1 cm) adenomas that may contain villous tissue or high-grade dysplasia are considered "advanced" adenomas and have an increased risk of malignant potential. Approximately 5–7% of patients with adenomas have high grade dysplasia and 3–5% have invasive carcinoma at the time of diagnosis. The risk of malignant potential correlates with increased adenoma size, villous histology, and patient age.

Colorectal adenomas result from molecular alterations in normal colonic cells that result in dysregulated cell growth. Accumulation of multiple molecular defects drives the histologic progression of early adenomas to late adenomas and then into cancers. Continued cell growth necessary for adenoma formation results from genetic alterations causing deregulated cell cycle checkpoints, loss of programmed cell death (apoptosis), and

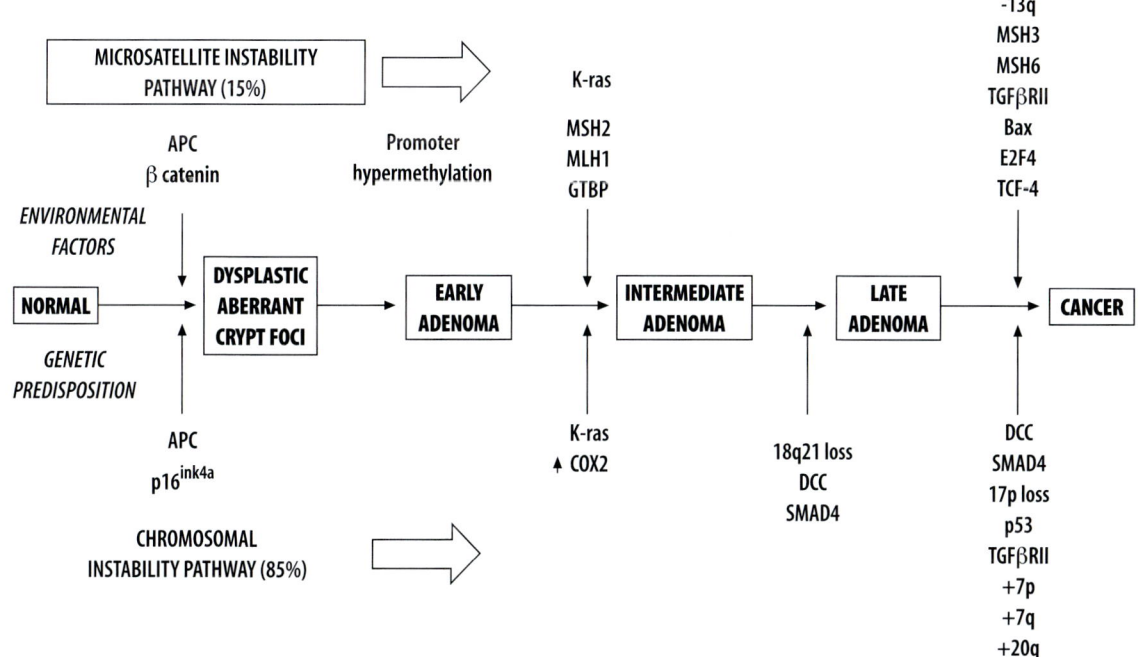

Figure 2
Molecular events in the adenoma to carcinoma sequence

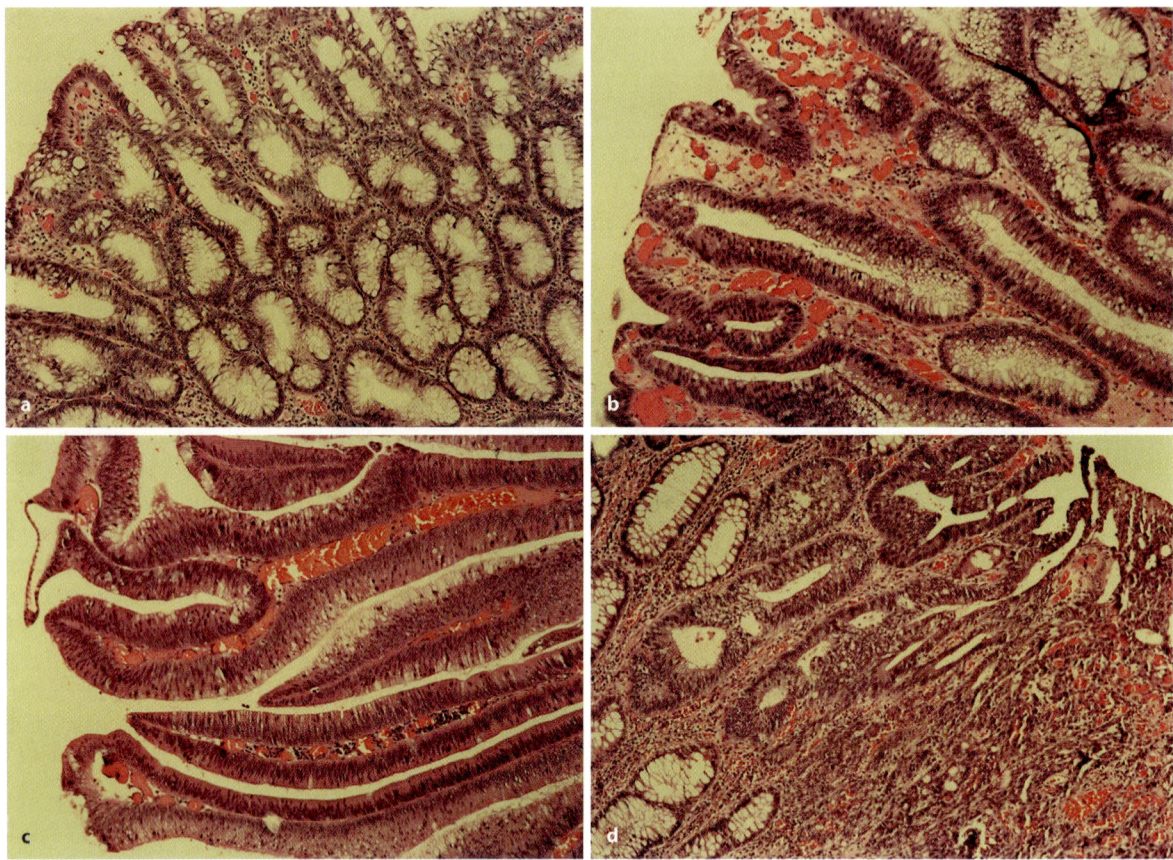

Figure 1a–d
Histology of colorectal adenomas. a Tubular adenoma (0–25% villous histology); **b** Tubulovillous adenoma (25–75% villous histology); **c** Villous adenoma (75–100% villous histology); **d** Tubulovillous adenoma with invasive carcinoma. All Photomicrographs taken with 10x objective (courtesy Dr. Stephen L. Ewing)

deregulated intracellular signalling pathways. These genetic alterations occur in two major classes of genes – proto-oncogenes and tumor suppressor genes. Activation of proto-oncogenes can occur by several mechanisms, including point mutations, gene amplification/rearrangement, or loss of promoter methylation. Only one allele of these genes needs to be altered in order to result in activation. Tumor suppressor genes inhibit cell growth. In general, both alleles of a tumor suppressor gene must be disabled by mutation, gene loss, or deactivation by promoter methylation for the cell to be affected.

Loss or inactivation of the adenomatous polyposis coli (*APC*) tumor suppressor gene is an early step in the

formation of sporadic adenomas. *APC* mutations have been shown to occur in dysplastic aberrant crypts, and ultimately are found in over 80% of sporadic colorectal cancers. *APC* mutations involve a truncated protein that loses all but one or two of the seven β-catenin binding/degradation sites. As a result, APC cannot downregulate β-catenin levels, resulting in increased translocation of β-catenin to the nucleus where it initiates transcription of genes involved in cell proliferation and prevention of apoptosis. The dysplastic aberrant crypt is characterized by persistant replication of dysplastic cells near the crypt surface, coupled with loss of apoptosis, leading to infolding and branching patterns in the crypt. Activating mutations of the *K-ras* proto-oncogene also occur at an early stage in adenoma formation, and are documented in approximately half of colonic neoplasms. Cyclooxygenase-2 (Cox-2) levels are increased in the majority of adenomas and cancers, whereas levels of cyclooxygenase-1 (Cox-1) remain unchanged. The mechanism by which increased Cox-2 activity promotes adenoma progression are unknown, but recent studies have implicated that the nuclear receptor PPARd may be activated by prostaglandins. Selective Cox-2 inhibitors have been shown to decrease polyp formation in patients with familial adenomatous polyposis.

Stepwise molecular alterations resulting in the progression of a small tubular adenoma to an advanced adenoma or cancer can occur in two types of pathways (Fig. 2). Approximately 85% of sporadic adenomas and cancers are characterized by chromosomal instability. These cancers display marked losses or gains in large portions of chromosomes. Tumor cells with abnormal quantities of DNA are termed aneuploid. In sporadic adenomas and cancers the most frequent reported chromosomal losses involve 5q, 18q, and 17p, whereas the most common gains involve 8q and 20q. Chromosomal instability is an early event in tumor formation that increases with tumor progression. The molecular basis for chromosomal instability is not clear, but may involve genes involved in kinetochore structure and function, centrosome and microtubule formation and behavior, chromosome condensation, sister chromatid cohesion, and cell cycle checkpoint control.

Inactivation of a component of the DNA mismatch repair system causes genomic instability by increasing the rate of polymerase-generated replication errors. This increases the error rate in DNA replication, particularly at microsatellite repeat sequences. Microsatellites is a term given to nucleotide repeat sequences (commonly An/Tn or CAn/GTn) that are distributed throughout the genome. Replication errors in dinucleotide repeats result in an increase in the numbers of these repeats in the tumor DNA, and is termed microsatellite instability. At least six genes have been identified that function in the human DNA repair system. Patients with hereditary non-polyposis colorectal cancer (HNPCC) have a germline mutation in a DNA mismatch repair gene, usually MSH2 or MLH1, resulting in cancers with microsatellite instability. Approximately 10–15% of sporadic colorectal cancers are also characterized by microsatellite instability. These cancers are diploid and do not have increased rates of chromosomal aberrations. Most patients with sporadic microsatellite instability cancers do not have mutations in the known DNA mismatch repair genes. In contrast, hypermethylation of the MLH1 promoter has been shown to occur in approximatley 70% of these cancers, resulting in inactivation of this mismatch repair gene. The molecular alterations that occur in the microsatellite mutator phenotype pathway are different from the chromosomal instability pathway. The most frequently mutated gene in the microsatellite pathway is the transforming growth factor-β receptor type II tumor suppressor gene, which occurs at the adenoma-carcinoma transition. β-catenin mutations are found in 16–25% of cancers with the microsatellite mutator phenotype, but are not common in microsatellite-stable cancers. Mutations of insulin growth factor 2 receptor; Bax and caspase 5, proteins that regulate apoptosis; E2F, a transcription factor; and MSH3 and MSH6 DNA mismatch repair proteins have been described in adenomas and cancers with the microsatellite mutator phenotype, but the timing of these events remains to be mapped. Colorectal cancers with the microsatellite mutator phenotype are more common on the right side of the colon, more poorly differentiated, may have a mucinous or signet-ring phenotype, and may have a better prognosis than other colorectal cancers.

Treatment

Synopsis

Small polyps detected by screening flexible sigmoidoscopy should be biopsied to determine if they are adenomatous. Data are conflicting as to whether small distal adenomas predict the presence of proximal advanced adenomas, therefore the decision to do colonoscopy must be individualized. A patient who has had successful colonoscopic excision of a large sessile polyp (=2 cm) should undergo follow-up colonoscopy in 3–6 months to determine whether resection was complete. If resection is not complete after two or three procedures, the good-risk patient should be referred for surgical resection. Malignant sessile polyps can be managed by colonoscopic polypectomy if the resected specimen has no prognostic features that may indicate an increased risk of residual cancer or nodal metastases.

Most patients with polyps detected by any means should undergo colonscopy to excise the polyp and search for additional neoplasms. When a small polyp is encountered during screening flexible sigmoidoscopy, it should be biopsied in order to determine if it is an adenoma. Hyperplastic polyps found during flexible sigmoidoscopy have not been shown to predict the presence of proximal adenomas, and hence are not an indication for colonoscopy. Several studies indicate that patients with one or two small tubular adenomas in the left colon are not at increased risk of subsequent colorectal cancer. Other studies give conflicting data regarding the risk of right sided adenomas in patients with one or two small adenomas in the left colon. On the other hand, patients with advanced adenomas in the left colon appear to have an increased risk for adenomas in the right colon. Therefore when a single small adenoma is found by flexible sigmoidoscopy, the decision to proceed with complete colonoscopic screening needs to be individualized.

Colonoscopic polypectomy alone is recommended for malignant polyps if the following criteria are met:

1. the polyp is considered to be completely excised;
2. the polyp is fixed and sectioned so that it is possible to determine the depth of invasion and completeness of excision;
3. the cancer is not poorly differentiated;
4. there is no vascular or lymphatic involvement;
5. the margin of excision is not involved.

Invasion of the stalk of a pedunculated polyp, by itself, is not an unfavorable prognostic finding. Patients with favorable prognostic criteria in a sessile polyp should undergo repeat colonoscopy in 3 months to check for residual abnormal tissue at the polypectomy site. If this is negative, then care can revert to standard surveillance. If a malignant polyp has poor prognostic features, the relative risks of surgical resection need to be weighed against the risk of death from metastatic cancer. The risk of death from elective colonic resection varies from 0.2% in young, healthy individuals to >5% in elderly patients. The risk of residual cancer or nodal metastases from endoscopically resected pedunculated or sessile polyps with favorable criteria are 0.3%–1.5%, respectively; whereas the risks associated with resected pedunculated or sessile polyps with poor prognostic features are 8.5%–14.4%, respectively.

Screening, Surveillance, Prevention

Screening

Screening of average risk populations using fecal occult blood testing or routine flexible sigmoidoscopies has been shown to decrease colorectal cancer incidence and mortality. A drawback of both of these techniques is the poor sensitivity of occult blood testing for advanced adenomas and the lack of accessing the right colon with flexible sigmoidoscopy. A multicenter Veterans Affairs Cooperative Study of asymptomatic patients between 50 and 75 years of age was performed to determine the efficacy of colonscopy in screening for colorectal neoplasia. A total of 3121 patients underwent colonoscopy, and 37.5% of patients were found to have one or more neoplastic lesions. Advanced adenomas were found in 9.5% of patients, and invasive cancer in 1.0%. Of the 1765 patients with no polyps in the left colon, 48 (2.7%) had advanced proximal neoplasms. Patients with adenomas in the distal colon were more likely to have advanced proximal neoplasms than were patients with no distal adenomas. However, 52% of the 128 patients with advanced proximal neoplasms had no distal adenomas. Ten patients (0.3%) had serious complications related to the procedure. Not surprisingly, these data indicate that screening colonoscopy can detect more advanced neoplasms compared with flexible sigmoidoscopy in asymptomatic adults. Further studies are needed to determine if routine colonoscopic screening is more effective than current screening methods for reducing the mortality rate from colorectal cancer.

Surveillance

In patients with a colorectal adenoma, the presence of synchronous polyps is 30–50%. Metachronous adenomas occur in 20–50% of patients, depending on the follow-up surveillance interval used. Several large patient series have found no increased incidence of cancer in patients after resection of small colorectal polyps (<1 cm) compared with local communities. These studies also have shown that patients with large (=1 cm) adenomas, adenomas with villous histology, or multiple adenomas have increased of subsequent adenomas. Data from the National Polyp Study showed that colonscopy performed 3 year after the initial colonscopic removal of adenomas detected advanced adenomas as effectively as follow-up colonoscopy performed after both 1 and 3 year. At 3 year only 3.3% of patients in each group had advanced adenomas. Therefore, current recommendations indicate that after complete clearing colonoscopy has been accomplished after an initial polypectomy, repeat colonscopy to check for metachronous adenomas should be performed in 3 years for patients with multiple (two or more) adenomas, a large =1 cm adenoma, or an adenoma with villous histology or high-grade dysplasia. Patients at low risk for metachronous adenomas can have a repeat colonoscopy in 5 years. These include patients with one or two small tubular adenomas and no family history of colorectal cancer. Further data indicates that after a patient has had one negative follow-up colonoscopy, the subsequent surveillance interval may safely be increased to 5 year. Selected patients at low risk for metachronous adenomas may not require follow-up surveillance, which needs to be individualized according to the age and co-morbidities of the patient.

Primary Prevention

A number of epidemiologic and animal studies have suggested that diets high in animal meat and total fat is linked to increased rates of adenoma and cancer formation. The National Cancer Institute has recommended that Americans eat a diet low in fat and high in fruits, vegetables, and fiber. A recent long term study employing dietary questionnaires in young female nurses showed no protective effect of total dietary fiber. Regular exercise that maintains a normal body weight can reduce the risk of colorectal neoplasia. Smoking and excessive alcohol intake has been linked to increased colorectal cancer rates, and should be avoided.

Numerous epidemiologic studies have shown a protective effect of aspirin and NSAIDs against adenomatous polyps, invasive cancer, or both. The Physicians Health Study evaluated the effects of aspirin (325 mg every other day) on cardiovascular events, and found that this dose did not lower the risk of colorectal adenomas or cancer. A recent prospective randomized trial by the Polyp Prevention Study Group, however, demonstrated a modest statistically significant reduction in recurrent adenomas in patients taking low-dose aspirin compared

to placebo. This effect was most pronounced for recurrent advanced lesions (adenomas one centimeter or greater, those with tubulovillous or villous histology, severe dysplasia or cancer).

Randomized controlled trials involving patients with prior adenomas have been conducted involving the use of beta carotenes and fiber supplements. No differences in the rate of adenoma or colorectal cancer formation was demonstrated in groups randomized to the supplements compared with controls. The Polyp Prevention Trial randomized over two thousand subjects with a history of colorectal adenomas to receive counseling together with a low-fat, high-fiber diet rich in fruits and vegetables, or to receive their usual diet alone. The incidence of recurrent adenomas at 1 and 4 years as determined by colonoscopy was similar in both groups. The Phoenix Colon Cancer Prevention Network found that administration of supplemental fiber as wheat bran also failed to affect the incidence of recurrent adenomas at a median follow-up of 34–36 months. One recent trial randomized patients after resection of one or more adenomas to 3 gm calcium carbonate daily or control over a 4 year period. The total number of recurrent adenomas was reduced 24% in the group taking calcium. Studies are underway to determine the efficacy of aspirin, rofecoxib, and celocoxib in preventing the recurrence of sporadic adenomas after polypectomy. Also under investigation is the combination of NSAIDs and folate, eflornithine, angiotensin-converting-enzyme inhibitors, statins, or calcium. Enthusiasm for the use of Cox-2 inhibitors is tempered by the possible risk of cardiovascular events due to a prothombotic potential.

Future Perspectives

Current screening and treatment strategies for colorectal adenomas have the promise of reducing colorectal cancer mortality; this will continue to improve with new technologic advances and continued basic science research. New diagnostic techniques for screening average and high risk populations will be developed. These include the use of radiologic "virtual" colonscopy and the use of molecular markers in blood and stool. Technologic advances in fiberoptic colonscopes will occur that will increase the efficacy, safety and comfort of colonoscopic procedures. Finally, increased understanding of the molecular pathways involved in adenoma formation and of predisposing genetic susceptibility genes will enable us to identify and tailor specific interventions to populations at greatest risk. Primary prevention of colorectal adenomas also holds the promise of preventing colorectal cancer.

References

1. Bond JH. Polyp guideline: Diagnosis, treatment, and surveillance for patient with colorectal polyps. Am J Gastroenterol 2000;95:3053–3063.
2. Terdiman JP. Genomic events in the adenoma to carcinoma sequence. Seminars Gastrointest Dis 2000;11:194–206.
3. Schatzkin A, Lanza E, Carlo D. Lack of effect of a low-fat, high-fiber diet on the recurrence of colorectal adenomas. N Engl J Med 2000; 342: 1149–55.
4. Alberts DS, Martinez ME, Roe DJ. Lack of effect of a high-fiber cereal supplement on the recurrence of colorectal adenomas. N Engl J Med 2000;342:1156–62.
5. Hennekens CH, Buring JE, Manson JE. Lack of effect of long-term supplementation with beta carotene on the incidence of malignant neoplasms and cardiovascular disease. N Engl J Med 1996;334:1145–9.
6. Winawer SJ, Stewart ET, Zauber AG et al. A comparison of colonoscopy and double-contrast barium enema for surveillance after polypectomy. National Polyp Study Work Group. N Engl J Med 2000;342:1766–72.
7. Winawer SJ, Zauber AG, Ho MN et al. Prevention of colorectal cancer by colonoscopic polypectomy. N Eng J Med 1993;329:1977–1981.
8. Netzer P, Binek J, Hammer B, Lange J, Schmassmann A. Significance of histologic criteria for the management of patients with malignant colorectal polyps and polypectomy. Scand J Gastroenterol 1997; 32: 910–6.
9. Haggitt RC, Glotzbach RE, Soffer EE, Wruble LD. Prognostic factors in colorectal carcinomas arising in adenomas: implications for lesions removed by endoscopic polypectomy. Gastroenterology 1985; 89: 328–36.
10. Volk EE, Goldblum JR, Petras RE, Carey WD, Fazio VW. Management and outcome of patients with invasive carcinoma arising in colorectal polyps. Gastroenterology 1995;109:1801–7.
11. Potter JD, Slattery ML, Bostick RM, Gapstur SM. Colon cancer: a review of the epidemiology. Epidemiol Rev 1993;15:499–545.
12. Winawer SJ, Zauber AG, O'Brien MJ et al. Randomized comparison of surveillance intervals after colonoscopic removal of newly diagnosed adenomatous polyps. The National Polyp Study Workgroup. N Engl J Med 1993;328:901–6.
13. Greenberg ER, Baron JA, Tosteson TD et al. A clinical trial of antioxidant vitamins to prevent colorectal adenoma. Polyp Prevention Study Group. N Engl J Med 1994;331:141–7.
14. Winawer SJ, Zauber AG, Gerdes H et al. Risk of colorectal cancer in the families of patients with adenomatous polyps. National Polyp Study Workgroup. N Engl J Med 1996;334:82–7.
15. Fenlon HM, Nunes DP, Schroy PC, et al. A comparison of virtual and conventional colonoscopy for the detection of colorectal polyps. N Engl J Med 1999;341:1496–1503.
16. Janne PA, Mayer RJ. Chemoprevention of colorectal cancer. N Engl J Med 2000;342:1960–8.
17. Lieberman DA, Weiss DG, Bond JH, Ahnen DJ, Garewal H, Chejfec G. Use of colonoscopy to screen asymptomatic adults for colorectal cancer. Veterans Affairs Cooperative Study Group 380. N Engl J Med 2000; 343: 162–8.

10 Hereditary Polyposis Syndromes

J.M. CARETHERS

Summary

The polyposis syndromes are a group of clinically distinct, autosomal dominantly inherited disorders characterized by the finding of multiple polyps in the gastrointestinal tract and a predisposition to cancer. There are two groups of syndromes. In the adenomatous polyposis syndromes, the polyps are dysplastic and the risk of colon cancer formation in patients with adenomas approaches 100%. These syndromes have provided key insights into the pathogenesis and genetics of sporadic, non-familial colorectal cancer. The second group is the hamartomatous polyposis syndromes in which mature but non-dysplastic and disorganized tissue characterizes the histology of the polyps. Some patients with hamartomatous syndromes may develop colon cancer, but extra-intestinal cancers may be more common, depending on the syndrome. Familiarity with these syndromes is paramount in patient management. The key management strategies include the surveillance and prevention of known complications of these syndromes. Many of the genes that are linked to these syndromes have now been described, which provides an avenue for genetic testing in individuals with a syndrome, as well as in family members prior to the development of signs of the syndrome.

Adenomatous Polyposis Syndromes

Familial Adenomatous Polyposis (FAP) and its Variants

Epidemiology

FAP, (also known as adenomatous polyposis coli) is an autosomal dominant inherited disorder characterized by hundreds to thousands of adenomatous polyps throughout the colon. All patients with this syndrome will develop colon cancer if left untreated. Because the genetic defect in the germ line of FAP patients has been characterized, it is now recognized that syndromes thought distinct from FAP are in reality part of the phe-notypic spectrum of FAP. Syndromes with a germ line mutation in the *adenomatous polyposis coli* (*APC*) gene include FAP, Gardner syndrome, some Turcot syndrome families, and Attenuated Adenomatous Polyposis Coli (AAPC) (Table 1).

FAP and its variants contribute 1% of the total colorectal cancer burden. FAP has been described in all races worldwide. It occurs between 1 in 7000 to 1 in 10,000 births, with a male:female ratio of 1:1. The average age of adenomatous polyp development is approximately 16 yrs, and the average age of colorectal cancer is approximately 40 yrs of age.

Etiology and Pathogenesis

The *APC* gene is a tumor suppressor gene that becomes inactivated as the initial step in the formation of an adenomatous polyp. Thus, the *APC* gene is considered the "gatekeeper" of colonic neoplasia. When mutated in the germ line (i.e. inherited), every cell in the affected person contains one mutated and one normal copy of *APC*. Mutation of *APC* almost always results in a truncated protein. In the colon, an event occurs that inactivates the remaining normal copy of *APC* (usually by mutation in FAP), thus completely removing APC's tumor suppressive function. This allows for the initiation of adenomatous polyp growth. Because every cell is affected by the germ line mutation, all colonic epithelial cells already have one APC allele mutated. Inactivation of the second APC allele is widespread in the colon, allowing numerous adenomas to develop.

Normal APC protein promotes apoptosis in colonic cells. Its most important function may be to sequester oncogenic β-catenin, a protein that transcriptionally accelerates growth in conjunction with TCF factors. Thus, loss of APC function would prevent apoptosis and allow β-catenin to accumulate intracellularly and stimulate cell growth. Clonal expansion of cells that lack APC function occurs, and these cells' rapid growth increases the possibility for other growth-advantageous genetic events to occur. Ultimately, enough genetic events hap-

Table 1
Polyposis syndromes and their associated germ line-mutated genes

Polyposis Syndrome	Chromosomal Location	Mutated Gene	Frequency in Germline [%]
Familial Adenomatous Polyposis	5q21	APC	100
Gardner's Syndrome (FAP Variant)	5q21	APC	100
Lynch Syndrome (HNPCC)	2p16	hMSH2	45
	3p21	hMLH1	49
	2p16	hMSH6	1
Muir-Torre Syndrome	2p16	hMSH2	100
Turcot's Syndrome			
– FAP Variant	5q21	APC	67
– Lynch Variant	7p22, 3p21	hPMS2, hMLH1	33
Hereditary Mixed Polyposis Syndrome	6q	unknown	-
Juvenile Polyposis (JPS)	18q21.1	SMAD4	21–50
	10q22.3	PTEN/MMAC1/TEP1	<10
	10q22	BMPR1A/ALK3	?50
Bannayan-Riley-Ruvalcaba (BRRS)	10q23	PTEN/MMAC1/TEP1	~60
Cowden Disease (CD)	10q22–23	PTEN/MMAC1/TEP1	>80
Peutz-Jeghers Syndrome	19p13.3	STK11/LKB1	70–90%

pen to allow the adenomatous polyp in FAP patients to become malignant, and this process is similar to that of sporadic adenomas.

Symptoms and Clinical Signs

The majority of FAP patients are asymptomatic until cancer development. In rare instances, nonspecific symptoms of unexplained anemia, rectal bleeding, diarrhea, or abdominal pain could be present. A careful family history and pedigree may suggest the possibility of FAP if there is a history of multiple adenomas and colorectal cancer, particularly if relatives are under the age of 40 yrs.

Congenital hypertrophy of the retinal pigment epithelium is pigmented ocular fundus lesions that range in size from 0.1 to 1.0 fundic disc diameters and are best seen by ophthalmologic slit lamp examination. In FAP, these are often bilateral and multiple, and often precede the polyposis in patients. The presence of these lesions correlates with mutations between exons 9 and 15 of the APC gene.

A number of extra-intestinal manifestations can be seen in FAP patients, and were used to define the Gardner's variant of FAP. Osteomas of the skull and mandible may be present. Dental abnormalities, including supernumerary teeth, unerupted teeth, dentigerous cysts, and odontomas may be found. Epidermoid cysts (often developed before puberty) located on the legs, face, scalp, and arms may be manifested. Fibromas may be located on the scalp, shoulders, arms, and back of an FAP patient. (Table 2).

Diagnostics

Because of the diffuse nature of the polyposis, a flexible sigmoidoscopy with visualization of >100 polyps in a patient is adequate to make the diagnosis of FAP. Colonoscopy is appropriate for suspected AAPC patients because of the reduction in the diffuse nature of the polyposis. Removal of some polyps by endoscopic polypectomy is needed to confirm the diagnosis of adenomatous polyps at histological examination.

Dental and skull x-rays for suspected osteomas and dental abnormalities may be used to aid in the diagnosis of FAP. Esophagogastroduodenoscopy, performed after a diagnostic sigmoidoscopy or colonoscopy, might be used to evaluate for the presence of duodenal and periampullary adenomas. Benign fundic gland polyps are often seen in the fundus and body of the stomach.

Germ line testing is available commercially for patients suspected of having FAP or AAPC. The tests available only require a peripheral blood sample in which the white blood cells have their RNA or DNA extracted. All genetic testing should be done after consultation with a trained genetic counselor. A truncated protein test (also called the *in vitro* protein synthesis assay) utilizes the extracted RNA, which is reverse transcribed ultimately into five overlapping segments of the APC protein. Because most mutations of this large gene cause truncation of APC, a shortened piece of the protein can often be detected to demonstrate the presence of a mutation. A second approach is to amplify APC DNA by the polymerase chain reaction from the blood sample, and directly sequence the product. With both approaches, the proband is tested first to confirm (or deny) the presence of a mutation. If the proband possesses a mutation, then other family members can be tested for the identical mutation after genetic counseling.

Histological Classification and Molecular Genetics

Patients with FAP and its variants have multiple adenomatous polyps upon histological examination. Since there are other syndromes that manifest with multiple polyps that are not adenomas, histological examination is important to confirm the diagnosis.

The progression of an adenoma to cancer is thought to occur through a series of mutations and loss of genes during clonal expansion within the polyp. After both alleles of APC are inactivated, mutations in oncogenic K-RAS are selected and allow the adenoma to grow as an exophytic growth. Mutation of the *P53* tumor suppressor gene on chromosome 17p and mutation of an 18q allele (presumably at the *DCC, SMAD2* or *SMAD4* loci) occur, followed by loss of the remaining normal alleles at these chromosomes, allowing malignant transformation that is recognized at the tissue level.

While all of the FAP variants have mutation of the APC gene by definition, there are historical differences as well as observed genotype-phenotype correlations among the variants. Gardner's variant and traditional FAP were historically identified separately, with extraintestinal manifestations defining the Gardner's variant. Both of these variants share similar mutational spectrums of the APC gene. Most mutations of APC are nonsense or frame shift mutations, leading to truncation of the APC protein, and occur in exon 15 between codons 1250 and 1464 (the middle portion of the gene). AAPC, which demonstrates fewer polyps in the colon and has an older age of cancer onset, has mutations of the APC gene that occur at the extreme 5' or 3' end of the gene. Approximately two-thirds of Turcot's variant families demonstrate mutations in APC that are not different

Table 2
Polyposis syndromes and their clinical and cancer associations.

Polyposis Syndrome	Non-Cancer Associations	Cancer Associations
FAP and variants	Congenital hypertrophy of the retinal pigment epithelium, desmoid, dental abnormalities, epidermoid cysts	Colorectal, duodenal ampullary, medulloblastoma
Lynch syndrome and variants	Sebaceous adenomas and carcinomas, keratoacanthomas (Muir-Torre)	Colorectal, endometrial, ovarian, kidney, ureter, bladder, stomach, small intestine, glioblastoma
JPS	Rare congenital abnormalities	colorectal, pancreas, gastric, duodenal
BRRS	Macrocephaly, visceral and cutaneous hamartomas, pigmentation of penis in males, Hashimoto's thyroiditis	? similar to Cowden disease ? similar to JPS
Cowden Disease	Facial trichilemmomas, mucocutaneous papules, goiter, fibrocystic breast disease, cerebellar gangliocytomatosis (Lhermitte-Duclos)	medullary thyroid, breast
Peutz-Jeghers syndrome	Mucocutaneous melanosis	Small intestine, stomach, pancreas, colorectal, esophagus, ovary, lung, uterus, breast
Hereditary Mixed Polyposis Syndrome	none	colorectal

from those in traditional FAP families. Since Turcot's variant was defined as the co-existence of adenomatous polyposis and brain tumors, the type of brain tumors associated with FAP and APC mutations were found to be medulloblastomas, and it was realized that all FAP patients have an elevated risk for this tumor (see Tables 1 and 2).

Treatment

In unoperated FAP, colonoscopic surveillance every 3 to 6 months with removal of large polyps is recommended. However, because of the diffuse nature of the polyposis and the inevitability of colorectal cancer, surgical therapy is ultimately required. Surgical therapy should occur before the typical onset of cancer. Colectomy with mucosal proctectomy and ileoanal pouch pull through has become the procedure of choice for many centers. This procedure allows the retention of rectal function. Other options include: subtotal colectomy with ileoanal anastomosis, and total proctocolectomy with ileostomy.

Prognosis

Untreated FAP has a life expectancy of 42 years of age. Since the risk of colorectal cancer is 100% in FAP, life expectancy is extended greatly in those treated with colectomy. The most common cause of death in colectomized FAP patients is upper gastrointestinal cancers and desmoids. The cumulative probability of non-colorectal cancer development of any type is 11% by age 50 years, and 52% by age 75 years, mostly due to periampullary tumors. The overall frequency for duodenal or periampullary adenocarcinoma in FAP is 4 to 12%. Desmoid formation can occur in 20% of FAP patients, and typically occurs post-colectomy. Other cancers that may rarely develop include medulloblastoma (Turcot's variant), hepatoblastoma, and thyroid and adrenal cancers.

Follow-Up

The FAP patient must be monitored closely for surveillance of cancer formation. Medical therapy, such as the NSAIDs sulindac or celecoxib, has no role as sole primary therapy in unoperated FAP. Neither sulindac nor celecoxib prevent or delay the onset of polyposis. However, in FAP patients who have had colectomy with ileoanal anastomosis, sulindac (or celecoxib) may be beneficial in reducing the size and number of adenomatous polyps in the remaining rectum. Sigmoidoscopic surveillance of retained rectum or ileal pouch in operated FAP should occur every 3 to 6 months. Endoscopic ablation of the rectal adenomas should be done. Eventual rectal resection is necessary in some because of the inability to control polyps medically.

Once the diagnosis of FAP is made, esophagogastroduodenoscopy every 1 to 3 years should be performed. Scrutiny of the papilla of Vater is best done accurately with a side-viewing endoscope.

Intra-abdominal desmoid tumors may respond to anti-estrogen therapy (i.e. tamoxifen) because of a suspected estrogen support for its growth. Sulindac may also be beneficial in slowing a desmoid's growth. Chemotherapy with doxorubicin and dacarbazine may be attempted if there is no response. Extra-abdominal desmoids may be resected with adequate margins. Resection of intra-abdominal desmoids is generally reserved for ureteral or intestinal obstruction.

Screening, Surveillance, Prevention

Patients with FAP should be educated on the need for cancer surveillance after colectomy.

Surveillance of family members of FAP patients should begin by age 12 years. Flexible sigmoidoscopy every 1–2 years until the age of 35 is adequate, then every 3 years thereafter. Genetic testing may eliminate the need for surveillance in some family members. Genetic counseling should be offered before any genetic testing is done. The patient and family members should be made aware of the limitations of genetic testing, and the consequences associated with genetic testing.

Lynch Syndrome (Hereditary Non-Polyposis Colorectal Cancer (HNPCC)) and its Variants

Epidemiology

Lynch syndrome is an autosomal dominantly inherited genetic disease characterized by an increased risk for cancers of the colon, rectum, and a number of other organs including the female reproductive and urinary tracts (see Table 2). Lynch syndrome is a cancer predisposition syndrome without apparent antecedent polyposis (thus the prior name of hereditary non-polyposis colorectal cancer). The apparent proportion of families with Lynch syndrome (based upon a history of multiple cancers in the family) is approximately 3–4% of all colo-rectal cancers. These estimates predict a prevalence in the population of approximately 1/300 to 1/500. The true estimate is not realized, given the lack of consideration of non-colonic cancer involvement in many studies, and the lower penetrance (70–80%) for the expression of the syndrome. A more realistic estimate for the frequency of HNPCC in the general population may be higher.

The average age of colorectal cancer development in Lynch syndrome is 40 years of age. This is 2 to 3 decades younger than the typical development of sporadic colo-rectal cancer. Multiple synchronous primary tumors develop 18% of the time, and metachronous tumors ac-cumulate at a 3 to 5% rate per year. Lynch syndrome-associated colon tumors demonstrate microsatellite instability (MSI, defined below), are significantly corre-lated with the tumor's location in the proximal (right) colon and have an overall increased survival compared to non-MSI tumors (despite having a histologically poor grade). The hyper-mutable phenotype associated with MSI appears to be a mechanism for rapid neoplastic progression in Lynch syndrome, making the finding of polyps challenging in this syndrome.

There are three additional Lynch syndrome variants recognized. Muir-Torre syndrome is characterized by Lynch syndrome-associated cancers together with skin tumors such as sebaceous adenomas, epitheliomas, kera-toacanthomas, and sebaceous carcinomas. Additionally, approximately one-third of Turcot's syndrome patients have mutations in the DNA mismatch repair (MMR) genes associated with Lynch syndrome and no mutation in APC. The brain tumors in this Turcot's variant of Lynch syndrome are glioblastomas, as opposed to the medulloblastomas seen in the Turcot's variant of FAP. Finally, an attenuated form of Lynch syndrome has been described in which patients present with cancer at an older age (61 yrs) and there is a tendency for endome-trial cancer predominance in women. This attenuated form is caused by mutations in the DNA MMR protein hMSH6, which has some redundant functions with another DNA MMR protein (hMSH3). This overlap in function is hypothesized to be responsible for the later onset of cancer.

Etiology and Pathogenesis

Lynch syndrome is associated with germ line mutation of one of the proteins that comprise the DNA MMR sys-tem (see Table 1). The DNA MMR system is an evolution-arily conserved system capable of repairing mispaired nucleotides and short mismatched loops in DNA, pre-sumably as a result of insertion mistakes made by DNA polymerases during replication. The mismatch repair system replaces the mispair on the newly synthesized daughter strand, as these proteins recognize the nicks present in the newly synthesized strand. Defects in the mismatch repair genes *hMSH2*, *hMLH1*, and *hMSH6* in humans have been linked to Lynch syndrome. As the DNA MMR proteins function as tumor suppressors, when the second allele is inactivated in a target tissue thus eliminating protein expression, nonrepair of poly-merase mistakes within the DNA strands ensues. This is detected in the laboratory as MSI, which represents the inability to repair frameshift alterations caused by loop formation at repetitive DNA sequences termed micro-satellites. Most microsatellites occur in non-coding re-gions of DNA. However, some genes have microsatellites in their coding regions, and the formation of cancer seems dependent on the cell's selection for these muta-tions. Genes commonly inactivated in Lynch associated colon tumors include the *transforming growth factor β receptor II* gene, the *activin A type II receptor* gene, *BAX*, the *insulin-like growth factor II receptor* gene, the *TCF-4* transcription factor, and two of the DNA mismatch re-pair genes, *hMSH3* and *hMSH6*.

There is clinical and genetic evidence for rapid pro-gression through an adenoma to carcinoma sequence in microsatellite unstable colorectal cancers. The genetic mishaps during this progression are different than those seen for FAP and most sporadic tumors, but still may require inactivation of the "gatekeeper" function of the APC/β-catenin/TCF-4 pathway. Given the improved sur-vival of patients with microsatellite unstable colon tu-mors, it is possible that there is some beneficial effect of the hyper-mutable phenotype to slow metastases once the cancer has formed.

Symptoms and Clinical Signs

Patients with Lynch syndrome are often asymptomatic until cancer formation occurs. Tumors of this syndrome often occur at uncharacteristically early ages compared to non-gene carriers. Colorectal cancer is the predominant feature of Lynch syndrome, and occurs in an approximately 80% of all gene carriers. The majority of colon cancers (60–70% of the tumors) occur proximal to the splenic flexure. Iron deficiency, abdominal pain or symptoms of colonic obstruction may be present after cancer formation. In women, endometrial cancer could be the presenting tumor, with pelvic pain and menorrhea.

Diagnostics

The diagnosis of Lynch syndrome is usually made by considering the family history. Even a single first-degree relative who develops a colorectal or endometrial cancer at a very young age raises this possibility. There is no pre-morbid clinical phenotype that identifies a Lynch syndrome patient antecedent to the development of cancer. Because of the lack of premorbid phenotype, clinical criteria were developed in Amsterdam, The Netherlands. These criteria originally stated that to clinically diagnose a Lynch syndrome kindred, there should be 3 relatives with histologically verified colorectal cancer, of which one is a first degree relative of the other 2, at least 2 successive generations affected, at least one colorectal cancer occurring before age 50, and FAP is excluded. These criteria proved to be exclusive of some families, and a revision was put forth later that included endometrial, small bowel, ureteral and renal pelvis cancer as part of the defining spectrum.

A subset of Lynch syndrome families has a constellation of findings termed the Muir-Torre Syndrome. This syndrome consists of all of the features of Lynch syndrome plus sebaceous gland tumors and keratoacanthomas. Basal and squamous cell carcinomas also occur in Muir-Torre Syndrome. Although these skin tumors are unusual manifestations of Lynch syndrome, this diagnosis should be considered in any patient who has more than one skin tumor of this variety.

Polyps or tumors from a suspected Lynch syndrome patient may be sent for MSI testing. In sporadic adenomatous polyps, it is rare to find MSI and thus its presence could indicate the possibility of Lynch syndrome. Colorectal cancers of Lynch syndrome patients almost always demonstrate MSI, but since approximately 15% of sporadic colorectal cancers also demonstrate MSI, it is not specific to Lynch syndrome. If a colorectal cancer does not demonstrate MSI, then it is very unlikely to have come from a Lynch syndrome patient. Thus, MSI testing could be used as a screen prior to genetic testing for mutated DNA MMR genes.

Direct sequencing of the exons in *hMSH2* and *hMLH1* is the most straightforward approach to diagnosing Lynch syndrome. At this time, the full spectrum of disease-producing germ line mutations and innocuous polymorphisms has not been catalogued, which may complicate the interpretation of DNA sequence data. The range of germ line mutations in *hMSH2* and *hMLH1* (the two most common genes mutated) is wide, and includes insertions, deletions, nonsense mutations, and missense mutations. Large deletions of genetic material that span part of a DNA MMR gene will not be identified by direct sequencing, and the patient may be classified as having no mutation present. Thus, clinical suspicion and family history may form the cornerstone of diagnosis in some families.

Histological Classification and Molecular Genetics

Colorectal neoplasms in Lynch syndrome occur at early ages, and most are in the proximal colon. Using typical pathological criteria, 37% of colorectal cancers are classified as poorly differentiated, which would suggest that the tumors would behave aggressively. Contrary to this, colorectal cancers in Lynch syndrome have a better outcome than sporadic tumors matched for stage. Colorectal cancers in Lynch syndrome are significantly more likely to be diploid or near diploid compared to sporadic tumors. Over 35% of colorectal cancers in Lynch syndrome are mucinous carcinomas. Approximately 40% of tumors have a lymphoid "Crohn's-like" reaction around the tumor. These pathological features may increase one's suspicion of Lynch syndrome when they are found in familial clusters of cancer.

The genetics of Lynch syndrome are somewhat complex, but follow the paradigms of other tumor suppressor genes. The evolutionarily conserved genes which comprise the MMR system and that have been found mutated in Lynch syndrome families include *hMSH2*, *hMLH1*, and *hMSH6*. Although other components of the MMR system have been identified (*hMSH3*, *hPMS2*, and *hPMS1*), germ line mutations have not been convincingly found in Lynch syndrome families. When a physical deformation remains in the newly replicated DNA double helix (caused by the mispairing of nucleotides or due to slippage and looping at microsatellite loci), a complex termed hMutSα (a heterodimer of hMSH2 and hMSH6 proteins) identifies the error and binds the DNA at this site. Subsequently, hMutSα recruits the hMutLα complex, a heterodimer of hMLH1 and hPMS2 proteins, which targets the newly synthesized, daughter DNA strand for "long patch" excision repair. It remains unclear how hPMS1 interacts within the complex. Loss of any of the components of the MMR system will inactivate or attenuate repair. Germ line mutations in the *hMLH1* and *hMSH2* genes account for the majority of Lynch syndrome families identified to date. One wild-type allele of a MMR gene is generally sufficient to maintain normal MMR function. For colon cancer to develop in Lynch syndrome patients, a second somatic event (in addition to the vertically transmitted mutant allele) must occur in the wild type allele of a colonocyte. This makes both of the MMR genes completely inactive and causes the hyper-mutable phenotype seen within Lynch syndrome tumors.

Treatment

When a Lynch syndrome patient presents with an invasive cancer, the appropriate treatment is to perform a subtotal colectomy with an ileosigmoid or ileorectal anastomosis. The increased risk for tumor development in the rest of the colon mandates aggressive surgical treatment, but the ability to screen the rectum for recurrent disease makes a total proctocolectomy unnecessary. If a patient should present with an invasive rectal cancer, a total proctocolectomy may be required.

There are no known medical treatments for patients with Lynch syndrome. Aspirin may play an important protective effect against the development of sporadic colorectal cancer, however its impact in Lynch syndrome is not known. No interventions other than diagnostic screening and prophylactic surgery have been demonstrated to have a beneficial effect in this disease.

Prognosis

A Lynch syndrome patient must be monitored closely for cancer formation in the absence of colectomy. Cumulative risk for colorectal cancer in Lynch syndrome has been estimated at 78%, and endometrial cancer has been estimated at 20–40%. Patients with Lynch syndrome develop colorectal cancer at an average age of 40 years. There is a propensity for multiple synchronous

and metachronous cancers to develop in the colon, and extracolonic tumors can develop metachronously as well.

Follow-Up

There is an increased risk of synchronous and metachronous cancers of the colon, rectum, and other organs, including the small bowel, stomach, the female reproductive tract and the urinary tract. Surveillance of the colon for unoperated Lynch syndrome patients should be done with colonoscopy every 1–2 years starting around 20 years of age or at least 10 years prior to the youngest cancer patient in the kindred. There appears to be no increase in risk for cancer of the lung, breast, prostate, bladder, bone marrow or larynx.

Screening, Surveillance, Prevention

To evaluate a potential Lynch syndrome kindred, a careful family history should be taken in all patients who develop a cancer. A full pedigree should be drawn, and critical information should include all relatives who develop tumors, the organs affected, the age of first cancer, the occurrence of multiple cancers, and the ages reached by individuals who did not develop cancer. When the Amsterdam criteria are met, Lynch syndrome is very likely. When available, tumor tissue from paraffin-embedded tissues can be assayed for MSI. If no MSI is found, the likelihood of Lynch syndrome is substantially reduced.

Once Lynch syndrome patients are identified, a screening program consisting of colonoscopy every 1–2 years significantly reduces the rate of tumor development and death in patients with Lynch syndrome.

Patients who are identified in the pre-symptomatic stage by genetic testing should be informed that their lifetime risk for colorectal cancer is probably 80–90% and that surveillance colonoscopy every three years can significantly reduce morbidity and mortality. Genetic testing after genetic counseling can be offered to confirm the diagnosis, and identify family members at risk which helps direct surveillance efforts. Once a mutation is identified in a Lynch syndrome patient, there is near 100% accuracy in identifying carriers and non-carriers in the kindred.

Further information on Lynch Syndrome can be found in the chapter written by Lynch et al.

Hamartomatous Polyposis Syndromes

Peutz-Jeghers (P-J) Syndrome

Epidemiology

P-J syndrome is an autosomal dominantly inherited disorder characterized by intestinal hamartomatous polyps in association with mucocutaneous melanocytic macules. The syndrome was named after Peutz, who first noted a relationship between the intestinal polyps and the mucocutaneous macules in 1921, and Jeghers' definitive description in 1944 and 1949.

P-J syndrome is rare, with a frequency encounter from polyposis registries one-tenth as often as FAP. This would place the range of occurrence from 1 in 70,000 to 1 in 200,000 people. P-J syndrome has been described in all races, and has a male to female ratio of 1:1. The average age of diagnosis is 23 years in men, and 26 years in women.

Etiology and Pathogenesis

The cause of P-J syndrome appears to be a germ line mutation of the *STK11* (*serine threonine protein kinase 11*, also called *LKB1*) gene, located on chromosome 19p13.3. Because the signaling pathway of the *STK11* gene product is currently not identified, the mechanism of hamartomatous polyp formation and mucocutaneous pigmentation is not known. There is some suggestion through murine models that STK11 is involved in vascular endothelial growth factor (VEGF) signaling.

Symptoms and Clinical Signs

Patients with P-J syndrome, have characteristic mucocutaneous pigmentary spots in association with intestinal hamartomatous polyps. Pigmentary macules (1–5 mm) are often in the perioral region and cross the vermilion border. These macules may fade after puberty.

The principal causes of morbidity in P-J syndrome stem from the intestinal location of the polyps (small intestine >>colon >stomach). These include small intestinal obstruction and intussuseption (43%), abdominal pain (23%), hematochezia (14%), and prolapse of a colonic polyp (7%), and typically occur in the second and third decades of life. As the P-J patient ages, the morbidity risk shifts to that of malignancy, particularly cancers

of the luminal GI tract, pancreas, female reproductive tract, lung and breast. Thus, patients may present with symptoms of cancer if the diagnosis was not previously made.

Diagnostics

A careful history and physical examination of the patient will often make the diagnosis of P-J syndrome, usually in association with the classic histological findings within a polyp. Clues from a patient's history may include episodes of repeated bouts of abdominal pain in a patient (particularly if less than 25 years old), unexplained intestinal bleeding in a young patient, prolapse of "tissue" from the rectum in a young patient, and menstrual irregularities in females (due to hyper-estrogenism from sex cord tumors with annular tubules). A family history of P-J syndrome may be present.

On physical examination, cutaneous pigmentation (1–5 mm macules) of the perioral region, crossing the vermilion border occurs in 94% of patients. The macules can be in the perinasal and perioral areas, and may be present on the fingers and toes, and on the dorsal and volar aspects of the hands and feet. These macules often fade with after puberty, and there is no malignant potential. There may be mucus membrane pigmentation, primarily the buccal mucosa (in 66% of patients), and rarely the intestinal mucosa. There may be gynecomastia and growth acceleration (due to a Sertoli cell tumor). A rectal examination may indicate a mass, or a testicular examination may yield a palpable mass.

Since the small intestine is the most common location for polyp formation, small bowel radiography is utilized to determine the presence of small intestinal polyps. Esophagogastroduodenoscopy is also used to assess for polyps in the upper GI tract.

Patients with P-J syndrome have a characteristic hamartomatous polyp that separates P-J from other hamartomatous syndromes (see below).

Genetic testing for mutant *STK11* is available to confirm the diagnosis of P-J syndrome.

Histological Classification and Molecular Genetics

The P-J polyp is distinctive in that it has an arborizing pattern of growth of the muscularis mucosa extending into the branching fronds of the polyp. Benign glands within the polyp may be surrounded by the arborizing smooth muscle, and may extend into the submucosa or muscularis propria. The glandular epithelium is often described as "pseudoinvading" into the deeper layers of the polyp.

P-J families have a germ line mutation of the *STK11* gene, located on chromosome 19p13.3. This gene is likely regulated by phosphorylation by a cAMP-dependent kinase, but the full regulation and spectrum of action of STK11 is not currently known. STK11 appears to be a classic tumor suppressor gene. Genetic analysis of P-J polyps demonstrates that both alleles of STK11/LKB1 are inactivated by mutation and loss of heterozygosity (LOH) in most polyps. In adenomatous tissue or adenocarcinoma from P-J patients, additional genetic lesions appear, such as LOH of 17p or mutation of p53 (located on chromosome 17p), LOH of 18q, and mutation of β-catenin. Nuclear localization of β-catenin, indicating an alteration in the APC/β-catenin/TCF-4 pathway, has been seen in P-J polyps within the epithelial cells. Based on a mouse knockout model of STK11/LKB1, the loss of STK11/LKB1 in P-J polyps may increase cancer risk by an increased angiogenic potential mediated by the increased expression of VEGF. These findings suggest multiple pathways for STK11/LKB1 involvement, and it may be the "gatekeeper" for the development of P-J polyps.

Treatment

Removal of hemorrhagic or large polyps (>5 mm) by endoscopic polypectomy should confirm the diagnosis of P-J syndrome and help control symptoms. Laparotomy and resection may be needed for repeated or persistent small intestinal intussusception, obstruction, or persistent intestinal bleeding.

Prognosis

Despite the average age of diagnosis in the mid 20's, younger P-J patients often present with obstructive symptoms of the small intestine (intussusception and abdominal pain) where the polyps occur most frequently, but the diagnosis is often not entertained. Laparotomy in P-J patients should only be used when necessary, as repeated abdominal surgeries can cause adhesions and intestinal obstruction or short bowel syndrome.

As the P-J patient ages, the morbidity risk shifts to that of malignancy. There is a 15 fold elevated relative risk of developing cancer, with 93% of P-J patients developing cancer by age 64 years. The major sites are in order of relative risk (RR) over the general population are: small intestine (RR 520), stomach (RR 213), pancreas (RR 132), colon (RR 84), esophagus (RR 57), ovary (RR 27), lung (RR 17), uterus (RR 16), and breast (RR 15.2). In addition, other reproductive site cancers have been associated with P-J syndrome, including adenoma malignum of the cervix, Sertoli cell tumors, and sex cord tumors with annular tubules.

Follow-Up

Management of P-J patients involves prevention of complications from the polyps, and cancer surveillance. Repeated removal of hemorrhagic or large polyps (>5 mm) by endoscopic polypectomy is often performed. An annual complete blood count to screen for anemia is also prudent.

Forty-eight percent of P-J syndrome patients will develop and die from cancer by the age of 57 years. Sites of cancer formation include small intestine, stomach, colon, pancreas, ovary, uterus, and breast (often bilateral disease), testes, and cervix. An annual physical examination that includes evaluation of the breasts, abdomen, pelvis, and testes is suggested. Small intestinal radiological examinations should commence by age 10 and be repeated every 2 years. Endoscopic examinations of the colon and stomach should begin by the second decade of life, and be repeated every 2–3 years. Imaging of the pancreas by ultrasound (or computed tomography) should begin by age 30 and be continued every 1–2 years. Breast examination by mammography and ultrasonographic examination of the female reproductive tract should begin by the mid 20's and be repeated every 2–3 years in a P-J patient. If feminizing features occur in a male P-J patient, a testicular ultrasound should be performed.

Screening, Surveillance, Prevention

The patient with P-J should be educated on potential symptoms of intestinal obstruction, and instructed on the need for cancer surveillance.

Offspring and relatives of patients with P-J syndrome should be evaluated clinically for the presence of the syndrome. Genetic testing is commercially available and is nearly 100% accurate for family members if a mutation is found in the proband.

Cowden Disease

Epidemiology

Cowden disease is a syndrome described in 1963 in which multiple hamartomas develop on the skin and mucous membranes, as well as throughout the gastrointestinal tract. Its hallmark is facial trichilemmomas, and there is a high risk for thyroid and breast disease. The true incidence of Cowden disease not known, but estimates are that it occurs in 1 in 200,000 individuals. Male and females are affected equally.

Etiology and Pathogenesis

The genetic cause for Cowden disease appears to be a germ line mutation in *PTEN* (also known as *MMAC1* and *TEP1*) (see Table 1), located on chromosome 10q23, which encodes a 403 amino acid dual-specific phosphatase (phosphoserine/phosphothreonine and phosphotyrosine residues) that can dephosphorylate proteins (focal adhesion kinase and others), and lipids (phosphatidylinositol phosphates). Nearly half of the mutations identified are in exon 5 of *PTEN*, the location encoding the phosphatase core motif. PTEN is a tumor suppressor protein that, by its dephosphorylating ability, contributes to programmed death of the cell, and inhibits the cell's ability to migrate and invade. PTEN's effects on lipids seem to be the most essential for tumor suppression. Mutational inactivation of PTEN would remove these phenotypes, and have the net effect of increasing cellular proliferation and enhancing cell migration and invasion.

Symptoms and Clinical Signs

The hallmark of Cowden disease is the development of facial trichilemmomas, which are small pinpoint to pea-sized, smooth or keratotic papules that develop on the bridge of the nose and around the mouth and eyes. They may also be observed on the distal extremities, including the palms and soles. The diagnosis of Cowden disease is often delayed until the second or third decade of life because the facial trichilemmomas may not develop until then.

The Cowden patient may have intestinal hamartomas throughout the GI tract (Fig. 1). Patients can present with a proteus syndrome when young, anemia, hema-

tochezia, or intestinal obstruction or intussuseption in rare cases if polyps become large.

A number of extra-intestinal hamartomas can develop. These include those of mucous membranes, such as flat or verrucous papules that develop on the tongue, gingiva, and oral mucosa. Additionally, other soft tissue tumors can develop, including lipomas, hemangiomas, lymphangiomas, neurofibromas, meningiomas, and uterine leiomyomas.

Two-thirds of Cowden disease patients will develop thyroid goiter, with a 10% incidence of thyroid cancer. More than 75% of patients will have breast lesions, including fibrocystic breast disease and fibroadenomas, and 50% will develop breast cancer. The breast cancer is often bilateral, and has a median age of diagnosis of 41 years of age.

A number of unusual phenotypic features may be present in a Cowden disease patient. These include a high arched palate, beaked nose, and mandibular, maxillary, and soft palate hypoplasia. Café-au-lait spots may be present, and some patients can develop retinal gliomas, odontitis, dental caries, adenoid facies, kyphoscoliosis, and pectus excavatum. A variant of Cowden disease, the Lhermitte-Duclos syndrome, shares the phenotype and genotype of Cowden disease and in addition has macrocephaly, ataxia and dysplastic cerebellar gangliocytomatosis as features.

Diagnostics

A careful history and physical examination of the Cowden patient will often suggest the diagnosis, but there has to be a high index of suspicion by the health care provider. Intestinal hamartomas, if present, could present at a young age and could be confused with "inflammatory polyposis" or other hamartoma syndromes because the histology of the polyps is not necessarily uniform (see below). Thyroid disease may also occur in the first decade of life, and this should increase the suspicion of this condition. Facial trichilemmomas will often develop in the second or third decade of life, although they are the hallmark of the disease. Confusion of Cowden disease with multiple endocrine neoplasia (MEN) type 2B may occur, because both syndromes share intestinal ganglioneuromas and thyroid disease in their phenotype. However, MEN2B's thyroid cancer is medullary, not follicular as seen in Cowden disease.

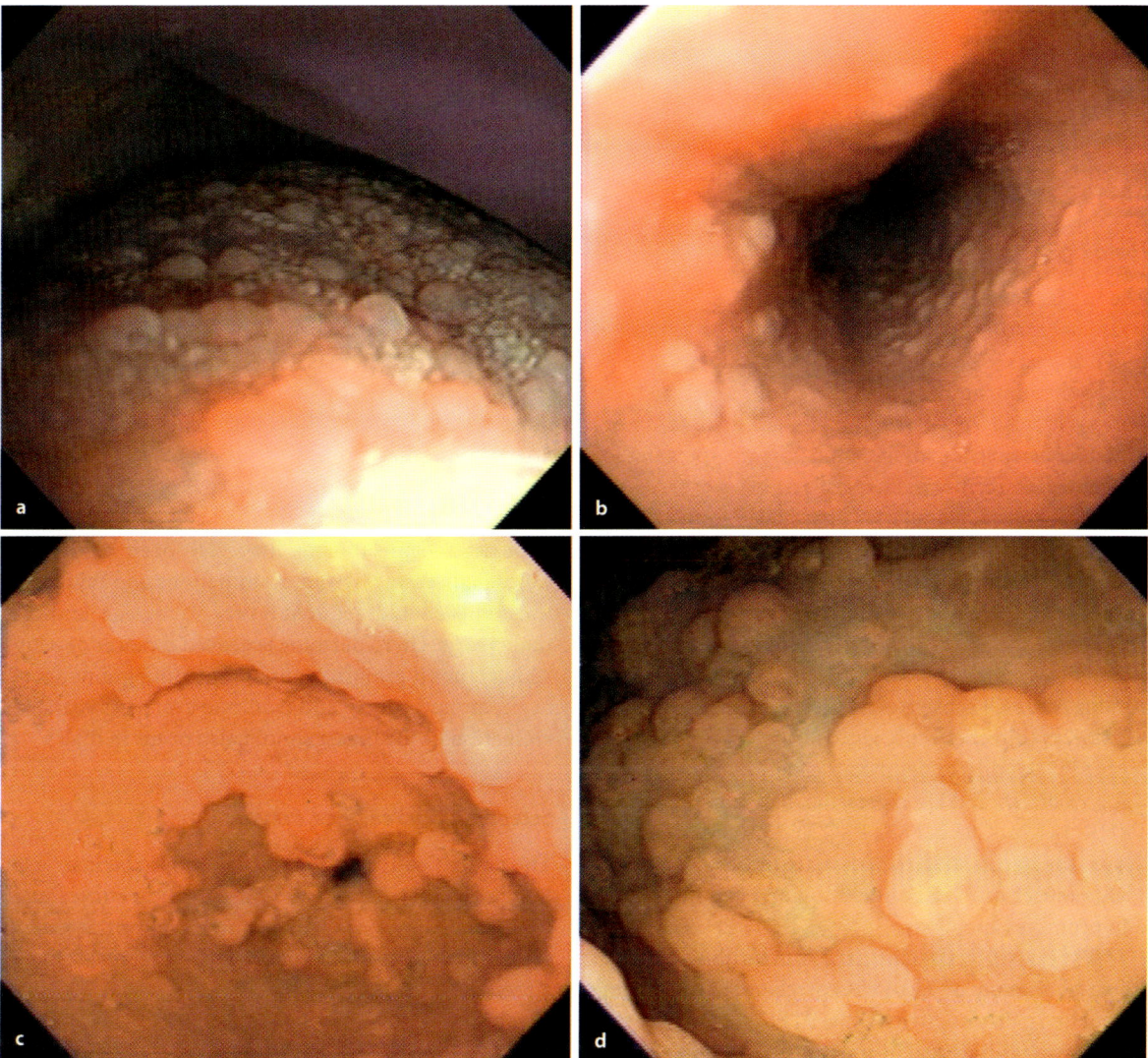

Figure 1a–d
Intestinal polyps in Cowden disease (also known as Multiple Hamartoma Syndrome). Hamartomatous polyps are distributed throughout the gastrointestinal tract as seen endoscopically here. Note that the tongue (**a**), the esophagus (**b**), the gastric antrum (**c**), and the rectosigmoid (**d**) are all affected by polyposis in this one patient

The International Cowden Consortium has suggested specific clinical diagnostic criteria for Cowden disease. Pathognomonic criteria include facial trichilemmomas, acral keratosis, papillomatous papules and mucosal lesions. The diagnosis can be made if 2 major criteria are met, which includes at least macrocephaly or Lhermitte-Duclos syndrome, and any of breast carcinoma, follicular thyroid carcinoma, or endometrial carcinoma. Minor criteria can also make the diagnosis of Cowden disease if 3 are present with 1 major criterion or if 4 minor criteria are present. Minor criteria include thyroid adenoma or goiter, mental retardation, gastrointestinal hamartomas, fibrocystic breast disease, lipomas, fibromas or the presence of a genitourinary tumor or malformation.

Genetic testing for mutant *PTEN* is available to confirm the diagnosis of Cowden disease. However, since *PTEN* mutations can occur in some other hamartomatous syndromes, Cowden disease is defined clinically. Cowden disease may be part of the spectrum of manifestations from a germ line *PTEN* mutation.

Histological Classification and Molecular Genetics

The hamartomatous polyps in Cowden disease demonstrate a broad range of histology; the most common polyp appears to be a protuberance of cytologically normal epithelium indigenous to the region from which the polyps arose. Hyperplastic polyps are also common. Lipomas, juvenile polyps, inflammatory polyps, ganglioneuromas, and lymphoid hyperplasia can occur.

PTEN germ line mutations have been found in 81% of Cowden disease kindreds. With wild type PTEN's ability to dephosphorylate phosphatidylinositol-3,4,5-triphosphate (PIP3), a key role of PTEN in the cell is to antagonize the effects of Akt/protein kinase B (PKB), which plays a major role in many tumors' pathogenesis. Among Akt/PKB substrates that regulate cellular activity are GSK3b (direct effect in glucose uptake, and involved with APC's ability to degrade β-catenin), c-myc, c-jun, c-fos, cyclin D1 and D3 expression, p27, Bad, Caspase 9, FKHR, IKK-α, CREB, FAK, PKC, and others. PTEN reverses the effects of these downstream targets of Akt/PKB, reduces cellular proliferation and cell migration, and promotes apoptosis.

PIP3 is a key molecule involved in insulin signaling. Phosphorylation of Akt/PKB correlates with insulin-stimulated glucose activity, while PTEN antagonizes this effect by inhibiting insulin-induced 2-deoxyglucose uptake and GLUT4 translocation. Indeed, a patient with Cowden disease has been demonstrated to have a more rapid clearance of glucose than controls, indicating insulin hypersensitivity in this patient.

Treatment

Removal of large polyps by endoscopic polypectomy should control symptoms related to the polyps in Cowden disease. There appears to be little risk of the development of colorectal cancer.

Prognosis

Patients with Cowden disease who have cancer surveillance and treatment may potentially live a normal life span.

Follow-Up

In addition to the intestinal hamartomas, two-thirds of Cowden patients have thyroid adenomas and goiters, and up to three-fourths will have fibrocystic breast disease and fibroadenomas. While an increase risk in gastrointestinal cancers has not been demonstrated, the two most common cancers that develop in Cowden patients are thyroid cancer in 10% of patients (typically follicular), and breast cancer in up to 50% of patients. Other cancers such as renal cell, Merkel cell carcinoma, lymphomas, and melanomas have also been reported in Cowden disease. Thyroid examinations and thyroid ultrasounds should begin at a very young age, and continue yearly. Thyroidectomy is needed if cancer develops. Annual breast examinations and mammograms should begin around age 25, and continue every 1–2 years. Examination of the breast should also occur in males.

Screening, Surveillance, Prevention

The patient with Cowden disease should be instructed on the need for thyroid and breast cancer surveillance. Genetic testing is available commercially after genetic counseling for family members, if a mutation is found in a proband.

Bannayan Riley-Ruvalcaba Syndrome (BRRS)
Epidemiology

BRRS, also known as Bannayan-Zonana syndrome, Ruvalcaba-Myhre-Smith syndrome, and Riley-Smith syndrome because of its phenotypic variability, is a rare congenital syndrome with features that include intestinal juvenile polyps and certain characteristic extraintestinal features such as pigmentary spotting of the penis, visceral and cutaneous hamartomas, and macrocephaly. The prevalence of BRRS syndrome is unknown. Patients reported with this syndrome represent sporadic occurrences as well as familial occurrences with an autosomal dominant pattern of inheritance.

Etiology and Pathogenesis

A proportion of BRRS patients (~60%) have germ line mutations in *PTEN*, the same mutated gene that is associated with Cowden syndrome (Table 1). Indeed, there are reports of BRRS and Cowden disease occurring in the same family, suggesting that the two might be one causal entity. Analysis of BRRS and Cowden disease patients with germ line *PTEN* mutations indicate a similar mutational spectra and a correlation of *PTEN* mutation and cancer or breast fibroadenoma in any given Cowden disease, BRRS, or BRRS/Cowden disease overlap family. There are probably uncharacterized genetic or epigenetic events in the manifestation of a germ line *PTEN* mutation's effects on the phenotype. While there is some overlap with the mutational spectra of *PTEN* between BRRS and Cowden disease, there are certainly unique mutations that occur in each syndrome. Signaling pathways involving PTEN may be differentially compromised depending on the mutation, which could have a direct bearing on the phenotype. The overall implication is that PTEN-mutation positive Cowden disease and BRRS may be different presentations of a single syndrome, and that both should receive equal attention with respect to cancer surveillance.

A number of BRRS patients do not have germ line mutation of *PTEN*. Some patients have gross chromosome deletions or rearrangements involving the *PTEN* locus on chromosome 10, thus making the patient haploinsufficient. Other patients, despite an exhaustive search for chromosomal deletions and mutation of *PTEN*, do not demonstrate abnormalities of *PTEN* or its locus. There is probably an additional germ line cause for BRRS, which may explain its phenotypic difference with Cowden disease.

Symptoms and Clinical Signs

In addition to intestinal juvenile polyps, patients with BRRS may manifest macrocephaly, subcutaneous and visceral lipomas and hemangiomas, cognitive and motor developmental delay, lipid storage myopathy, Hashimoto's thyroiditis, and pigmentary spotting of the penis in males. Many of these features are recognized early in life, and the constellation of these signs should suggest BRRS. Intussuseption can also complicate this syndrome.

Diagnostics

BRRS is diagnosed clinically, usually after recognition of some of the features and having a high index of suspicion.

Histological Classification and Molecular Genetics

BRRS patients harbor intestinal hamartomatous polyps, typically of the juvenile polyp variety.

Sixty percent of BRRS families harbor a germ line mutation in the *PTEN* tumor suppressor gene. While some patients have gross chromatin loss at chromosome 10q23, the site of *PTEN*, there are some patients described without any chromatin loss or genetic mutation of *PTEN*. Because of the genetic similarity with Cowden disease, some have suggested that BRRS is a subset of Cowden disease.

Treatment

Removal of large polyps by endoscopic polypectomy should control symptoms related to the polyps in BRRS. The risk for the development of colorectal cancer is not known.

Prognosis

Because of the rarity of this syndrome, the prognosis is not known, particularly relative to cancer risk.

Follow-Up

With a similar genotype to Cowden disease, patients with BRRS should be screened for thyroid and breast disease in a similar fashion to Cowden disease.

Screening, Surveillance, Prevention

Genetic testing for germ line *PTEN* mutations is available commercially, particularly for family members of a proband, or for sporadic cases to confirm the diagnosis. BRRS is identified generally after clinical suspicion, and due to allelism, may be seen in Cowden disease families as well.

Juvenile Polyposis Syndrome (JPS)

Epidemiology

JPS is a congenital syndrome in which 10 or more juvenile polyps occur in the gastrointestinal tract. Unlike solitary sporadic juvenile polyps, familial juvenile polyps almost always recur after removal. Patients present by age 30, with the mean age of presentation being 9.5 years. This syndrome is diagnosed by the exclusion of extra-intestinal lesions seen with the other hamartomatous syndromes. An estimate for prevalence in the population is 1 in 250,000 individuals.

Patients with JPS have a twelve-fold elevated risk for developing colorectal carcinoma. Other cancers associated with JPS include pancreatic, gastric, and duodenal cancers.

Etiology and Pathogenesis

There appears to be heterogeneity in the genetic cause of JPS. Two cases of deletions involving chromosome 10q23 have been reported. Subsequently, germ line mutations in *PTEN*, located on 10q23 and mutations of which are also associated with Cowden disease and BRRS, were found in four families (see Table 1). The clinical diagnosis of JPS might be in doubt in the young patients who have not yet developed other features of Cowden disease, but seem clear in older patients who have had time to develop extra-intestinal manifestations that would exclude JPS. However, linkage mapping in eight informative JPS families excluded chromosome 10q22–24 as the susceptibility locus for JPS, and no *PTEN* mutations were detected in 14 families and 11 sporadic cases in another study.

Linkage analysis in families without *PTEN* mutations revealed a second gene on chromosome 10q23, *BMPR1A*, which is mutated in the germ line of some JPS families (see Table 1). The mutations found result in premature truncation of the protein. BMPR1A is a 532 amino acid, cellular transmembrane protein that mediates bone morphogenic protein (BMP) signaling. It is a type I receptor of the TGF-β superfamily, with a cysteine-rich extracellular domain, an intracellular glycine-serine-rich domain near the plasma membrane and an intracellular kinase domain. Several BMP ligands bind to specific type II BMP receptors. The type II receptors, after ligand binding, activate the type I receptors through their glycine-serine rich domains. Subsequently, BMPR1A, activated by the type II receptor, phosphorylates SMAD1, SMAD5, and possibly SMAD8, which then associate with SMAD4 to form a heteromeric complex. The SMAD4-SMAD 1, 5, or 8 complexes then translocate from the cytoplasm to the nucleus, associate with DNA-binding proteins and regulate transcription of genes that may regulate apoptosis and mesoderm formation. The demonstration of germ line mutation of BMPR1A in JPS patients is the first evidence that BMPs may play a role in controlling colonic epithelial growth and neoplasia.

A separate large kindred with JPS demonstrated linkage to chromosome 18q21.1. Subsequently, 3 familial and 2 sporadic JPS cases out of nine total demonstrated germ line mutations in the *SMAD4* gene at chromosome 18q21.1, whose gene product encodes a key intracellular signal transducer and transcriptional regulator for the TGFβ superfamily of ligands and receptors (see Table 1). The most common *SMAD4* mutation was a four-bp deletion from codons 414–416; a 2 bp deletion from codon 348 and a 1-bp insertion at codon 229 have also been reported. All of these mutations are predicted to cause a truncated SMAD4 protein and prevent homotrimerization at its carboxyl terminus.

Symptoms and Clinical Signs

The classical symptom is rectal bleeding, but with a large number of polyps, patients can present with protein loss, malnutrition, cachexia, and failure to thrive, typically in the first decade of life. Large polyps can cause obstruction or altered bowel habits. The average age for colorectal cancer presentation is 34 years, so anemia and obstruction from tumor can be presenting symptoms later in life.

There are other rare features described for JPS, particularly congenital conditions. These include cardiac abnormalities, hydrocephalus, malrotation of the bowel, Meckel diverticulum, mesenteric lymphangioma, cranium abnormalities, cleft palate, and polydactyly.

Diagnostics

The finding of multiple juvenile polyps in the GI tract, particularly if there are more than 10 in the colon, in the absence of extra-intestinal manifestations that define other hamartomatous syndromes is generally adequate to make the diagnosis. Germ line testing for *PTEN*, *BMPR1A*, and *SMAD4* mutations can be performed to confirm the diagnosis. In the case of *PTEN* mutations, careful consideration for Cowden disease may be particularly important, if the patient is too young for pathognomonic features to have developed.

Histological Classification and Molecular Genetics

JPS patients harbor classic juvenile polyps. The polyps can range from several millimeters to several centimeters in size. Larger polyps may demonstrate alternating red and white patterns visible on the surface, the white areas representing dilated glandular cysts filled with mucin near the polyp surface (Fig. 2). Within a juvenile polyp, there is a greatly expanded lamina propria with multiple mucin-filled, single-layer, epithelial-lined cysts. It is not clear if the cysts form a network within the polyp or are individual.

In JPS patients, there is a clearly demonstrated risk for malignancy to occur from within their juvenile polyps. Thirty-one percent of familial juvenile polyps demonstrated dysplasia, with no dysplasia occurring in solitary, sporadic juvenile polyps. Within dysplastic polyps, 79% had abnormal coexpression of the proliferative marker Ki-67 and the cyclin-dependent kinase inhibitor p21$^{WAF1/CIP1}$, suggesting loss of proliferative control within the dysplastic epithelium. Somatic mutations of the *APC* gene, detected by an *in vitro* transcription/translation assay, were also found in half of the dysplastic familial juvenile polyps. This suggests that one potential mechanism for dysplasia (adenoma formation) to occur is through mutation of the *APC* gene.

Treatment

Some JPS patients can be managed with repeated polypectomies, particularly if symptoms are not severe or if there is a small number of polyps. With severe symptoms such as failure to thrive, colectomy with ileoanal anastomosis may become necessary. For cancer, colectomy is the therapy of choice, given the increased risk of metachronous cancers that may develop. After colectomy, continued surveillance of the remaining rectum is necessary to remove recurrent polyps.

Prognosis

Patients with JPS are predisposed to juvenile hamartomatous polyps and gastrointestinal cancer, with a 15% incidence of colorectal carcinoma in young patients and a cumulative risk of 68% by 60 years of life. Colorectal cancer occurs at a mean age of 34 years. Surveillance and treatment of cancers found greatly extend the life expectancy. Other cancers that may occur rarely in JPS patients include pancreatic, gastric, and duodenal cancers.

Follow-Up

Because of the greatly elevated colorectal cancer risk, colonoscopy is recommended to begin with symptoms, or in the early teenage years if no symptoms occur. Colonoscopy should be repeated every 1–3 years, depending on the number of observed polyps. Because there may be an increased risk for cancers of the stomach and duodenum, and to identify and remove large polyps, an upper GI endoscopy may be performed beginning in the teenage years and repeated every 1–3 years. There is no specific recommendation to survey the pancreas at this time.

Screening, Surveillance, Prevention

Genetic testing for germ line *PTEN*, *BMPR1A*, and *SMAD4* mutations is available commercially, particularly for family members of a proband or for sporadic cases, to confirm the diagnosis.

Hereditary Mixed Polyposis Syndrome (HMPS)

Epidemiology

HMPS is a recently described syndrome in which affected family members have atypical juvenile polyps, hyperplastic polyps, colonic adenomas, and colonic adenocarcinomas.

Etiology and Pathogenesis

Although this syndrome can present with atypical juvenile polyps, its gene has been linked to chromosome 6q in one extended family and not at the chromosomal sites

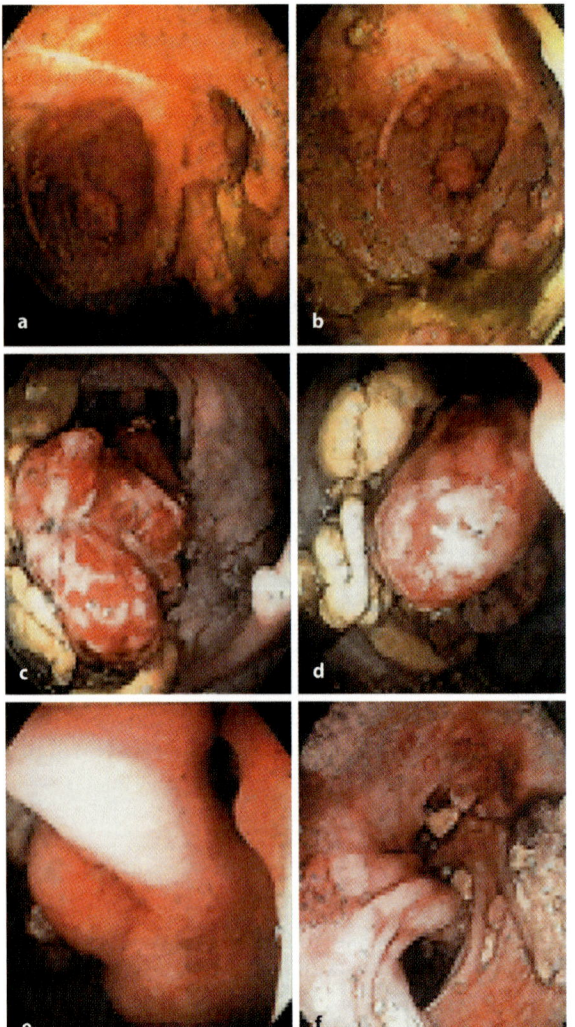

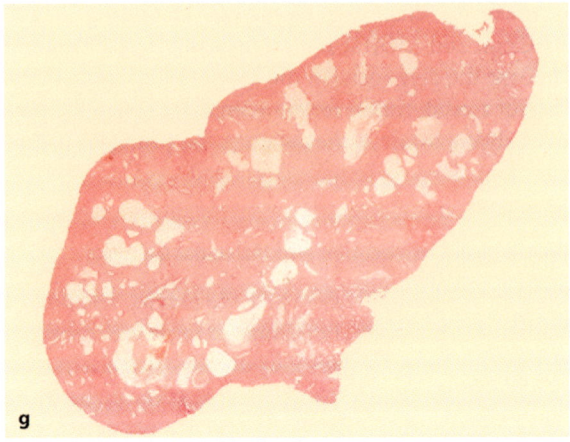

Figure 2a–g
Intestinal polyps in juvenile polyposis. In (a–f), gross endoscopic view of polyps. Some large polyps feature the alternating red and white patches that are characteristic of juvenile polyps (middle panels). In (g), low power magnification (40X) of a sectioned juvenile polyp demonstrating dilated epithelial cysts that contain mucin, and surrounded by a greatly expanded lamina propria

that have been implicated for BRRS, JPS, and Cowden's disease. Thus, the genetic cause for this syndrome remains obscure. There was no linkage to the *APC* site on Chromosome 5q, nor linkage to chromosome 10q23, the site for *PTEN* and *BMPR1A*, suggesting that HMPS is a distinct entity.

Symptoms and Clinical Signs

The median age of symptomatic presentation was 40 years of age from a large kindred, and the youngest patient in that kindred developed polyps at age 23 years.

There are no extra-intestinal findings. Symptoms are related to the polyps in the colon and may include anemia, occult blood loss, hematochezia, or obstruction.

Diagnostics

Patients with HMPS typically have 15 or fewer polyps at colonoscopy. The diagnosis is made from the family history, and the finding of multiple histological findings that feature different types of polyps.

Histological Classification and Molecular Genetics

Some patients have polyps of more than one histological type, while other individuals demonstrated mixed histology within individual polyps.

Treatment

Colonoscopy with removal of the polyps usually controls symptoms and helps to make the diagnosis.

Prognosis

The median age of diagnosis of colorectal cancer was 47 years of age, and there is a 30% lifetime risk for developing colorectal cancer.

Follow-Up

Colonoscopic surveillance for colorectal cancer is recommended every 2 years in HMPS, and should begin by age 25, or 10 years younger than the youngest patient with colorectal cancer.

Screening, Surveillance, Prevention

Identification of family members who have HMPS rests on analysis of the family pedigree, and identification of the characteristic polyps in the colon.

Future Perspectives

The human polyposis syndromes represent the extreme end of a spectrum of phenotypic expression when a gene is mutated in the germ line leading to haploinsufficient single gene expression. These syndromes may "exaggerate" similar sporadic conditions and give clues to the pathogenesis of a relatively common disease.

Certainly this has been the case with FAP and Lynch syndromes, which have helped characterize sporadic colorectal cancer tumorigenesis. While this is not clear in the case of hamartomatous polyposis syndromes, the germ line defects found in these syndromes will undoubtedly have implications in the pathogenesis of colorectal and perhaps other cancers. Major questions still to be answered are what defines or characterizes the hamartomatous polyposis syndromes, what determines their phenotypic expression, what determines organ-specific cancer risk, and what are the steps for cancer to form in those organs? These questions are being addressed in a number of laboratories throughout the world.

References

1. Giardiello FM, Brensinger JD, Tersmette AC, Goodman SN, Petersen GM, Booker SV, Cruz-Correa M, Offerhaus JA. Very high risk of cancer in familial Peutz-Jeghers syndrome. Gastroenterology 2000;119:1447–1453.
2. Zigman AF, Lavine JE, Jones MC, Boland CR, Carethers JM. Localization of the Bannayan-Riley-Ruvalcaba syndrome to chromosome 10q23. Gastroenterol 1997;113:1433–1437.
3. Huang SC, Chen CR, Lavine JE, Taylor SF, Newbury RO, Pham T-TT, Ricciardiello L, Carethers JM. Genetic heterogeneity in familial juvenile polyposis. Cancer Res 2000;60:6882–6885.
4. Whitelaw SC, Murday VA, Tomlinson IPM et al. Clinical and molecular features of the hereditary mixed polyposis syndrome. Gastroenterol 1997;112:327–334.
5. Hamilton, SR; Liu, B; Parsons, RE et al. The molecular basis of Turcot's syndrome. New Eng J Med 1995;332:839–47.
6. Giardiello, FM; Hamilton, SR; Krush, AJ et al. Treatment of colonic and rectal adenomas with sulindac in familial adenomatous polyposis. New Eng J Med, 1993;328:1313–6.
7. Marra G and Boland CR. Hereditary Nonpolyposis Colorectal Cancer (HNPCC): The Syndrome, the Genes, and an Historical Perspective. J Natl Cancer Inst 87:1114–1125, 1995.
8. Liaw D, Marsh DJ, Li J, Dahia PLM et al. Germline mutations of the PTEN gene in Cowden disease, an inherited breast and thyroid cancer syndrome. Nat Genet 1997;16:64–67.
9. Powell, SM; Petersen, GM; Krush, AJ et al. Molecular diagnosis of familial adenomatous polyposis. New Eng J Med, 1993;329:1982–7.
10. Luce MC, Marra G, Chauhan DP et al. *In vitro* transcription/translation assay for the screening of *hMLH1* and *hMSH2* mutations in familial colon cancer. Gastroenterology 109:1368–1374, 1995.

11 Hereditary Nonpolyposis Colorectal Cancer (Lynch Syndrome)

H.T. LYNCH, J.F. LYNCH

Summary

The diagnosis and management of hereditary nonpolyposis colorectal cancer (HNPCC), also referred to as the Lynch syndrome, is dependent upon knowledge of its medical-genetic features and its natural history, a well-orchestrated family history, evidence for MMR mutations and an understanding of their significance, all in concert with its phenotypic and genotypic heterogeneity. From the clinical standpoint, variable expressivity of the phenotype is a well-established phenomenon in virtually all hereditary disorders, inclusive of HNPCC. Phenotypic variability may be a function of the differences in the expressivity of a single gene or it may occur in concert with modifier genes, and/or environmental factors. However, a full understanding of these events in HNPCC remains elusive. Nevertheless, important surveillance and management implications may emerge from translation of this knowledge into the clinical practice setting.

Epidemiology

Colorectal cancer (CRC) is common in the United States wherein its annual incidence is approximately 148,300 (72,600 males; 75,700 females), with a mortality of 56,600 (27,800 males; 28,800 females). The general population lifetime CRC risk is about 5–6%. A familial risk (two or more first- and/or second-degree relatives with CRC) accounts for approximately 20% of all CRCs, while approximately 5–10% will have a documented autosomal dominantly inherited syndrome. Hereditary nonpolyposis colorectal cancer (HNPCC), also known as Lynch syndrome, the subject of this chapter, is a prime example of hereditary CRC, and is the most common hereditary CRC-prone disorder.

Multiple risk factors have been ascribed for CRC wherein increasing age is perhaps the most important. Host susceptibility factors include gender, race, and, in particular, family history. Contributing environmental risk factors are diet (high-fat, low-fiber), habit patterns such as smoking and alcohol consumption, as well as a decreased amount of physical activity. Molecular genetic events play a prominent role in many of the hereditary forms of CRC, as evidenced by mutations in the *APC* gene that predispose to the time-honored familial adenomatous polyposis (FAP) syndrome and its attenuated FAP variant (AFAP).

Etiology and Pathogenesis

Understanding the importance of colonic adenomas, particularly number, size, pathology features, age of the patient, and cancer proclivity in HNPCC have posed a vexing problem [1]. Lindgren et al. [2] performed a retrospective cross-sectional study over a ten-year period on 304 subjects at increased risk for CRC. This included an ongoing surveillance program with regular colonoscopies. Patients were classified as follows: "Families with HNPCC; families with hereditary CRC (HCC, non-Lynch syndrome); and a third group of families with an increased empirical risk for CRC based on a family history of two close relatives (TCR) with CRC." There were 195 colonic adenomas and six CRCs detected among 85 individuals. When comparing adenomas from the entire risk population with the general population, the relative risk (RR) was 2.6. Patients from TCR families had the most adenomas, while those from HNPCC had the least. There was a shift from proximal adenomas to distal carcinomas in families with HCC and TCR which suggested an increased cancer risk in distal adenomas. Importantly, families with HNPCC showed an earlier age at adenoma onset with adenomas showing a higher degree of dysplasia. Furthermore, there was a similar localization of adenomas and carcinomas in HNPCC, thereby suggesting an increased risk of cancer in all adenomas. These authors concluded that there was an "...overrepresentation of adenomas in all three family types compared with the reference population. In HNPCC, we found earlier onset of adenomas and faster progression to cancer. Families with HCC, and even more so TCR subjects, had a later onset and lower risk of cancer from proximal adenomas...".

Reasoning that CRCs in HNPCC arise from adenomas, and that CRCs occur predominantly in the proximal colon, Rijcken et al. [3] investigated whether this proximal CRC predominance was due to a proximal predominance of adenomas. In addition, they pursued whether there was a difference in malignant transformation rates in these adenomas relevant to differences between distal and proximal colon location of the adenomas.

They studied 100 HNPCC adenomas and compared them with 152 sporadic adenomas for location, size, and dysplasia. *MLH1* and *MSH2* mutations were present in 25 adenomas from patients with a mismatch repair germline mutation. They found that, "...HNPCC adenomas were more often located proximally (50% *v* 26%; p = 0.018) and were smaller in comparison with sporadic adenomas. They were similarly dysplastic. However, all proximal HNPCC adenomas ≥5 mm were highly dysplastic compared with 17% of the larger proximal sporadic polyps (p<0.001). They were also more often highly dysplastic than larger distal HNPCC adenomas (p<0.001). Small HNPCC adenomas were, except for their location, not different from sporadic adenomas. Fifteen of the 25 "known mutation" adenomas showed loss of expression of either MLH1 or MSH2 ...".

Therefore, the authors concluded that adenomas in HNPCC were located mainly in the proximal colon. The progression to high-grade dysplasia was more common in proximal as opposed to distal HNPCC adenomas. This indicated a faster transformation rate from early adenoma to cancer in the proximal colon. Furthermore, they concluded that, "... MMR gene malfunction probably does not initiate adenoma development but is present at a very early stage of tumorigenesis and heralds the development of high grade dysplasia."

Accelerated carcinogenesis of CRC occurs in HNPCC, wherein a tiny adenoma may progress into a carcinoma within two to three years, as opposed to the eight to ten years for this same process in the general population [1, 4]. The reason carcinogenesis in HNPCC occurs at such a rapid rate remains elusive. However, this knowledge is extremely important and therein mandates our recommendation for more frequent colonoscopic surveillance, i.e., annual colonoscopy initiated at age 25.

Symptoms and Clinical Signs

Lynch Syndrome I

Clinical features of HNPCC of the Lynch syndrome I variant include transmission of CRC through succeeding generations, diagnosed at an early age (~44 years) with right-sided predominance (~70% proximal to the splenic flexure), and a significant excess of synchronous and metachronous CRCs. Approximately 25–30% of patients will have a second primary CRC within 10 years of surgical resection for initial CRC, if the surgery was anything less than a subtotal colectomy.

Lynch Syndrome II

Lynch syndrome II is characterized by all of the aforementioned Lynch I features but, in addition, includes a significant excess of extracolonic cancers, foremost of which is endometrial carcinoma, followed by carcinoma of the ovary, stomach, small bowel, hepatobiliary tract, pancreas, upper uro-epithelial tract, brain and breast. In addition, sebaceous adenomas/carcinomas, and multiple keratoacanthomas occur in the Muir-Torre syndrome (MTS) variant of Lynch syndrome II in some families.

Diagnostics

Synopsis

Criteria for identifying HNPCC families

Amsterdam I criteria
At least 3 relatives should have histologically verified CRC:
▸ One should be a first degree relative of the other two;
▸ At least two successive generations should be affected;
▸ At least one of the relatives with CRC should be diagnosed at <50 yrs. of age;
▸ FAP should be excluded.

Amsterdam II criteria

At least 3 relatives should have an HNPCC-associated cancer (CRC, endometrial, stomach, ovary, ureter/renal pelvis, brain, small bowel, hepatobiliary tract, and skin [sebaceous tumors]):

▸ One should be a first degree relative of the other two;

▸ At least two successive generations should be affected;

▸ At least one of the HNPCC-associated cancers should be diagnosed at <50 yrs. of age;

▸ FAP should be excluded in any CRC cases;

▸ Tumors should be verified whenever possible.

Bethesda guidelines

Persons fulfilling Amsterdam criteria and/or fulfilling one of the following:

▸ Persons with 2 HNPCC cancers;

▸ CRC and FDR with HNPCC cancer <45 years or FDR with adenoma <40 years;

▸ CRC or endometrial cancer <45 years;

▸ Right-sided CRC, undifferentiated <45 years;

▸ Signet ring CRC <45 years;

▸ Adenomas <45 years.

The terms familial, hereditary, and sporadic, are relatively crude descriptions of the occurrence of CRC in families (or its absence in families), and are operationally defined as follows:

Sporadic

Sporadic implies that none of the CRC-affected subjects first-degree or second-degree relatives manifest CRC. Nevertheless, the definition will remain crude since the penetrance of many hereditary variants is incomplete, and the classification may be significantly enhanced by the association of CRC with other varieties of cancer.

Familial

Familial is also an imprecise term and is operationally defined by us as any index CRC case who has one or more first- and/or second-degree relatives with CRC wherein at least two of these cases are histologically verified. Therefore, every attempt must be made to extend the pedigree in the search for cancer phenotypic identifiers (all anatomic sites) and/or non-cancer phenotypic features, such as multiple colonic adenomas.

When extended, the pedigree might show a pattern of vertical transmission of colon cancer and other associated cancers (considering penetrance concerns) that would reveal a hereditary etiology, thus eliminating the so-called familial definition.

Hereditary

Hereditary CRC implies that there is a pattern of cancer occurrences (CRC and other anatomic sites) segregating within the extended pedigree wherein three or more first- and/or second-degree relatives manifest CRC. At least two CRC cases must be histologically verified. So-called site specific hereditary CRC is characterized by the following: 1) CRC is manifested from one generation to the next in a site-specific pattern throughout the extended pedigree. 2) Other cancers known to have an integral association with CRC, such as endometrial and ovarian cancer, may signify HNPCC. 3) The *sine qua non* for hereditary CRC's diagnosis would be the presence of a germline mutation that segregates in affected individuals, e.g., mutations in mismatch repair genes (*MSH2, MLH1*) in HNPCC or the *APC* mutated gene in FAP.

Cancer Family History

The first and most important step in the diagnosis of HNPCC is gathering genealogy information and general medical history in concert with the history of cancer occurrences in the family. This history must focus on cancer of *all* anatomic sites, given the fact that there are multiple integrally-associated extracolonic cancers in HNPCC [1].

It is rarely necessary to extend the information beyond the modified nuclear pedigree (Fig. 1). This includes a detailed description of the proband (index case) with pathology verification of cancer. Family history with as much documentation as possible should then proceed to the proband's siblings, progeny, and both maternal and paternal sides of the family. When extending the history to both maternal and paternal aunts and uncles and both sets of grandparents, one is dealing with older individuals and they, therefore, will have passed through the cancer risk age and be more genetically informative. With this much information, one is often capable of establishing a presumptive hereditary CRC

PATIENT'S MODIFIED NUCLEAR PEDIGREE

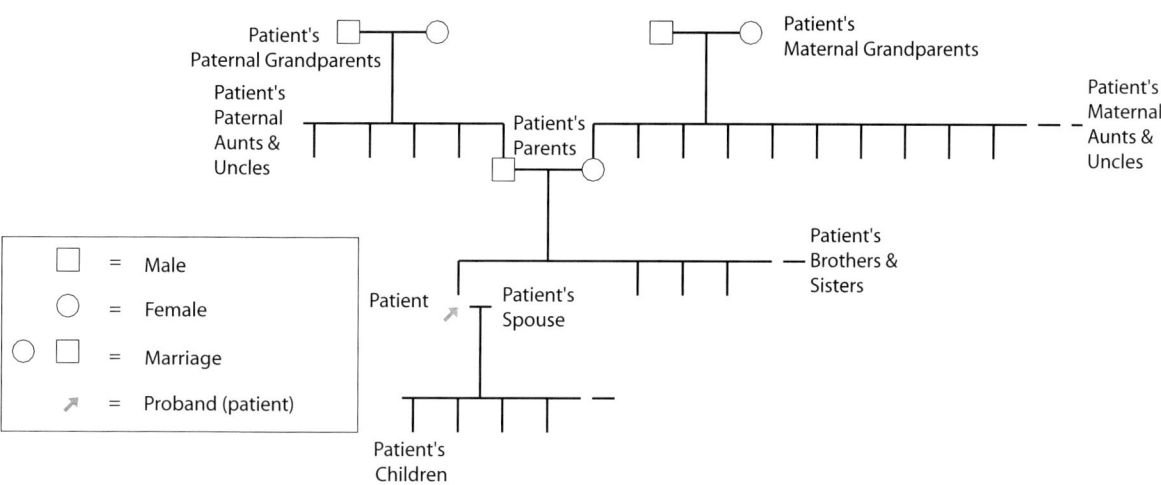

Fig. 1
Diagram portraying a modified nuclear pedigree, the minimum information needed to evaluate cancer family history. (Updated and republished by permission from Lynch et al. Surv Dig Dis 2:244–260, 1984)

diagnosis, if it exists within the family. If a known germline mutation is available for the particular CRC syndrome, such as the *APC* gene for FAP or *MSH2* or *MLH1* mismatch repair genes for HNPCC, one should then pursue this molecular genetic approach to high-risk family members by giving careful attention to their positions in the pedigree.

The initial mutation testing should be done on the most informative affected individual. In the case of HNPCC, this would include a young family member with CRC, particularly if diagnosed at an early age (<50 years) and ideally with proximal colonic location, and who is in the direct genetic lineage. It could include a patient with early-onset endometrial cancer, or any patient with *both* endometrial cancer and CRC or combinations with any other integral HNPCC extracolonic cancers.

The identification of a germline mutation in a particular family, particularly when segregating in high-risk and/or cancer-affected patients, will be the *sine qua non* for diagnosis. The proband's consenting high-risk relatives would be candidates for genetic counseling and DNA testing. Surveillance measures may then be melded

to the disorder's natural history in the interest of reduction of cancer's morbidity and mortality [1]. Although physicians' knowledge about cancer genetics is improving, several studies have shown the need for better understanding in this area. This is important, since identifying germline mutation carriers provides an opportunity to focus surveillance measures on those individuals. Alternatively, those who are negative for the deleterious mutation will not need to go through the extensive screening but will revert to general population surveillance measures.

The following pedigrees (Figs. 2–5) depict clinical and genetic features in concert with clinical variation in HNPCC families.

Family A (Fig. 2): This family shows HNPCC syndrome cancers through five generations. Cancers that are less common in HNPCC but are present in this family include bile duct (IV-3), small bowel (IV-25), and breast (III-13, III-20, IV-10).

Family B (Fig. 3): This family shows all of the criteria of an HNPCC family as well as carcinoma of the urologic system. Patient II-10 had papillary adenocarcinoma of

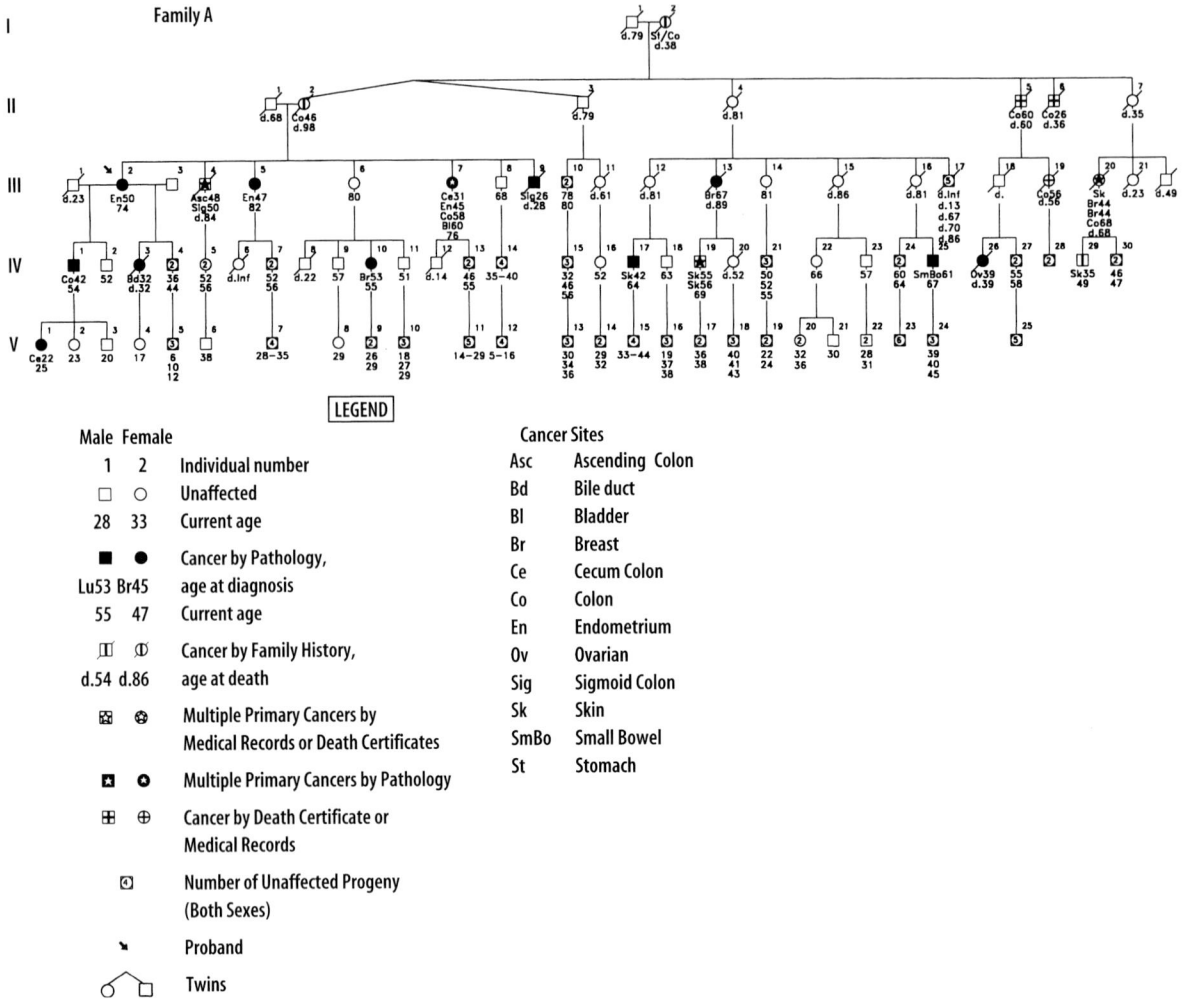

Figure 2
Pedigree of family manifesting some cancers that are less common in HNPCC. (Updated and published with permission from Lynch et al. Am J Gastroenterol 83:741–747, 1988)

the renal pelvis when he was 54 years old and transitional cell carcinoma of the ureter at age 56, as well as CRC at 69 years. Patient III-5 had transitional cell carcinoma of the ureter when she was 57 years old and carcinoma of the cecum at age 60.

Family C (Fig. 4): Adenocarcinoma of the small bowel is one of the HNPCC-associated cancers. It is rare and accounts for about one percent of all gastrointesti-

nal tract cancer. Two patients in Family C had adenocarcinoma of the jejunum. One was a male (IV-7) with adenocarcinoma of the ascending colon at age 31 and carcinoma of the jejunum at age 44. His maternal aunt (III-7) had numerous primary carcinomas of the colon, a carcinoma of the renal pelvis (transitional cell carcinoma) and ovary at age 54 and a carcinoma of the jejunum at age 54.

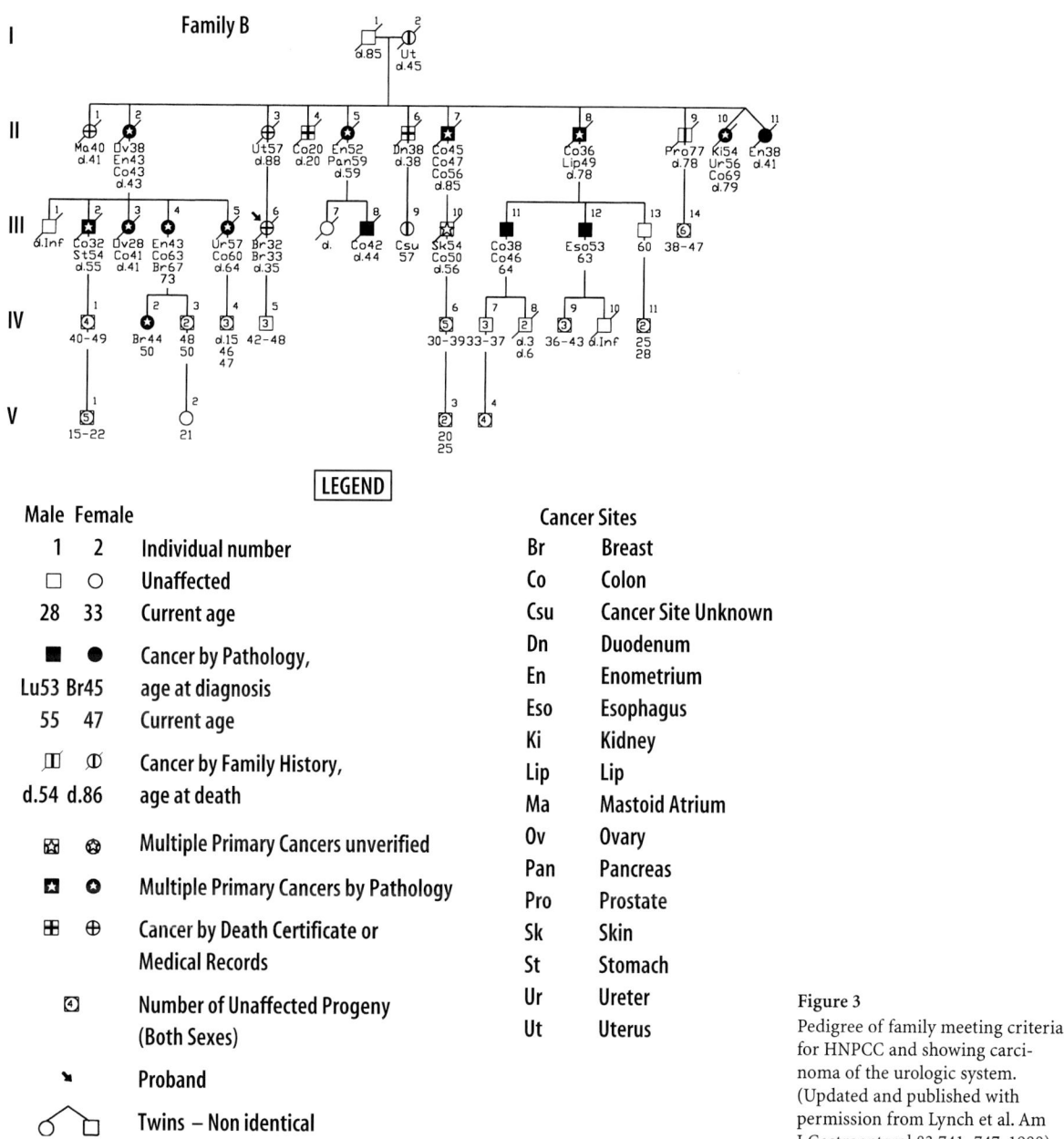

Figure 3

Pedigree of family meeting criteria for HNPCC and showing carcinoma of the urologic system. (Updated and published with permission from Lynch et al. Am J Gastroenterol 83:741–747, 1988)

Family D (Fig. 5): This family was first reported by us in 1985 because of the occurrence of cutaneous signs which are associated with the Muir-Torre syndrome. We postulated at that time that these lesions could represent a possible variant of HNPCC. Since then, other HNPCC families have been documented with Muir-Torre lesions. In family D, patients III-8, III-19, III-29, IV-4, IV-12, have the Muir-Torre cutaneous phenotype and all of them

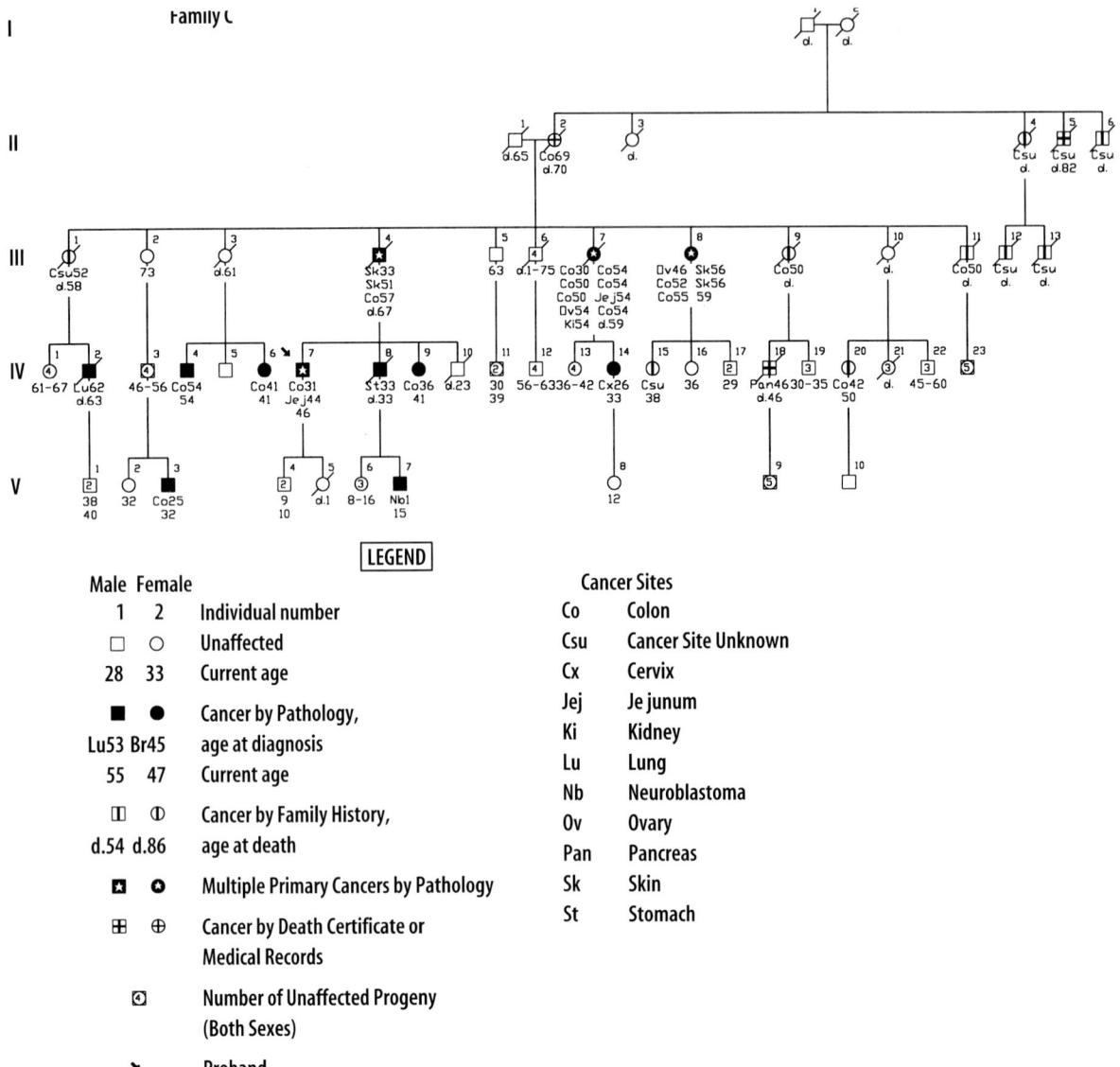

Figure 4
Pedigree of HNPCC family with two patients having adenocarcinoma of the small bowel. (Updated and reprinted with permission from Lynch et al. Cancer 64:2178–2183, 1989)

except IV-12 have had malignant solid tumors. For example, the proband, III-29, has had multiple keratoacanthomas, sebaceous adenomas, squamous cell carci-

nomas of the skin, and transitional cell carcinoma of the renal pelvis and bladder, carcinoma of the colon and of the prostate. He is alive at age 72.

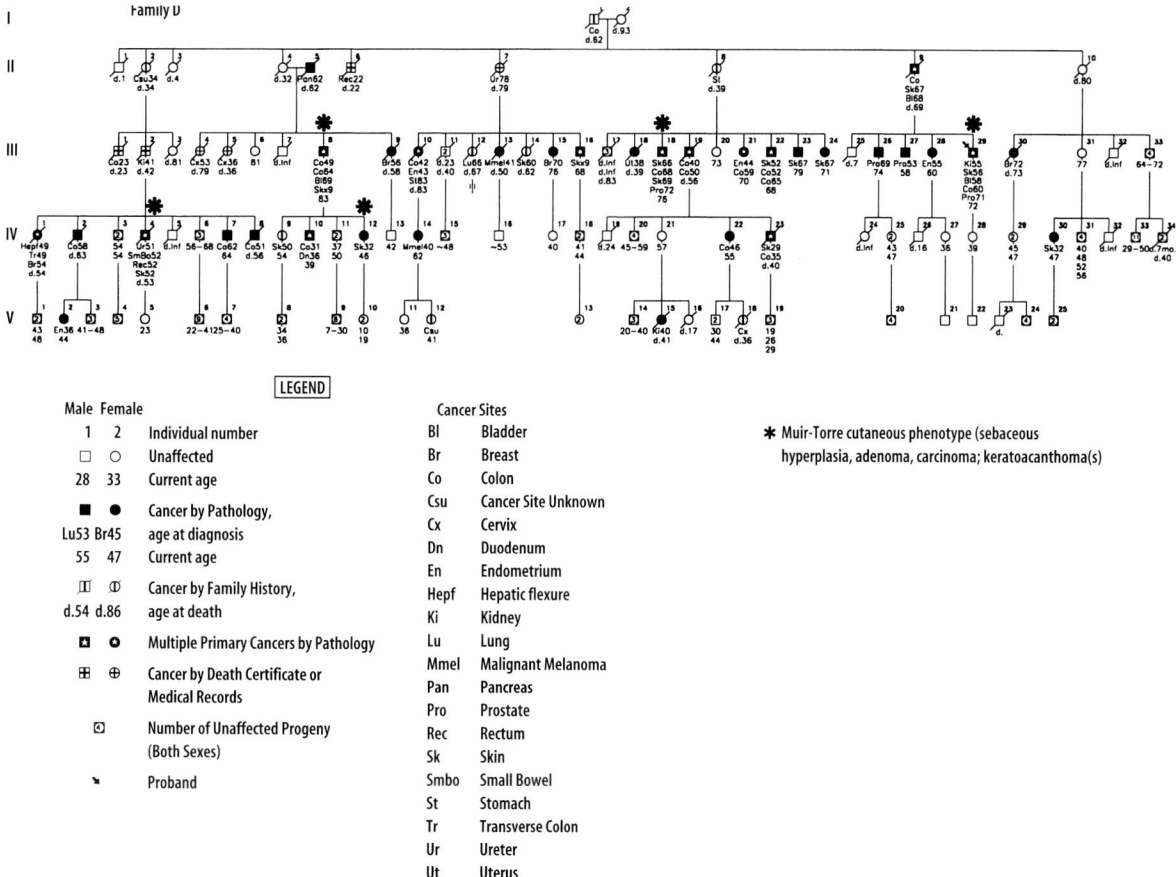

Figure 5
Pedigree of family showing Muir-Torre syndrome variant of HNPCC. (Updated and republished from Lynch et al. Br J Dermatol 113:295–301, 1985)

HNPCC Definitions: Amsterdam I and II Criteria:

Original definitions of HNPCC were by clinical and pedigree criteria such as the more stringent Amsterdam I criteria, or the newer Amsterdam II criteria which are less stringent because they allow for consideration of integral extracolonic cancers (see above synopsis under Diagnostics).

When applying these criteria to patients and/or their families, one must appreciate the fact that there are many situations where pattern recognition of cancer expression may be utilized, especially in small families. Therein cancer of markedly early onset, the pattern of multiple primary cancers, even in a single family member, or the presence of the cutaneous features of MTS, should alert the clinician to the possibility of HNPCC (Fig. 5).

The differential diagnosis of hereditary CRC is extensive, and is driven in a major way by its marked phenotypic and genotypic heterogeneity. Table 1 depicts the complexity of this problem when considering an HNPCC diagnosis.

Table 1
Hereditary form of colorectal cancer (CRC). (Adapted with permission from Lynch et al., Eur J Cancer 31A:1039–1046, 1995)

Type	Inheritance pattern	Gene	Polyps	Cancer	Noncancer features	Screening	Surgical management and/or prophylaxis	Presymptomatic DNA testing	Genetic counseling
Familial adenomatous polyposis (FAP)	AD	APC gene at chromosome 5q, mutation distal to 5^c	Adenomatous, often start in distal colon/rectum; usually >100 polyps; adenomas may occur in small bowel; gastric polyps common, usually fundic gland polyps	CRC, average age at onset 39 years; many cases in teens and twenties; cancer of small bowel; stomach (particularly in Japan), papillary thyroid cancer, periampullary carcinoma, sarcoma, brain tumor	Gardner's variant – epidermoid cysts of skin, osteomas of mandible, congenital hypertrophy of the retinal pigment epithelium; desmoid tumors (intra-abdominal) do not metastasize but may kill by direct extension and may be initiated by surgery (dissected surfaces); adrenal adenomas	If positive for APC germline mutation: baseline flexible sigmoidoscopy at age 10–12 years and annually thereafter; upper endoscopy every 1–3 years starting when colonic polyps first appear; screen remaining rectal segment (annually) after surgical prophylaxis; if at risk but not tested for APC: follow same strategy; if eventually found to be APC negative: baseline sigmoidoscopy at age 15–20 years and, if sigmoidoscopy is negative, revert to general population screening recommendations	Prophylactic subtotal colectomy with low ileorectal anastomosis when phenotype (florid polyposis) identified; consider rectal mucosectomy with ileal pouch anal anastomosis if too many rectal polyps to manage or if compliance for rectal segment follow-up is poor; consider chemoprevention with sulindac (while reducing polyps, cancer may still occur)	Test for APC germline mutation as early as age 10–12 years	Initiate in preteens, include parents
Attenuated familial adenomatous polyposis coli (AFAP)	AD	APC gene at chromosome 5q, mutation proximal to 5^c	Ordinary adenomas but also flat adenomas with proximal colonic predominance; may be few (5–10), sometimes >100	CRC with average age at onset 55 years; occasional periampullary carcinoma	Fundic gland polyps in stomach; adenomas in duodenum	Colonoscopy and upper endoscopy, beginning at age 20 yrs and annually for APC germline-positive patients or every 2 yrs if at genetic risk but not tested for APC	Prophylactic subtotal colectomy if too many polyps to manage; consider chemoprevention with sulindac	Test for APC germline mutation at age 20 years	Initiate at age 20 years, include parents

Table 1 *continued*

Type	Inheritance pattern	Gene	Polyps	Cancer	Noncancer features	Screening	Surgical management and/or prophylaxis	Presymptomatic DNA testing	Genetic counseling
Ashkenazi Jewish I1307K mutation	AD	I1307K mutation in *APC*	Occasional adenomatous colonic polyps	CRC, "young" age at onset but average age of onset not known	None known	Full colonoscopy, starting at age 30-35 years in gene carriers	Standard CRC surgery	Ashkenazi *APC* mutation	Initiate at age 25 years
Turcot's syndrome (HNPCC, FAP)	AD	Both FAP (*APC*) and HNPCC, *hPMS2*, *hMLH1*, mutation variants	Multiple colonic adenomas, but may not be florid	CRC and central nervous system, particularly brain tumors; in *APC* (FAP families) cerebellar medulloblastomas; in *hMLH1* and *hPMS2* (HNPCC families) glioblastoma multiforme	Rare examples of multiple café-au-lait spots and pigmented nevi but not clear if truly integral to the syndrome	Baseline flexible sigmoidoscopy at age 10–12 years and annual flexible sigmoidoscopy thereafter; consider CT scan or MRI of brain	Prophylactic subtotal colectomy if colonic polyps present, as in FAP; in HNPCC variant, colonoscopy	Two DNA variants: (1) *APC* gene with predominance of cerebellar medulloblastoma; (2) *hMLH1* or *hPMS2*, with predominance of glioblastoma multiforme	Initiate at age 10–12 years, include parents
Juvenile polyposis coli	AD	Protein tyrosine phosphate gene (*PTEN*) SMAD4/DPC4	Diffuse hamartomatous polyps (may have adenomatous component) in colon, but may occur in small bowel and stomach	CRC	Children may manifest diarrhea (may be severe)	Initiate colonoscopy at age 10–12 years	Prophylactic subtotal colectomy when phenotype present with too many polyps to manage	Tyrosine phosphate gene (*PTEN*)	Initiate pre-teens, include parents
Peutz-Jeghers syndrome	AD	Gene encoding Peutz-Jeghers serine threonine kinase (STK11) on chromosome 19p13.3 LKB1/ STK11	Peutz-Jeghers polyps (may have adenomatous features) in stomach, small bowel, and colon	Stomach, small bowel, colon, sex cord tumors of ovary and testes	Mucocutaneous melanin pigmentation	Baseline colonoscopy and upper endoscopy, initiate at age 20 yrs; flexible sigmoidoscopy annually thereafter	Consider prophylactic subtotal colectomy if too many polyps to manage and if mixed adenomatous features	Serine threonine kinase (STK11) on chromosome 19p13.3	Initiate in teens, include parents

Table 1 *continued*

Type	Inheritance pattern	Gene	Polyps	Cancer	Noncancer features	Screening	Surgical management and/or prophylaxis	Presymptomatic DNA testing	Genetic counseling
Hereditary mixed polyposis syndrome (HMPS)	AD	Unknown; possible site on chromosome 6q	Atypical colonic juvenile polyps, adenomatous and hyperplastic polyps; usually <15 colon polyps	CRC	None known	Colonoscopy, initiate at age 20 years, every 2–3 years thereafter	Polypectomy; consider prophylactic colectomy if polyps too many to manage	None known	Initiate in teens
Discrete colonic adenomatous polyps and CRC of Burt	AD; may be similar to pattern of some familial CRC	Unknown	Occasional (never florid) adenomatous colonic polyps	CRC, average age in accord with population expectations	None known	Initiate baseline flexible sigmoidoscopy at age 40 and every 3 years thereafter	Standard surgical procedure for CRC	None known	Initiate at age 25–30 years
Hereditary nonpolyposis colorectal cancer (HNPCC)	AD	Germline mutations of any of the mismatch repair genes: hMSH2 at chromosome 2p; hMLH1 at chromosome 3p; hPMS1 at chromosome 2q; hPMS2 at chromosome 7q	Occasional colonic adenomas that are on average larger and more villous and at younger age than in general population. Colonic polyps no more frequent than in general population	CRC most common, with proximal predominance and an excess of synchronous and metachronous CRC. Others include cancer of the endometrium, ovary, small bowel, and stomach, and transitional-cell carcinoma of the ureter and renal pelvis. Average age of cancer onset is 44 years; may show rapid progression from adenoma to CRC	Muir-Torre syndrome variant shows cancer features of HNPCC but includes sebaceous adenomas, sebaceous epitheliomas, basal cell epitheliomas with sebaceous differentiation, meibomian gland carcinomas, and sebaceous carcinomas; single or multiple keratoacanthomas	Colonoscopy, initiate at age 20–25 years, annually for germline mutation carriers; every other year when mutation studies are lacking; endometrial aspiration biopsy at the same time as colonoscopy	Subtotal colectomy for initial CRC; consider prophylactic option of prophylactic subtotal colectomy for germline carriers; consider prophylactic total abdominal hysterectomy and bilateral salpingo-oophorectomy for patients with initial CRC who do not want future pregnancies	Test for germline mutations no earlier than age 18–20 years	Initiate at age 18 years, prior to any consideration for gene testing

Table 1 *continued*

Type	Inheritance pattern	Gene	Polyps	Cancer	Noncancer features	Screening	Surgical management and/or prophylaxis	Presymptomatic DNA testing	Genetic counseling
Familial CRC	Empirical risk 3-fold increase for CRC in patients with one or more first-degree relatives with CRC; likely multifactorial and/or low penetrant genes	Unknown	In accord with population expectations	CRC, comparable to general population for age of onset and colonic location	None	Baseline flexible sigmoidoscopy at age 35, repeat every 3 years; if two first-degree relatives affected or one at age <50 years, risk is 4–6-fold increased, and full colonoscopy every 3–5 years is indicated	Standard surgical procedure for CRC	None known	Initiate at age 30–35 years
Inflammatory bowel disease (ulcerative colitis [UC] and Crohn's disease [CD])	Unknown; possible AD in some families; polygenic also likely	Tentative findings of linkage to chromosomes 16 (IBD$_1$) and 12 (IBD$_2$)	Pseudopolyps (non-adenomatous)	CRC; lymphoma of GI tract	UC: Arthritis, pyoderma gangrenosum, annular erythemas, and vascular thromboses, sclerosing cholangitis. CD: Features similar to UC but small-bowel involvement prominent; may involve colon	UC: Colonoscopy, annual in patients with chronic pancolitis of ≥8 years duration; check for high-grade dysplasia of colonic mucosa; CD: BE may help; x-ray of small bowel may show rigidity, narrowing submucosal edema, or stenosis, inflammation, "cobblestoned appearance." May see clinical and genetic overlap in UC and CD	Subtotal colectomy for CRC; consider prophylactic subtotal colectomy for patients with persistent high-grade dysplasia of colonic mucosa in UC. Proctocolectomy if IBD mandates	None known	Initiate at age 18–20 years

AD autosomal dominant; *CRC* colorectal cancer; *IBD* inflammatory bowel disease; *UC* familial ulcerative colitis; *CD* Crohn's disease; *BE* barium enema.

Histological Classification and Molecular Genetics

Synopsis

The histology of CRC in HNPCC tends to vary from that of sporadic CRC. Mutations in mismatch repair (MMR) genes have been found to be etiologic in HNPCC. However, known MMR mutations can be found in only 40–60% of HNPCC families, indicating that etiologic mutations still remain to be identified in other genes. Also being investigated is HNPCC's genotypic and phenotypic heterogeneity.

CRC tumors in HNPCC are more often poorly differentiated, with an excess of mucoid and signet-cell features, show a Crohn's-like reaction, and contain a significant excess of infiltrating lymphocytes within the tumor [5]. Microsatellite instability (MSI) is found in most CRC tumors in HNPCC [1].

Mutations in six different mismatch repair (MMR) genes have been identified as etiologic in HNPCC patients: *MLH1*, located on chromosome 3p21.3; *MSH2* and *MSH6*, both located on 2p21; *PMS2*, located on 7p22; *MLH3*, located on 14q24.3; and possibly *PMS1*, located on 2q31-q33 [1, 6]. However, only 40–60% of HNPCC patients harbor such identifiable germline mutations, most common of which are *MSH2* and *MLH1* mutations [6]. Other MMR genes as well as non-MMR genes are likely to be identified as etiologic for HNPCC and will eventually account for an unknown set of typical as well as atypical HNPCC-like kindreds. Common environmental carcinogenic exposures may also be responsible for certain occurrences of HNPCC [1].

Penetrance of a mutated MMR gene is in the range of 70–90%. This compares to the penetrance of CRC-prone germline mutations which may be extremely low, as in the case of the I1307 K *APC* Ashkenazi mutation, to almost complete penetrance in familial adenomatous polyposis (FAP), which also involves mutations in the *APC* gene.

Microsatellite instability (MSI) is a phenomenon found in the DNA of CRCs but absent in normal mucosa, and has been found in approximately 90% of HNPCC cases and in 12–17% of so-called sporadic CRC. MSI testing of a colorectal tumor is indicated as a screening test for HNPCC.

These advances have led to new hypotheses about cancer control through our understanding of the molecular genetic pathways which appear to drive the multistep process of carcinogenesis in colonic mucosa. This knowledge has been heralded in a major way by pioneering molecular genetic investigations by of Vogelstein and Kinzler [7]. Herein, we now consider it axiomatic that a form of genomic instability contributes to the sequential accumulation of those molecular genetic alterations that lead to CRC.

Molecular advances in the understanding of genetic factors in CRC have increased almost logarithmically during the past decade. These include microarray systems, genomics, proteomics, high-throughput screening, and bio-informatics. Collectively, greater precision in the molecular profiling of CRC is expected to occur through technological advances in these systems. However, within such biotechnology systems, one must question whether or not certain of these elements may be impacted by those unique molecular characteristics of mismatch repair genes such as *MLH1* and *MSH2* in HNPCC. *A priori*, the phenotypic differences between tumor expression of *MSH2* and *MLH1* suggest that this may be the case [8]. Therefore, it becomes important to identify the differences in the biology of mismatch repair genes, their origin, and international distribution.

Partial evidence for genotypic and phenotypic heterogeneity in the Lynch syndrome has been elucidated by Vasen et al. [8]. Herein, the lifetime risk of developing cancer of any site was significantly greater for *MSH2* mutation carriers as opposed to *MLH1* mutation carriers ($p<0.01$). Of the several families in their investigation, *MSH2* mutation carriers were found to have a significantly greater risk of developing urinary tract cancer ($p<0.05$). Clearly, this is the type of clinical knowledge that needs to be developed when assessing the significance of germline mutations not only in HNPCC but in *all* hereditary cancer syndromes wherein causal germline mutations have been identified.

Staging

Synopsis

Staging of colorectal cancer in the setting of HNPCC is the same as that for sporadic colorectal cancer

Since HNPCC encompasses cancer of many anatomic sites, the staging for a particular type of cancer would be the same as in its sporadic counterpart. Uniform staging is best done based on the tumor-node-metastases (TNM) staging system of the American Joint Committee on Cancer (AJC).

Treatment

Synopsis

Since HNPCC is a syndrome that includes cancer of varying anatomic sites, the treatment would generally follow the accepted treatment for each cancer's sporadic counterpart. Exceptions have been noted. However, a standard of care for the treatment of CRC or any of the extracolonic cancers that are integral to the Lynch syndrome does not exist at this time.

Surgery

Subtotal colectomy for initial CRC, when control of this lesion is possible, is recommended because of the extremely high rate of metachronous CRC. However, aggressive endoscopic surveillance of the rectum is indicated following abdominal colectomy for HNPCC affecteds. Rectal cancer has been shown to develop in 8 (11%) of 71 patients at a median of 158 months, with a range of 38–282 months, following their primary surgical procedure for CRC [9]. Herein, the risk for developing rectal cancer in one such study was estimated to be approximately 12% at 12 years (1% per year) following abdominal colectomy.

Prophylactic surgery in the Lynch syndrome remains controversial. Nevertheless, we consider it prudent to discuss the options for prophylactic colectomy and prophylactic total abdominal hysterectomy and bilateral salpingo-oophorectomy with those patients who harbor mismatch repair germline mutations, of which *MSH2* and *MLH1* would be the most common [1], or with those who are at high risk based upon their position in the pedigree. Candidates for surgical prophylaxis are those high-risk patients who have one or more colonic adenomas, who may be noncompliant with colonoscopy, or who have cancer phobia with poor quality of life due to worry about CRC and who, in turn, would prefer pro-phylactic colectomy to the alternative of frequent life-long colonoscopy.

The risk for CRC in HNPCC is not significantly different from that in FAP, a disorder for which the use of prophylactic colectomy is orthodoxy. For example, in FAP the average age of CRC onset is about 39 years, while in HNPCC it is about 44 years. CRC occurs with approximately the same frequency in germline carriers of the two syndromes, where the only difference is that in FAP we have the florid polyposis phenotype to guide us. One must therefore ponder why prophylactic colectomy is non-controversial in FAP but is controversial in its Lynch syndrome counterpart with such strikingly similar CRC risks. One point which has been raised is the fact that the penetrance for CRC is virtually 100% in FAP compared to only 70–90% in HNPCC.

Endoscopy (Resection/Palliation)

Endoscopic resection of colorectal adenomas is performed during surveilance colonoscopy (see below). Endoscopic therapy for cancer, including use of the nyodynium-yttrium-aluminum-garnet (Nd:YAG) laser or photodynamic therapy is considered palliative as for sporadic cancer, and is reserved for patients who are poor risks for surgery.

Radiotherapy

Radiotherapy of rectal cancer in the setting of HNPCC is the same as that for sporadic cancer.

Chemotherapy

Chemotherapy of colorectal cancer in the setting of HNPCC is the same as that for sporadic cancer.

Radiochemotherapy

Adjuvent multimodality therapy (radiation plus chemotherapy) and radiation therapy for advanced rectal cancer in the setting of HNPCC is the same as that for sporadic colorectal cancer.

Immunotherapy

Immunotherapy and immunotargeted therapy of colorectal cancer in the setting of HNPCC is similar to that of sporadic cancer, and is considered to be of limited proven efficacy.

Others

Genetic Counseling

Genetic counseling is an essential part of the medical management of all high-risk patients. We initiate genetic counseling in HNPCC by age 18, at which age we offer DNA testing. The high-risk family member should be counseled again prior to disclosure of test results. Counseling can be initiated in a general educational program offered as a group Family Information Service (FIS). However, disclosure of genetic test results must be done on an individual basis. An exception may be made for those patients who may elect to have a close relative, spouse, or significant other attend the individual genetic counseling session for emotional support.

Genetic counselors need to be psychologically versed and oriented, compassionate, and knowledgeable about HNPCC's differential diagnosis, natural history, surveillance, and management strategies, and the significance of those MMR gene mutations responsible for HNPCC, including variation in gene penetrance, and of the potential for laboratory error. Patients must be told about the potential for employment or insurance discrimination, although it is exceedingly rare. Many high-risk patients nevertheless harbor the perception that such discrimination is common. Patients must be assured of the strict confidentiality code. This code must be meticulously followed for all pertinent but potentially vulnerable information, including cancer genetic risk status. Problems such as fear, anxiety, concern about family discord, and survivor guilt must be dealt with during this counseling process.

Prognosis

Survival from CRC in HNPCC is significantly better than in its sporadic counterpart.

Follow-Up

Screening must be significantly more intensive in HNPCC than in its sporadic counterpart.

Screening, Surveillance, Prevention

The Standard Task Force, the American Society of Colon and Rectal Surgeons, and The Collaborative Group of the Americas on Inherited Colorectal Cancer, provide guidelines for addressing the recognition, testing, and screening of CRC-prone families with FAP and HNPCC. Emphasis has been given to the preventable aspects of hereditary CRC through early diagnosis, through early detection of asymptomatic cancers, and through removal of colonic adenomas.

Surveillance

In HNPCC, given the right-sided predominance of CRC, the presence of accelerated carcinogenesis, and early age of cancer onset, we recommend an annual full colonoscopy, initiated between ages 20 and 25, in those family members with *MLH1*, *MSH2*, or *MSH6* germline mutations and/or obligate gene carriers by virtue of their positions in the pedigree. Patients at 50% risk, again by their positions in the pedigree, also merit intensive surveillance until proven that they are negative for the deleterious germline mutation. Endometrial cancer screening includes annual transvaginal ultrasound and pelvic examination with endometrial aspiration beginning at age 30. Transvaginal ovarian ultrasound and CA-125 analysis may be helpful for ovarian cancer surveillance; however, given the low sensitivities and specificities of these methods for early diagnosis of ovarian cancer, the patient must realize their limitations. Screening must be considered for other organ sites such as the upper uro-epithelial tract and stomach (particularly in natives of Korea or Japan, where gastric cancer occurs frequently in HNPCC, and/or when an excess of these extracolonic sites occur within a particular family).

Jarvinen et al. [10] evaluated the efficacy of CRC screening in HNPCC in a controlled clinical trial extending over 15 years. The incidence of CRC was compared in two cohorts of at-risk members of 22 HNPCC families. One hundred thirty-two subjects had colonic screening at three-year intervals while 118 of their high-risk relatives (controls) had no screening. CRC developed in eight screened subjects (6%), compared with 19 controls (16%; $p = 0.014$). The CRC rate was reduced by 62%. In mutation positive cases, CRC rates were 18% in screened vs. 41% in controls ($p = 0.02$). All CRCs in the screened group were local, causing no deaths, compared with nine deaths caused by CRC in the controls. The overall death rates were 10 vs. 26 subjects in the study and control groups ($p = 0.003$); in mutation-positive subjects, the rates were 4 vs. 12 ($p = 0.05$). It was concluded that CRC screening at three-year intervals more than halves the risk of CRC, prevents CRC deaths, and decreases overall mortality by about 65% in HNPCC families.

Cost Effectiveness for Colonoscopic Screening

Identifying HNPCC harbors a lifesaving potential through early cancer detection. This was also evidenced by Ramsey et al. [11] in a computer-driven model investigation of MSI screening which also was proven to be highly cost effective. These authors used the National Colorectal Cancer Registry data and the Creighton University International Hereditary Colorectal Cancer Registry, Medicare claims records and published literature, and patients with newly-diagnosed CRC, where their siblings and children provided the target population. Eligibility for initial office-based screening was based upon their personal and family cancer history, followed by testing of the tumor for MSI. Those who were positive for MSI were then offered germline testing. The siblings and children of those found to be mutation positive were offered genetic testing, and those who were positive for the mutation received life-long colorectal cancer screening. Results showed significant cost-effectiveness of screening. Specifically, "...When only the patients with cancer were considered, cost-effectiveness of screening was $42 210 per life-year gained. When patients with cancer and their siblings and children were considered together, cost-effectiveness increased to $7556 per life-year gained." Thus, this study showed that among patients with newly-diagnosed CRC, screening for HNPCC was cost-effective, particularly when the benefits to their immediate relatives (siblings and children) were considered [11].

Non-Invasive Screening

Traverso et al. [12] utilized purified DNA from stool samples containing exfoliated tumor cells in order to determine the feasibility of detecting *APC* mutations in fecal DNA employing newly-developed molecular methods. They studied stool samples from 28 individuals with nonmetastatic CRC, and from 18 other individuals with colonic adenomas that were at least 1 cm in diameter, and 28 controls who did not have neoplastic disease. Findings disclosed that, "... *APC* mutations were identified in 26 of the 46 patients with neoplasia (57%; 95% confidence interval, 41–71%, and in none of the 28 control patients (0%; 95% confidence interval, 0–12%; $p<0.001$). In the patients with positive tests, mutant *APC* genes made up 0.4–14.1% of all *APC* genes in the stool." These authors concluded that *APC* mutations can be readily identified in fecal DNA from patients with early CRC, thereby providing a new and highly practical approach for early diagnosis of CRC.

Traverso et al. [13] also examined microsatellite markers in stool from sporadic cancers with mismatch repair deficiencies, tumors which nearly always occur in the proximal colon, as an adjunct to sigmoidoscopy, which detects only distal colorectal lesions. Their objective was to determine feasibility, sensitivity, and specificity of these tests.

Using a sensitive method for MSI mutation detection, they found 18 of 46 cancers to harbor MSI alterations, while identical mutations could be identified in the fecal DNA of 17 of these 18 cases. They concluded that *BAT26* seems to be substantially more specific, thereby precluding a need for follow-up colonoscopies in many patients with false-positive fecal occult blood tests. On a very practical matter, there was no need to change dietary habits before testing, nor to provide several fecal samples, potentially increasing compliance. However, cost is high. The test needs validation with a larger sample. Sigmoidoscopy is not an appropriate comparison, since full colonoscopy is essential in HNPCC. The method used in this study may be appropriate for the general population, given epidemiologic evidence of increasing proximal CRC.

In another noninvasive screening approach, Ahlquist et al. [14] investigated freezer-archived stools in a blinded fashion from 22 patients with CRC, 11 not manifesting cancer but having adenomas ≥1 cm, and 28 who had endoscopically normal colons. Following isolation of DNA from stool, assay targets included point mutations in K-*ras*, *p53*, and *APC* genes; Bat-26, a MSI marker; as well as highly amplifiable DNA. They were able to derive analyzable DNA from all of the stool samples. Results showed, "... Sensitivity was 91% (95% confidence interval, 71%–99%) for cancer and 82% (48%–98%) for adenomas ≥1 cm with a specificity of 93% (76%–99%). Excluding K-*ras* from the panel, sensitivities for cancer were unchanged but decreased slightly for adenomas to 73% (39%–94%), while specificity increased to 100% (88%–100%) ..." These investigators concluded that their assay of altered DNA held promise as a stool screening approach for colorectal neoplasia, and they recommended larger clinical investigations.

It is clear that such an approach could have enormous benefit when applied to patients at inordinately high CRC risk, such as those with HNPCC. This would be particularly important for those individuals who otherwise would not participate in a colonoscopic screening program. Importantly, these patients must be advised that this fecal testing is not a substitute for colonoscopic screening.

Future Perspectives

Molecular genetics, proteomics, and micro-array technology are on the "cutting edge" of new technology for the diagnosis and management of all varieties of hereditary CRC, inclusive of the Lynch syndromes [1, 6, 7]. These new techniques will also be extremely helpful in sorting out the nosology of CRC. These molecular advances may also help to define CRC's prognosis and may even predict efficacy of chemotherapy and/or radiation therapy.

New Molecular-Based Diagnostic and Designer Drug Discoveries

It is essential to comprehend the underlying biology and pathogenesis of cancer with particular attention to the responsible multifaceted molecular genetic events underlying this biology so that highly-targeted pharmacologic therapy responsive to these events, can be produced. Such research must target the proteins which are translated by the gene. If the drug can successfully in-

hibit such deleterious alterations, then, conceivably, the progression to cancer may be halted. This entire process is directed toward the production of designer drugs that are responsive to the molecular genetic and endogenous idiosyncrasies of the cancer predisposition for a specific patient. Although the creation of such highly-targeted molecular based drugs are conceptually sound, they will require intensive investigations "at the bedside." Hereditary cancer-prone subjects, as in the case of HNPCC, particularly those who harbor cancer-prone germline mutations, will be prime candidates for drug studies.

Chemoprevention

What is the evidence to date that chemoprevention will be effective? An increasing number of epidemiological studies have shown that long-term use of nonsteroidal anti-inflammatory drugs (NSAIDs), particularly aspirin, can lead to a reduction in the incidence of colorectal adenomatous polyps and, ultimately, CRC. For example, the NSAID sulindac was found to regress colorectal adenomas in a placebo-controlled trial of patients with FAP. Celebrex has also been found to be effective in FAP [15].

Ruschoff et al. [16] demonstrated that microsatellite instability (MSI) in CRC cells that are deficient for a subset of mismatch repair (MMR) genes is markedly reduced following exposure to aspirin or sulindac. This effect "... was reversible, time and concentration dependent, and appeared independent of proliferation rate and cyclooxygenase function. In contrast, the MSI phenotype of a hPMS2-deficient endometrial cancer cell line was unaffected by aspirin/sulindac. We show that the MSI reduction in the susceptible MMR-deficient cells was confined to non-apoptotic cells, whereas apoptotic cells remain unstable and were eliminated from the growing population. These results suggest that aspirin/sulindac induces a genetic selection for microsatellite stability in a subset of MMR-deficient cells and may provide an effective prophylactic therapy for hereditary nonpolyposis colorectal cancer kindreds where alteration of the hMSH2 and hMLH1 genes are [*sic*] associated with the majority of cancer susceptibility cases." This was an *in vitro* study in a cell culture model, but it nevertheless has important implications for HNPCC.

At the clinical level, there is a paucity of data from chemoprevention studies in HNPCC or, for that matter, in any of the familial nonpolyposis colorectal cancer syndromes. The multiple high-risk target organs in these high-risk patients represent ideal candidates for cancer prevention trials. The goal of cancer prevention is not only to reduce cancer risk but also to improve the patient's quality of life.

Chemopreventive agents cannot be recommended at this time for individuals in the general population who are at average risk and/or those with sporadic colorectal tumors. Rather, chemoprevention efforts should be focused on those individuals who are at inordinately high risk, inclusive of those with FAP and HNPCC [15]. As in the mentioned noninvasive strategies employing DNA from exfoliated tumor cells in stool, chemoprevention cannot be considered as a substitute for colonoscopy.

References

1. Lynch HT, de la Chapelle A (1999) Genetic susceptibility to non-polyposis colorectal cancer. J Med Genet 36:801–818.
2. Lindgren G, Liljegren A, Jaramillo E, Rubio C, Lindblom A (2002) Adenoma prevalence and cancer risk in familial non-polyposis colorectal cancer. Gut 50:228–234.
3. Rijcken FEM, Hollema H, Kleibeuker JH (2002) Proximal adenomas in hereditary non-polyposis colorectal cancer are prone to rapid malignant transformation. Gut 50:382–386.
4. Jass JR, Stewart SM (1992) Evolution of hereditary non-polyposis colorectal cancer. Gut 33:783–786.
5. Smyrk TC, Watson P, Kaul K, Lynch HT (2001) Tumor-infiltrating lymphocytes are a marker for microsatellite instability in colorectal cancer. Cancer 91:2417–2422.
6. de la Chapelle A (2002) Microsatellite instability phenotype of tumors: genotyping or immunohistochemistry? The jury is still out. J Clin Oncol 20:897–899.
7. Vogelstein B, Kinzler KW (eds) (1998) The Genetic Basis of Human Cancer. McGraw-Hill, New York.
8. Vasen HFA, Stormorken A, Menko FH et al. (2001) *MSH2* mutation carriers are at higher risk of cancer than *MLH1* mutation carriers: a study of hereditary nonpolyposis colorectal cancer families. J Clin Oncol 19:4074–4080.
9. Rodriguez-Bigas MA, Vasen HFA, Pekka-Mecklin J et al., International Collaborative Group on HNPCC (1997) Rectal cancer risk in hereditary nonpolyposis colorectal cancer after abdominal colectomy. Ann Surg 225:202–207.
10. Jarvinen HJ, Aarnio M, Mustonen H, Aktan-Collan K, Aaltonen LA, Peltomaki P, de la Chapelle A (2000) Controlled 15-year trial on screening for colorectal cancer in families with hereditary nonpolyposis colorectal cancer. Gastroenterology 118:829–834.
11. Ramsey SD, Clarke L, Etzioni R, Higashi M, Berry K, Urban N (2001) Cost-effectiveness of microsatellite instability screening as a method for detecting hereditary nonpolyposis colorectal cancer. Ann Intern Med 135:577–588.
12. Traverso G, Shuber A, Levin B et al. (2002) Detection of *APC* mutations in fecal DNA from patients with colorectal tumors. N Engl J Med 346:311–320.
13. Traverso G, Shuber A, Olsson L et al. (2002) Detection of proximal colorectal cancers through analysis of faecal DNA. Lancet 359:403–404.
14. Ahlquist DA, Skoletsky JE, Boynton KA, Harrington JJ, Mahoney DW, Pierceall WE, Thibodeau SN, Shuber AP (2000) Colorectal cancer screening by detection of altered human DNA in stool: feasibility of a multitarget assay panel. Gastroenterology 119:1219–1227.
15. Steinbach G, Lynch PM, Phillips RKS et al. (2000) The effect of celecoxib, a cyclooxygenase inhibitor, in familial adenomatous polyposis. N Engl J Med 342:1946–1952.
16. Ruschoff J, Wallinger S, Dietmaier W, Bocker T, Brockhoff G, Hofstadter F, Fishel R (1998) Aspirin suppresses the mutator phenotype associated with hereditary nonpolyposis colorectal cancer by genetic selection. Proc Natl Acad Sci USA 95:11301–11306.

12 Colorectal Cancer in Inflammatory Bowel Disease

V. CROOG, S.H. ITZKOWITZ

Summary

Patients with inflammatory bowel disease (IBD) affecting the colon are at increased risk of developing colorectal cancer (CRC) compared to the general population. Both duration and extent of colitis are important risk factors for CRC, as is the presence of primary sclerosing cholangitis (PSC), family history of CRC, and (in some studies) early age at diagnosis of colitis. Efforts to reduce this risk have focused on colonoscopic surveillance as the best alternative to the more definitive but less appealing approach of prophylactic colectomy. Though surveillance has benefits that probably include decreased CRC mortality, its efficacy has not been firmly established and is limited by problems of patient dropout, sampling error when too few biopsies are taken at endoscopy, and difficulty in histopathological interpretation of dysplasia. High false negative rates at endoscopy have led to the recommendation that colectomy be considered for dysplasia of any grade.

Epidemiology

CRC that develops in the background of IBD constitutes less than 1% of all CRC cases, but because it accounts for one-sixth of all deaths in UC patients, it warrants attention. Several factors have been associated with an increased risk for CRC in patients with IBD (Table 1). Increasing duration of colitis is an important risk factor; after 10 years of disease, 0.5% of patients per year develop CRC, and this risk increases to 1% of patients per year after 20 years of disease. A recent critical review of 116 studies representing a total of 54,478 patients revealed that the risk of CRC in UC is 2% at 10 years, 8% at 20 years, and 18% at 30 years [1]. After 40 years of disease, 25–30% of patients with pancolitis will have developed CRC [2]. While the risk of CRC associated with Crohn's disease was previously underestimated, newer studies

have established a similar risk profile and similar biologic and pathologic features for CRC in both Crohn's colitis and UC [3]. Anatomic extent of colitis is one of the most significant determinants of risk for colonic neoplasia in IBD. While patients with proctosigmoiditis do not differ in risk compared with the normal population, those with more extensive colitis are at a substantially greater risk for developing carcinoma. Standardized incidence ratios for CRC risk have been estimated at 1.7 (95% CI, 0.8–3.2) for patients with proctitis, 2.8 (95% CI, 1.6–4.4) for patients with disease beyond the rectum but no further than the hepatic flexure, and 14.8 (95% CI, 11.4–18.9) for patients with disease extending beyond the hepatic flexure [4].

The presence of PSC in patients with UC carries with it an increased risk of CRC that approaches 50% after 25 years of colitis. Although PSC is present in only 2 to 4% of patients with UC, it is important to realize that 70 to 80% of patients with PSC have underlying UC that must be deliberately looked for by colonoscopy and biopsy, since these patients often lack symptoms of colitis. A

Table 1
Factors associated with risk of colorectal cancer in IBD

Factors associated with increased risk:
Longer disease duration
Greater anatomical extent of disease
Personal history of primary sclerosing cholangitis
Family history of colorectal cancer
Young age of colitis onset (some studies)
Factors associated with decreased risk:
Surveillance colonoscopy
Regular doctor visits
Use of 5-aminosalicylates
Use of oral steroids (not recommended for primary chemoprevention)
Folate supplements (suggestive effect)
Ursodeoxycholic acid (effect seen in PSC patients only)

family history of colon cancer is associated with a two- to three-fold increase in risk of CRC in UC patients. Some studies have identified younger age of onset of UC as a risk factor; one group found that patients diagnosed with colitis before the age of 15 years had a 50% risk of developing CRC by age 50. Disease activity has not been associated with an increased risk of CRC; in fact, it is the patient with quiescent disease, who has not undergone colectomy for severely active disease, who carries the increased risk of CRC and who may be lost to follow-up, potentially leading to missed dysplasia or cancer.

Etiology and Pathogenesis

Colorectal cancer, in both the sporadic and colitis setting, develops from a dysplastic precursor lesion (Fig. 1). Dysplasia is defined as unequivocal neoplastic change of the colonic epithelium. In sporadic CRC, the dysplastic precursor lesion is typically a discrete polypoid mass, referred to as an adenomatous polyp. In colitis, dysplastic epithelium can be polypoid or flat. Moreover, in inflamed colonic epithelium, histological features associated with tissue repair can mimic dysplasia, making it difficult for even expert pathologists to distinguish between reactive atypical and dysplasia. In 1983, in order to address this diagnostic dilemma and to provide stan-

dardization to the field, the IBD Morphology Study Group established histological criteria for classifying dysplasia as indefinite for dysplasia (ID), low-grade dysplasia (LGD), high-grade dysplasia (HGD), or carcinoma (CRC). Since the introduction of these criteria, more accurate diagnoses of dysplasia have permitted more focused management decisions, yet considerable interobserver variability remains, even among experienced histopathologists, particularly in the diagnosis of LGD.

Symptoms and Clinical Signs

In IBD patients, carcinomas present much as they do in patients with sporadic CRC. They may be silent, especially at earlier stages, or they may present with bleeding, change in bowel habits, or obstructive symptoms (particularly cancers of the descending and sigmoid colon). While such symptoms are helpful and typically worrisome indicators of an aberration in patients without IBD, to the patient with colitis these symptoms are all too familiar and may not prompt a call to action, especially in someone with continuous smoldering colitis symptoms or intermittent moderate-to-severe flares. Likewise, patients who are generally asymptomatic may be less likely to comply with the recommended surveillance practices and are at risk of presenting after years of absenteeism with an advanced-stage cancer.

Diagnostics

Synopsis

Definitive diagnosis of colorectal carcinoma is based on the histopathological analysis of specimens obtained an endoscopic exam or at the time of colectomy.

Histological interpretation of tissue specimens represents the most reliable method for establishing the diagnosis CRC in IBD patients. For the most part, carcinomas that develop in IBD are preceded by characteristic premalignant histological changes, termed dysplasia. Dysplasia can be detected by sampling the colonic mucosa at colonoscopy. Accordingly, programs of colon-

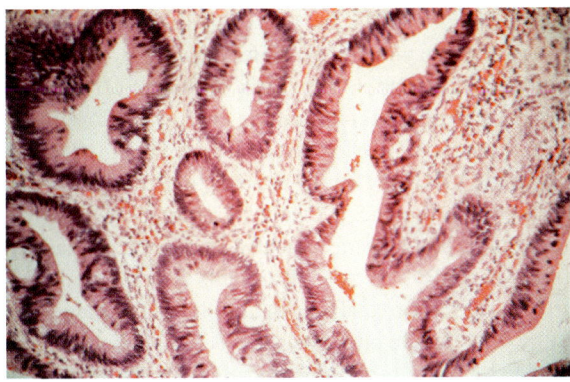

Figure 1
Dysplastic colonic mucosa in the setting of ulcerative colitis. Glands are irregularly branched and crowded together. Cell nuclei are hyperchromatic with occasional mitoses, and occur at different levels, displaying a pseudopalisading or "picket-fence" appearance. (courtesy of Robert S. Bresalier, M.D.)

oscopic surveillance have been recommended starting after 8 to 10 years of disease (when cancer risk begins to rise) in the hope of finding a dysplastic lesion or early cancer and preventing the development of a more advanced CRC. Dysplasia may occur in a visible lesion, sometimes referred to as a dysplasia-associated lesion or mass (DALM), but it can also lie within apparently normal "flat" mucosa, evading the eye of even the best endoscopists. For this reason, surveillance should entail taking a series of random biopsies throughout the mucosa of the large bowel, including any suspicious lesions. It is worth noting that some studies have found carcinomas at colectomy without any previous detection of dysplasia, suggesting a possible non-dysplastic pathway in the development of CRC in colitis, and highlighting a pitfall of relying completely on dysplasia as a detectable marker of cancer risk.

Histological Classification and Molecular Genetics

Compared to sporadic CRC, IBD-associated cancers often demonstrate a different biology, with a distinct timing and pattern of molecular alterations [4]. Presumably, the chronic inflammation at play in IBD creates a different substrate for carcinogenesis. Neoplasms arising in colitis are more often multifocal, mucinous or poorly differentiated. DNA aneuploidy and microsatellite instability have been associated with findings of dysplasia and cancer in patients with UC, suggesting that chromosomal instability and impaired DNA repair play an early role in carcinogenesis. Mutations in $p53$, a late event in sporadic CRC, occur earlier in the UC carcinogenesis pathway and have been correlated with DNA aneuploidy. The APC mutations commonly seen as early, if not essential, changes in sporadic CRC are relatively rare and late events in UC-associated cancers. Activation of the K-ras oncogene commonly found in sporadic CRC, appears to be uncommon in colitis-associated neoplasia.

Staging

The staging of CRC in patients with IBD follows that of sporadic CRC. Cancers are staged according to whether the tumor cells invade into or through the colonic wall,

and whether lymph nodes are involved. Once a diagnosis of cancer or HGD is made at colonoscopy, most surgeons are comfortable proceeding directly to colectomy without the need for prior imaging studies such as CT scans, endoscopic ultrasound or other procedures.

Treatment

Surgery

Once cancer is detected by colonoscopy, surgery is the initial treatment of choice unless the patient is considered to be a very poor operative candidate. Unlike sporadic CRC, where only the region of colon involved by cancer is removed, in the colitis patient, total proctocolectomy is necessary because of the high risk of metachronous cancer if colonic mucosa is left in place. Therefore, subtotal colectomy with ileorectal anastomosis is to be avoided. The two main surgical options for IBD patients are total proctocolectomy with either end-ileostomy or an ileal pouch-anal anastomosis (IPAA). The former is the procedure of choice for older patients or patients with poor anal sphincter function to minimize problems associated with frequent bowel movements and fecal incontinence. Complications of this procedure include irritation, infection, or herniation at the stoma site as well as the psychosocial impact of a permanent ileostomy.

Ileal pouch-anal anastomosis is often the preferred procedure for younger patients because it avoids the need for a permanent ileostomy. If the cancer involves the rectum, IPAA should not be performed, and many would argue likewise for dysplasia involving the rectum. There is a 5% failure rate of the ileal pouch requiring the formation of an end-ileostomy. Frequent bowel movements and incontinence are also known complications of IPAA, and up to 25% of patients develop pouchitis that is generally treatable with antibiotics but may prove to be disabling. In addition, there is a small but real risk of CRC in any remaining rectal mucosa, prompting many investigators to suggest continued surveillance of the pouch and any rectal cuff.

It is generally accepted that finding HGD during surveillance warrants colectomy given the high (approximately 40%) risk of concurrent cancer [5]. Debate continues as to whether colectomy should be performed if LGD is detected by surveillance colonoscopy. A retrospective review of studies performed prior to the mid-1990's disclosed a high (19%) concurrence rate of CRC for biopsy-positive LGD, although this was based on small numbers of patients. Since then, several groups have found a 16% to 54% rate of progression from LGD to either HGD or CRC [5]. Consequently, many experts recommend colectomy for a patient with any grade of definite dysplasia – a policy that may explain the somewhat lower rate of CRCs found in some surveillance series (such as Scandinavia).

The often segmental nature of Crohn's colitis presents a controversy when cancer or dysplasia is detected. Many surgeons (and patients) would opt to remove the lesion in question by performing segmental resection or subtotal colectomy rather than total proctocolectomy in these patients. The risk of metachronous neoplasia in any residual colonic mucosa has not been well studied.

Endoscopy

Some patients with IBD have discrete, polypoid lesions that resemble common sporadic adenomas. Studies have demonstrated that if such lesions can be completely resected endoscopically, and there is no other evidence of dysplasia either in the mucosa surrounding the base of the polyp or anywhere else in the colon, these lesions can be safely treated with polypectomy alone, followed by regular colonoscopic follow-up, without resorting to proctocolectomy (6). So far, these lesions are classified based only on gross endoscopic appearance (discrete, well-defined sessile or pedunculated polypoid lesions) because histologically they are indistinguishable from more ominous DALMs. Efforts have been made to distinguish adenoma-like polyps from DALMs based on molecular alterations, but to date, the sensitivity and specificity of such analyses precludes their use in clinical practice.

A finding of ID should be followed-up with repeat endoscopy in 6 months, at which time an increased number of biopsies should be taken at the site of the previous ID finding and throughout the colon. Some experts feel that any active inflammation should be aggressively treated prior to re-scoping, to minimize any confusion between reactive and dysplastic tissue.

Prognosis and Follow-Up

The prognosis of IBD patients with CRC is similar to those without a history of colitis, with an overall 5-year survival rate of approximately 50%. Prognosis is based on cancer stage at the time of diagnosis. Some studies that have reported a somewhat worse survival for patients with IBD-associated CRC found that there were more advanced stage cancers among the IBD patients. This reflects, in part, delays in diagnosing colon cancer because symptoms of cancer overlap those of colitis, and inaccuracies inherent in surveillance colonoscopy may also contribute.

Screening, Surveillance, Prevention

Undergoing prophylactic total proctocolectomy before 8–10 years of colitis, when the cancer risk starts to rise, is certainly the most definitive way to eliminate the risk of CRC. This approach to CRC prevention is reasonable for a young person facing several decades of surveillance with all of its inherent imperfections, and is often more acceptable for those with chronic bothersome symptoms or intermittent moderate-to-severe flare-ups. A published model of life expectancy found that prophylactic colectomy would add 2 to 10 months of life per patient compared with any surveillance scheme and 1.1 to 1.4 years compared to no surveillance [7]. Physicians should discuss with those patients considering an early operative course the issue of quality of life after colectomy. In a questionnaire-based study comparing surgery with continued medical therapy, bowel movements were more frequent in the surgical group, but urgency was worse in the medically treated patients. Overall function and quality of life was better in those who had surgery than in those who pursued a non-operative course [8].

Still, many patients opt to keep their colons and undergo colonoscopic surveillance, especially if the colitis is relatively asymptomatic. No randomized controlled trial has been performed to assess the efficacy of colonoscopic surveillance for reducing CRC mortality, and no such trial is likely to occur given the reluctance of patients and physicians to accept a no-surveillance option. However, data from case-control studies suggest that the use of colonoscopy almost certainly lowers CRC mortality in UC patients, and patients who partake in at least some form of surveillance have a better prognosis than

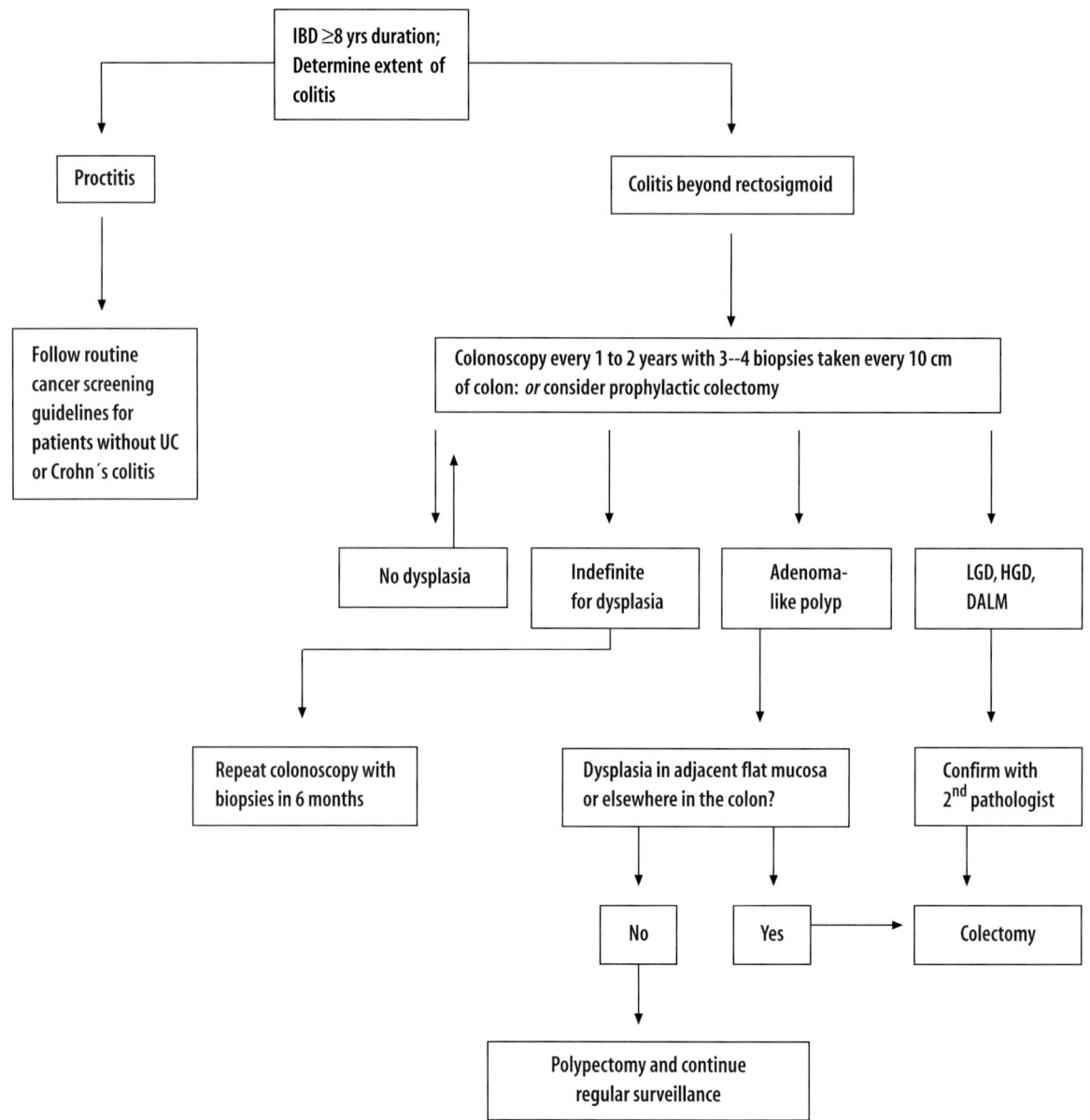

Figure 2
Suggested algorithm for CRC surveillance in IBD

those who leave surveillance or never comply [2]. The benefits of a surveillance program extend beyond just the colonoscopic procedure itself, since regular doctor visits are also beneficial. Colonoscopy is a rather safe procedure with few complications even in the IBD population.

The usual protocol in UC is to begin surveillance after 8 to 10 years of colitis in patients with disease extending beyond the sigmoid colon (see suggested algorithm in Fig. 2). Exams should be performed thereafter at 1- to 2-year intervals. Ideally, a surveillance colonoscopy involves a thorough inspection of the entire colonic mucosa, from ileocecal valve (and terminal ileum when possible) to anus. Random biopsies should be taken in groups of 3 or 4 at 10 cm intervals. Since the sigmoid and rectum have higher rates of CRC in UC, some authorities recommend taking an increased number of biopsies at these distal sites. It has been estimated that 33 biopsy specimens are needed for 90% certainty of ruling out dysplasia. While very little is known about surveillance in Crohn's colitis, it is useful to apply the same recommendations to patients with long-standing Crohn's colitis that involves at least one-third of the colon.

The goal of surveillance is ideally to detect neoplasia while it is still in its early stages. However, it is important to realize that once dysplasia is detected, there is a chance that more advanced neoplasia is either already present elsewhere in the colon, or may subsequently develop. It has been estimated that at immediate colectomy for the diagnosis of LGD, DALM, or HGD, the frequency of finding cancer is 19%, 43% and 42%, respectively [5]. Furthermore, 16 to 29% of patients who pursued a non-operative course after a finding of LGD progressed to DALM, HGD or cancer. Other investigators have found the rate of progression from LGD to more advanced pathology to be approximately 50% at five years [9].

It is crucial that doctors understand the pitfalls of surveillance and discuss them with their patients at the initiation of surveillance and at times throughout follow-up. In particular, patients should know that if dysplasia is found on a surveillance exam, it is possible that a cancer is already present. Some patients will have a cancer found at colonoscopy or colectomy despite recent negative surveillance colonoscopies. Other limitations of surveillance relate to the difficulty in detection and interpretation of dysplasia. There can be considerable interobserver variability, especially in cases of ID and LGD. Any histological ambiguity should be resolved between two experienced pathologists, particularly before recommending colectomy for a finding of dysplasia at colonoscopy. As with any long-term preventive program, patient compliance is a problem that further limits the efficacy of surveillance colonoscopy. Patients with relatively quiescent disease are at greatest risk of being lost to follow-up. Physicians must encourage their patients to stay with this lifelong plan or else consider prophylactic colectomy. Studies are presently underway to identify specific molecular markers in blood or stool samples that might supplement histology as a screening technique in patients with long term UC or Crohn's colitis.

The possible role of chemoprevention in IBD has received increased attention in recent years, fueled mostly by positive findings in the sporadic adenoma and carcinoma literature. The most promising results to date suggest a role for 5-aminosalicylate (5-ASA) compounds in CRC chemoprevention in UC. A case-control study by Eaden and colleagues in the UK found that the use of 5-ASA compounds was associated with a 75% decreased risk of CRC (95% CI, 0.13–0.48) [10]. Mesalamine use was associated with the greatest degree of protection, while sulfasalazine use was associated with a less protective effect that was statistically significant only at doses of 2 g/d or more. If the suggested protective effect of 5-ASA agents is due to their ability to suppress inflammation, it should follow that other types of anti-inflammatory agents commonly employed in the treatment of UC and Crohn's disease may provide some protection as well. While few studies have investigated this question, systemic (but not topical) steroids have been associated with a significant reduction in CRC. Nonetheless, given the high complication rate of chronic steroid use, these medications cannot be endorsed as chemopreventive agents.

In sporadic CRC, folate deficiency is a risk factor for the development of neoplasia and folate use protects against neoplastic progression. The paucity of data in UC patients suggests, but does not prove, that folate use is associated with a trend toward decreased risk of finding cancer or dysplasia in UC patients under surveillance. Folate supplementation should be offered to all UC patients, given the possibility of a protective effect, its low cost and excellent side effect profile. Ursodeoxycholic acid (ursodiol) use has been associated with a decreased risk of CRC in the high-risk group of UC patients with PSC. Whether this effect translates beyond this high-risk group to the general UC population is currently under investigation.

Future Perspectives

The epidemiology of colorectal cancer in inflammatory bowel disease has been reported, and its development from dysplastic mucosa well described. Further understanding of the molecular evolution of neoplasia in the setting of inflammatory bowel disease will be important, however, in helping to determine who will go on to develop dysplasia and eventually carcinoma. Why some individuals, but not others develop colorectal cancer is not well understood, but recent evidence suggests that carcinoma in this setting is associated with an underlying genetic instability of the colonic mucosa. This is associated with subcellular abnormalities including shortening of telomeres, the protective ends of chromosomes. Future studies will no doubt concentrate on an increased understanding of the molecular underpinnings of cancer in ulcerative colitis and Crohn's disease. This understanding will aid in the clinical management of patients with inflammatory bowel disease, including determining optimal Surveillance intervals for dysplasia and colorectal cancer.

References

1. Eaden JA, Abrams KR, Mayberry JF (2001)The risk of colorectal cancer in ulcerative colitis: a meta-analysis. Gut 48:526–35.
2. Ekbom A, Helmick C, Zack M, Adami HO (1990) Ulcerative colitis and colorectale cancer. A population-based study. N Engl J Med 323:1228–33.
3. Bansal P, Sonnenberg A (1996) Risk factors of colorectal cancer in inflammatory bowel disease. Am J Gastroenterol 91:44–8.
4. Itzkowitz SH (1997) Inflammatory bowel disease and cancer. Gastroenterol Clin North Am 26:129–39.
5. Bernstein CN, Shanahan F, Weinstein WM (1994) Are we telling patients the truth about surveillance colonoscopy in ulcerative colitis? [see comments]. Lancet 343:71–4.
6. Rubin PH, Friedman S, Harpaz N, Goldstein E, Weiser J, Schiller J, Waye JD, Present DH (1999) Colonoscopic polypectomy in chronic colitis: conservative management after endoscopic resection of dysplastic polyps. Gastroenterology. 117:1295–300.
7. Provenzale D, Kowdley KV, Arora S, Wong JB (1995) Prophylactic colectomy or surveillance for chronic ulcerative colitis? A decision analysis [see comments]. Gastroenterology 109:1188–96.
8. Sagar P, Lewis W, Holdsworth P, Johnston D, Mitchell C, MacFie J (1993) Quality of life after restorative proctocolectomy with a pelvic ileal reservoir compares favorably with that of patients with medically treated colitis. Dis Colon Rectum 36:584–92.
9. Ullman TA, Loftus, E.V.Jr, Kakar S, Burgart LJ, Sandborn WJ, Tremaine, WJ (2002) Fate of Low-Grade Dysplasia in Ulcerative Colitis. Am J Gastroenterol 97:922–7.
10. Eaden J, Abrams K, Ekbom A, Jackson E, Mayberry J (2000) Colorectal cancer prevention in ulcerative colitis: a case-control study. Aliment Pharmacol Ther 14:145–53.

Anal Canal

V

13 Anal Carcinoma

J.C. EGGENBERGER

Summary

Anal canal carcinoma is rare, accounting for less than 2% of all GI tract malignancies. Originally thought to be a consequence of chronic anal canal inflammation, it is now considered a result of infection by human papilloma virus, a sexually transmitted disease. Prior to the 1970s, anal cancer was treated by abdominoperineal resection with permanent colostomy. However, for the past thirty years, sphincter-preserving chemoradiation has been the standard of care, with survival superior to that resulting from primary surgical therapy. Although highly curable, anal carcinoma frequently presents late due to misdiagnosis or delay in presentation. Future improvements in the management and prognosis of this uncommon malignancy will likely be realized through the screening of high-risk groups, improvement in the treatment of venereal warts and the optimization of both radiation and chemotherapeutic regimens.

Epidemiology

Traditionally, a discussion of anal cancer has addressed both anal canal and anal margin malignancies. Although similar in presentation, they differ markedly in their anatomy, treatment and prognosis. Anal margin cancers arise in the hair-bearing stratified squamous epithelium distal to the anal verge (defined by the most distal aspect of the internal anal sphincter). Biologically, they behave like skin cancers and are treated by local excision. Anal margin cancers will be referred to only briefly, as the primary focus of the chapter will be anal canal carcinoma.

Although comprising only 1.5% of all GI tract cancers and 1–6% of all anorectal malignancies in the United States, anal canal carcinomas have increased in incidence over the past thirty years, coincident with an increase in the incidence of human papilloma virus infection [1, 2]. The incidence of anal cancer among the general population is approximately 0.8 per 100,000 men and women in the United States [3]. They present most often in the fifth and sixth decades of life and exhibit a marked female predominance in a ratio of 5:1, except in areas with large high-risk male populations where the female to male ratio approaches 1:1 and the age of presentation is the third and fourth decades of life.

Etiology and Pathogenesis

Until recently, anal cancer was thought to result from chronic inflammation of anal canal tissues in patients with symptomatic hemorrhoids, fistulae, fissures and inflammatory bowel disease. There has never been any scientific evidence put forth to support this theory. Primarily based upon accumulating epidemiological data, the development of anal cancer is strongly tied to infection by human papilloma virus (HPV) [2]. Its development closely parallels the known progression and relationship between HPV and carcinoma of the cervix. Carcinoma of the anus and cervix are biologically similar in many ways. Both share a similar histology, arise in areas of cellular transition from columnar epithelium to squamous type and have been strongly linked to infection with HPV subtypes 16 and 18 (viral DNA from HPV 16 has been found in a high proportion of anal neoplasms) [1, 2]. Additionally, they are often seen in association with squamous intraepithelial lesions (SIL) previously termed dysplasia, and long known to be the precursor of cervical cancer [3]. Similarly, it is likely that anal SIL is the precursor to anal carcinoma.

Although integral to the development of anal cancer, HPV infection is not the only risk factor for its development. Anal carcinoma is more common in men who have sex with men (MSM), patients with a history of sexually transmitted diseases (STD) (especially herpes simplex, chlamydia and gonorrhea), those with multiple sex partners, women with a prior history of cervical/vulvar/vaginal cancer and patients chronically immunosuppressed as a result of HIV infection, chemotherapy or solid organ transplantation [2].

The role of HIV infection in the development of anal cancer is not well understood. What is known is that HIV positivity increases the likelihood of HPV infection, which in turn increases the likelihood of anal cancer development [4]. Whether HIV infection has a direct effect on the pathogenesis of anal cancer is unknown.

As with cervical cancer, a history of smoking increases the risk of anal cancer 2–5 fold. Interestingly, this relationship may be reciprocal as lung cancer is twice as likely in those with a history of anal cancer compared to the general population [2].

Symptoms and Clinical Signs

The most common presenting symptom in patients with anal cancer is anal outlet bleeding, occurring in at least one-half of patients [1]. Anal pain and the sensation of an anal or rectal mass occur in up to one-third of patients. As many as one-fifth of patients are asymptomatic. Other symptoms include anal pruritus, discharge, and tenesmus. Change in bowel habits, fecal incontinence, pelvic pain and a vaginal discharge suggesting the presence of an anovaginal fistula are symptoms of advanced disease, often with sphincter involvement.

Physical exam will most often reveal a firm, indurated mass on digital exam. Peri-anal, intra-anal, perivaginal or vaginal condyloma may be seen, especially in high-risk populations. Locally advanced lesions can present with a visible mass at the anal orifice or anal stenosis on digital exam. Fifteen percent of patients at presentation will have palpable inguinal or femoral adenopathy.

Diagnostics

Synopsis

Standard diagnostic and imaging techniques for the detection and staging of anal cancer

▸ Digital rectal exam
▸ Incisional biopsy of anal mass
▸ Aspiration or excisional biopsy of palpable adenopathy
▸ Endoanal ultrasonography
▸ Chest X-ray
▸ Abdominopelvic CT

Evaluation should also include a detailed history to elucidate risk factors for anal cancer such as a prior history of HPV infection, HIV disease, history of anal intercourse, multiple sex partners, history of other HPV associated malignancies (cervical, vulvar or vaginal cancer) or chronic immunosuppression other than that due to HIV disease.

Despite the accessibility of the anus, the diagnosis of anal cancer can be difficult. Associated symptoms can be attributed to benign conditions, even after an apparently thorough anorectal examination. Definitive diagnosis of anal cancer is made via incisional biopsy, either as an office procedure via anoscopy or proctoscopy, or as a surgical procedure under conscious sedation with local or regional anesthesia. Palpable inguinal or femoral lymph nodes should undergo aspiration or excisional biopsy as an aid to diagnosis and staging of the tumor. Inconclusive results after office attempts to make a diagnosis warrant an examination under anesthesia to allow for a more thorough evaluation and additional biopsies. Laboratory evaluation can be limited to a complete blood count.

Endoanal ultrasonography can provide assessment of depth of tumor penetration, involvement of contiguous structures (prostate, sphincter mechanism) and local adenopathy. Abdominopelvic CT scan and chest radiography are also helpful in staging the primary tumor as between 5 and 8% of patients will have liver metastases at presentation [1]. Finally, colonoscopy or barium enema should be performed to exclude more proximally associated pathology (Figs. 1 and 2).

Histological Classification and Molecular Genetics

Synopsis

The vast majority of anal canal cancers are of epidermoid/epithelial origin, the most common type being squamous cell carcinoma (SCC). However, because their clinical behavior, response to treatment and prognosis are similar, they are classified together. Other histologic types originating within the anal canal include melanoma, adenocarcinoma, small cell type, undifferentiated and leiomyosarcoma (Fig. 3).

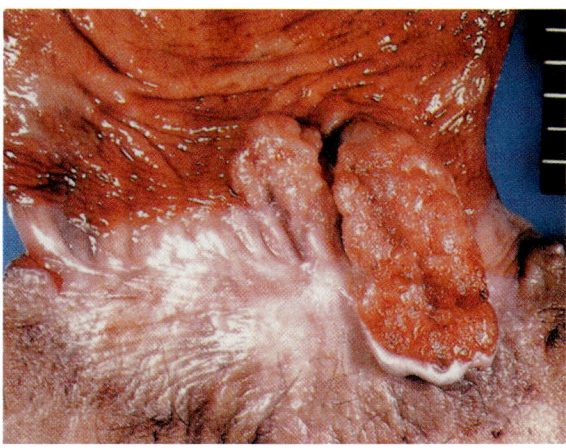

Figure 1
Anal canal carcinoma. (From Fenoglio-Preiser, editor. Gastrointestinal Pathology, p. 827 fig. 22.8C. Lippincott-Raven Publishers, 1989. With permission)

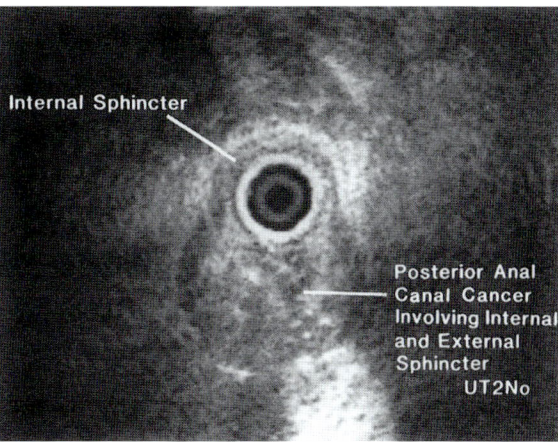

Figure 2
Anal ultrasound demonstrating a UT2N0 anal cancer. (From Cohen and Winawer, editors. Cancer of the Colon, Rectum and Anus, p. 1018, fig. 102—6. McGraw-Hill Publishers, 1995. With permission)

A discussion of anal cancer histology would not be complete without a thorough understanding of anal anatomy. The following text is based upon a joint statement of the American Joint Commission on Cancer (AJCC) and the Union Internationale Contre le Cancer (UICC) [1]. The anal canal is approximately 4 cm in length and denotes the termination of the intestinal tract. It extends from the anorectal ring (ARR) to the anal verge (AV) and is lined by both keratinizing and non-keratinizing squamous epithelium. The ARR is the muscular thickening formed by the confluence of the internal anal sphincter, external anal sphincter, puborectalis and the distal aspect of the longitudinal muscle of the rectum. The AV corresponds to both the distal most aspect of the IAS and the junction of stratified squamous epithelium (non-hair bearing) with perianal skin (hair-bearing). The anal margin is defined as that portion of perianal skin distal to the AV.

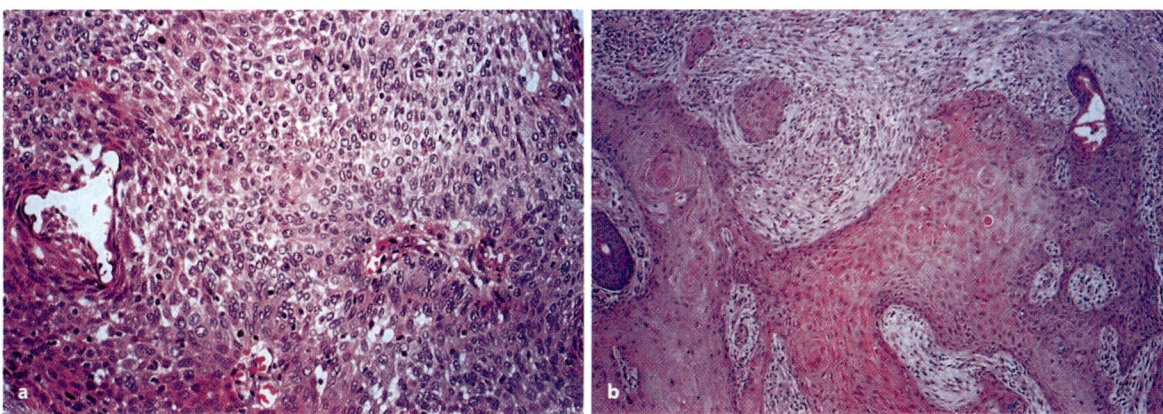

Figure 3a,b
a Non-keratinizing squamous cell carcinoma of the anus. b Keratinizing squamous cell carcinoma of the anus. (From Fenoglio-Preiser, editor. Gastrointestinal Pathology, p. 829 figs. 22.9, I and E. Lippincott-Raven Publishers, 1989. With permission.)

The dentate line is defined by the anal columns (of Morgagni) that separate the anal transitional zone of the lower rectum from the squamous epithelium of the anal canal. The anal transition zone is 6–12 mm in length and is located between the colonic mucosa of the distal rectum and the squamous epithelium of the anal canal. The transition zone is marked by histologic variability and contains columnar, transitional (urothelial-type) and non-keratinizing squamous epithelium. The dentate line separates the vascular and lymphatic supply of the proximal and distal anal canal. Anal canal tissues above the dentate line receive blood from the superior and middle rectal arteries and drain to the portal venous system. The area below the dentate line is supplied by the middle and inferior rectal arteries and drains to the systemic venous system. Lymph and neoplasms originating above the DL drain to the perirectal, superior rectal and para-aortic nodes and to the inguinal-femoral nodes if arising below the DL (Fig. 4).

As alluded to above, the histology of malignancies found within the anal canal is quite varied. The majority is classified as squamous cell carcinomas (SCCA), with the keratinizing type accounting for 50% of all anal canal cancers and originating below the dentate line [1].

Several non-keratinizing types originate above the dentate line within the transitional zone and account for 25% of anal cancers [1]. Historically, non-keratinizing SCCAs have been subdivided into cloacogenic and transitional cell types. However, these subtypes are felt to be variants of the general class of SCCA of the anus because their biological behavior, response to treatment and prognosis are similar to the keratinizing SCCAs.

Adenocarcinomas, although rare, have been described within the anal canal and originate from glandular elements either within the transitional zone (rectal-type), anal ducts or an anal fistula [5]. Histologically, these three variants can be very difficult to distinguish from one another.

Melanoma, although rarely found in the anal canal, constitutes the third most common primary site after skin and eyes [6]. It originates from melanocytes both above and below the dentate line. The majority of anal melanomas are lightly pigmented or amelanotic and can be misdiagnosed as polyps or other histologic types of anal cancer [6].

Other rare neoplasms of the anal canal include small cell carcinoma, undifferentiated type and leiomyosarcoma.

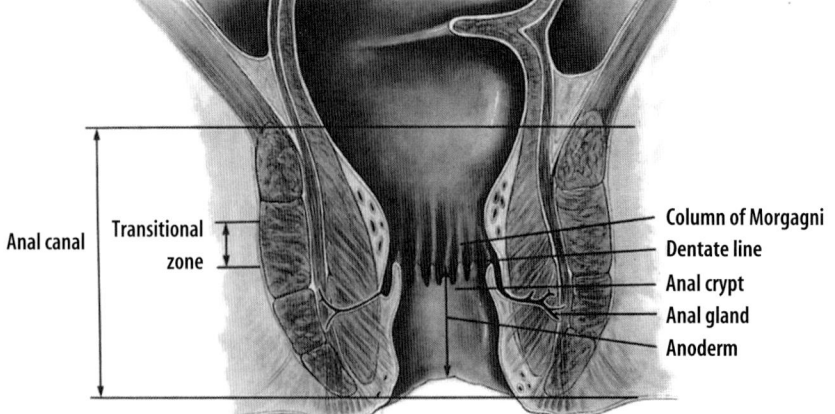

Figure 4
Anal canal anatomy. (From Gordon PH and Nivatvongs S, editors. Principles and Practice of Surgery for the Colon, Rectum and Anus, 2nd edition, p. 12, fig. 1.6. Quality Medical Publishing, 1999. With permission).

Staging

Synopsis

TNM classification of cancers of the anal canal

T   Primary tumor
TX   Primary tumor cannot be assessed
T0   No evidence of primary tumor
Tis Carcinoma in situ
T1   Tumor 2 cm or less in greatest dimension
T2   Tumor more than 2 cm but not more than 5 cm in greatest dimension
T3   Tumor more than 5 cm in greatest dimension
T4   Tumor of any size invades adjacent organs e.g. vagina, urethra, bladder (involvement of the sphincter muscles alone is not classified as T4)
N   Regional lymph nodes
NX   Regional lymph nodes cannot be assessed
N0   No regional lymph node metastasis
N1   Metastasis in perirectal lymph nodes(s)
N2   Metastasis in unilateral internal iliac and or inguinal lymph node(s)
N3   Metastasis in perirectal and inguinal lymph nodes and/or bilateral internal iliac and/or inguinal lymph nodes
M   Distant metastasis
MX   Distant metastasis cannot be assessed
M0   No distant metastasis
M1   Distant metastasis

Stage groupings	T	N	M
Stage 0	TIs	N0	M0
Stage I	T1	N0	M0
Stage II	T2	N0	M0
	T3	N0	M0
Stage IIIa	T1	N1	M0
	T2	N1	M0
	T3	N1	M0
	T4	N0	M0
Stage IIIb	T4	N1	M0
	Any T	N2	M0
	Any T	N3	M0
Stage IV	Any T	Any N	M1

Prior to the establishment of chemoradiation as the standard first line treatment of anal cancer, staging was surgical and similar to that of colorectal cancer. In 1987, the AJCC and the UICC established the clinical staging system delineated above [1]. Staging of adenocarcinoma of the anal canal is according to the TNM system for colon and rectal cancer. Staging systems for melanoma, small cell carcinoma, undifferentiated carcinoma and leiomyosarcoma do not exist due to their rare occurrence and poor prognosis. Anal margins tumors are staged as skin cancers.

Treatment

Synopsis

See Algorithm page 174

The treatment of anal cancer changed radically in the early 1970's when chemoradiation was added to abdominoperineal resection to reduce the incidence of surgical failure. Developed by clinicians at Wayne State University and commonly referred to as the Nigro protocol, treatment involved a combination of 5-FU, mitomycin C and external beam radiotherapy given over a thirty-five day period (Table 1). At the time of APR (abdominoperineal resection), patients were found to have had complete responses without either gross or microscopic

Table 1
The Nigro protocol (From Gordon PH and Nivatvongs S, editors. Principles and Practice of Surgery for the Colon, Rectum and Anus, 2nd edition, p. 462. Quality Medical Publishing, 1999.)

External irradiation:
3000 rads to the primary carcinoma and pelvic/inguinal nodes starting day 1 (200 rads/day)
Systemic chemotherapy:
5-fluorouracil 1000 mg/meter squared/24 hr. as a continuous infusion for 4 days starting on day 1.
Mitomycin C 15 mg/meter squared as an intravenous bolus on day 1 only.
5-fluorouracil repeated as a 4-day infusion starting on day 28.

Synopsis

Staging procedures ⟶ Stage IV disease ⟶ Clinical trials

Stage IV disease ⟶ Palliation

Staging procedures ⟶ Locoregional disease

Locoregional disease ⟶ Nigro protocol

Nigro protocol ⟶ Persistent disease ⟶ Modified Nigro Protocol*

Nigro protocol ⟶ Complete response

Modified Nigro Protocol* ⟶ Persistent disease

Persistent disease ⟶ APR

Complete response ⟶ Follow-up

APR ⟶ Follow-up

Follow-up ⟶ Local recurrence

Local recurrence ⟶ APR

Local recurrence ⟶ Modified Nigro protocol*

Modified Nigro protocol* ⟶ Follow-up

Local recurrence ⟶ Regional lymph node recurrence

Regional lymph node recurrence ⟶ Lymph node dissection

*Modified Nigro Protocol – boost of external beam radiotherapy combined with cisplatin

residual tumor, thus ushering in combined modality therapy as first line treatment for epithelial cancers of the anal canal [7]. Subsequent randomized trials (UK-CCCR, EORTC) comparing radiation alone vs. radio-chemotherapy utilizing 5-fluorouracil and mitomycin demonstrated the superiority of combination therapy in terms of reduced local recurrence rates, overall recur-rence rates and lower risk for colostomy due to persis-tent disease. These studies also demonstrated improved survival in patients treated with combination therapy when compared to APR alone [1]. The addition of mito-mycin C to 5-FU conferred lower rates of local recur-rence and improved disease-free survival in a study con-ducted by the RTOG and ECOG [2].

With the development of drug treatments resulting in prolongation of life in HIV positive patients, the incidence of anal cancer in this high-risk population is likely to increase. Currently, there is a lack of consensus regarding the management of such patients, although in general, these patients tolerate combination therapy as long as doses of both chemotherapy and radiation are reduced. Patients intolerant of combination therapy or those whose underlying immunosuppression makes them too high a risk for such treatment can be considered either for radiation alone or APR with its attendant higher peri/post-operative morbidity and mortality.

Melanoma of the anal canal is resistant to both chemotherapy and radiation and is therefore treated surgically. Controversy exists as to which procedure, local excision or APR, is most optimal. The prognosis following either operation is dismal with 5-year survivals less than 20%, as most patients die due to distant metastases [6]. The author favors local excision provided normal continence can be maintained. If this is not possible, an APR should be performed.

Adenocarcinomas of the anal canal are treated surgically. Those that arise within the transitional zone (rectal-type) are first staged with transrectal ultrasound. If they meet accepted criteria for local treatment (well-differentiated, UT1 stage, less than 1/3 of the circumference, non-ulcerated), wide local excision is an acceptable alternative to APR. Adenocarcinomas arising from the anal glands or within a chronic anal fistula are treated with APR due to their deeply invasive nature, often into the sphincter musculature. The role of chemoradiation has not been defined, but its use seems appropriate in advanced tumors (UT3 or UN1) to decrease local recurrence.

Ten to twenty percent of patients with anal canal carcinoma will develop distant metastatic disease (liver is the most common site) [1]. The prognosis is poor. Such patients do not benefit either from surgery or chemoradiation and therefore should be enrolled in clinical trials.

Surgery

Surgery still does play a role in the treatment of anal canal cancer, but primarily as salvage treatment for patients with persistent or recurrent disease following chemoradiation. Abdominoperineal resection is the procedure of choice, although local excision in highly selected patients has been reported. As noted above, a second course of combined modality treatment using cisplatin instead of mitomycin C has been utilized successfully as an alternative to APR. The overall survival following curative-intent APR approximates 50% [8].

APR is also indicated for severe complications of chemoradiation, especially fecal incontinence and for those patients who are deemed unsuitable or intolerant of chemoradiation, such as those with AIDS.

The management of anal margin tumors has been alluded to previously. They are staged and treated as skin cancers with wide local excision.

Endoscopy (Resection/Palliation)

Has no role in the treatment of anal canal.

Radiotherapy

The role of radiotherapy in the treatment of anal carcinoma has been discussed above in the context of standardized protocols.

Chemotherapy

The role of chemotherapy in the treatment of anal carcinoma has been discussed above in the context of standardized protocols.

Radiochemotherapy

The role of radiochemotherapy in the treatment of anal carcinoma has been discussed above in the context of standardized protocols.

Immunotherapy

No established or experimental role in the treatment of anal cancer.

Prognosis

Like most other malignancies, stage at diagnosis is the most important prognostic factor in patients with anal canal cancer. Size, specifically tumors greater than 5 cm in diameter (T3) are associated with significantly lower survival (40% v. greater than 50%) rates [1]. The presence of positive regional lymph nodes (N1–3) also substantially reduces survival (40–45% v. greater than 70%) compared to patients with negative nodes at the time of diagnosis [1]. The reported overall survival at three years following combination therapy for anal cancer varies from 65–72% [2].

Follow-Up

Although no standard follow-up protocol has been agreed upon, it is critical that regular follow-up be maintained, as treatment failures and recurrences can be treated successfully for cure when detected without delay. The author recommends the initial follow-up visit at six weeks following completion of treatment at which time a thorough history and baseline physical exam is performed. Any findings suggestive of persistent disease mandate either office or operative biopsy. Thereafter, visits are at three-month intervals for 2–3 years and then at six-month intervals until five years post-treatment. Currently, tumor markers for anal cancer do not exist. Endoanal ultrasound may play a limited role in the eval-

uation of patients with suspected recurrent cancer although radiation effects can make image interpretation difficult.

Screening, Surveillance, Prevention

The recognition of the role that HPV plays in the pathogenesis of anal canal cancer will allow for the identification and screening of high-risk individuals. Populations at high risk for the development of anal cancer include both HIV positive and negative men who have sex with men (MSM), men and women with a history of anogenital warts, women with a prior history of high grade dysplasia or carcinoma of the cervix and HIV positive men and women with CD4 counts less than 500 [2].

Primary prevention occurs as a result of educating the general public, particularly those identified as high-risk groups, of the association between HPV and anal cancer. Promoting safe sexual practices among those at-risk populations can reduce the spread of HPV and the subsequent development of anal cancer.

Based upon the similar pathogenesis and biologic behavior of cervical and anal cancer and the success of cervical cancer screening in reducing morbidity and mortality in sexually active women, investigators have proposed a parallel screening program for individuals at high risk for the development of anal cancer [3]. Components of such a program include a complete history with questions designed to detect symptoms associated with both SILs and anal cancer, and a focused physical exam of the perineum, anus and regional lymphatics. Digital rectal exam should be deferred until after anal cytology is performed as cytology is more accurately interpreted prior to anal canal lubrication. Anal cytology is initiated by inserting a cytette brush to the upper anal canal. It is then withdrawn, rotating it against the walls of the anal canal. The collected cells are smeared, fixed on a slide with alcohol and stained according to Papanicolou methods. Abnormal cytology warrants high-resolution anoscopy with microscope magnification after the application of 3% acetic acid to the anal canal mucosa. This is performed in the operating room under regional or general anesthesia. Those areas that are consistent with high-grade squamous intraepithelial lesions are surgically excised, cauterized or destroyed with laser. Palefsky et al., utilizing a high-risk population (MSM) has proposed the screening algorithm detailed in figure 5 below [3].

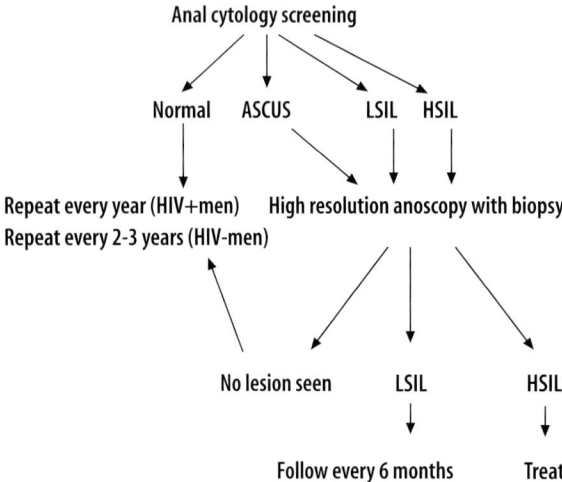

Figure 5
Screening protocol of ASIL in HIV positive and negative men who have sex with men. (From Palefsky JM. Anal squamous intraepithelial lesions in human immunodeficiency virus-positive men and women. Seminars in Oncology 27(4): 471–479. WB Saunders Publishing. With permission). *ASCUS* atypical squamous cells of uncertain significance; *LSIL* low grade SIL; *HSIL* high grade SIL, squamous intraepithelial lesion

The rationale for following rather than treating LSIL is based upon the high spontaneous regression rate of similar lesions in the cervix.

Goldie et al. [9], utilizing the above schema and a Markov model, demonstrated that screening HIV-negative homosexual men with anal cytology every two or three years resulted in a prolongation of life at a cost comparable to other preventive strategies currently employed in clinical medicine. Screening at two year intervals resulted in a cost of $15,100 per quality-adjusted life year (QALY) gained and at three-year intervals, cost $7,000 per QALY.

Future Perspectives

The widespread application of screening programs for high-risk populations will potentially have the greatest impact on the future management of anal cancer. Screening will allow for both the prevention and earlier diagnosis of the disease. Clinical studies in the future will need to focus on optimizing the delivery of currently available treatment modalities and exploring the use of different chemotherapy based regimens. Expanded mole-culogenetic research may lead to novel treatment techniques. Finally, the known association between HPV and anal cancer should lead to the development of new drug treatments to eradicate established HPV infection.

References

1. Chawla AK, Willett CG (2001) Squamous cell carcinoma of the anal canal and anal margin. Hematology/Oncology Clinics of NA 15(2):321–44
2. Ryan DP, Compton CC, Mayer RJ (2000) Carcinoma of the anal canal. NEJM 342 (11):792–99
3. Palefsky JM (2000) Anal squamous intraepithelial lesions in human immunodeficiency virus-positive men and women. Seminars in Oncol 27 (4):471–79
4. Palefsky JM (2000) Human papillomavirus-related tumors. AIDS 14 (suppl 3): 5189–95
5. Perkowski PE, Sorrells DL, Evans JT, Nopajaroonsri C, Johnson LW (2000) Anal duct carcinoma: case report and review of the literature. Amer Surgeon 66:1149–52
6. Felz MW, Winburn GB, Kallab AM, Lee JR (2001) Anal melanoma: an aggressive malignancy masquerading as hemorrhoids. Southern Med J 94(9):880–85
7. Nigro ND, Vaitkevicuis VK, Considine B (1974) Combined therapy for cancer of the anal canal: a preliminary report. Dis Colon Rectum 17: 354–56
8. Allal AS, Laurencet FM, Reymond MA, Kurtz JM, Marti M (1999) Effectiveness of surgical salvage therapy for patients with locally uncontrolled anal carcinoma after sphincter-conserving treatment. Cancer 86(3): 405–9
9. Goldie SJ, Kuntz KM, Weinstein MC, Freedberg KA, Palefsky JM (2000) Cost-effectiveness of screening for anal squamous intraepithelial lesions and anal cancer in human immunodeficiency virus-negative homosexual and bisexual men. Am J Med 108:634–41.

Pancreas

VI

14 Neoplastic Lesions of the Pancreas

H.G. BEGER, M. SIECH

Summary

Most of the patients suffering from pancreatic cancer complain about upper abdominal pain, back pain, weight loss and change of bowel movements. The following signs and symptoms are suspected to be caused by pancreatic cancer: weight loss and back pain in the lower spinal column managed by orthopedic measures without improvement, upper abdominal pain continuing after cholecystectomy and unexplained abnormal glucose tolerance. Patients in cancer stage UICC I+II have survival benefits from oncological resection. However many patients are diagnosed in a very advanced stage with metastasation and/or cancer infiltration into retropancreatic vessels and the mesentery of the small and large bowel. Subgroups of patients with unresectable cancer have benefits from palliative chemotherapy and continuous pain management in regard to maintenance of quality of life and prolongation of survival.

Adenocarcinoma of the Pancreas

Epidemiology and Etiology

The incidence of pancreatic cancer increases worldwide, not only as a consequence of improvements in diagnostic sensitivity [1]. The incidence is related to age: at the age of 50–65 years the incidence is 10/100000 per year whereas 20/100000 per year are registered at >80 years. With regard to the gender, the frequency is 1.5 to 1, male to female respectively. 10–15% of pancreatic cancers are discovered during autopsy.

Etiological investigations disclosed a relation of risk between long-lasting alcohol consumption as well as cigarette smoking and pancreatic cancer. Recent studies revealed a significant increase of cancer risk in patients suffering from chronic pancreatitis. 2–3% of patients with alcoholic chronic pancreatitis develop cancer of the pancreas after 10 years. In comparison to a healthy control group, patients with chronic pancreatitis have a 16-fold increased pancreatic cancer risk [2]. An early onset of diabetes mellitus is considered to be linked to development of pancreatic cancer. In about 5% of patients with pancreatic cancer a genetic determination has been discovered [3].

Molecular Genetics and Prognosis

In spite of increased knowledge about molecular mechanisms, in the carcinogenesis of pancreatic cancer we are not able to identify molecular prognostic markers. Certain genetic alterations are important for the prognosis of pancreatic cancers. Mutations of the k-ras oncogen occur in about 90% of pancreatic cancers. An overexpression of growth factors: epidermal growth factor, transforming growth factors (α and β), the fibroblast growth factors (a + b) and the growth factor receptors, C-erbB-2 and -3 and TGFR have frequently been shown in pancreatic cancer [4]. Cell cycle control genes such as p53, p16, p21, SMAD4 and cyclin D1 are found with high mutation levels [5]. The expression of several of the growth factors and their receptors has been shown to be associated with poorly differentiated tumors, diagnosed in an advanced stage and linked to a decreased survival. Inactivation of cell cycle control genes like p16, p53 and p21 and the expression of several apoptotic genes such as bax and bcl-2 have not been found to be of prognostic significance. The expression of the wild type p53, p16 and k-ras genes are associated on the other hand with an increased survival after Ro resection [6]; the expression of wild type p53 gene seems to predict responsiveness to chemotherapy.

Symptoms and Clinical Signs

To achieve the best possible diagnostic result a multidisciplinary approach is necessary, taking into account staging of the tumor, dissemination pattern of the cancer and the patients morbidity (Table 1).

Table 1
Ductal pancreatic cancer: Cancer cell dissemination

Lymphogenous	Lymphnodes
	Lymphvessels
Perineural	Intrapancreatic nerves
	Perivascular nerves
	Extrapancreatic nerve plexus
Hematogenous	Liver
	Bone marrow
Intraperitoneal	Free cancer cells in peritoneal cavity
Local	Common bile duct
	Duodenum, stomach
	Portal vein, splenic vein, superior mesenteric vein
	Peritoneum: lesser sac

More than one third of the patients are older than 65 years at the time of diagnosis. The most frequent symptoms caused by pancreatic cancer are weight loss, pain in the upper abdomen and the back, nausea and vomiting, icterus and changes in the bowel movements. Loss of appetite and fatigue are frequently observed in association with pancreatic cancer. In regard to the pain syndrome, many of the patients have upper abdominal pain with radiation into the back; every third patient with pancreatic cancer had been treated for pain localized in the lower spinal column by orthopedic measures. The changes in bowel movements are observed as diarrhea and/or obstipation; meteorism is frequent.

In every second patient physical investigation of the abdomen reveals objective clinical signs e.g. palpable gallbladder (Courvoisier's sign), jaundice, increased liver size and ascites. Nonspecific laboratory investigations reveal in 2/3 of the patients anemia; in 1/3 a pathologic glucose metabolism and frequently an increase of the tumor marker CA19–9 in serum. Elevated levels of CA 19–9 are often seen in cholestasis caused by lesions other than cancer. However, 97 of 100 patients with a serum concentration of more than 1000 U/ml (cutoff value of 37 U/ml) suffer from a malignant tumor (mainly pancreatic or cholangiocellular carcinoma).

There are patients complaining about specific symptoms caused by pancreatic cancer e.g. icterus without pain, epigastric fullness with vomiting and diarrhea. Patients with an early onset of diabetes mellitus should always be fully investigated for pancreatic cancer like patients who recently had a cholecystectomy without relief of abdominal complaints.

Diagnostics

The main goal of diagnostic measures is the early discovery of the malignant lesion. The first line of instrumental investigations is percutaneous ultrasonography, which has a high sensitivity and specificity in experienced hands. A jaundiced patient should have an ERCP for identification of the obstruction of the common bile duct. Preoperative biliary stenting of the tumor stenosis is frequently performed. It alleviates symptoms related to cholestasis and should be done if the indication for resection is not yet clear at the time of ERCP. However, it confers no advantage with regard to the surgical procedure; on the contrary, it has been associated with a higher incidence of cholangitis and delayed postoperative wound healing in some studies.

The most important diagnostic investigation is contrast enhanced, helical computed tomography (CT) or Angio magnetic resonance tomography (MRT) (Fig. 1).

The contrast enhanced Angio-CT has a sensitivity of above 85%. The Angio CT or magnetic resonance tomography (MRT) in combination with angiography offer the highest sensitivity to determine the degree of vascular wall involvement (Fig. 2) [7].

For preoperative staging of the cancer, it is necessary to diagnose liver and peritoneal metastasation (Fig. 3).

However small liver metastases and peritoneal seedings up to a diameter of 5–8 mm are frequently not detected by CT or MRI. To detect small liver metastases and peritoneal seedings in the upper and lower abdomen, a laparoscopic investigation is indicated in 8–15% of the patients [8]. Such diagnostic laparoscopy yields the histological diagnosis and the stage of metastasation in cancer stages UICC III and IVa and in non-resectable cases.

In most patients a conventional angiography is unnecessary because of the high sensitivity and specificity for vascular wall involvement detectable by contrast enhanced CT or Angio MRT. PET investigation for diagnosis of pancreatic cancer has a limited benefit. The most important differential diagnosis for pancreatic cancer is chronic pancreatitis with inflammatory mass in the

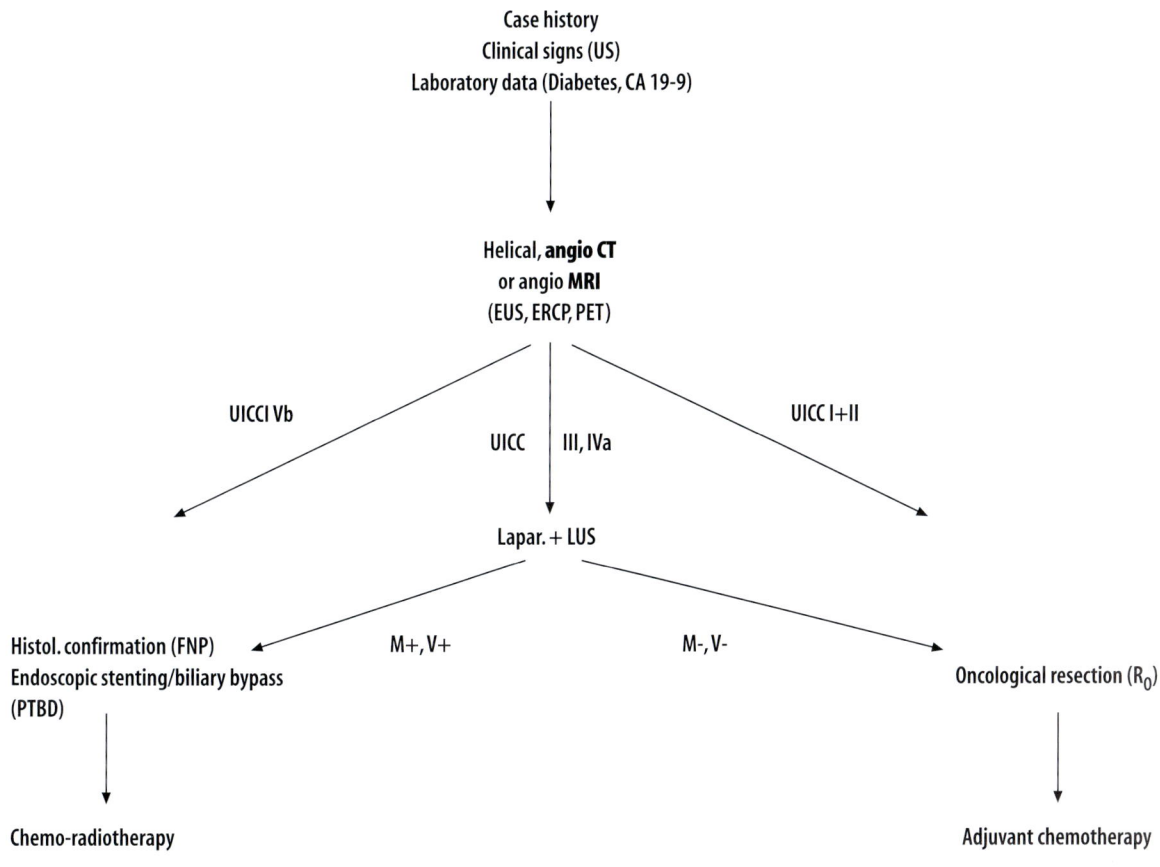

Figure 1
Pancreatic cancer – Diagnostic algorithm

head. In patients with a long-lasting case history of chronic pancreatitis, an additional ERCP contributes only little to the discrimination of chronic pancreatitis from a neoplastic lesion. In a subgroup of patients with chronic pancreatitis (4–6% of the patients) there is an association between chronic pancreatitis and pancreatic cancer; here a US-guided fine needle puncture or a laparoscopic guided puncture of the tumor is recommended.

Dissemination Pattern of Ductal Pancreatic Cancer and Staging

Ductal adenocarcinoma of the pancreas shows intrapancreatic but also – early in the growth of the malignant lesion – extrapancreatic tumor spread. In addition to infiltration into non-pancreatic tissue e.g. common bile duct, wall of the duodenum and portal vein, pancre-

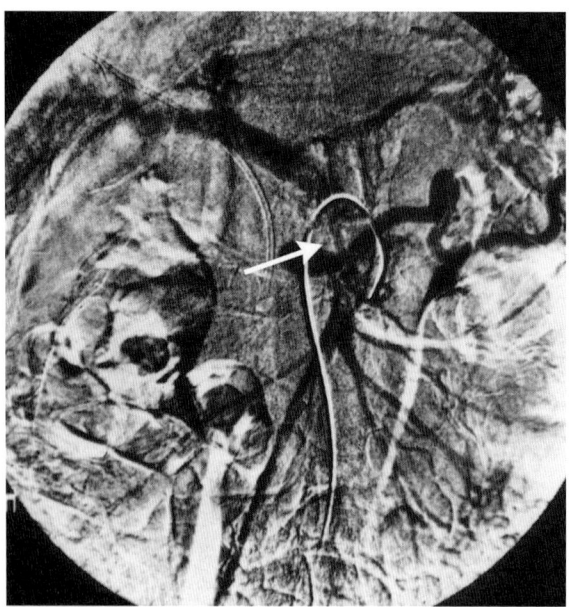

Figure 2
Digital subtraction angiography in a patient with carcinoma in the uncinate processus of the pancreas. Long-distance stenosis of the superior mesenteric vein marked by the arrow (Courtesy of H-J Brambs, Dept. of Diagnostic Radiology, University of Ulm, Germany)

atic cancer early in its course involves lymph tissue compartments, e.g. lymph nodes and lymph vessels around the pancreas (Table 2).

One-third of the patients operated on for resection show intraoperatively viable free tumor cells in the peritoneal washing. About 60% of the patients investigated after resective surgical treatment of advanced pancreatic cancer have intra- and extrapancreatic neural and perineural invasion including the perivascular neuroplexus around the portal and superior mesenteric vein and the extrapancreatic nerve plexus [7]. A correlation has been shown between extrapancreatic nerve involvement and the outcome after resection. The frequency of ductal pancreatic cancer without lymph node involvement, using histopathological investigations is below 10% and observed only in UICC stage I cancer. Even in patients with a small malignant lesion (tumor diameter <2 cm) a Japanese collective series showed lymph node involvement in 30%, extrapancreatic retroperitoneal cancer dissemination in 20% and serosal involvement in 10% as well as vascular wall infiltration in 6% [9]. In recent studies, several authors have investigated the prognostic significance of the detection of micrometastasis in lymph

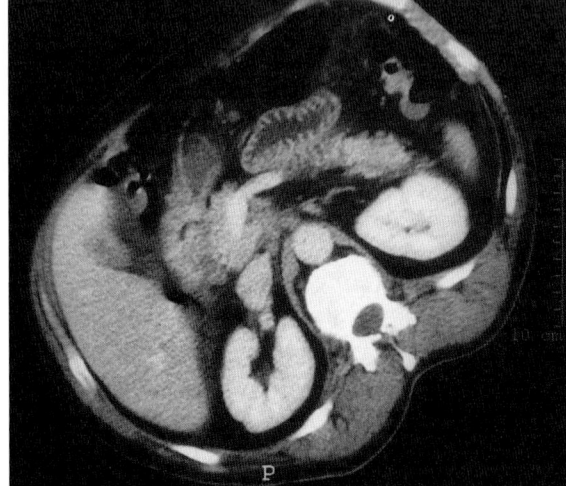

Figure 3
Contrast-enhanced CT scan of the upper abdomen showing carcinoma of the head of pancreas with liver metastasis, histologically ductal-type carcinoma. (Courtesy of H-J Brambs, Dept. of Diagnostic Radiology, University of Ulm, Germany)

Table 2
Staging of pancreatic malignancy (UICC 1998)

Tis	Carcinoma in situ
T1	≤2 cm, limited to pancreas
T2	≥2 cm
T3	Cancer infiltrates duodenum, CBD, peripancreatic tissue
T4	Cancer infiltrates stomach, spleen, colon, vessels
N0	No lymph node (LN) involvement histopathologically (>10LNs investigated)
N1	local LN metastasation
N1a	one LN cancer cell positive
N1b	two and more LNs involved

Stage groupings			
UICC 0	Tis	N0	M0
UICC I	T1/2	N0	M0
UICC II	T3	N0	M0
UICC III	T1/2/3	N1	M0
UICC IVa	T4	N+	M0
UICC IVb	T1–4	N+	M+

nodes, bone marrow and peripheral blood; clinical significance of micrometastasis in bone marrow in terms of prognosis has been demonstrated. In 40–70% of the lymph nodes which were histomorphologically cancer cell-negative, micrometastasation was detected by using PCR based assays. In a multivariate analysis, the presence of micrometastasis in histologically cancer-free lymph nodes was a prognostic factor.

Tumor Related Prognosis

Pancreatic cancer is the fourth most common cause of cancer-related death. 85% is the ductal type of pancreatic cancer; most of these patients die in the year after diagnosis [10]. For patients suffering from cyst-adenocarcinoma, the prognosis is probably better after resection than in ductal cancer. Patients with a left side pancreatic cancer are frequently diagnosed in a very advanced stage with metastasation.

In the subgroup of patients who may have survival benefits from oncological resection, factors have been determined which favorably influence the outcome (Table 3).

Size of the malignant lesion below 2 cm, absence of lymph node metastasis on the basis of histomorphological investigation and absence of vessel wall and extrapancreatic nerve infiltration are oncologic criteria favorably influencing the short- and long-term outcome. Additional positive prognostic signs are DNA diploid status, tumor cell differentiation (well) and absence of mutations of p53, DPC4, p21 and k-ras genes.

Table 3
Tumor biology and stage influencing long-term survival after oncological resection

Tumor size	< 2 cm	Tsuchiya	1988 [11]
Lymph node involvement	negative	Cameron	1991 [12]
Nerve infiltration	negative	Nagakawa	1996 [13]
Vascular wall infiltration	negative	Ishikawa	1988 [14]
Cell differentiation	G1 (well)	Geer + Brennan	1993 [15]
DNA content	diploid	Yeo + Cameron	1999 [16]
Cancer genes	wild type: p53, p16, DPC4	Rozenblum + Kern	1997 [5]

Table 4
Pancreatic head cancer. Survival after R0 resection

	R0 resection		R1 resection	
		Pts. [n]	Actuarial 5 year-survival	Pts. [n]	Actuarial 5 year-survival
Yeo/Cameron [17]	1995	143	26%	58	8%
Nitecki/Sarr [18]	1995		12%		0%
Trede [19]	1996	134	30%	92	0%
Hanyu [20]	1996	167	27%		0%
Fortnagel/ Beger [21]	2000	135	28%	90	0%

R0: resection margins cancer free after histopathological investigation; R1: resection margins microscopically cancer cell positive

The most important prognostic factor in regard to long-term survival is the achievement of an oncological (R0) resection. The absence of a residual tumor after cancer resection results in an actuarial 5-year survival between 10% and 30% (Table 4).

Treatment

Synopsis

80% of patients diagnosed with pancreatic cancer are in an advanced stage. Pancreatic cancer without cancer cell dissemination into lymph nodes is observed on the basis of histomorphological investigations in less than 10% of cases. Tumor size (up to 6 cm) is not a limitation for surgical resection. In about 60% of patients, metastases are found along the extrapancreatic nerves and in the adjacent nerve plexus. Patients with ductal adenocarcinoma of the body and tail of the pancreas usually have macroscopically and microscopically a stage of metastasation and infiltration into the retroperitoneal spaces. Resection of left sided ductal pancreatic cancer contributes to pain control but usually has no benefit for prolongation of survival.

Surgical Treatment

Patients in a cancer stage UICC I and II should have surgical resection. However only 8–15% of patients suffering from pancreatic cancer are in the stage without lymph node metastasation, based on preoperative staging (Table 5).

Table 5

Indications and contraindications for surgical resection

Indications	UICC I + II (T1–2, N0, M0)
	UICC III (T3, N+, M0)
	Resection not excluded:
	Tumor size < 6 cm
	LN involvement N2–3
	Infiltration of duodenum, stomach
	Limited vascular wall involvement
No benefit from resection	Liver metastasation
	Peritoneal metastases
	Pleura carcinosis
	Ascites
	Infiltration in mesentery of the intestine
	Circular encasement of vessels

Table 6

Pancreatic head resections – morbidity and mortality

Early postoperative morbidity	427 patients after resections	
	Patients [n]	Frequency [%]
Without any local/systemic complications	252	59.0
With minor local/systemic complications	111	26,0
With major local/systemic complications	44	10,3
Reoperation	10	2,3
Hospital mortality	10	2,3

5/1982–3/2001 Department of General Surgery, University of Ulm

Table 7

Survival after resection and radio-/chemotherapy of stage I cancers only (AJCC). National cancer database: 4787 patients, USA. (From Sener, J Amer Cell Surg 1999; 29)

	Actuarial survival [%]		
	1 year	3 years	5 years
Whipple resection	69,6	39,7	32,8
Surgery + Radiotherapy + Chemotherapy	68,3	34,9	24,3
Radiotherapy only	41,4	8,6	7,2
Chemotherapy only	38,2	6,5	5,4
Radiotherapy + Chemotherapy	51,5	13,1	8.4
Best supportive care	33,5	11,6	8,1

Patients with preoperative cancer stage III – tumor with lymph node metastasation – are candidates for surgical resection depending on the severity of comorbidity. The benefit of surgical resection is based on the degree of cancer dissemination and the application of an Ro resection.

The major achievement of surgery for treatment of pancreatic cancer is the low morbidity and low hospital mortality. In high-volume centers, hospital mortality is below 3–5% (Table 6).

The long-term morbidity after resection is related to diabetes mellitus, cholangitis and clinical implications of a decreased exocrine pancreatic function. However the most important long-term morbidity is related to development of local and systemic recurrence of cancer.

Patients in cancer stage I and II have long-term survival benefits after oncological resections. Patients with liver and peritoneal metastasation as well as circular encasement of vessels have no benefit from surgical resections. It has been observed that patients with adherence of portal and superior mesenteric vessel wall have in 50% of the cases no wall infiltration of the cancer. Patients with adherence of the tumor to portal and superior mesenteric vein are therefore candidates for surgical resection.

In pancreatic head cancer the Kausch-Whipple resection has been the standard resection in the past (Table 7).

Many European and American centers are currently using the pylorus preserving resection. With regard to radicality there is no difference between the surgical techniques. The pylorus preserving resection is considered to be beneficial in the first postoperative year as regards nutrition and weight gain. Both surgical techniques include the resection of the pancreatic head, the extrahepatic biliary tree, cholecystectomy and the resection of the flexura duodenojejunalis. The dissection of lymph nodes in the lig. hepatoduodenale, along the hepatic artery and between the infrahepatic cava and aorta are not included in the protocols of standard radical pancreatico-duodenectomy. Extended lymph node dissection has not been demonstrated to be superior to standard dissection techniques as regards 3 and 5 year survival.

Palliative Treatment and Pain Control

The objectives of palliative treatment are to improve the prognosis, avoiding obstruction of the biliary tract and duodenum and improve the quality of life, e.g. decreasing pain, the incidence of itching, vomiting and hospitalization times. Patients with a very advanced cancer and a survival expectation of up to 3 months should not undergo a palliative surgical procedure.

Patients who require relief of bile duct obstruction and are not candidates for intended curative resection should undergo endoscopic stent placement. There is a controversy as to whether to implant a plastic or expandable metal stent. Plastic stents continue to dominate in biliary endoscopy because of low cost and the ease of stent exchange. However, even the use of large diameter (10 F) plastic stents is limited by clogging after 3–6 months. This results in a higher frequency of cholangitis and rehospitalizations. The observation that an increase in stent diameter results in increased patency rates has prompted the development of expandable metallic stents which are not removable. These much more expensive endoprotheses will also occlude after 6 to 12 months, due to tumor ingrowth and overgrowth, mucosal hyperplasia, biliary sludge, and food impaction. New developments in stent technology (e.g., removable metallic stents, bioresorbable materials, drug coating) may overcome some of these problems in the future. In patients with advanced pancreatic cancer and the indication for palliative or neoadjuvant radiochemotherapy placement of metallic stents is not indicated.

Regarding palliative surgical procedures, a combination of biliary bypass and gastrojejunostomy should be considered in patients without liver metastasation. A biliary bypass should be indicated in patients with recurrent cholangitis or cholangiosepsis due to stenting and a life expectancy of 6–12 months. A gastric bypass is indicated in patients with a gastric outlet-syndrome caused by an increasing tumor compression of the duodenum [11]. Surgical bypass has become a treatment with low surgical morbidity and mortality by the use of laparoscopic techniques. Sohn [12] has reported that no difference in surgical morbidity was seen between those with and without additional gastrojejunostomy. The endoscopic placement of expandable metallic stents into the descending part of the duodenum awaits further evaluation.

For pain control, the patients undergoing a surgical bypass should have a combination with a neural block of the celiac plexus. For patients suffering from continuous severe pain, a thoracoscopic splanchnicectomy has been confirmed to be an effective method [13].

Multiple reports are published about relapse rates, disease-free survival and overall survival times for advanced pancreatic cancer. Recurrence after resective surgical treatment occurs in 80% of the patients as local tumor growth with perineural invasion, lymph node tumors and soft tissue infiltrations. Most of the patients have additionally liver metastasation; distant peritoneal seedings contribute in 40–60% to the clinical pattern of recurrence. After extended radical oncological resection of an UICC stage I+II cancer, liver metastasation but not local recurrence is the leading clinical location of cancer relapse. Careful follow-up studies after pancreatic cancer resection revealed however that one third of the patients die following septic complications. Many of the patients are undernourished, which contributes to the reduced nutritional state and quality of life. Besides palliative or adjuvant chemotherapy, attention has to be paid to supportive care, including enteral administration of a high-energy diet and continuous pain medication. In selected patients with pancreatic cancer and inability to eat, home parenteral nutrition may be indicated.

Palliative Chemotherapy

For palliative treatment of advanced pancreatic cancer, gemcitabine, an inhibitor of nucleic acid synthesis, has recently been introduced as a standard protocol. Stornioli [14] reported in 1999 a collected series of more than 3000 patients. The median survival in patients with cancer stage II+III was 6.6 months and in cancer stage IV 4.8 months. The one year survival rate was 15%, the overall response rate 12%. Japanese [15] and Italian [16] groups have reported the results of phase II trials with docetaxel and of a phase II trial with weekly chemotherapy using cisplatin (CDDP), 5-FU, epirubicin and leucovorin. Both trials showed low response rates, indicating a weak effectiveness in pancreatic cancer (Table 8).

Biological therapy is employed clinically in a single series. In 33 patients with resected pancreatic cancer, Nukui compared 16 patients who were treated according to the protocol of the Gastrointestinal Tumor Study Group (GITSG) and 17 patients receiving chemoradiation, combining 5-FU, CDDP and Interferon-α plus 45–54 Gy extracorporal radiation. They reported a 2-year survival rate in the 17 patients of 84% while the 2-year survival rate in the 16 patients in the GITSG-group was 54% [17]. Scheithauer used a combination of gemcitabine, epi-

Table 8
Results after palliative chemotherapy: Gemcitabine*. (Storniolo, Cancer 85; 1261; 1999; 14)

Median survival (2380 pts)	6,6 m (stage II/III)
	4,8 m (stage IV)
Survival probability (2012 pts)	6 m: 41%
	9 m: 22%
	12 m: 15%
Response (982 pts)	CR: 1,4%
	PR: 10,6%
Treatment related symptome improve	18,4%

*1000 mg/m² weekly, 30 min i.v. Stage II+III: 472 pts; stage IV: 1863 pts.

Table 9
Neoadjuvant treatment of advanced pancreatic cancer [19]. RT + FSP, radiotherapy combined with polychemotherapy (5-fluorouracil, streptozotocin, cisplatin = FSP protocol)

	Study period 1989–1997	
	RT + FSP (68 pts)	Surgery alone (91 pts)
Survival (median)	23,6 m	14 m p<0,006
Survival 20 pts downstaged after oncological resection	32,3 m	–
Survival adjuvant treatment yes	–	16,2 m
Survival adjuvant treatment no	–	10,5 m >0,025

rubicin and granulocyte colony stimulating factor for 66 patients with distant metastases. They reported 1 patient with complete response and 13 patients with partial response (an overall response of 21%); the median survival was 7.8 months and 43% had symptom improvement [18].

Synopsis

The cure of ductal pancreatic cancer is observed only after oncological resection. After R0 resection patients have an actuarial survival chance of 60% for 1 year and 10–30% for 5 years. However cure of pancreatic cancer is observed in less than 3% of all patients. After oncological resection of an advanced cancer, combination with adjuvant chemotherapy resulted in a median survival time of 12–24 months in a single institutional series. In unresectable cases, palliative radiochemotherapy may result in a survival expectation of 6–14 months. At present no standard protocols for palliative chemotherapy proved by controlled clinical trials are available.

Adjuvant and Neoadjuvant Chemotherapy

Several groups demonstrated survival benefits in adjuvant chemotherapy using 5-FU and radiotherapy in combination. After oncological resection of the pancreatic head, cancer patients with adjuvant radiochemotherapy had significant higher actuarial 1, 3 and 5-years survival [12].

Only a few data are presently available about the benefits of neoadjuvant treatment. In a prospective trial including 68 patients, Snady combined radiotherapy with chemotherapy, using 5-FU/folinic acid, streptozotocin,

and cisplatin. The median survival of the neoadjuvant treated patients was significantly higher in comparison to the surgical group; most impressive were the results of the downstaged patients after oncological resection. One third of the neoadjuvant treated patients were downstaged and had an oncological resection, their median survival was 32 months [19] (Table 9).

Again this group demonstrated that adjuvant chemotherapy in patients after oncological resection has a significant survival benefit as regards median survival time.

Cystic Carcinoma of the Pancreas

Cystic tumors comprise a variety of gastrointestinal tumors that occur within the pancreas. In 1978, Compagno and Oertel set the basis for pathological differential diagnosis of these lesions [20]. They described two different entities [21]: one the microcystic or glycogen-rich adenoma (also known as serous cystadenoma), which is almost universally benign, and the other mucinous cystic neoplasm, which encompasses a spectrum that ranges from benign but potentially malignant lesions to carcinomas with a very aggressive behavior [21]. In 1996, Klöppel et al. defined all benign and malignant tumors of the pancreas for the first time in the new WHO classification [22]. This classification allowed for a better interpretation of the information generated by the use of CT and ultrasound, which have disclosed an increasing number of cystic tumors in asymptomatic or minimally symptomatic patients. These neoplasms comprise 1% of all pancreatic tumors and about 10% of cystic lesions.

The most common cystic pancreatic tumors are serous cystadenomas and mucinous cystic neoplasms (about 80%) [23]. However, there are other varieties (Table 10).

While serous cystic tumors are frequently benign, about 4–50% of mucinous cystic tumors are malignant [24].

Diagnosis

Cystic tumors of the solid pancreas can be distinguished from the more common pseudocysts by the presence of components, septa and loculations on CT and ultrasound. Calcification can be found in approximately 30% of cystic tumors. CT displays a cystic tumor in 98% of all patients; however, in about 10% the ERCP findings are completely normal. PET revealed an increase glucose metabolism in the area of the tumor in cystic tumors, regardless of the histological typing. Small tumors (<2 cm) are found in 15–28%, independently of the histological type [24]. Angiography shows that tumors are often hypervascular. In about 30% of the patients with cystic lesions, the tumor shows an impact on the arterial vessels [24].

The large veins (portal vein, splenic vein, superior mesenteric vein) are frequently encased, obstructed or draped in about 30% of all patients. Yamaguchi et al. performed an ERCP in 17 patients with cystic tumors, in ten of them, communication between the cystic spaces and the pancreatic ducts was documented.

The most important differential diagnosis is to exclude pancreatic pseudocysts. Warshaw et al. [25] found false diagnoses of pseudocyst mistreated by cystojejunostomy in 37% of cases. In our own experience, 10 of 51 cases (19%) were falsely diagnosed as pseudocysts. (Table 11).

Because the treatment of the two diseases is completely different, frozen section investigation of the wall of each pseudocyst that is treated surgically is strongly recommended.

Treatment

Half of the patients with mucinous tumors have malignancies. Extensive histologic sampling cannot be achieved until the tumor is excised. Therefore, all mucinous cystic neoplasms should be considered malignant and treated with radical resection. If metastases are present and resectable, they should be excised with the tumor. Early results even after extensive resections are satisfying. Most frequent complication after resection is pancreatic fistula which occurs in between 9 and 15% of cases. Long-term prognosis of resected mucinous cystic neoplasms is good. For resected cystadenocarcinomas, long-term survival rates are achieved in 50–76% [23, 24].

Intraductal Papillary Tumor of the Pancreas

In 1986, a subtype of mucinous cystadenomas was first described in 5 Japanese patients [25]. In 1996, mucinous ductal ectasia was separated from mucinous cystic adenomas and defined as intraductal papillary cystic tumor of the pancreas. Until now whether this new nomenclature has clinical consequences has not been determined. There are few data available about the prognosis and whether a different concept of treatment is necessary.

Table 10
Cystic neoplasms of the pancreas

Benign/borderline	Malignant
Serous cystadenoma	Serous cystadenocarcinoma
Mucinous cystadenoma	Mucinous cystadenocarcinoma
Mucinous ductal ectasia	
Intraductal papillary mucinous tumor (IPMT)	IPMT-carcinoma
Cystic islet-cell tumor	
Solid pseudopapillary tumor	Acinar cystadenocarcinoma
Cystic teratoma	
Lymphangioma	
Hemangioma	
Paraganglioma	

Table 11
Differential diagnostics of pseudocysts (according to AI, AJ, AX)

History	Acute and chronic pancreatitis in the history
ERCP	Mucinous delivery out of the papilla – IPMT
Communication with the ductal system?	preoperative fine needle aspiration (amylase, lipase), content of the fluid
Intraoperatively	Sample out of the cystic wall investigated by frozen section intraoperatively in all operations for pseudocysts

Table 12

Symptoms of 23 patients with mucinous cystadenoma or intraductal papillary mucinous tumor of the pancreas (AX) [24]

Symptom	All	Mucinous cystadenoma	Intraductal papillary mucinous tumor
	n=23	n=15	n=8
Pain	20/23 (87%)	12/15 (80%)	8/8 (100%)
Nausea, vomiting	2/23 (9%)	1/15 (7%)	1/8 (12%)
Diarrhea	1/23 (4%)	0/15	1/8 (12%)
Jaundice	1/23 (4%)	1/15 (7%)	0/8

The mucinous ductal ectasia in IPMT-tumors is characterized by dilatation by filling of the main pancreatic duct or its side branches with thick, viscid mucus. The hyperplastic columnar epithelium of the duct, which is responsible for the overproduction of mucus, is arranged in papillary projections and may or may not be seen as granular, papillary tumors projecting into the duct volume. The epithelium may be completely normal in appearance, have atypia, carcinoma *in situ*, or infiltrating carcinoma. Characteristically, the tumor grows along the duct before invading the parenchyma (Fig. 4) [26].

Invasion of the duodenum, as well as metastasis to lymph nodes has been recorded.

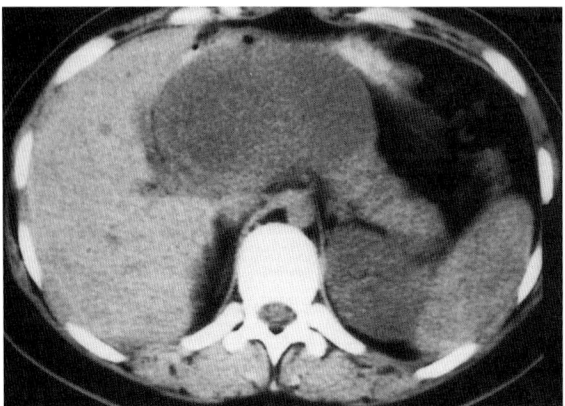

Figure 4

CT scan of the upper abdomen revealing solid pseudopapillary tumor of the pancreas with papillary cystic mass in the pancreatic head; advanced intraductal papillary mucinous tumor (IPMT). (Courtesy of H-J Brambs, Dept. of Diagnostic Radiology, University of Ulm, Germany)

Diagnosis

Many patients report recurrent acute pancreatitis or symptoms that mimic chronic pancreatitis, including exocrine and endocrine insufficiency. The leading symptom is pain in 100%, after that nausea, vomiting and diarrhea are unspecific symptoms (Table 12).

Diagnosis is made by CT and ERCP. In many instances mucus is extruding out of the ampulla of Vater and the pancreatogram always shows a dilated ductal system, with filling defects of varying sizes which correspond to mucus plugs, which are difficult to wash out.

Treatment

Because IPMT is a premalignant lesion, surgery is mandatory. Current evidence suggests that the natural history of IPMT is progression from hyperplasia to atypia, carcinoma *in situ* and infiltrating carcinoma. Because of the tendency of IPMT to grow along the duct some have suggested total pancreatectomy as surgical treatment. Since most of the tumors are located in the head of the pancreas, a pylorus-preserving pancreatoduodenectomy is appropriate. Because of the tendency to spread, it is important to ensure that the surgical margin is free of disease.

Synopsis

In general, intraductal papillary mucinous tumors of the pancreas have a favourable prognosis. The IPMT is classified into 4 groups, including benign adenoma, borderline tumors with moderate dysplasia and carcinomas (non-invasive and invasive). Some cases of invasive carcinomas of this type show rapid progression and frequent distant metastases after resection and have a poor prognosis. A cystic neoplastic lesion of the pancreas should be considered as an indication for local extirpation respectively oncological resection. Patients with a serous cystadenoma have an increased risk of development of carcinoma and should be considered for local surgical treatment.

Other Tumors

These include papillary cystic, neoplasm, cystic paragangliomas [27], dermoids (also known as cystic teratomas) and lymphangiomas. The latter, of which more than 30 cases have been reported, has a honeycomb appearance, similar to that of serous cystadenoma. Confusion between the two IMPTs has been reported. Interestingly, lymphangioma of the pancreas occurred more frequently in females (70% of the cases); the mean age at diagnosis was 46 years.

Solid Pseudopapillary Tumor of the Pancreas

According to the WHO classification this tumor is a borderline tumor [22]. It was first described by Frantz et al. in 1959 [28]. This tumor is very rare (approximately 70 cases in the literature). It occurs most frequently in young females.

Because the tumor is almost in all instances asymptomatic, it is diagnosed at large diameters between 8 and 10 cm. Sometimes an abdominal mass might be palpated. CT-scan shows a solid tumor in 45%, solid and cystic in 40% and cystic alone in 15%. Endoscopic retrograde pancreatography quite often shows displacement of the duct [29]. Communication between the ductal system and the cystic components of the tumor has never been observed. Angiography may show either a hypo-vascular or hypervascular tumor. A very few cases in the literature demonstrate that papillary cystic neoplasm may take a malignant course. For surgical treatment, a partial pylorus-preserving duodenopancreatectomy is recommended. Because there is no safety margin and some of the tumors may become malignant, we rather suggest a resection providing a safety margin.

References

1. DiMagno EP, Reber HA, Tempero MA (1999) American Gastroenterological Association Medical Position Statement: Epidemiology, diagnosis, and treatment of pancreatic ductal adenocarcinoma. Gastroenterology 117;1463–1484
2. Lowenfels AB, Maisonneuve P, Cavallini G et al (1993) Pancreatitis and the risk of pancreatic cancer. N Engl J Med 328; 1433–1437
3. Ghane P, Katscha A, Evans JD, Neoptolemos P, Molecular prognositic markers in pancreatic cancer. (2002) J Hepatobiliary Pancreat Surg 9; 1–11
4. Korc M, Chandrasekar B, Yamanaka Y, Friess H, Büchler M, Beger H (1992) Overexpression of the epidermal growth factor receptor in human pancreatic cancer is associated with concomitant increase in the levels of epidermal growth factor and transforming growth factor alpha. J. Clin Invest 90; 1352–1360
5. Gansauge F, Gansauge S, Schmidt E, Müller J, Beger HG (1998) Prognostic significance of molecular alterations in human pancreatic carcinoma – an immunohistological study. Langenbeck's Arch Surg383;152–155
6. Rozenblum E, Schutte M, Goggins M (1997), Tumor suppressor pathways in pancreatic carcinoma. Cancer Res 57; 1731–1734
7. Friedrich J M (1996) Computed tomography and magnetic resonance imaging in pancreatic cancer. In: Diagnostic procedures in pancreatic diseases Ed.P. Malfertheimer et al., Springer p 349–357
8. Fernandez-Castillo C, Rattner DW, Warshaw AL (1998) Further experience with laparoscopy and peritoneal cytology in the staging of pancreatic cancer. Br J Surg 82; 1127–1129
9. Tsuchiya R, T Noda, N Harada et al (1986) Collective review of small carcinomas of the pancreas. Ann. Surg. 203; 77–82
10. Gudjonsson B (1996) Treatment and survival in 13,560 patients with pancreatic cancer, and incidence of the disease, in the west Midlands: an epidemiological study. Br J Surg 83; 874
11. Pitt H, Gomes A, Luis JF (1985) The preoperative percutaneous biliary drainage reduce operative risk or increase hospital cost? Ann Surgery 201,545–553
12. Sohn TA, Lillemoe KD, Cameron JL et al (1999) Surgical palliation of unresectable periampullary adenocarcinoma. J Am Coll Surg 188; 658–669
13. Peitralina A, Vistoli F, Carobbi A et al (2000), Thoracoscopic splanchnicectomy for pain relief in unresectable pancreatic cancer. Arch Surg 135; 332–335
14. Stornioli AM, Enas NH, Brown Ca et al (1999) An investigational new drug treatment program for patients with gemcitabine. Cancer 85; 1261–1268
15. Okada S, Sataka Y, Matsuno S et al (1999) Phase II study of docetaxel in patients with metastatic pancreatic cancer. Br J Cancer 80; 438–443
16. Cascim S, Frontini L, Comella G et al (1999) Intensive weakly chemotherapy is not effective in advanced pancreatic cancer patients. Br J Cancer 79; 491–494
17. Nukui Y, Picozzi VJ, Traverso LW (2000) Interferon based adjuvant chemoradiation therapy improves survival after pancreaticoduo-denectomy for pancreatic cancer. Am J Surg 179; 367–371
18. Scheithauer W, Kornek GV, Raderer M et al (1999) Phase II trial of gemcitabine, epirubicin and granulocyte colony-stimulating factor in patients with advanced pancreatic cancer. Br J Cancer 80; 1797–1802
19. Snady H, Bruckner H, Copermann A, Paradiso D, Kiefer L (2000) Survival advantage of combined chemoradiotherapy compared with resection as the initial treatment of patients with regional pancreatic carcinoma. Cancer 89; 314–327
20. Compagno J, Oertel JE. (1978) Mucinous cystic neoplasms of the pancreas with overt and latent malignancy (cystadenocarcinoma and cystadenoma). AM J Clin Pathol; 69: 573–580
21. Compagno J, Oertel JE. (1978) Microcystic adenomas of the pancreas (glycogen-rich cystadenomas). Am J Clin Pathol, 69: 289–298
22. Klöppel G, Solcia E, Longnecker DS, et al. Histological typing of tumors of the exocrine pancreas. In: World Health Organization International Histological Classification of Tumours. 2nd ed. Springer, Berlin Heidelberg New York; 1996; 11–20
23. Warshaw AL, Compton CC, Lewandrowski K, Cardenosa G, Mueller PR. Cystic tumors of the pancreas: new clinical, radiologic, and pathologic observations in 67 patients. Ann Surg 1990; 212: 432–445
24. Siech M, Tripp K, Schmidt-Rohlfing B, Mattfeldt T, Widmaier U, Gansauge F, Gorich J, Beger H G. (1998) Cystic tumours of the pancreas: diagnostic accuracy, pathologic observations and surgical consequences, Langenbecks Arch Surg, 383: 56–61
25. Warshaw AL, Compton CC, Lewandrowski K, Cardenosa G, Mueller PR. (1990) Cystic tumors of the pancreas: new clinical, radiologic, and pathologic observations in 67 patients. Ann Surg; 212: 432–445
26. Obara T, Maguchi H, Saitoh Y, Ura H, Koike Y, Kitazawa S, Namiki M. (1991) Mucin-producing tumor of the pancreas: a unique clinical entity. Am J Gastroenterol; 86: 1619–1625
27. Bartley O, Ekdahl PH, Hulten L. (1966)Paraganglioma simulating pancreatic cyst. Acta Chir Scand; 132: 289–297
28. Frantz VK (1959) Tumor of the pancreas. In: Hartmann WH (ed) Atlas of tumor pathology. VII, fascicles 27 and 28. Armed Forces Institute of Pathology, Washington, DC, p 32
29. Siech M, Merkle E, Mattfeldt T, Widmaier U, Brambs HJ, Beger HG. (1996) Solid-pseudopapilläre Tumoren des Pankreas; Chirurg, 67: 1012–1015

30. Skogseid B, Eriksson B, Lundqvist G, Lorelius LE, Rastad J, Wide L, Akerstrom G, Oberg K. (1991) Multiple endocrine neoplasia type 1: a 10-year prospective screening study in four kindreds. J Clin Endocrin Metab 73: 281–287

31. Zollinger RM, Ellison EH. (1955)Primary peptic ulceration of the jejunum associated with islet cell tumors of the pancreas. Ann Surg 142: 709–728

32. Gregory RA, Tracy HJ, French JM, Sirus W. (1960) Extraction of a gastrin-like substance from a pancreatic tumor in a case of Zollinger-Ellison syndrome. Lancet i: 1045–1048

33. Ellison EH, Wilson SD. (1964) The Zollinger-Ellison syndrome: reappraisal and evaluation of 260 registered cases. Ann Surg 160: 512–530

34. Wolfe MM, Jensen RT. (1987) Zollinger-Ellison syndrome, current concepts in diagnosis and management. N Engl J Med 317: 1200–1209

35. Meko JB, Norton JA. Gastrinoma. In: The Pancreas, edited by Beger HG, Warshaw AL, Büchler MW, Carr-Locke DL, Neoptolemos JP, Russell C, Sarr MG; (1998) Vol. 2, Blackwell science, p 1228–1253

36. Norton JA. (1994) Neuroendocrine tumors of the pancreas and duodenum. Curr Probl Surg 31:77–164

37. Pipeleers-Marichal M, Somers G, Willems G, Foulis A, Imrie C, Bishop AE, Polak JM, Hacki WH, Stamm B, Heitz PU. (1990) Duodenal gastrinomas as the source of hypergastrinemia and Zollinger-Ellison syndrome in patients with MEN-I. N Engl J Med 322: 723–727

38. Arnold R, Frank M, Bülchmann G. Insulinoma and persistent neonatal hyperinsulinemic hypoglycemia (nesidioblastosis). In: The Pancreas, edited by Beger HG, Warshaw AL, Büchler MW, Carr-Locke DL, Neoptolemos JP, Russell C, Sarr MG. Vol. 2, Blackwell science, 1998; p 1187–1202

39. van Heerden JA, Edis AJ, Service FJ. (1979) The surgical aspects of insulinomas. Ann Surg 189: 677–682

40. McEntee GP, Nagorney DM, Kvols LK, Moertel CG, Grant CS. (1990) Cytoreductive hepatic surgery for neuroendocrine tumors. Surgery 108: 1091–109

Neuroendocrine Gastro-Entero-Pancreatic Tumors

VII

15 Neuroendocrine Gastro-Entero-Pancreatic (GEP) Tumors

R. Arnold, R. Göke, M. Wied, Th. Behr

Summary

Neuroendocrine gastro-entero-pancreatic (GEP) tumors are rare but present with variable, sometimes dramatic clinical syndromes. The majority of these tumors is non-functioning and most functioning and non-functioning tumors are malignant. This chapter describes the various clinical entities, has a special focus on histopathology of these tumors as a reliable source for prognosis and summarizes current state and new trends in diagnosis and treatment of these tumors. The management of neuroendocrine GEP-tumors needs a multidisciplinary approach. Therefore, diagnostic and therapeutic aspects of this chapter recognize the important contributions of surgery, pathology, radiology, nuclear medicine and gastrointestinal endocrinology.

Definition

Several terms for endocrine tumors of the gastrointestinal tract are currently applied to describe the same pathological entity: "carcinoid", "neuroendocrine tumor", "neuroendocrine carcinoma", "APUDoma", "gastro-entero-pancreatic (GEP) tumor", "islet cell tumor" (in case of pancreatic origin). The term "carcinoid" was introduced by S. Oberndorfer in 1907 to distinguish carcinoids as less rapidly growing and well-differentiated epithelial tumors of the small intestine from the more aggressively growing adenocarcinoma of the gut and, thus, recognizing the decisive difference to carcinomas which is the very slow growth of most endocrine tumors and which is frequently associated with an uncompromized life quality. Strictly speaking is the term "carcinoid" reserved for endocrine tumors of the gastrointestinal tract (Table 2) and not for those of the pancreas (Table 1). Endocrine pancreatic tumors are assumed to arise from islets of Langerhans although their origin from the diffuse endocrine cell system scattered within the mucosa of the gastrointestinal tract and the pancreatic duct system cannot be excluded. At least in vertebrates, the islets of Langerhans arise within an independent islet organ which melts together with the exocrine pancreas during ontogenesis. The blurredness of the term "carcinoid" results from its histological features which are almost identical with those of endocrine pancreatic tumors. Therefore, even pathologists frequently use the term "carcinoid" to describe an endocrine pancreatic tumor. To avoid the dilemma, the term "carcinoid" should be used only for well-differentiated endocrine tumors of the gut and the term "malignant carcinoid" to designate the corresponding well differentiated endocrine carcinoma [1]. If a "carcinoid" is associated with a clinical syndrome as a Zollinger-Ellison syndrome in the case of a gastrin-producing endocrine tumor of the duodenum, the respective "carcinoid" should better be called gastrinoma.

The term "neuroendocrine" reflects the origin of the endocrine cells of the gastrointestinal tract fom the embryonic neural crest. They have been designated as "Helles Zellenorgan" by F. Feyrter. The acronym "APUDoma" (amine precursor uptake and decarboxylation) describes the potency of endocrine tumors to synthesize in addition to hormones biogenic amines as serotonin and other peptides characteristic to cells originating from the neural crest first described by A.E.G. Pearse.

Endocrine tumors of the gastrointestinal tract are epithelial tumors and differ histologically from neuronal tumors as neuroblastomas, pheochromocytomas and paragangliomas which also arise from the diffuse neuroendocrine system and are, therefore, of neural crest origin.

Amphicrine and mixed endocrine-exocrine tumors will not be discussed within this survey since their prognosis and biological features are determined by the exocrine cell department with a predominantly unfavourable prognosis.

Table 1
Classification and leading symptoms of the most frequent endocrine tumors of the gastrointestinal tract

Name (Syndrome)	Leading Symptoms	Responsible Hormone	Other Hormones in the Tumor	Malignancy (%)	Localization of primary	Extra-pancreatic Localization
Insulinoma	Hypoglycaemia	Insulin	Glucagon, PP	5–10	Pancreas	very rare
Gastrinoma (Zollinger-Ellison syndrome)	Peptic Ulcers, Diarrhea, Reflux Disease	Gastrin	Insulin, PP, Glucagon, ACTH, Somatostatin, Chromogranin A	>90	Pancreas	Duodenum, Stomach, Mesenterium
Carcinoid syndrome	Flush, Diarrhoea, Bronchial Obstruction	Serotonin	Tachykinins, Prostaglandins, Chromogranin A	100	Ileum	Pancreas (rare)
VIPoma (Verner-Morrison syndrome), Pancreatic Cholera	Intractable Diarrhea, Hypokalemia	VIP, PHI	PP, Glucagon, Somatostatin, Chromogranin A	75	Pancreas	
Glucagonoma	Erythema necrolyticans migrans, Diabetes	Glucagon	PP, Insulin, Somatostatin, Chromogranin A	50	Pancreas	Rare
Somatostatinoma	Diabetes, Steatorrhea, Gallstones	Somatostatin	PP, Insulin, Calcitonin	50	Pancreas	Duodenum
GHRHoma	Acromegaly	GHRH	Somatostatin, Gastrin, Insulin, Chromogranin A	100	Pancreas	Lung
CRHoma, ACTHoma	Cushing's syndrome	CRH	Gastrin, PP, Chromogranin A	>90	Pancreas	Lung

ACTH Adreno-corticotrophic hormone; *CRH* Corticotropin releasing hormone; *GHRH* Growth hormone releasing hormone; *PHI* Peptide histidine isoleucine; *PP* Pancreatic peptide; *VIP* Vasoactive intestinal polypeptide.

Table 2
Characteristics of extra-pancreatic endocrine gastrointestinal tumors ("carcinoids")

Localization	% of all carcinoids	Peptides and hormones	Functional activity	Endocrine cell type	Malignancy
Esophagus	0.04	Chromogranin A	rarely	Grimelius positive, NSE positive	>50%
Stomach	2–3	Chromogranin A (histamine, gastrin), Ghrelin, VMAT-2	very rarely	ECL-cells, rarely EC-cells, rarely G-cells	highly variable
Duodenum and proximal jejunum	22	5-HT, gastrin, somatostatin, PP, calcitonin, ACTH	Zollinger-Ellison syndrome or functional inactive	EC-cells, G-cells, somatostatin-cells	50%
Distal jejunum and ileum	23–28	Chromogranin A, serotonin, substance P, tachykinins, others	mostly inactive; carcinoid syndrome in 5–7%	EC-cells	>50% in tumors larger then 1 cm
Appendix	19	Serotonin, GLP-1, GIP-2, PP/PYY	mostly inactive; carcinoid syndrome extremely rare	EC-cells, L-cells	risk factor size >2 cm and invasion of mesoappendix
Cecum	8	Serotonin	carcinoid syndrome in 5%	EC-cells	> 50%
Ascending Colon	8	GLP-1, GLP-2 PP/PYY		L-cells	
Rectosigmoid	20	Serotonin,	no	EC-cells	15% depends on tumor size and invasion
Rectum	20	GLP-1, GLP-2 PP/PYY		L-Cells	

Classification

Endocrine GEP tumors can be subdivided according to their origin into those originating from the foregut (esophagus, stomach, duodenum, proximal jejunum, pancreas), midgut (distal jejunum, ileum, appendix, cecum, right-sided colon) and hindgut (left-sided colon and rectum). This classification is based on the embryologic assignment of the different parts of the gut. Vary rarely endocrine tumors of the same histology can arise in the ovary, extrahepatic bile ducts, the liver, the kidney, testis, spleen, breast and larynx and other organs as the broncial system and thymus.

Clinically more relevant is a classification according to the functional activity of endocrine GEP tumors. Most benign and malignant endocrine GEP tumors are functionally inactive and patients commonly present with abdominal pain, weight loss, obstructive jaundice and intestinal obstruction depending on the localization and size of the tumor. Noteworthy, many tumors are asymptomatic even in the presence of metastases and are discovered incidentally during routine imaging procedures.

Survival of patients with GEP tumors is even in the metastatic state much more favourable than in patients with other malignancys and depends on the site of the primary tumor and the extent of metastatic spread. Of pancreatic endocrine tumors the best prognosis is associated with insulinomas which are in more that 95% of patients solitary and benign. In contrast, most of the other pancreatic entities are malignant (see Table 1).

As shown in Tables 1 and 2 the majority of functionally active endocrine tumors arise within the pancreas (see Table 1) whereas functionally active tumors within the gastrointestinal tract can cause the Zollinger-Ellison syndrome if originating from the duodenum or cause a Carcinoid syndrome due to a metastatic tumor of the ileum.

Endocrine GEP tumors may be benign or malignant. The majority of endocrine pancreatic tumors are malignant and present with metastases mostly to the liver (see Table 1). The malignancy rate of endocrine tumors within the gastrointestinal tract is highly variable and mostly depending on the size of the carcinoid.

Endocrine GEP tumors can arise sporadic or as part of the Multiple Endocrine Neoplasia (MEN) syndromes (Table 3). MEN-I syndrome is an autosomal dominantly inherited disorder characterized by the synchronous or metachronous occurrence of tumors in multiple endocrine organs, predominantly the pancreas, parathyroid, pituitary and duodenum. The genetic locus was ascribed to a segment of the long arm of chromosome 11, where the menin gene – a tumor suppressor gene – is located which is in MEN-I syndrome mutated [2, 3]. MEN-I syndrome is present in 20% of patients with gastrinoma

Table 3
MEN syndromes

Syndrome	Affected organ	Alterations
MEN-1 (Wermer's syndrome)	Parathyroid gland	Hyperplasia, multiple adenomas
	Pancreas	Islet cell tumors (insulinoma, gastrinoma, VIPoma, glucagonoma)
	Pituitary (anterior)	Adenoma (prolactin, ACTH, STH, GH, non-funtioning)
MEN-2A (Sipple's syndrome)	Thyroid gland	C-cell hyperplasia, medullary thyroid carcinoma
	Adrenal medulla	Phaeochromocytoma
	Parathyroid gland	Hyperplasia, multiple adenomas
MEN-2B	Thyroid gland	C-cell hyperplasia, medullary thyroid carcinoma
	Adrenal medulla	Phaeochromocytoma
	Mucosa	Neuromas
	Other abnormalities: Marfanoid habitus, Megacolon	

[4], 4% of patients with insulinoma [5] and 13–17% of patients with glucagonoma [6]. However, in MEN-I syndrome most endocrine pancreatic tumors are non-functional containing mostly pancreatic polypeptide or glucagon [5].

Epidemiology

Endocrine GEP tumors are rare events. The exact incidence and prevalence of these tumors is difficult to ascertain because many are asymptomatic. From autopsy studies an annual incidence of 8.4 gastrointestinal endocrine tumors (carcinoids) per 100.000 people has been calculated [7, 8] (Table 4). 90% of these tumors were incidental autopsy findings. For endocrine pancreatic tumors an annual incidence of 0,1–0,4 tumors per 100.000 has been reported. [8]. Table 4 summarizes the published annual incidence rates for the most common gastrointestinal (carcinoids) and pancreatic endocrine tumors. Endocrine tumors originating in the midgut encompass by far the majority of all endocrine tumors followed by the pancreatic endocrine tumors.

Almost all endocrine tumors originating within the hindgut are asymptomatic and do not create symptoms as a consequence of hormone overproduction. The reason for that is unknown since many of these tumors contain peptides and hormones which are also pro-

Table 4

Epidemiological data of endocrine GEP tumors

Localization	Incidence cases per 100.000 people per year	Remarks (% of all gastro-intestinal carcinoids)	Mean age [years] (range)
Stomach	0.002–0.1	(11–14%)	50–60
		type I: 74%	63 [15–88]
		type II: 6%	50 [28–67]
		type III: 13%	55 [41–61]
		poorly differentiated: 6%	
Duodenum		(22%)	59 [30–90]
		Gastrin-producing: 62%	
		Somatostatin-producing: 21%	
		Gangliocytic pasaganglioma: 9%	
		Undefined tumors: 5,6%	
Proximal Jejunum		(1%)	
Distal Jejunum/Ileum [30–99]	0.28–0.89	(28%)	60–70
Appendix [6–80]		(19%) more frequent in females	32–45
Colon	0.07–0.21	(right-sided colon: 8%)	58
		(left-sided colon: 20%)	
Rectum	0.14–0.76		60
Pancreas			
all	0.01 – 0.3		
Insulinoma	0.1–0.2		47 [8–82]
Gastrinoma	0.05–0.15		[33–53]
VIPoma	0.005–0.02		
Glucagonoma	0.001–0.01		

duced in tumors responsible for the carcinoid syndrome. The same is true for most gastric carcinoids and carcinoids arising in the distal ileum. Even in metastatic tumors a hormone mediated symptomatology is mostly absent. Of the endocrine pancreatic tumors almost 50% are functionally inactive as well [8]. The incidence rates of the functionally active tumors with insulinoma as the most frequent tumor are listed in table 4.

According to an analysis of 8305 cases of carcinoid tumors identified by the "Surveillance, Epidemiology, and End Results" (SEER) program of the American National Cancer Institute (NCI) from 1973 to 1991 and by an earlier NCI program 5-year survival of patients was 50.4% [7]. The presence of regional and distant metastases reduced survival rate to 21,8%. If survival rates are calculated separately for tumors arising in the foregut, midgut and hindgut 5-year survival rates were 44.5%, 61% and 72% respectively [7]. Most favourable survival have appendiceal carcinoids with 85.9%. Surveillance rates for endocrine GEP tumors of specific localizations will be discussed in more detail later in this chapter.

Etiology

The etiology of endocrine GEP tumors is unknown. It is comprehensible to assume that they originate from cells or rather precursor cells of the diffuse neuroendocrine cell system. Endocrine tumor cells display certain cytochemical properties with endocrine cells scattered within the mucosa of the gastrointestinal tract and with the constituents of the islets of Langerhans as the expression of neuron-specific enolase, synaptophysin and chromogranin A and C [1, 16]. Chromogranins are acidic glycoproteins present in almost all endocrine and neuronal tissues. They are released into the circulation and can serve as tumor markers since they are found in more than 90% of patients with endocrine GEP tumors. Although endocrine pancreatic tumors are also called "islet cell tumors" it is unproven that pancreatic insulinomas, gastrinomas, VIPomas etc. originate from the islets of Langerhans. In favour of this assumption are findings in experimental settings which clearly demonstrate that insulinomas in rats can under defined conditions arise from islets. However, some endocrine pancreatic tumors produce hormones and peptides as gastrin or VIP which are not synthesized from islet cells

after birth. Therefore, it is conceivable to assume that islet tumors originate from endocrine pancreatic multipotent precursor cells which are constituents of the pancreatic duct epithelium [13].

General Pathophysiology

The key event occurring in functionally active endocrine GEP tumor cells is the loss of capacity to store their hormonal product as insulin in insulinomas, gastrin in gastrinomas etc. within the tumor cell. Therefore, inappropriately released hormones and peptides not responding to the physiological feedback inhibition are responsible for the clinical manifestation of the disease. According to the concept of an impaired storage capacity of tumor cells, it has been shown, that insulinoma cells contain less insulin than normal β-cells, and the mean total insulin content of insulinomas was even lower than the mean insulin content of the whole pancreas of the respective patient [14]. Very similar is the gastrin content of the majority of gastrinomas lower compared to the gastrin content of the whole antral mucosa which contains more gastrin-producing cells than the tumor [15].

Histopathology

Most endocrine GEP tumors display a solid, trabecular or glandular arrangement of well-different (Fig. 1a–c) [1, 16]. However, not in every case these features permit recognition of the endocrine nature of the tumor. In these tumors special staining methods as silver methods or immunohistochemical staines for general endocrine markers as chromogranins (Fig. 1e), synaptophysin or neuron-specific enolase are needed for tumor identification [1, 16]. To characterize the tumor cell further with regard to their hormone/peptide production specific antibodies against polypeptide hormones are needed to identify a tumor cell as insulin-, gastrin-, glucagon- or other hormones producing cell (Fig 2a, b) [16]. Endocrine tumors with predominant insulin production can be classified as insulinoma, those with predominant glucagon- or gastrin production as glucagonoma or gastrinoma. This does not indicate that a tumor which histologically has been diagnosed as insulinoma or glu-

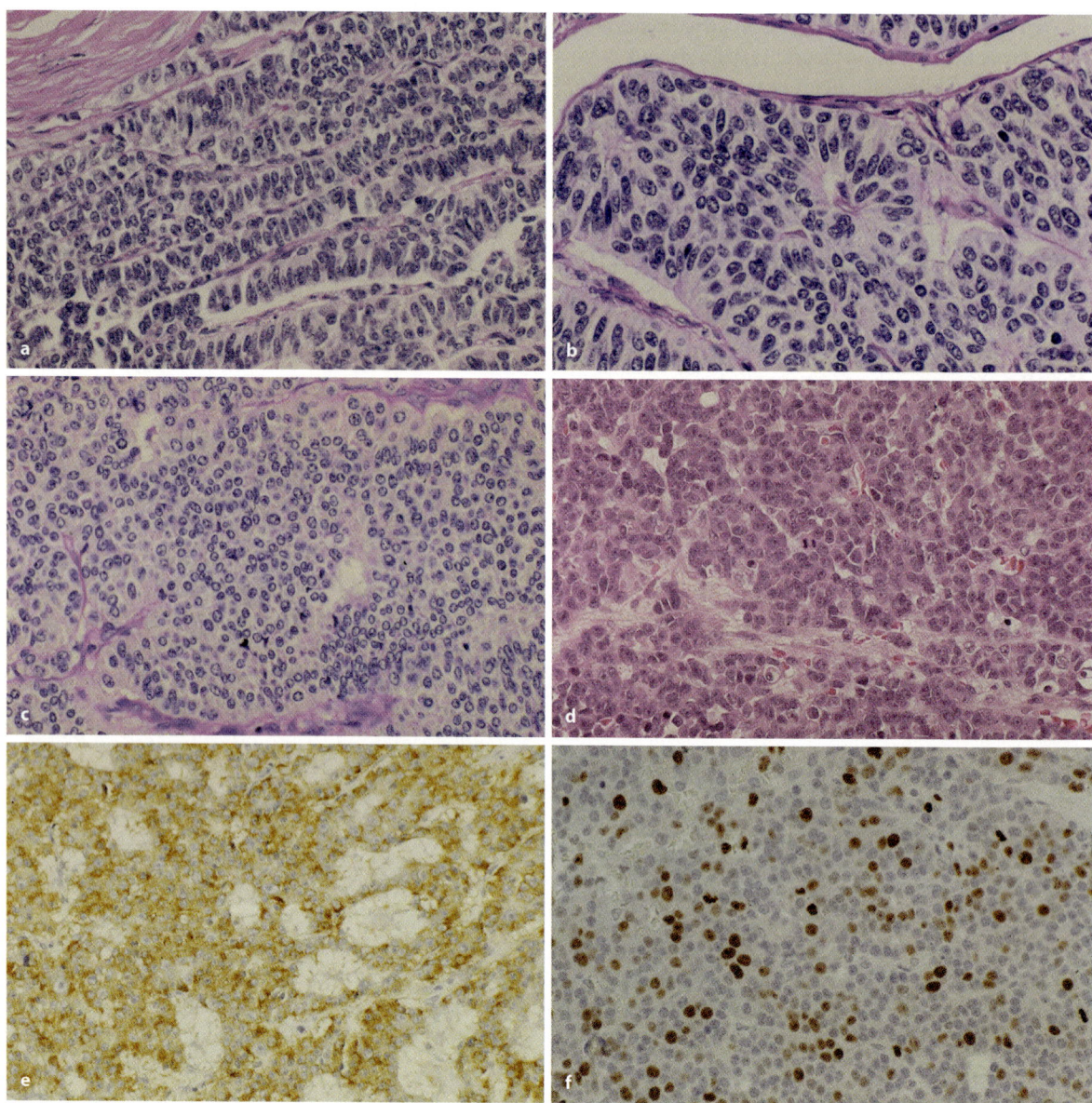

Figure 1a–f
Histopathological patterns in pancreatic endocrine tumors. a trabecular pattern; PAS staining; **b** glandular pattern; PAS staining; **c** solid pattern; PAS staining; **d** poorly differentiated neuroendocrine tumor; PAS staining; **e** staining with the endocrine marker chromogranin A; **f** staining with an antibody against the proliferation marker Ki-6

cagonoma acts as a functionally active endocrine tumor responsible for hypoglycemic attacks in the case of an insulinoma or giving rise to the typical symptoms of a glucagonoma syndrome. Functional activity or inactivity cannot be deducted from histology. Correspondingly and most characteristicly, many endocrine tumors as part of the MEN-I syndrome are functionally inactive [18].

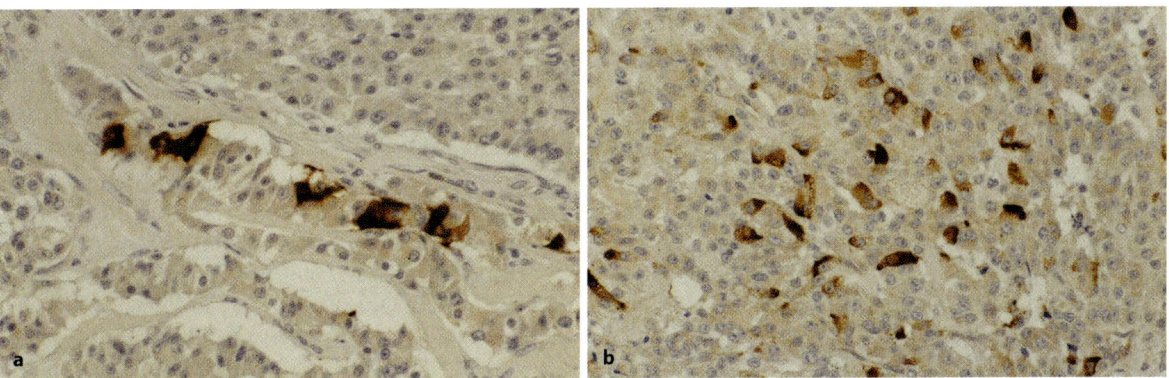

Figure 2a,b
Demonstration of several hormones present within the same endocrine Pancreatic tumor. **a** immunohistological staining for insulin; **b** immunohistological staining for gastrin

Most endocrine tumors are composed of more than one cell type. An endocrine pancreatic tumor with predominant insulin-producing cells can contain additional somatostatin- or glucagon- or pancreatic polypeptide-producing cells [15]. This feature is independent on the functional status of the tumor and can be observed in functionally active and inactive tumor [15]. It is unclear, why in the presence of multiple hormones within a single endocrine tumor only one or no clinical syndrome occurs. Nevertheless, in few patients, a second clinical syndrome can be present initially or develop later. This occurs preferably in patients with metastatic endocrine pancreatic tumors or in patients with MEN-I syndrome and multiple endocrine pancreatic tumors [4]. According to own observations which are in accordance with reports from the literature the combination of ectopic ACTH-producing and gastrin-producing pancreatic tumors giving rise to a combination of Cushing's syndrome and Zollinger-Ellison syndrome is frequent, although the condition itself with two functionally active tumors is a rare event.

Since most endocrine tumors are well-differentiated, their mitotic index visualized by the Ki67 labelling (Fig. 1f) index [9] is low which is in accordance with their slow growth behaviour. Therefore, it is difficult to predict the biological behaviour of well-differentiated tumors using classical histopathological malignancy criteria as cellular or structural atypia, necrosis, mitotic activity or microscopic invasion. A panel of international pathologists has, therefore, proposed to classify benign and malignant endocrine tumors into the categories listed in table 5 [1]. The basis for distinguishing a well-differentiated endocrine tumor from a well-differentiated endocrine carcinoma is the presence of metastases and/or evidence for local invasion. Benign or low risk endocrine tumors are distinguished from tumors with greater risk of malignancy on the basis of a combination or features such as tumor size, local extension, angioinvasion, cellular atypia, proliferative activity and the expression of hormones regularly found in the specific organ ("eutopic" hormone production) or the expression of "ectopic" hormonal products (as ACTH in an endocrine pancreatic tumor).

Poorly differentiated small cell carcinoma (Fig. 1d) is for experienced pathologists easy to distinguish from well-differentiated endocrine tumors on the basis of cellular atypia, the presence of markedly hyperchromatic nuclei, a high nuclear/cytoplasmic ratio, focal necrosis and high mitotic activity. To classify such an indifferentiated tumor as endocrine, tumors must react for

Table 5
General endocrine tumor categories

1	Well-differentiated endocrine tumor
2	Well-differentiated endocrine carcinoma
3	Poorly differentiated endocrine (small cell) carcinoma
4	Mixed exocrine-endocrine tumor
5	Tumor-like lesions

cytosolic neuroendocrine markers as synaptophysin and neuron-specific enolase [1]. However, these tumors are frequently negative for markers of endocrine granules as chromogranin and for specific hormonal products.

Additional histopathologic characteristics and tumor classifications will be discussed later when specific tumors are described in more detail.

Molecular Pathogenesis

Sporadic GEP Tumors

In sporadic pancreatic endocrine tumors (PETs) an allelic deletion of the tumor-suppressor gene MEN-I located on chromosome 11q13 has been found very frequently [3, 17]. However, the mutational frequency of MEN-I is different in functional and non-functional PETs: 30% of functional but only 8% of non-functional PETs showed mutations of the MEN-I gene [17, 18]. Furthermore, there are differences within the group of functional PETs: Alterations in MEN-I have been found in 54% (15/28) of gastrinomas, 50% (4/8) of VIPomas, 2/3 glucagonomas, 1/1 somatostatinoma but only in 7% (4/54) of insulinomas [17]. While such findings support the relevance of MEN-I for the pathogenesis of endocrine neoplasms, it is important to note that the incidence of MEN-I alteration is obviously tumor-type related and found more frequently in gastrinomas and non functional PETs than in insulinomas. Other frequent genetic abberations found in 25–50% of PETs analyzed are chromosomal deletions on 3p, 3q, 6q, 10q, 11q, 11p, 16p, 20q, 21q, 22q, Xq and Y. In up to 25% of PETs gains on chromosomes 5q, 7q, 7p, 9q, 12q, 17p and 20q were found.

The p53 tumor suppressor gene located on chromosome 17p13 encodes a nuclear protein which is involved in multiple cellular processes like cell cycle, DNA repair, replication, transcription, apoptosis and cell differentiation. p53 alterations are detectable in almost all cancers but are extremely rare in PETs. However, increased p53 protein concentrations were found in malignant insulinomas most likely due to inactivating mutations resulting in an increased stability or posttranslational events leading to overexpression [19].

The p16 (INK4a, MTS1) gene located on chromosome 9p21 encodes a protein that binds to cyclin-dependent kinase 4 inhibiting its interaction with cyclin. p16 alterations do not play a role in non-functional PETs and insulinomas. Since p16 was found abnormal in 42% of 8 gastrinomas analyzed [20] it might play a role in gastrinoma tumorigenesis. However, further studies are necessary to confirm this assumption.

DPC4/Smad4 is a tumor suppressor gene located on chromosome 18q21 encoding a protein which is involved in the TGF-β signaling pathway. Previous data suggested that Smad4 mutations seem to be common in non-functional PETs [21]. However, based on a more recent study it is unlikely that Smad4 plays a role in tumorigenesis of endocrine tumors.

Of the oncogenes c-myc, c-fos, K-ras and c-erbB-2 only K-ras was found to be overexpressed in PETs. However, only 10 of 90 PETs analyzed in the literature showed a ras mutation indicating that this is a rare event in these tumors. Most PETs with ras mutations were malignant insulinomas suggesting that alterations of ras might play a role in the pathogenesis of these tumors.

Recent data indicate that losses of sex chromosomes are common in PETs and are associated with presence of metastases, local invasion and poor survival.

Up to date the pathogenesis of neuroendocrine tumors of the gastrointestinal tract is not well characterized. Allelic loss of the MEN-I gene located on chromosome 11q13 was identified in type II ECL cell tumors and carcinoids of the jejunum and ileum. In type I ECL cell tumors abnormal RegIalpha gene was observed. In poorly differentiated neuroendocrine neoplasms allelic loss of p53 located on chromosome 17p13 were found in 4 of 9 cases suggesting a role for p53 in the development of these aggressive tumors.

Multiple Endocrine Neoplasia-Type 1

Multiple endocrine neoplasia-type 1 (MEN-I; Wermer's syndrome) is characterized by a combined occurrence of primary hyperparathyroidism, pancreatic endocrine tumors and pituitary adenomas [5]. The development of additional tumors in other endocrine or non-endocrine tissues indicates that the protein menin encoded by the MEN-I gene might have a function in a wide variety of tissues. Most MEN-I patients (90%) exhibit primary hy-

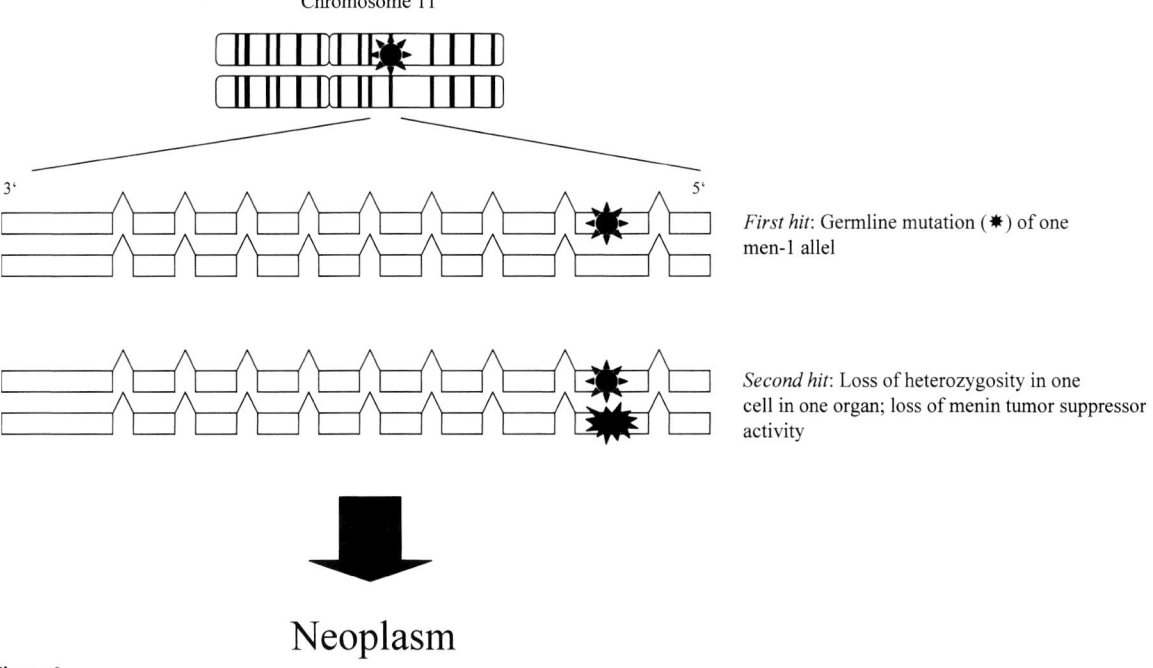

Chromosome 11

3'   5'

First hit: Germline mutation (✳) of one men-1 allel

Second hit: Loss of heterozygosity in one cell in one organ; loss of menin tumor suppressor activity

Neoplasm

Figure 3
Tumorigenesis in MEN-1 according to the two hit model described by Knudson. Patients show a germline mutation of the MEN-1 gene. Later they acquire another mutation in the wild-type allele resulting in an loss of suppressor function of the gene

perparathyroidism. Pancreatic endocrine tumors occur in ~60% and are usually benign and non-functional [5]. The most common functional tumors are insulinomas and gastrinomas. The prevalence of pituitary adenomas is between 15–50%. A recent large study including 324 MEN-I patients showed pituitary adenomas in 42% of the cases which were larger in size and more aggressive than without MEN-I.

MEN-I is an autosomal dominant inherited syndrome and is related to mutations of the MEN-I gene located on chromosome 11q13 [2, 3]. The tumorigenesis of MEN-I is supposingly a process according to the two hit model by Knudson (Fig. 3). Patients inherit a mutated MEN-I gene and later aquire another mutation in the wild-type allel (loss of heterozygosity) in vulnerable endocrine tissue. This results in a loss of the tumor suppressor function of the MEN-I gene. The MEN-I gene contains 10 exons encoding the protein menin consiting of 610 amino acids [2]. Two transcripts have been identified which are most likely due alternative splicing.

A 2.9 kb transcript was detected in all tissues while a 4.2 kb transcript was found in pancreas, stomach and thymus only [2]. Menin contains two nuclear localization sites and is predominantly a nuclear protein. However, during cell cycle menin was shown to shuttle from nucleus to cytoplasm.

In Ras-transformed NIH3T3 cells overexpression of menin resulted in decreased proliferation, suppression of clonogenicity in soft agar and inhibition of tumor growth in mice. Menin directly interacts with JunD, a transcriptional factor of the AP-1 complex, via three JunD interacting domains and inhibits JunD activation of transcription [22]. However, since JunD inhibits growth of Ras-transformed NIH3T3 cells the repressive effect of menin should result in enhanced growth. This indicates that the mechanism of action of menin is more complex than we know today and probably involves other genes and proteins. This assumption is supported by a recent observation that menin interacts with NF-κB proteins and inhibits NF-κB-mediated transactivation).

Up to date more than 400 mutations of the MEN-I gene have been identified. Most mutations were unique but some occurred twice or more in unrelated families (107, 110–112). Of 262 mutations observed in MEN-I patients between 1997 and 1999 approximately 22% are nonsense mutations, 48% frameshift deletions and insertions, 8% inframe deletions and insertions, 5% donor-splice site mutations and 17% missense mutations. The majority of mutations result in an inactivation of the MEN-I gene. There is no genotype-phenotype correlation in MEN-I. However, most patients with agressive phenotypes show truncating mutations.

Multiple Endocrine Neoplasia-Type 2

The term multiple endocrine neoplasia-type 2 (MEN-2) describes the combined occurrence of inherited forms of medullary thyroid carcinoma (MTC) with other malignomas. In MEN-2A (Sipple's syndrome) MTC is combined with pheochromocytoma and primary hyperparathyreoidism. MEN-2B (Gorlin's syndrome) is characterized by the occurrence of MTC, pheochromocytoma, neurinomas of the gastrointestinal tract and a marfanoid habitus [23].

Men-2 is caused by germline mutations of the RET gene located on chromosome 10q11–2 encoding a transmembrane tyrosine kinase receptor with cadherin-like and cystein-rich extracellular domains and a tyrosine kinase intarcellular domain [23]. RET genomic size is 60 kb and the gene contains 21 exons. GDNF (glia cell line-derived neurotrophic factor), neurturin, artemin and persephrin act as RET protein ligands inducing homodimerization through the cystein-rich region resulting in an activation of the tyrosine kinase domain and the Ras-MAP-kinase pathway. 95% of MEN-2A patients show mutations of the cystein-rich extracellular domain. The most common mutation affects codon 634 (Cys→Arg/Tyr/Gly). Missense mutations have also been identified in codons 609–611, 618 and 620. Approximately 98% of MEN-2B patients exhibit mutations in the intracellular tyrosine kinase domain (codon 918; Met→Thr). While mutations in the cystein-rich region result in the formation of constitutive active RET dimers, mutations in the intracellular tyrosine kinase domain lead to a switch to an abnormal signalling pathway.

Germline RET mutations were observed in approximately 100% of men-2 families. Therefore, genetic analysis of RET is advisable to identify young asymptomatic gene carriers and perform prophylactic thyroidectomy.

Other Inherited Syndromes Associated with GEP Tumors

In a recent report 12% of 158 patients with von Hippel-Lindau (VHL) syndrome had neuroendocrine tumors [24]. These patients showed no symptoms due to hormonal hypersecretion suggesting that the endocrine tumors were non-functioning. The VHL syndrome is caused by a germline mutation of the VHL gene which is located on chromosome 3p35–36 coding for a 213-aa protein. The VHL gene product is a component of an Skp1-Cdc53-F-box-like ubiquitin-ligase complex targeting the α-subunits of the hypoxia-inducible factor heterodimeric transcription factor for polyubiquitylation and proteasomal degradation. Somatostatinomas have been described in patients with von Recklinghausen's neurofibromatosis. Neurofibromatosis is caused by alterations of the NF1 gene located on chromosome 17q11.2 coding for neurofibromin which is a 2485-aa protein.

Growth Characteristics and Metastatic Spread and Secondary Non-Endocrine Malignancies

As recognized as early as in 1907 by S. Oberndorfer who introduced the term "carcinoid", endocrine GEP tumors grow slowly even in the metastatic state compared to adenocarcinomas of the gastrointestinal tract. However, the spontaneous tumor growth varies from one patient to another. Some tumors remain unchanged in size for months or even years without therapy, others grow slowly independent of any antiproliferative measures and still others exhibit exploding growth. The latter tumors are poorly differentiated and mostly small cell carcinomas. Even spontaneous tumor regression without any treatment has been reported in well-differentiated tumors. A schematic presentation, how malignant GEP tumors can grow is shown in fig. 4.

Unfortunately the use of proliferative markers and immunostaining of tumors for oncoproteins, tumor suppressor genes, and adhesion molecules gave contradic-

% Tumor growth

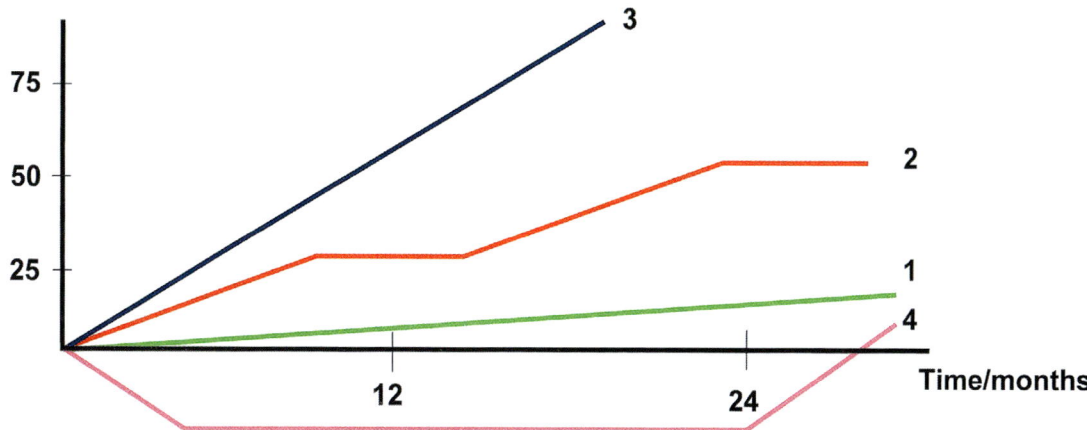

Figure 4
Schematic presentation how endocrine GEP tumors can grow. Some tumors grow so slowly that they do not meet the 25% increase according to the accepted NIH criteria of tumor progression even after 18 months (*1*). Tumor (*2*) displays an intermediate tumor growth. Tumor (*3*) grows very rapidly corresponding to its histology of a small cell neuroendocrine carcinoma. Tumor (*4*) decreased spontaneously in size, remained constant for 2 years and started to grow after 24 months of observation without any treatment

tory results. One study was performed in gastrointestinal carcinoid tumors and indicated that expression of p53, cyclin D1, Rb, bcl-2 and Ki-67 does not correlate with malignant behaviour, whereas p21 overexpression did. Others concluded from studies in bronchial carcinoid tumors and in gastrointestinal carcinoid tumors that high expression of ki-67, a tumor size >3 cm and a high mitotic index (in the case of ECL cell tumors of the stomach) is malignancy predictive. Possibly, these findings are dependent on the site of the primary tumor since in carcinoid tumors of the duodenum and ampulla of vater an aggressive behaviour of the tumor was not associated with higher proliferative indices as proliferating cell nuclear antigen (PCNA), Ki-67 and p21.

Malignant GEP tumors can spread in almost all organs: lymphnodes, peritoneal spread, liver, spleen, kidney, lung, skin, brain and bones. Table 6 is an example of the metastatic spread of patients with malignant gastrinoma and patients with carcinoid syndrome observed in the institution of the authors.

It is noteworthy that patients with malignant endocrine GEP tumors tend to synchronous and metachronous non-endocrine malignancies. In a 20-year retrospective study of 150 patients with gastrointestinal

Table 6

Metastatic spread in different endocrine GEP tumors (own data, values in percent)

Site	Non-functioning tumor	Carcinoid syndrome	Gastrinoma
Lymph nodes	64	76	54
Liver	61	88	57
Bones	13	17	11
Lung	9	14	7
CNS	2	0	4
Peritoneal	17	23	4
Other	28	24	4

carcinoids followed up for a median of 66 months 22% developed synchronous non-carcinoid tumors and 10% metachronous tumors. In another retrospective study on 69 patients with gastrointestinal carcinoid tumors 42% hat synchronous and 4% metachronous tumors. The most common site for the secondary primary malignancy was the gastrointestinal tract with carcinoma of the colon and rectum. Patients with colorectal carcinoids have, in addition, an increased risk for cancer in the colon, ano-rectum, small bowel, esophagus, stomach, lung, urinary tract and prostate.

Staging of Endocrine GEP Tumors

Staging of tumors is a useful and essential tool in oncology to define tumor size, invasion and infiltration into adjacent tissues and metastatic spread into regional lymph nodes, liver and other organs. This is important for further management using surgical, radiotherapeutic and chemotherapeutic approaches. For this, TNM classification has been elaborated for specific tumor entities as published by the AICC Cancer Staging Manual and UICC. No corresponding TNM classifications exist for endocrine GEP tumors and their malignant variants because management of endocrine tumors depends even in metastatic tumors primarily on growth behaviour (see Fig. 4) and functional activity. Insulinomas must be removed because they produce life-threatening symptoms independent on the size of the tumor which may be too small to be visualised by available imaging techniques. Metastatic insulinomas have to be partially resected if possible to reduce tumor burden and, thus, to facilitate control of hypoglycemic symptoms. In patients with very slowly growing metastatic GEP tumors the beneficial effect of many therapeutic measures is unsettled. The same applies for non-functioning small endocrine pancreatic tumors in patients with MEN-I syndrome for whom resection has not been shown to influence patient's outcome.

In an attempt to classify endocrine GEP tumors not having metastasized at diagnosis a panel of pathologists has recently proposed a classification of endocrine GEP tumors and assigned the tumors according to the categories summarised in table 5 [1]. The basis of distinguishing well differentiated endocrine carcinomas from other well differentiated endocrine tumors was usually the presence of metastases and/or evidence of local invasion. Benign or low risk endocrine tumors were distinguished from tumors with greater risk of malignancy on the basis of a combination of features such as tumor size and site, local extension, angioinvasion, cellular atypia and proliferative activity. Differentiation of poorly differentiated endocrine small cell carcinoma from well-differentiated endocrine tumors was performed by conventional histological characteristic featurs including high-grade cellular atypia, markedly hyperchromatic nuclei, focal necrosis and high proliferation.

In tables 7–11 these major principles have been transferred to endocrine tumors arising in different organs of the GI tract as the pancreas (Table 7), stomach (Table 8), the duodenum and upper jejunum (Table 9), the ileum, cecum, colon and rectum (Table 10) and the appendix (Table 11).

Clinical Entities: Symptoms and Laboratory Findings

Insulinoma

Epidemiology

Around 40% of endocrine pancreatic tumors are insulinomas. Based on a review of 224 insulinoma patients over a 60-year period the medium age was 47 (range 8–82) years and 41% of patients were male [25]. The yearly incidence is 0,5 to 4 per one million population and 5,8% had malignant insulinoma [25]. In 7,6% of patients the insulinoma was part of the MEN-I syndrome [4, 25]. Almost all insulinomas are situated in or close to the pancreas. 1–3% of insulinomas have been reported to arise in the duodenum, ileum and lung [26]. Insulinomas are evenly distributed within the pancreas [26]. Based on a study in 1067 cases most insulinomas are small: 5% smaller then 0.5 cm, 34% were 0.5 to 1 cm, 53% 1 to 5 cm and only 8% larger then 5 cm in size. With the exception of the rare malignant insulinomas prognosis of patients with a benign insulinoma and curative resection is excellent. For definition of "benign" insulinoma see Table 7.

Table 7
Clinicopathological staging of endocrine tumors of the pancreas. (Mod. according to [1])

1	Well-differentiated endocrine tumor
1.1	Benign behaviour: confined to the pancreas, nonangioinvasive, <2 cm in size*, ≤2 mitoses and ≤2% Ki67 positive cells/10HPF
1.2	Uncertain behaviour: confined to the pancreas ≥2 cm in size, >2 mitoses, >2% Ki67 cells/10 HPF, or angioinvasive
2	Well-differentiated endocrine carcinoma
2.1	Low grade malignant with gross local invasion and/or metastases
3	Poorly differentiated endocrine carcinoma – small cell carcinoma, high grade malignant

*<2 cm in size implies close to 100% probability of benign behaviour, >3 cm corresponds to 90% probability of malignancy. Functioning, associated with pertinent clinical syndrome of endocrine hyperfunction; nonfunctioning, not associated with pertinent clinical syndrome, irrespective of hormone detection in blood or tumor tissue.

Table 9
Clinicopathological staging of endocrine tumors of the duodenum and upper jejunum. (Mod. according to [1])

1	Well-differentiated endocrine tumor – carcinoid
1.1	Benign behaviour: nonfunctioning, confined to mucosa-submucosa, ≤1 cm in size, nonangioinvasive
1.1.1	Gastrin-producing tumour (proximal duodenum)
1.1.2	Serotonin-producing tumor
1.1.3	Gangliocytic paraganglioma, any size and extension (ampullary region)
1.2	Uncertain behaviour: confined to mucosa-submucosa >1 cm in size or angioinvasive
1.2.1	Gastrin-producing tumor, functioning (Zollinger-Ellison syndrome) or nonfunctioning, sporadic, or MEN-1-associated
1.2.2	Somatostatin-producing tumor (ampullary region) with or without Recklinghausen disease
1.2.3	Serotonin-producing tumor, nonfunctioning
2	Well-differentiated endocrine carcinoma – malignant carcinoid
2.1	Low grade malignant. extending beyond submucosa or with metastasis
2.2	Gastrin-producing carcinoma, functioning (Zollinger-Ellison syndrome) or nonfunctioning, sporadic, or MEN-1-associated
2.3	Somatostatin-producing carcinoma (ampullary region) with or without Recklinghausen disease
2.4	Serotonin-producing carcinoid, nonfunctioning or functioning (any size or extension) with carcinoid syndrome
2.5	Malignant gangliocytic paraganglioma
3	Poorly differentiated endocrine carcinoma – small cell carcinoma
4	High grade malignant (ampullary region)

Table 8
Clinicopathological staging of endocrine tumors of the stomach. (Mod. according to [1])

1	Well-differentiated endocrine tumor – carcinoid
1.1	ECL-cell carcinoid
1.1.1	ECL-cell carcinoid type I associated with type A gastritis
1.1.2	ECL-cell carcinoid type II associated with Zollinger-Ellison syndrome
1.1.3	Sporadic ECL-cell carcinoid
1.2	ECL-cell carcinoid
1.3	G-cell carcinoid
2	Small cell carcinoma – poorly differentiated endocrine tumor
3	Tumor like lesions: Hyperplasia, Dysplasia

Table 10
Clinicopathological staging of endocrine tumors of the ileum, cecum, colon and rectum. (Mod. according to [1])

1	Well-differentiated tumor – carcinoid
1.1	Benign behaviour: confined to mucosa-submucosa, nonangioinvasive, ≤1 (small int.) or ≤2 cm (large int.) in size
1.2	Uncertain behaviour: nonfunctioning, confined to mucosa-submucosa, >1 cm (small int.) or >2 cm (large int.) in size, or angioinvasive
2	Well-differentiated endocrine carcinoma – malignant carcinoid, low grade malignant, deeply invasive (muscularis propria or beyond), or with metastases
3	Poorly differentiated endocrine carcinoma – small cell carcinoma, high grade malignant
4	Mixed exocrine-endocrine carcinoma – moderate to high grade malignant

Table 11
Clinicopathological staging of endocrine tumors of the appendix. (Mod. according to [1])

1	Well-differentiated endocrine tumor – carcinoid, benign behaviour, nonfunctioning, confined to appendiceal wall, nonangioinvasive, ≤2 cm in size
1.1.1	Serotonin-producing tumor
1.1.2	Enteroglucagon-producing tumor – uncertain behaviour, nonfunctioning, confined to subserosa, >2 cm in size, or angioinvasive tumor
2	Well-differentiated endocrine carcinoma – malignant carcinoid
2.1	Low grade malignant, invading the mesoappendix or beyond, and/or with metastasis
2.2	Serotonin-producing carcinoid with or without carcinoid syndrome
3	Mixed exocrine-endocrine carcinoma
3.1	Low grade malignant – goblet-cell carcinoid

Pathophysiology

Insulinoma cells fail to respond adequately to low blood glucose levels. This is indicative of a defective negative feedback which maintains euglycemia in healthy subjects. In addition, the storage capacity of insulinoma cells is impaired, resulting in an inappropriate insulin release [14].

Symptoms

Insulinoma symptoms are the consequence of neuro-hypoglycemia and superimposed by symptoms which are the consequence of adrenergic counter regulation as sweating, tremulousness, palpitation (Table 12). As a rule, the frequently nonspecific symptoms are associated with fasting and occur more often after muscular exercise and during late night or early morning and when a meal is delayed. Whipple's triad is highly suggestive of an insulinoma and comprises of hypoglycemic symptoms, a parallel demonstration of low blood glucose levels less then 50 mg/dl (2.8 mmmol/l) and improvement of symptoms after administration of glucose [12, 25, 26]. There is often a long-lasting delay between onset of clinical signs and diagnosis, because symptoms listed in table 12 are unspecific and do not appear in a clear sequence. The mean duration of symptoms prior to diagnosis varies between 15 months and more then 3 years [12, 25]. Each patient displays his/her own pattern of symptoms which differ from patient to patient. Since regular food intake prevents the occurrence of symptoms, patients are used to eat regularly and often gain weight. If misinterpreted, severe and longer lasting hypoglycemia can progress to seizure and permanent brain damage. Some insulinoma patients are diagnosed only in psychiatric hospitals, having been admitted with misdiagnosed symptoms.

Differential Diagnosis

In addition to insulinoma hypoglycemia can have several causes which are summarised in table 13. Factitious hypoglycemia secondary to self-administration of insu-

Table 12
Clinical symptoms in patients with insulinoma

Symptoms of neurohypoglycemia	Symptoms of adrenergic cate-cholaminergic response
Diplopia	Anxiety
Blurred vision	Sweating
Confusion	Tremulousness
Abnormal behaviour	Hunger
Weakness	Nausea
Amnesia	Fatique
Aphasia	Tremor
Transient motor defects	Palpitation
Dizziness	
Speech difficulty	
Headache	
Seizure	
Memory loss	
Lethargy	
Disorientation	
Mental change	
Convulsion	
Coma	
Obesity	

Table 13
Other causes of hypoglycemia

Insulin or insulin-like-mediated	Factitious hypoglycemia (153)
	Tumor associated hypoglycemia (151, 152)
	insulin autoantibodies (154)
	Transient hypoglycemia of infancy
	Nesidioblastosis
Postprandial (reactive) hypoglycemia	Previous gastric surgery (Billroth I and II gastrectomy)
	Idiopathic
Food stimulated	Ethanol
	Unripe kakee fruit (159)
Hormone deficiency	Addison's disease
	Growth hormone deficiency
	Hypothyroidism
Hepatic diseases	End-stage liver failure
	Glycogen storage disease
	Glycogen synthetase deficiencies
	Fructose-1,6-disphosphate deficiency
Metabolic diseases	Severe malnutrition
	Sepsis
Drugs	Sufonylureas (155)
	Quinine (156)
	Disopyramide (157)
	Haloperidol (158)

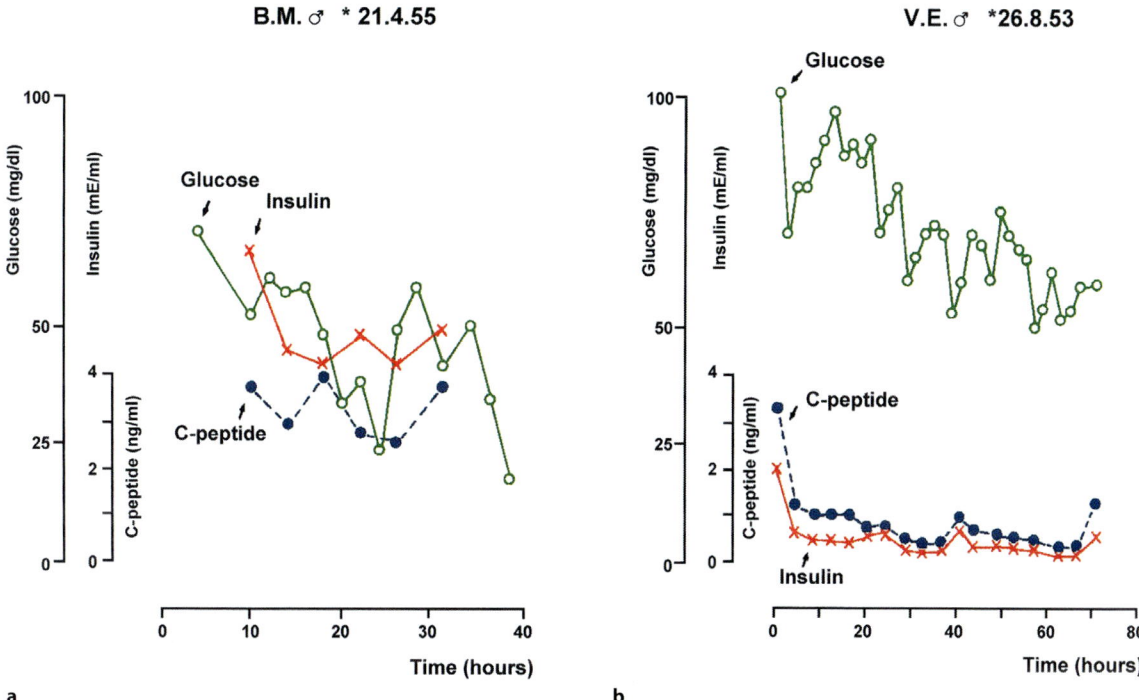

Fig. 5a,b
Blood glucose, insulin and C-peptide levels during a 40 h fast, suggesting an insulin producing tumor since insulin and C-peptide levels remained inadequately elevated despite low blood glucose levels (**a**). In **b** insulin and C-peptide levels dropped down to very low levels during a 72 hour fast

lin or oral intake of hypoglycemic agents should be considered if an insulinoma cannot be ascertained by diagnostic measures. In the author's institution the following conditions are mostly the cause of hypoglycemic episodes if an insulinoma could be excluded: postprandial hypoglycemia (late dumping syndrome) even in the absence of gastric resection (Billroth I and II resection) due to rapid gastric emptying; mesenchymal tumors, such as fibrosarcoma, liposarcoma, rhabdomyosarcoma, hemangiopericytoma, mesothelioma, leiomyosarcoma, IGF-II-producing tumors; endstage of liver cirrhosis.

Diagnosis

Biochemical testing. The gold standard for the diagnosis of an insulinoma is the "72 h fast" test. About 75% of insulinoma patients will develop symptoms and blood glucose levels of <40 mg/dl (2.2 mmol/l) within the first

24 h of the fast (Fig. 5), 90% within 48 h, and 100% within 72 h. The test should be performed using a standardised protocol as follows:

1. begin the test immediately after the last meal (breakfast); insert a capped intervenous cannula;
2. allow intake of calorie-free fluid ad lib (water);
3. encourage physical activity (walking);
4. analyze plasma glucose, insulin and C-peptide in the same specimen every 6 h until blood glucose drops to <60 mg/dl; then increase sampling to every 1–2 h;
5. terminate the test when the patient develops symptoms of hypoglycemia *and* glucose is <40 mg/dl. If the patient is asymptomatic, prolong the test until suggestive symptoms appear; sample always blood glucose, insulin and C-peptide at the end of the test;
6. when symptoms arise, give 10% glucose intravenously or orally until the patient is asymptomatic.

The pathophysiologic background of the prolonged fast test is that steadily decreasing blood glucose levels signal to the normal b-cell of the islets of Langerhans to turn down insulin and C-peptide levels which decrease to either not measurable or very low levels. In insulinoma patients insulin and C-peptide are inadequately suppressed despite even lower blood glucose levels then observed in healthy controls (see Fig. 5). Importantly, plasma insulin in insulinoma patients go rarely beyond levels normally found in the fasted and fed state of normal subjects; however, they are inappropriately high for the prevailing blood glucose concentration. Therefore, plasma insulin and C-peptide levels must always be assessed in relation to the corresponding blood glucose levels. Some authors have advised to calculate a ratio of insulin to glucose because borderline low levels of insulin have been reported in some patients with proven insulinoma in association with hypoglycemia. However, also these ratios do not reliably differentiate between insulinoma patients and healthy subjects since there is not in every subject a linear correlation of insulin and glucose levels. Normal subjects rarely exceed a ratio of plasma insulin (in µU/ml) to glucose (in mg/dl) of 0.3 which is based on the observation that insulin levels are in normals less than 6 µU/ml when blood glucose levels decrease to less than 40 mg/dl. For example: if plasma insulin measures 8 µU/ml and blood glucose is 40 µg/dl, than the ration is 8: 40=0.2. However, neither this ratio or an amended variation of such a ratio do reliably discriminate between insulinoma patients and healthy subjects because there is not in every patient a clear linearity between plasma insulin and glucose levels.

Some experts recommend estimation of proinsulin in insulinoma patients which is elevated in most insulinoma patients to more than 20% of the total plasma insulin levels. Indeed, some insulinomas produce and secrete predominately proinsulin.

In previous literature, various stimulatory and suppressive tests have been recommended because they are believed to facilitate the diagnosis of an insulinoma as C-peptide suppression test, tolbutamide test, glucagon test, calcium infusion test, euglycaemic clamp procedure and others. These tests are neither specific nor sensitive and due to the possibly harmful side effects of prolonged hypoglycemia in case of the tolbutamide and calcium infusion not favoured in the more recent literature.

Figure 6a–f

Localization of endocrine GEP tumors by various imaging techniques. **a** Endoscopic ultrasound showing a small (11 mm) pancreatic insulinoma; **b** CT imaging of desmoplastic reaction in a patient with carcinoid syndrome due to an ileum carcinoid; **c** OctreoScan showing wide metastatic spread in a patient with a non-functioning endocrine pancreatic tumor; **d** MRT imaging of liver metastases in a patient with non-functioning endocrine pancreatic tumor; **e** MRT imaging of two brain metastases in a patient with malignant gastrinoma; **f** endoscopic demonstration of a rectal carcinoid. Notice *yellow colour* ▶

To exclude other causes of hypoglycemia as factitious hypoglycemia or postprandial hypoglycemia measurement of plasma sulfonylurea should be performed to exclude surreptitious use of these drugs and an oral glucose load with estimation of blood glucose and insulin levels in 30 minutes intervals for 3 h should be considered if reactive hypoglycemia is considered.

Localization. Imaging studies to localize an insulinoma should only be performed once the diagnosis of an insulinoma is highly suggestive by biochemical testing. Experienced surgeons claim that the most sensitive localization instrument is the finger of the skilled surgeon during intraoperative abdominal exploration and recommend no preoperative localization procedures. Indeed, almost all insulinomas are situated in the pancreas and only 1–3% found ectopically. On the other side, there is no localization procedure available with an 100% detection rate. At the institution of the authors, 50 patients with biochemically proven insulinoma had undergone operative exploration within the last 10 years and all insulinomas have been identified at the first operation (R. Rothmund, personal communication). These results have been confirmed by some but not all authors. The latter claim that 10–27% of insulinomas remained undetected and advocated, therefore, the need for preoperative localization procedures.

The most accurate and sensitive imaging procedure to localize and to stage (see table 7) an insulinoma is endoscopic ultrasound (EUS) which localizes an insulinoma in up to 85% and thus being superior to other imaging studies as CT, MRT, conventional ultrasound and arteriography (Fig. 6a). Of course, detection rate is mostly dependent on the experience of the investigator and expert investigators will detect tumors less than 0.4 cm in diameter. In such institutions EUS will be the

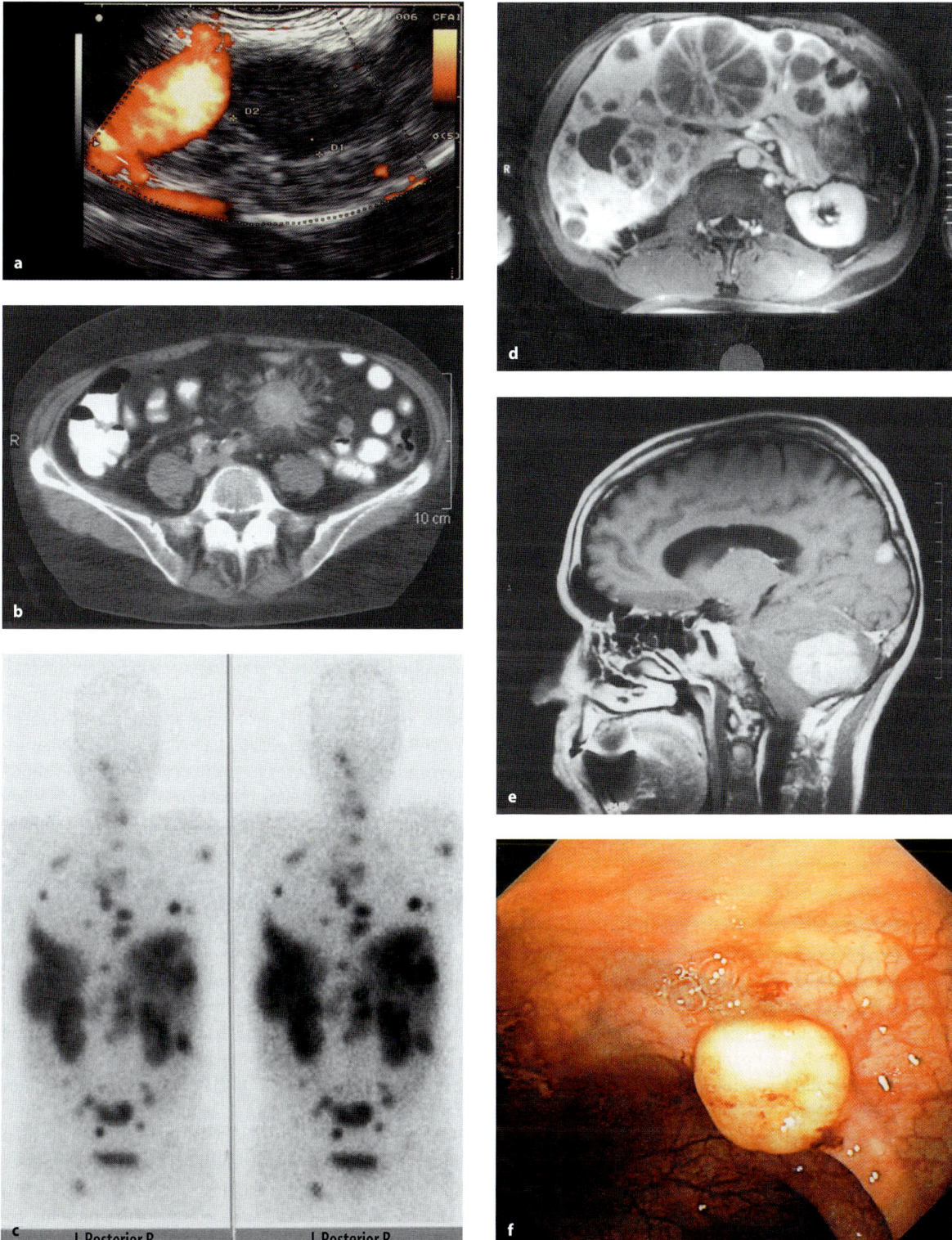

Table 14

Sensitivity of imaging studies in the detection of endocrine GEP tumors

	SRS [%]	CT [%]	MRI [%]	EUS [%]
Gut tumors	72–96%	33%	n.d.	-
Pancreatic tumors	58–100%	25–38%	24–71%	58–86%
Insulinoma	12–50%	29%	13%	81–94%

primary and exclusive diagnostic modality for tumor imaging. Sensitivity of other imaging procedures are summarised in table 14. Angiography was for many years the preferential method in localising insulinomas due to the characteristic high blood supply of the tumor. In earlier reports successful tumor localization of up to 90% has been described whereas more recent data indicated a sensitivity of only 30–50%. The method is invasive, expensive and requires considerable experience in data interpretation. Therefore, both computed tomography (CT) with rapid-sequence spiral CT, with oral and intravenous contrast enhancement and magnetic resonance imaging (MRI) with the use of dynamic gadolinium enhancement and fat suppression have replaced angiography in many centers that prefer an exact preoperative tumor localization. Somatostatin receptor szintigraphy which recognizes high numbers of somatostatin receptors present on most endocrine GEP tumors detects, in contrast to other GEP tumors, only 50% of insulinomas due to the inconsistant frequency of somatostatin receptor subtype 2 on insulinomas. Therefore, negative somatostatin receptor scintigraphy does not exclude the presence of an insulinoma.

Treatment. The primary treatment option in patients with a biochemically proven insulinoma is surgery. Once the tumor is localized pre- and intraoperatively surgeons will decide whether the tumor can be enucleated or whether proximal or distal pancreatic resection is the perferred method. Total pancreatectomy or "blind" distal resection should be avoided if the insulinoma cannot be identified intraoperatively. In this case laparotomy should be terminated and tumor localization repeated. Surgery is also indicated in metastatic insulinoma since operative tumor debulking has been shown to provide long-lasting symptomatic improvement. Symptomatic

antisecretory therapy is indicated in the pre-operative phase and in metastatic disease. To prevent hypoglycemic events regular intake of carbohydrates in required and a light carbohydrate meal in the late evening is important. If diet does not prevent hypoglycemia, oral administration of diazoxide and subcutaneous long-acting somatostatin analogues are the therapeutic priciples of choice to prevent hypoglycemia whereas β-blocking agents, glucocorticoids, calcium-channel blockers and phenytoin have been used earlier but with limited therapeutic effects.

Diazoxide is a non-diuretic benzothiadizine that inhibits the release of insulin from the secretory granules of normal β-cells and of insulinoma cells. Unfortunately, not all insulinoma patients respond to diazoxide but it should be tried with starting dosages of 25 µg b.i.d. and the dose can be escalated up to 200 µg t.i.d. Side effects including cardiac arrhythmia, cardiomyopathy, bone marrow depression, sodium retention and peripheral edema should be noticed and can force to discontinue therapy.

Also long-acting somatostatin analogues (Fig. 7) as octreotide and lanreotide suppress insulin secretion. They have been first introduced for the treatment is disabling acromegaly and later for functionally active endocrine GEP tumors to supress hormone secretion [27]. Octreotide, lanreotide and octreotide LAR are modifications of the naturally occuring somatostatin (Fig. 7). Lanreotide and octreotide-LAR bound to polylactidglycolide microspheres permit sustained release allowing single subcutaneous injections of lancreotide every 2 weeks and of octreotide-LAR every 4 weeks. Somatostatin and its analogs act through a family of at least 5 receptors (sstr 1–5). Most encocrine GEP tumors express sstr 2, whereas the other 4 sstr are less frequently or not expressed (179). Unfortunately, long acting somatostatin analogs are effective in only 50% of insulinoma patients since sstr 2 is only expressed in 50% of insulimas. Therefore, the hypoglycemia preventing effect of somatostatin analogs is unpredictable. Importantly, somatostatin analogs can even aggravate hypoglycemic symptoms because they suppress also the counter regulatory hormone glucagon. Therefore, insulinoma patients must be monitored carefully if somatostatin analogs are considered to prevent hypglycemia. Treatment should be started with 50 µg short-acting octreotide b.i.d. and increased to 200 µg t.i.d. according to the patients re-

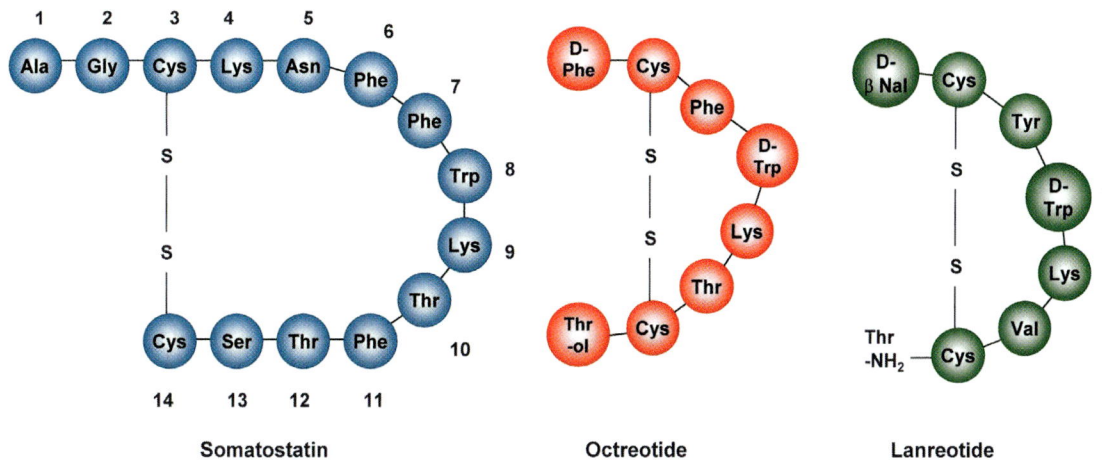

	Somatostatin	Octreotide	Octreotide LAR	Lanreotide	Lanreotide autogel
Dosing	3.5 µg/kg/h i.v.	50-200 µg s.c.	10-30 mg i.m.	30 mg s.c.	60 mg s.c.
Interval	continous	8h	28 days	14-28 days	28 days
Preferential receptors	sstr1-5	sstr2, (sstr5)	sstr2, (sstr5)	sstr2, (sstr5)	sstr2, (sstr5)

Figure 7
Structure and characteristics of native somatostatin and its long-acting analogues octreotide and lanreotide

sponse. If they respond adequately to the short lasting somatostatin formulations, the longer lasting octreotide-LAR and lanreotide-LAR which have to be administered only every 2 weeks (lanreotide-LAR) or every 28 days (octreotide LAR) can be offered.

In patients with malignant and metastatic insulinoma several therapeutic options have to be considered including palliative surgery, embolisation of liver metastases and chemotherapy with streptozotocin combinations (for further details see "General aspect of management" under "Medical treatment of symptoms")

Persistent Neonatal Hyperinsulinemic Hypoglycemia (PNHH).
Persistent neonatal hyperinsulinemic hypoglycemia was earlier called "nesidioblastosis" and originally described by Laidlow in 1938 [28]. He called cells which originated from the pancreatic ductal epithelium nesidioblasts, their proliferation nesidioblastosis and the resulting tumor nesidioblastoma. Today, the term "nesidioblastosis" is substituted by the term "persistent neonatal hyperinsulinemic hypoglycemia (PNHH). This entity is characterized by the occurrence of hyperinsulinemic hypoglycemia in the absence of an endocrine pancreatic tumor. As in insulinomas hypoglycemia occurs in the fasting state and insulin secretion is not adequately suppressed. The disease affects newborn children within the first 6 months of life and only very rarely adults [28]. The term nesidioblastosis is misleading since it implies general islet cell hyperplasia which does not exist. The pancreas of the newborn enfant has physiologically much more and smaller islets of Langerhans compared to the situation in later life. The morphological abnormalities of the endocrine pancreas that underly PNHH are heterogeneous and encompass small endocrine tumors (insulinoma), unifocal or multifocal adenomatosis characterized by local and excessive proliferation of islet

cells, hyperplasia of islets of Langerhans and frequently even no recognizable pathomorphological abnormalities [28]. In the latter situation, a functional defect of the pancreatic β-cells is assumed to cause unrestrained insulin release. PNHH occurs in a sporadic and a familial autosomal recessive form [28]. In the familial variant of PNHH a genetic defect has been identified on the short arm of chromosome 11p14–15.1. The respective gene codes for the sulfonylurea receptor which is mutated in the familial form of PNHH. This mutation results in abnormal insulin secretion and altered sensitivity of the β-cell to glucose. The genetic defect responsible for the sporadic form of PNHH is also identified. A recent report suggests a dysfunction in the adenosine triphosphate-sensitive potassium channel present in the plasma membrane of pancreatic β-cells [29].

Clinically, the respective infants present with nonspecific symptoms resulting from neuroglucopenia. Medical management includes continuous glucose infusion via a central venous catheter, diazoxide and long-acting somatostatin analogs. Recently, it has been demonstrated that calcium channel blocking agents can be used with efficacy and safety to control hypoglycemia in PNHH. However, definitive cure requires in most patients subtotal pancreatectomy.

Adult onset PNHH is very rare and requires the same multimodal therapeutic approach as in the infantile form.

Gastrinoma

Epidemiology and Prognosis

Gastrinomas are as insulinomas very rare tumors. The yearly incidence is 0,5 to 3 per one million population [4, 8]. The mean age at diagnosis is 50 years. Unlike insulinomas, the majority of gastrinomas is malignant. Gastrinomas are in 30–50% part of the MEN-1 syndrome [8]. In a recent study with 151 patients with surgically removed non-metastasised gastrinoma, of whom 128 were part of MEN-1 syndrome, it has been shown that 34% of patients with sporadic gastrinoma but none of patients with MEN-1 syndrome were disease free after 10 years [30]. This demonstrates that in sporadic gastrinoma definitive cure can be achieved in a substantial proportion by surgery. In contrast, patients with gastrinoma as part of MEN-1 syndrome have either multiple gastrinoma or have metastatic disease at operation.

Whereas insulinomas are almost exclusively located in the pancreas and are not located in a special part of the pancreas, the vast majority of gastrinomas occur in the "gastrinoma triangle". This region is defined by the junction of the neck and body of the pancreas, the junction of the second and third part of the duodenum and the confluence of the cystic and common bile duct. 50% of gastrinomas are located in the duodenum. Very rarely, gastrinomas arise in the antrum, omentum, liver, lymph node or elsewhere [8]. In MEN-1 gastrinomas are more frequently located in the duodenum where they are mostly very small and multifocal. Sporadic gastrinomas, in contrast, occur more frequently in the pancreas. The malignant potential of sporadic gastrinomas and those arising in patients with MEN-1 syndrome is not uniform. Recent studies indicate that approximately one fourth of patients with sporadic gastrinomas persue an aggressive growth pattern, with a 10-year survival of 30%, whereas in the remaining 75% of patients gastrinomas display a less aggressive growth pattern with a 10 year survival of 95% [30]. Similarly, in patients with metastatic gastrinomas to the liver aggressive growth was demonstrated only in a minority of patients whereas the majority displayed indolent growth [30]. Tumor related deaths occur almost entirely in the aggressive growth group. According to a recent investigation in patients with gastrinoma and MEN-1 syndrome growth behaviour is also not uniform. 23% of patients with gastrinoma and MEN-1 syndrome developed liver metastases and 14% had an aggressively growing gastrinoma. Aggressive growth of the primary gastrinoma but not of liver metastases growing less aggressively was associated with decreased survival [30]. High serum gastrin levels, a primary tumor size of >3 cm and the presence of bone and liver metastases were associated with an aggressive gastrinoma growth [30].

Pathophysiology

The pathophysiological events occurring in patients with Zollinger-Ellison syndrome are summarized in Fig. 8. Hypergastrinemia as the result of unrestrained hormone release from the tumor displays two effects: stimulation of gastrid acid secretion from the parietal cell and stimulation of parietal and ECL-cells both located in the oxyntic mucosa of the proximal stomach. The consequences of gastric acid hypersecretion are summarized in Fig. 8. All patients with gastrinoma develop diffuse,

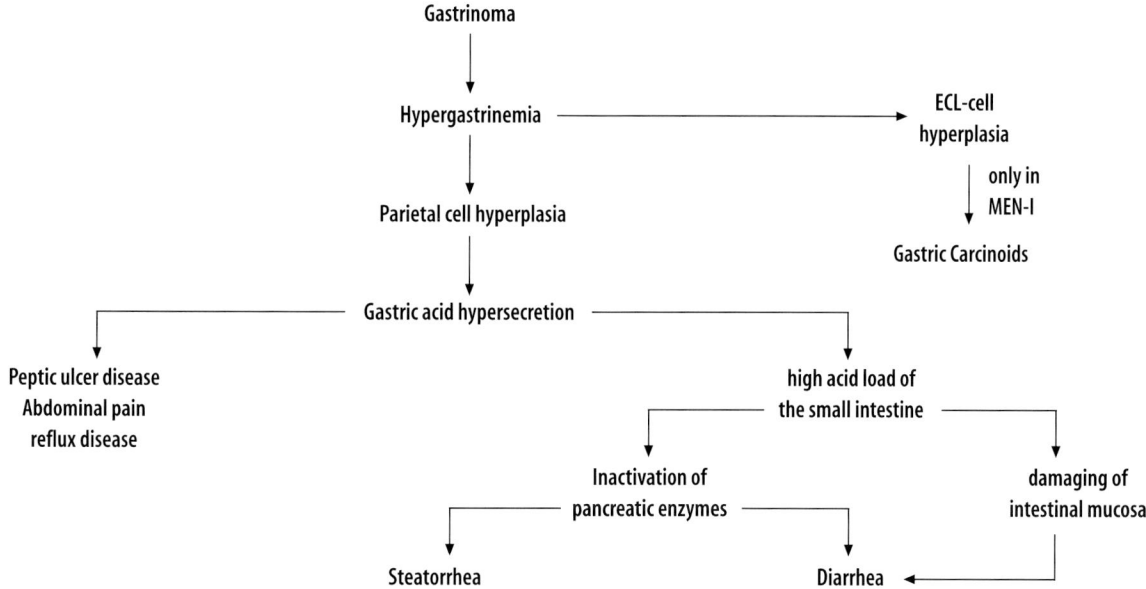

Figure 8
Pathophysiology of Zollinger-Ellison syndrome

linear and micronodular ECL-cell hyperplasia but gastric carcinoids arise almost exclusively in patients with MEN-1 syndrome. This indicates that a genetic trait must be present together with the trophic action of high serum gastrin levels.

Symptoms

Clinical presentation of patients with Zollinger-Ellison syndrome has changed considerably in the last two decades mainly due to the availability of potent antisecretory drugs. Before the discovery of H_2-blockers and proton pump inhibitors patients presented with severe relapsing peptic ulcer disease and its sequelae: lifethreatening bleeding and perforation. Patients died from complications and not from the tumor itself. This has dramatically changed. Most patients with gastrinoma present today with severe and medically resistant reflux disease requiring higher than standard dosages of PPIs. More then 90% of gastrinoma patients suffer from epigastric discomfort and peptic ulcer disease. Most ulcers are situated in the duodenal bulb or the distal stomach, whereas ulcers located in atypical sites (distal to the

duodenal bulb, jejunum) are the exception. 30% of gastrinoma patients have helicobacter pylori infection, but eradication has virtually no influence on peptic ulcer relapse rate. 5–10% of patients do not have peptic ulcer disease and present with secretory diarrhea (Fig. 8). Patients report on watery stools arising during late night and early morning with some improvement after intake of meals. Secretory diarrhea is present in more than 50% of gastrinoma patients. A history of nephrolithiasis and the presence of hypercalcemia are suspicious for hyperparathyroidism as part of MEN-1 syndrome. The association between Zollinger-Ellison syndrome and Cushing's syndrome due to ectopic ACTH production by the endocrine pancreas tumor is rare and patient's survival depends mainly on the control of hypercorticism (see later).

Differential Diagnosis

Differential diagnosis of Zollinger- Ellison syndrome encompass few states of relapsing ulcer disease, hypergastrinemia and gastric acid hypersecretion. Antral G-cell hyperfunction is are rare event and results, ac-

Table 15
Differential diagnosis of hypergastrinemia

With gastric acid hypersecretion	With hypo- or achlorhydria
Antral G-cell hyperfunction	Typ-A gastritis
Massiv resection of small bowel	Renal insufficiency
"excluded antrum"	Prolonged acid-suppressive medication

cording to recent reports, from *H. pylori* infection. In these patients *H. pylori* inhibits antral somatostatin release much more powerfully then in other *H. pylori* infected individuals and leads to hypergastrinemia because antral gastrin producing G- and somatostatin-producing D-cells are situated in close vicinity. After food intake serum gastrin increases in patients with antral G-cell hyperfunction to much higher levels then in patients with normogastrinemic ulcer disease. Cure of infection prevents further peptic ulcer relapse and fasting and postprandial hypergastrinaemia normalize.

The "excluded antrum syndrome" is currently extremely rare and was more frequent in earlier decades when patients with peptic ulcer disease have been subjected to distal gastric resection (Billroth II). In this condition, a small part of the distal antrum adjacent to the duodenal bulb was inadvertently left on the blind loop. Hypergastrinemia results from the neutral environment of this part of antral mucosa and produces acid hypersecretion with the consequence of relapsing ulcer disease in the remaining stomach or around the gastro-jejunal anastomosis.

Diagnosis

Biochemical Testing. The triad: "excessive gastric acid hypersecretion, intractable peptic ulcer disease and the presence of a non-insulin-producing pancreatic endocrine tumor" was recognized as entity in 1955 by Zollinger and Ellison. Biochemically, diagnosis of a Zollinger-Ellison syndrome is based on the simultaneous presence of elevated serum gastrin levels and low intragastric pH. Elevated serum gastrin levels alone do not prove a gastrinoma since it can be found in several conditions mostly as consequence of reduced or absent gastric acid. Examples are the intake of PPIs, the presence of chronic atrophic gastritis (type A gastritis) and severe *H. pylori*

associated chronic gastritis (Table 15). Therefore, diagnosis of Zollinger-Ellison syndrome is easily made if elevated serum gastrin levels combined with gastric acid hypersecretion exists. Since most patients with Zollinger-Ellison syndrome are under long-term PPIs, treatment should be stopped and shorter lasting H_2-blockers offered. Ten days after discontinuation of PPI-treatment basal acid secretion and serum gastrin should be studied after 12 hours withdrawal of H_2-blockers. A serum gastrin level of greater 500 pg/ml in the absence of conditions summarized in table 14 but in the presence of elevated basal acid output (BAO) are highly suggestive of Zollinger-Ellison syndrome. BAO is generally above 10 mEq/hr in an intact stomach and above 5 mEq/hr in patients after Billroth I and II resection. If serum gastrin levels are in the upper normal range or only moderately elevated Zollinger-Ellison syndrome can be confirmed by a secretin provocative test. After intravenous rapid injection of 2 U/kg secretin, serum gastrin rises "paradoxically" within 15 minutes by more then 50% or 200 pg/ml in patients with Zollinger-Ellison syndrome. Blood for gastrin measurement should be taken at times – 5 min and immediately before secretin and after 2, 5, 15 and 30 minutes post secretin. The mechanism of gastrin increase after secretin is not completely understood. There are no other conditions with gastrin increase after secretin. In contrast, hypergastrinemia due to chronic atrophic gastritis or "excluded antrum" declines after secretin (Fig. 9). The sensitivity of the secretin test is below 100% since in some gastrinoma patients no or only small increases of serum gastrin occur.

Localization. During the past decade significant advances in the localization of endocrine GEP tumors could be achieved. Imaging studies in patients with gastrinoma are focused on the detection of the primary (pancreas, duodenum, elsewhere) and to the presence of metastases. As other malignant endocrine tumors malignant gastrinomas tend to metastasize into lymph nodes, liver, bones and other sites as skin and brain. Somatostatin receptor szintigraphy using [111]indium-labelled octreotide (OctreoScan) has changed the imaging strategies of gastrinomas and other endocrine pancreatic tumors since somatostatin subtype 2 (sst_2) receptors have been demonstrated in approximately 90% of gastrinomas using in vitro autoradiography. It could be shown that OctreoScan has a sensitivity of 71–75% and a specificity of up to 82% (see Fig. 7c). According to a recent report in which OctreoScan was compared with conventional imaging procedures in 80 gastrinoma patients, OctreoScan was the most sensitive modality for detection of primary and metastatic gastrinoma. However, size of the primary gastrinoma was an important factor and tumors smaller then 0.5 cm could not be visualized. According to this study 33% of primaries, especially small duodenal gastrinomas that could be detected later intraoperatively, were missed by OctreoScan [8]. Somatostatin receptor szintigraphy and MRI were the most sensitive imaging procedures to detect bone metastases and OctreoScan was the only method to distinguish small liver metastases from small hemangiomas. Therefore, OctreoScan is presently the imaging procedure of choice to localize the primary and to define the extent of metastatic spread. As in insulinomas endoscopic ultrasound is highly accurate in the localization of small pancreatic and duodenal gastrinomas whereas contrast medium enhanced CT and MRT have been shown to have sensitivities of approximately 80–85% [32].

The most important questions which have to be answered are:
▸ Is the biochemically and clinically highly suggestive gastrinoma sporadic or part of the MEN-1 syndrome?
▸ Is the gastrinoma malignant and has spread to lymph nodes, to the liver and elsewhere?
▸ What is the potential benefit of surgical intervention?

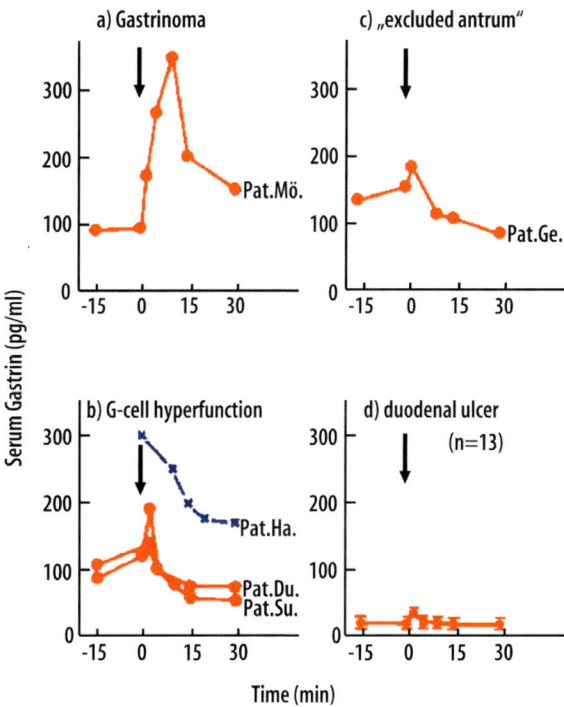

Figure 9a–d

Serum gastrin levels after secretin injection in patients with **a** Zollinger-Ellison syndrome; **b** antral G-cell hyperfunction; **c** patient with "excluded antrum"; **d** patients with regular duodenal ulcer disease

If the size of a gastrinoma is greater then 2 cm in case of a pancreatic tumor (see Table 7) and greater then 1 cm in case of a duodenal tumor (see Table 9) malignant behaviour is likely and the effect of surgical intervention with respect to cure the disease uncertain. In patients with MEN-1 syndrome frequently more then only 1 endocrine pancreatic tumor can be visualized. In this condition it is almost impossible to identify the tumor which is responsible for the Zollinger-Ellison syndrome.

For practical reasons one should always start with OctreoScan. If the primary as well as metastatic spread have been detected by OctreoScan the findings should be further confirmed by contrast-medium enhanced CT or MRT (see Fig. 7e). If a solitary gastrinoma, no primary and no metastases are found by OctreoScan and upper abdominal CT and/or MRT careful upper gastroduodenoscopy should be performed to confirm the presence of a duodenal primary. Endoscopic ultrasound should complete endoscopy. In case of a solitary primary

and if no primary and no metastases exist laparotomy is indicated to localize and to remove the primary tumor within the "gastrinoma triangle".

Treatment. The sequelae of gastric acid hypersecretion as reflux disease, peptic ulceration and watery diarrhea can be effectively controlled by proton pump inhibitors (PPI). They have completely substituted surgical procedures as total gastrectomy and vagotomy. They are superior to all available histamin-H_2-blockers. For all currently available PPIs a comparable therapeutic efficacy and safety has been demonstrated. However, the exact dosage necessary for symptomatic control and for inhibition of gastric acid secretion has to be determined for every individual patient. The dosage can range from normal and 3–4 times elevated dosages. One should start with the regular PPI dose bid (2×20 mg Omeprazole; 2×30 mg Lanzoprazole; 2×40 mg Pantoprazole; 2×40 mg Rabeprazole etc.) and increase the dosage until patients are symptom-free and BAO decreased to less then 5 mEq/hr in patients with intact stomach. BAO should be studied prior to the next scheduled dose. If BAO is around 0 mEq/hr PPI dosage should be reduced if desired.

There is no place for long-acting somatostatin analogs which have to be administered subcutaneously and which do not control acid secretion as reliably as PPIs.

In case of a sporadic non-metastasized gastrinoma, surgical removal should always be desired [31]. In patients with a gastrinoma as part of MEN-1 syndrome available data do not indicate whether removal of the primary has an survival advantage for the patient. In addition it is difficult to define which of several pancreatic tumors is the tumor responsible for the Zollinger-Ellison syndrome. Therefore, laparotomy in Zollinger-Ellison syndrome and MEN-1 syndrome is a controversial issue.

For management of metastatic disease see under "General aspect of management".

Glucagonoma

Definition, Epidemiology and Prognosis

Glucagonomas are endocrine pancreatic tumors that contain predominantly glucagon. However, only some of these tumors secrete excessive amounts of glucagon into the circulation and cause the glucagonoma syndrome. The latter tumors are malignant, sized 5 cm in diameter and even larger, frequently solitary but they can spread to the liver, lymphnodes, bone and other sites. Most glucagonomas, especially small tumors found in most patients with MEN-1 syndrome are non-functioning and not associated with a clinical syndrome. Their malignant potential is small.

All glucagonomas whether functionally inactive or active encompass less then 1% of all endocrine tumors of the GEP system. Whereas functionally inactive small and benign glucagonomas are found not only in patients with MEN-1 syndrome but even by chance at autopsy the glucagonoma syndrome is rare if compared with insulinoma and gastrinoma.

The prognosis of small functionally inactive glucagonomas is likely favourable whereas in the malignant variant as cause of the glucagonoma syndrome prognosis depends on the aggressiveness of tumor growth and the response to antiproliferative measures.

Pathophysiology

Elevated glucagon levels have metabolic consequences which explain some but not all clinical features in patients with glucagonoma syndrome. Weight loss results from the catabolic effects of glucagon and from a recently described anorectic substance found in animals with transplantable glucagonoma. Glucagon stimulates glycogenolysis and gluconeogenesis leading to impaired glucose tolerance and diabetes mellitus as found in most Patients with glucagonoma syndrome. Since exogenous administration of glucagon decreases erythropoiesis in animals anemia which is frequently observed in these patients can be attributed to glucagon hypersecretion. However, the role of hyperglucagonemia in the pathogenesis of thromboembolic complications including pulmonary embolism is poorly understood. The necrolytic migratory erythema (Fig. 10) is believed to be related to hypoaminoacidemia present in most but not all patients and not the consequence of hyperglucagonemia. Skin lesions disappear despite high glucagon levels if plasma amino acid levels normalize. They are similar to those observed in patients with zink deficiency and zink suplementation has been shown to improve skin lesions in some patients as well. According to the authors experience skin lesions can disappear after resection of the primary without normalization of hyperglycagonemia and hypoaminoacidemia due to metastases to the liver suggesting a still undetected substance released by the tumor as cause of the necrolytic migratory erythema.

Symptoms

Main symptoms in patients with glucagonoma syndrome are skin lesions, diabetes mellitus, weight loss and anorexia present in up to 90% of patients with glucagonoma syndrome. Less frequently normochromic and normocytic anemia, venous thrombosis and pulmonary embolism occur. Diarrhea and steathorhea are present in 14% of patients. Their etiology is unclear. Rare clinical features include, in addition, psychiatric disturbances including depression and complex neurologic symptoms with dementia and optic atrophy, possible related to protein hypercatabolism that can recover after treatment with long-acting somatostatin analogs.

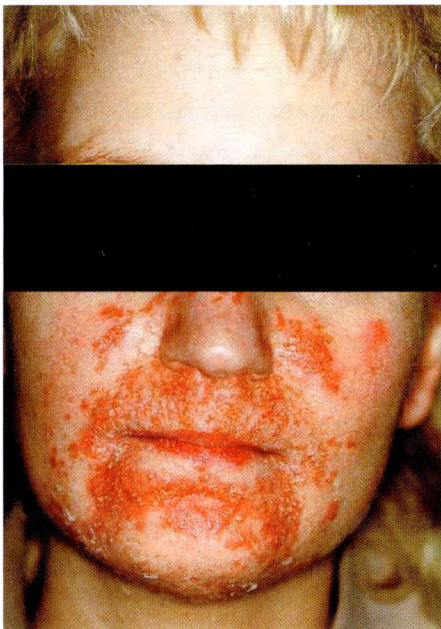
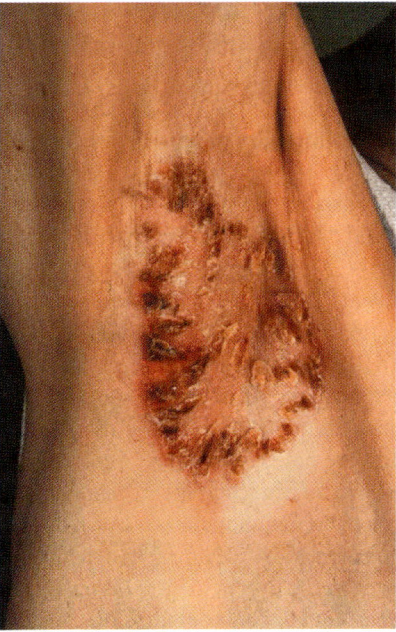

Figure 10
Necrolytic migratory erythema
in two patients with glucagonoma
syndrome

The necrolytic migratory erythema is one of the most impressive clinical symptoms in patients with glucagonoma syndrome. Skin lesions involve the lower abdomen, groin perineum, face, armpits (Fig. 10) and distal extremities. They start with an erythematous lesion which becomes papular. The erythema spreads peripherally and becomes raised with superficial central blistering. Lesions begin to heal in the center with a raised erythematous ring. Healing is followed by hyperpigmentation. The sequence of skin manifestations take 1–2 weeks while new lesions appear elsewhere. Skin lesions frequently precede the diagnosis of the syndrome for many years and are misdiagnosed as acrodermatitis enteropathica, psoriasis, contact dermatitis and other skin disorders.

Diagnosis

Diagnosis is based on the presence of a mostly large pancreatic tumor with and without metastases to the liver or elsewhere, clinical symptoms described in detail in "Symptoms" and the demonstration of high plasma glucagon levels. Total plasma aminoacids should be determined and support the diagnosis if they are markedly decreased. In most patients the pancreatic tumor can be visualized by conventional US. Fine-needle biopsy proves the endocrine nature of the tumor. Somatostatin receptor szintigraphy, CT and MRT imaging are helpful in evaluating tumor burden outside the pancreas [32].

Treatment

Surgical removal of the primary and of resectable liver metastases should always be considered because tumor debulking has been shown to have a favourable effect on clinical symptoms including skin lesions.

Medically, long-acting somatostatin analogs have been shown to be currently the medical principle of choice in the control of skin lesions, to improve symptoms as weight loss, anemia and diarrhea. Most studies recommend 200–600 µg per day or 10–20 mg octreotide-LAR every 28 days. Unfortunately, long-acting somatostatin analogs are not effective in up to 50% of patients. In these individuals debulking operation, embolization of liver metastases and chemotherapy with streptozotocin combinations or dacarbazine should be considered. For details see "General aspect of management".

Verner-Morrison Syndrome (VIPoma)

Epidemiology and Prognosis

An endocrine tumor mostly located within the pancreas and responsible for a syndrome characterized by extreme watery diarrhea, hypochlohydria and hypokalemia was first discribed by Priest and Alexander in 1957 and by Verner and Morrison in 1958. Alternative acronyms are "Verner-Morrison syndrome", "VIPoma" (due to the hormone vasoactive intestinal polypeptide responsible for the diarrhea), "WDHH (watery diarrhea, hypokalemia, hypochlorhydria) syndrome" and "Pancreatic Cholera". In adults VIPomas are mostly located in the pancreas and rarely outside the pancreas in the retroperitoneum, liver, small intestine and bronchial system. In children, a ganglioneuroma or an ganglioneuroblastoma can cause a VIPoma syndrome. Most VIPomas are malignant and have metastasized to the liver at diagnosis. VIPomas are as glucagonomas, somatostatinomas and endocrine pancreatic tumors with ectopic hormone production very rare. Prognosis of this malignant tumor was prior to the availability of long-acting somatostatin analogues unfavourable and patients died from the consequences of excessive watery diarrhea as dehydratation and pulmonary embolism. Presently, prognosis depends on the aggressiveness of tumor growth which differs between VIPomas and their responsiveness to chemotherapy.

Pathophysiology

Although VIPomas produce frequently several hormones as Peptide Histidine-Methionine-28 (PHM-27), secretin, pancreatic polypeptide and prostaglandines, vasoactive intestinal polypeptide (VIP) which is elevated in all patients with Verner-Morrison syndrome is the cause of watery diarrhea and electrolyte disturbances. VIP induces massive small intestinal net secretion of water and ions, especially potassium with an inconsistent effect on water absorption in the colon. If VIP is infused intravenously in healthy individuals in amounts reflecting circulating VIP-levels in patients with Verner-Morrison syndrome, subjects develop massive secretory diarrhea, hypokalemia and hypochloremic metabolic acidosis. VIP reduces water and sodium absorption

from the colon and induces potassium secretion, thus explaining hypokalemia which may induce secondary hypoaldosteronism. In addition, VIP inhibits gastric acid secretion. Fluid secretion from the small intestine is attributed to activation of adenylate cyclase and cyclic adenosine monophosphate in intestinal cells. Some patients develop hypercalcemia which is attributed to the stimulation of bone osteolytic activity by VIP.

Symptoms

Patients with Verner-Morrison syndrome present with excessive watery diarrhea up to 5–10 L per day. Chronic diarrhea is a constant feature in 50% of patients but may be intermittent in others. Diarrhea decreases only slightly during fasting or exclusive parenteral nutrition proving its secretory nature. Untreated diarrhea leads to dehydration, weight loss, hypkalemia and hypomagnesemia resulting in paresthesia, muscle weakness and cardiac arrhythmia. Before the availability of long-acting somatostatin analogs patients died from the consequences of dehydration and electrolyte loss as cardiac arrhythmia and pulmonary embolism. 25% of patients report flushing episodes.

Differential Diagnosis

Secretory diarrhea of other origin as diarrhea in patients with Zollinger-Ellison syndrome, carcinoid syndrome, medullary carcinoma of the thyroid is mostly less pronounced compared to diarrhea in VIPoma patients. A stool volume of less then 700 ml per day excludes a VIPoma and is suggestive for other causes of secretory diarrhea. The most important differential diagnosis is laxative abuse and Münchhausen's syndrome. Repeatedly normal VIP-levels should induce search for laxatives in stool and urine.

Diagnosis

The combination of excessive watery diarrhea, hypokalemia and elevated plasma VIP-levels together with a pancreatic mass visualized by conventional US or CT/MRT imaging are highly suggestive for a VIPoma. The endocrine nature of the tumor can be ascertained by fine needle biopsy.

Treatment

Surgical intervention should always be considered if the primary is resectable and liver metastases could be removed with tenable risk for the patients. Medical therapy and patient's prognosis have been dramatically changed through the currently available long-acting somatostatin analogs. They substituted a number of drugs tried earlier to control diarrhea as loperamide, prednisone, clonidine, phenothiazines, indomethacin, lithium and others. Octreotide is in most patients effective and doses of 200–600 µg per day in two to three single injections are recommended. If the short lasting formulations are effective, long-acting depot formulations as octreotide-LAR 20 mg every 28 days can be offered. Unfortunately, some patients escape from treatment with long-acting somatostatin analogs after an initial longer lasting response. The mechanisms behind tachyphylaxis and/or desensitisation are not completely understood. Treatment should be terminated and started again after few weeks.

Somatostatinoma

Epidemilogy and Prognosis

Somatostatinoma is an endocrine tumor containing somatostatin as shown by immunihistology and arises either in the pancreas or in the duodenum where it is located close to the ampulla vateri. Most duodenal somatostatinomas are solitary and small (<1,5 cm) whereas pancreatic somatostatinomas tend to be larger. Malignancy rate in large tumors is 50–90% and metastases to liver, lymph nodes and bones have been described. According to table 9 duodenal somatostatinomas tend to metastasize if they are larger then 2 cm.

Approximately 90% of these tumors are functionally inactive and only 10% are cause of the somatostatinoma syndrome. Non-functional somatostatinomas located in the region of ampulla vateri are associated with von Recklinghausen's disease. Small pancreatic somatostatinomas of the pancreas can be part of MEN-1 syndrome. Prognosis of somatostatinomas seems to be favourable in small, non-metastasized tumors. In larger tumors it depends on the aggressiveness of tumor growth.

Pathophysiology

Somatostatin inhibits the release of gastrointestinal hormones as CCK and gastrin, inhibits basal and simulated gastric acid secretion and stimulated pancreatic secretion and inhibits the absorption of food constituents from the intestine. Through inhibition of CCK release somatostatin inhibits gallbladder emptying. Inhibition of pancreatic secretion is believed to cause diarrhea and steatorrhea in the somatostatinoma syndrome. Since somatostatin inhibits insulin release impaired glucose tolerance is a frequent finding in patients with somatostatinoma syndrome.

Symptoms

Leading symptoms in patients with somatostatinoma syndrome are cholecystolithiasis, diabetes mellitus, diarrhea and steatorrhea, hypochlorhydria and as a consequence of a tumor situated close to the ampulla vateri obstructive jaundice. However, the reported symptoms are rarely present in all patients with somatostatinoma syndrome. Other symptoms are epigastric pain, weight loss and nausea.

Since symptoms in patients with somatostatinoma syndrome can arise although in other conditions as cholecystolithiasis, diabetes mellitus and diarrhea and steatorrhea some authors question the existence of this entity.

Treatment

Medical treatment should be directed to correct symptoms associated with cholecystolthiasis, diabetes mellitus and diarrhea. Few observations suggest that diarrhea and diabetes mellitus can improve by exogenous somatostatin. But this suggestion is clearly experimental. Surgery should considered to be reduce tumor burden.

Tumors with Ectopic Hormone Production

Epidemiology, Classification and Prognosis

Most benign and malignant endocrine GEP tumors produce more then one hormone within the same tumor. Insulinomas contain next to insulin frequently somatostatin-producing and glucagon-producing cells, gastrinomas additional pancreatic-polypeptide-, insulin- and somatostatin-producing cells (see Fig. 2). As a rule the additional hormones are not released into the circulation and do not produce hormone-mediated symptoms. In patients with MEN-1 syndrome, however, two clinical syndromes from two independent pancreatic or one pancreatic and one duodenal endocrine tumor can arise, mostly the combination of a gastrin-producing tumor situated in the duodenal bulb with the clinical symptoms of Zollinger-Ellison syndrome and a pancreatic functionally active insulinoma. In the latter condition additional endocrine pancreatic tumors exist, mostly glucagonomas and somatostatinomas which are functionally inactive.

Apart from tumors producing multiple hormones regularly synthetized in the normal islets of Langerhans of adults (insulin, glucagon, pancreatic polypeptide, somatostatin) or during fetal life (gastrin) (eutopic hormone production) endocrine pancreatic tumors can produce hormones uncommon for the endocrine pancreas (ectopic hormone production) as growth hormone-releasing factor (GRF), ACTH or corticotropin-releasing factor (CRF) and parathyroid hormone-related peptide (PTH-RP) or an unknown hypercalcemic substence mimicking the action of PTH. These tumors are mostly malignant and very rare. In addition, few patients with neurotensin-producing tumors have been described. Tumor prognosis depends on the aggressiveness of tumor growth and the success of antiproliferative measures.

Clinical Symptoms, Pathophysiology and Diagnosis

GRFoma. The association of acromegaly with endocrine bronchial, intestinal and pancreatic tumors is rare and approximately 150 patients with this syndrome have been described. Pancreatic GRFomas are mostly large but multiple GRFomas have also been reported. They are part of MEN-1 syndrome. Different from pituitary adenoma GRFomas arise 3 times more frequent in females then in males. They can be associated with other endocrine syndromes as gastrinoma, insulinoma, Cushing's syndrome and pheochromocytoma. In 30–40% metastatic disease which spreads mostly to the liver is present.

Clinically, patients present with characteristic signs indistinguishable from pituitary derived acromegaly with elevated GH and IGF-1 levels. If GRFomas are associated with other endocrine functionally active tumors, symptoms of acromegaly could be blurred by hypoglycemia resulting from an insulinoma etc.

Treatment includes surgical resection of the primary and debulking procedures and, medically, the suppression GRF levels by long-acting somatostatin analogs.

ACTH-Producing Tumors. According to a recent report from the Mayo Clinic in 106 patients ectopic ACTH or CRF production results in 25% from bronchial carcinoids, 16% from malignant islet cell tumors, 16% from medullary thyroid carcinoma, 11% from small cell carcinoma of the lung, 7% from disseminated neuroendocrine tumors with unknown primary source, 5% from thymic carcinoids and 3% from pheochromocytoma. Whereas in MEN-1 syndrome Cushing's disease results from a pituitary adenoma ectopic ACTH-production in the case of an islet cell tumor has been found mostly in sporadic gastrinomas. In the latter condition the gastrinoma is metastatic and the prognosis poor.

In a recent prospective study Cushing's syndrome in patients with Zollinger-Ellison syndrome due to a solitary malignant gastrinoma was an independent predictor for poor survival. Patients with ectopic ACTH syndrome differ from those with pituitary adenoma because they present with muscle waisting and weight loss which is more frequently observed then the classic features of Cusing's syndrome.

Possibly, symptom differences in patients with ectopic and eutopic ACTH-production result from a different processing of pro-piomelanocortin with the release of high amounts of ACTH precursors and less intact ACTH in the circulation in patients with ectopic hormone production. However, symptoms may overlap those seen in pituitary dependent Cushing's disease. Ectopic ACTH-producing endocrine tumors are more resistant to chemotherapy and the severe hypercortisolism is responsible for a high rate of life-threatening complications.

Treatment is frequently difficult since only few tumors respond to long-acting somatostatin analogs. If ketoconazoles, animogluthetimide or mifepristone do not control hypercortisolism and curative or palliative resection of the primary tumor and its metastases is not possible, patients are likely to benefit from bilateral adrenalectomy. For additional antiproliferative measures see "general aspects of management" (below).

PTH-RP-Producing Tumors. Few endocrine pancreatic tumors present with hypercalcemia and secret parathyroid hormone-related peptide (PTH-RP) or not identified hypercalcemic substances mimicking the action PTH. According to a recent review of 19 patients common features were hypercalcemia, normal or low PTH levels associated with extremely vascular, large and usually malignant tumors (17 of 18) displaing positive stains for PTH-RP. Some patients respond favourably to long-acting somatostatin analogs and to streptozotocin combinations if tumor resection is not possible.

Nonfunctioning Endocrine Pancreatic Tumors

Epidemiology, Classification and Prognosis

Nonfunctioning endocrine pancreatic tumors can be subdivided into benign and small tumors as part of the MEN-1 syndrome and large, malignant tumors which mostly spread into lymph nodes, liver, bones, and elsewhere. The latter can or cannot secret hormonal products into the circulation. Pancreatic polypeptide or neurotensin are released by some tumors but do not produce a clinical syndrome. Other functionally inactive tumors do not secret any products with hormonal activity. However, they release chromogranin A, a constituent of the secretory machinery of endocrine cells. Exact incidence rates for malignant non-functioning tumors are missing but according to own experiences they are at least as frequent as all functionally active endocrine pancreatic tumor together. By histology and immunohistology functioning PETs cannot be distinguished from nonfunctioning tumors.

Clinically, tumors and their metastases are either found incidentally at routine abdominal check-up, by the patient itself who realizes the presence of an upper abdominal mass or by obstructive jaundice due to a pancreatic head tumor. Most patients report no or only little upper abdominal discomfort and few present with more severe abdominal pain and weight loss. Frequently, tumors are misdiagnosed as endocrine pancreatic carcinomas but the unrestricted life quality of patients and hypervascular lesions identified by imaging procedures lead the correct diagnosis. Other patients present during routine US investigations with cystic liver lesions misdiagnosed as benign liver cysts. Prognosis of patients with non-functioning malignant tumors depends on the aggressiveness of tumor growth which can vary considerably from exploding tumor growth to long intervals of stable disease even in the absence of any treatment.

Diagnosis

The correct diagnosis requires histology which can mostly be obtained by ultrasound or CT-guided fine-needle biopsy. If the endocrine nature of the primary tumor or of its metastases is ascertained, OctreoScan should be performed to identify tumor load and the presence of distant metastases as in bones. If the primary is not identified within the pancreas upper and lower endoscopy and careful CT/MRT examinations of the chest should be performed to localize the primary within the fore-, mid- and hindgut (Fig. 6d). Because tumors do not produce a hormone-mediated syndrome, expensive hormone analyses are not helpful and should be avoided. However, chromogranine A should be estimated which is elevated in most metastatic tumors and serves as tumor marker. Some tumors produce, in addition, pancreatic polypeptide which serves as tumor marker as well.

Treatment

Treatment should follow the principles of other endocrine pancreatic malignancies. If resectable, non-metastatic primaries should be removed either by Whipple's procedure or partial pancreatectomy. In metastatic diseases several antiproliferative measures are available which are summarized under "general aspect of management".

Endocrine Tumors of the Stomach and Gut

Gastric Carcinoids

Epidemiology, Classification. Endocrine tumors of the stomach are nonfunctioning. As shown in table 8 there are 4 types of tumors:
▸ ECL-cell carcinoids;
▸ EC-cell carcinoids;
▸ Gastrin-cell tumors;
▸ poorly differentiated or small cell endocrine carcinomas [9, 10].

With the exception of the latter tumor most endocrine tumors of the stomach are well differentiated. Gastric carcinoids have been reported to occur with an incidence of 0,002–0,1 per 100.000 population per year and account for 11–41% of all gastrointestinal carcinoids from the esophagus to the rectum. The most frequent endocrine tumors of the stomach are gastric ECL-cell carcinoids representing 74% of gastric endocrine tumors and occuring more frequently in females. The mean age of detection is 63 years. Small cell undifferentiated carcinomas represent 6% of endocrine tumors of the stomach. EC-cell and Gastrin-cell carcinoids are extremely rare.

ECL-Cell Carcinoids. *Clinical and histopathological aspects and prognosis:* ECL-cell carcinoids can be subdivided into three entities:

▶ type I ECL-cell carcinoids are associated with type A-gastritis (autoimmune chronic atrophic gastritis) present in the oxyntic and fundic part of the gastric mucosa. Due to the loss of parietal cells type I ECL-cell carcinoids are always associated with achlorhydria and – as a consequence of achlorhydria – with massive hypergastrinemia of antral origin achieving levels comparable to that observed in Zollinger-Ellison syndrome. Carcinoids in type A-gastritis are usually small and multiple.

▶ type II ECL-cell carcinoids arise in patients with hypergastrinemia due to a Zollinger-Ellison syndrome, mostly as part of MEN-1 syndrome. In contrast to type I carcinoids oxyntic mucosa is hyperplastic due to the trophic action of gastrin but without any atrophic changes.

▶ type III (sporadic) ECL-cell carcinoids are neither associated with type- A atrophic gastritis although gastritis is present nor with hypergastrinemia. They arise in areas without ECL-cell hyperplasia which is a prerequisite for the formation of type-I and type-II ECL-cell carcinoids. Clinically, type III tumors present with relatively large (1–3 cm) tumors that are usually aggressive with local invasion and the formation of metastases to adjacent lymphnodes and the liver. They are mostly non-functioning but can be the source of gastric hemorrhage and obstruction. In rare cases they can be associated with an atypical carcinoid syndrome with red long-lasting flushing episodes but without diarrhea. These tumors secrete histamine and 5-hydroxytryptophane.

ECL-cell carcinoids arise from ECL-cells that are physiologically present in the oxyntic and fundic mucosa and contain histamine which stimulates gastric acid secretion via specific receptors on the parietal cells. They can proliferate by two mechanisms: both chronic atrophic gastritis and the trophic action of hypergastrinemia lead to ECL-cell hyperplasia which can further proliferate to type I ECL-cell carcinoids. Histologically ECL-cell hyperplasia consists of linear, diffuse, micronodular and adenomatoid ECL-cell hyperplasia (Fig. 11). The next step in tumor formation is dysplasia with enlarging and fusing micronodules, microinvasion and newly formed stroma. Nodules greater than 0.5 mm and invading into submucosa are called carcinoids. Smaller and multiple

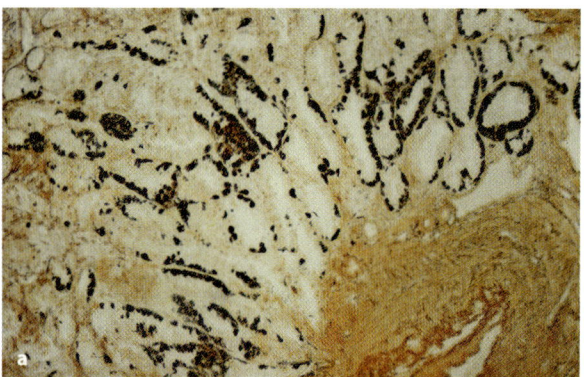
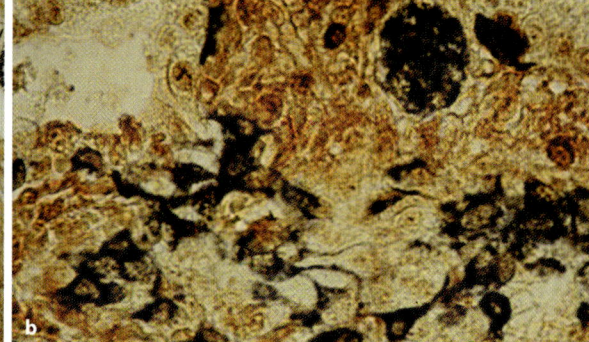

Figure 11
Histology of ECL-cell hyperplasia

nodules together with linear and diffuse ECL-cell hyperplasia a constituents of microcarcinoidosis. All these events are found in type A chronic atrophic gastritis and the ultimate step is the formation of type I carcinoids.

An identical spectrum of ECL-cell growth from ECL-cell hyperplasia to carcinoid formation is present in gastrinoma patients as part of MEN-1 syndrome. In contrast, sporadic gastrinoma patients develop ECL-cell hyperplasia but likely not ECL-cell carcinoids. This indicates the importance of a genetic trait (MEN-1) essential for the formation of type II carcinoids or the presence of severe atrophic gastritis as prerequisit for type I carcinoid formation through the trophic action of hypergastrinemia present in both.

Prognosis of type I and II ECL-cell carcinoids is excellent and favourable prognostic factors are: tumors confined to mucosa and submucosa, size <1 cm, low mitotic activity (Ki-67) and lack of angioinvasiveness. In contrast, angioinvasion, a size >1 cm, invasion of muscularis propria and beyond and high mitotic activity indicate a more aggressive behaviour. Metastatic spread into lymph nodes and to the liver is rare (5% rsp. 2.5% in type-I carcinoids) and slightly greater in type-II carcinoids.

Treatment: ECL-cell carcinoids (type I) in type-A chronic atrophic gastritis are mostly small and should be endoscopically excised. Yearly controls are recommended for further surveillance. If carcinoids are larger than 1 cm endoscopic US should estimate whether or not invasion of muscularis propria is present. In case of invasion local surgical excision is recommended. No agreement exists between experts whether or not antrectomy should be offered to remove the gastrin source as the trophic principle responsible for carcinoid formation.

Type II ECL-cell carcinoids should be handled as type I tumors but patients' prognosis depends mostly on the aggressiveness of underlying Zollinger-Ellison and MEN-I syndrome.

Type III ECL-cell tumors (sporadic carcinoids) should be removed according to the principles for non-endocrine gastric adenocarcinomas. No proven strategy exists if metastatic spread occurred. Tumors are mostly insensitive to available chemotherapeutic strategies.

EC-Cell Carcinoid. EC-cell carcinoids are very rare and always malignant. They present with rapid growth and are functionally inactive.

Gastrin-Cell Tumor. These very rare tumors are mostly well differentiated and small. They are found incidentally at endoscopy as small muscosal/submucosal nodules. They can and can't present with Zollinger-Ellison syndrome.

Small Cell Carcinoma (Poorly Differentiated Endocrine Neoplasm). These very rare tumors display exploding tumor growth similar to small cell carcinomas of the lung and of other origin.

Endocrine Tumors of the Duodenum and Proximal Jejunum

Epidemiology, Classification and Prognosis

Duodenal carcinoids account to 22% of all gastrointestinal carcinoids (see Table 9). In contrast, jejunal carcinoids are very rare. Most endocrine tumors of the duodenum are gastrinomas which in 7–21% are part of MEN-1 syndrome. Not all gastrinomas are cause for a Zollinger-Ellison syndrome and present as non-functional tumors. Gastrinomas can arise at multiple sites (15%) and are mostly small (<1 cm). Non-functioning gastrinomas have a more favourable prognosis as tumors associated with Zollinger-Ellison syndrome that have a higher incidence of metastases. However, compared to pancreatic gastrinomas duodenal gastrinomas have significantly less frequent metastases to the liver (5% versus 52%). Ten years survival of patients with duodenal gastrinoma is significantly better then those of pancreatic origin (59% versus 9%).

Somatostatinomas account for 21% of endocrine tumors in the upper small intestine and are located at, or very close to, the ampulla of vater. They are larger as gastrinomas (>2 cm) and can cause obstructive jaundice, pancreatitis and intestinal obstruction. Histologically, tumors contain characteristic concentrically laminated psammoma bodies. They are mostly malignant, with local invasion into surrounding tissues (sphincter of Oddi, head of the pancreas) and spread into paraduodenal lymph nodes and to the liver. Duodenal somatostatinomas are mostly non-functioning and genetically associated with neurofibromatosis von Recklinghausen.

Gangliocytic paragangliomas are very rare events characterized by an admixture of three cell types: spindle cells, epithelial cells and ganglionic cells. The spindle cells are neural in nature. They are usually benign but can be larger then 2 cm in size.

Treatment

Duodenal gastrinomas should be surgically removed either by local excision or Whipple's procedure. In cased of metastatic spread surgery should be avoided. The place of radical surgery in patients with duodenal and/or pancreatic endocrine tumors as part of MEN-1 syndrome is controversial even between experienced surgeons. Somatostatinomas and gangliocytic paragangliomas should be resected if possible. In case of metastatic spread, see "General aspect of management" under "Control of tumor growth in malignant and metastatic tumors".

Endocrine Tumors of the Distal Small Intestine (Jejunum, Ileum)

Epidemiology, Classification and Prognosis

The incidence of carcinoids arising in the distal small bowel has been reported to be 0,28–0,89 per 100.000 population and year. Most gastrointestinal carcinoids are localized in this area (see Table 10). Carcinoids of this site have been observed in equal proportion in males and females with and age peak in the 6th and 7th decade. Histologically, tumors are EC (enterochromaffine)- cell carcinoids containing serotonin. A minority of carcinoids consists of glucagon-like peptides- or pancreatic polypeptide- and peptide YY producing cells. EC-cell carcinoids can be multiple and are in 15% associated with other malignancies as gastrointestinal adenocarcinoma, breast cancer and others. The majority of tumors is located in the distal ileum close to the ileocecal valve. Only 5–7% of EC-cell carcinoids are functionally active and cause of the carcinoid syndrome. The primary is mostly situated in the ileum. Despite most EC-cell carcinoids are functionally inactive patients present with intermittent lower abdominal cramps due to incomplete intestinal obstruction and desmoplastic reaction of the mesenterium. Occasionally, small ileal carcinoids are incidentally detected during routine colonoscopy.

Prognosis of carcinoids arising in the distal jejunum and ileum is generally unfavourable if compared to that for duodenal, gastric (ECL-cell carcinoids) and rectal carcinoids since endocrine tumors arising in the distal small intestine frequently lead to metastases. 10 year survival is approximately 43% and more favourable if the primary tumor is removed and liver metastases absent. Therefore, patients with even small ileal carcinoids found incidentally during routine colonoscopy should be recommended right-sided hemicolectomy since metastatic spread into regional lymph nodes occurs early and is independent on the size of the primary.

Pathophysiology and Symptoms

Non-Functioning EC-Cell Tumors. Even tumors less than 1 cm, confined to the mucosa and submucosa discovered incidentally during colonoscopy and intubation of the terminal ileum are frequently malignant with metastatic spread to regional lymph nodes (see Table 10). They present very rarely with gastrointestinal bleeding.

Tumors measuring >1 cm in diameter are mostly malignant with metastases to the regional lymph nodes and later to the liver, bone and elsewhere. Patients frequently report on intermittent abdominal discomfort existing sometimes for years. Later, complaints worsen and diagnosis will be made if intermittent intestinal obstruction occurs. The latter is assigned to the role of growth factors secreted by the tumor cell as PDGF, TGFα, bFGF and others which stimulate neighburing fibroblasts which lead to new stroma formation and later to the typical desmoplastic reaction of the mesenterium. The consequence is angulation of the bowel with subsequent obstruction. Since also vasculature is affected by the stroma formation, ischemia develops in the involved segment and surgeons find the respective bowel dark-blue. Gastrointestinal bleeding is also in larger EC-cell tumors rare. Desmoplastic reaction can easily be detected by high-resolution MRT.

Functioning EC-Cell Tumors and Carcinoid Syndrome. EC-cell tumors responsible for the carcinoid syndrome do not different histologically from non-functioning tumors. However, carcinoid syndrome apperars only in patients with metastases to the liver. The symptoms are the consequence of unrestrained release of hormones and other mediators [11]. Flushing is present in up to 94% of patients and is characterized by red to purple discoloration of face, neck and upper chest. Duration of episodes is mostly short (few minutes) but can continue for hours. Frequently, patients themselves do not notice flushing and their attention will be drawn by others. Occasionally, flushing is associated with unpleasant sensations of lacrimation, warmth, facial and conjunctival edema. The hormonal mediator of flushing has not been identified with certainty. The elevation of blood serotonin during flushing does not prove its causal relationship. In addition, serotonin antagonist as methysergide and odansetone have only little effect. A more likely mediator are tachykinins as substance P and related peptides as neurokinins.

Serotonin is synthesized and secreted from carcinoid tumor cells. It arises from the amino acid tryptophan which is hydroxylated to 5-hydroxytryptophan and decarboxilated to 5-hydroxytryptamin (serotonin). Through several enzymes as monoamine oxidase and aldehyde dehydrogenase sterotonin is converted to 5-hydroxyindolacetic acid (5-HIAA) and excreted into urine.

Diarrhea with watery bowel movements is a common symptom and present in up to 85% of patients. It is possibly related to serotonin production but other mediators as prostaglandins have been suggested to contribute to diarrhea as well. Diarrhea responds better to serotonin antagonists then flushing.

The most important consequence of long-standing carcinoid syndrome is carcinoid heart disease, present in 45–77% of patients. Heart disease threatens patients with carcinoid syndrome at least by the same extent then the tumor itself and patients can die from carcinoid heart disease despite tumor growth is well controlled. Carcinoid heart disease involves mostly tricuspidic valve, pulmonary valve and rarely mitral and aortic valve. The mediator responsible for carcinoid heart disease is unknown. Several studies suggest the concept that serotonin is involved by reporting higher serotinin levels in plasma and 5-HIAA levels in urine in patients with compared to those without heart involvement. However, anorectic factors as well are discussed to be involved. Typically, the affected valves are thickened, shortened and retracted by fibrous transformation leading to tricuspid and pulmonary valve insufficiency which can be easily visualized by two-dimensional echocardiography.

Additional symptoms in carcinoid syndrome encompass bronchoconstriction, Pellegra-like skin changes and abdominal pain. The latter can result from diffuse liver enlargement or desmoplastic mesenterial reaction (see Fig. 7b). Pellegra-like skin reactions are the consequence of niacin deficiency which is due to the formation of serotonin from 5-hydroxytryptophan.

Carcinoid crisis is a rare exacerbation in patients with carcinoid syndrome mostly arising during anesthesia or surgery if patients are not under continuous somatostatin treatment. Flushing, hyper- and hypotension, severe bronchospasm and cardiac arrhythmias are the main features and subsequent death is not uncommon.

Diagnosis

In non-functional tumors, incidental detection of an ileal carcinoid during colonoscopy and in case of intestinal obstruction surgery uncovers the responsible carcinoid, which, in the latter situation, has mostly metastasized into regional lymphnodes. Non-functioning liver metastases from an ileal carcinoid are frequently detected by US during routine check-up. Most sensitive measures to estimate total tumor burden are Octreo Scan, CT and MRT. Biochemically, chromogranin A serves as most reliable tumor marker. Diagnosis of carcinoid syndrome is based on the demonstration of high 5-HIAA levels in the urine and elevated plasma serotonin and chromogranin A levels in the presence of liver metastases from an neuroendocrine tumor. CT, MRT and OctreoScan define total tumor burden and mostly the site of the primary. All patients deserve careful cardiologic diagnosis with two-dimensional echocardiography to prove or disprove cardiac involvement.

Differential Diagnosis

Some patients with non-functional ileal carcinoids develop diarrhea after right-sided hemicolectomy. They are later misdiagnosed as having carcinoid syndrome and somatostatin treatment will be started to prevent diarrhea. However, somatostatin treatment can even worsen diarrhea which is not hormone mediated but the consequence of bile acid loss into colon or bacterial overgrowth.

Treatment

Surgery is the treatment of choice to remove the primary and its local metastases reponsible for the desmoplastic reaction and subsequent abdominal pain. Surgery should further be considered in case of few and large liver metastases. In addition, right-sided hemicolectomy should be offered to patients with small ileal carcinoids detected incidentally during routine colonoscopy. Symptom control in patients with carcinoid syndrome was difficult before the availability of long-acting somatostatin analogs which are currently the principle or first choice to control flushing and diarrhea. They are indispensable in the treatment and prevention of bronchial obstruction and carcinoid crisis. They have, therefore, to be administered perioperatively and during laparotomy.

Their effects on carcinoid heart disease and its progression have not yet been demonstrated. Octreotide should be started at doses of 2–3×50 µg, but higher doses up to 3×500 µg may be necessary in some patients. If effective, LAR formulations should be offered (Octreotide-LAR 20 mg every 28 days). Long-acting somatostatin analogs are safe. One of the most frequent side effects is the formation of gall stones since somatostatin inhibits the release of CCK and by this mechanism gallbladder contraction. In few patients, somatostatin analogs induce diarrhea which can be as severe as diarrhea restulting from carcinoid syndrome. In these patients and those with tachyphylaxis to long-acting somatostatin analogs diarrhea should be controlled by serotonin receptor blockade. $5-HT_1$ (methysergide)-, $5-HT_{1+2}$ (cyproheptadine)-, $5-HT_2$ (ketanserin)- and $5-HT_3$ (ondansetron)-receptor antagonists have been recommended. But they do not completely stop diarrhea. To substitute niacin deficiency, patients should be offered niacin orally. Cardiac failure should be treated by conventional pharmacologic therapy.

Endocrine Tumors of the Appendix

Incidence rates of appendiceal carcinoids account for 0.075 new cases per 100.000 population and year. 19% of all gastrointestinal carcinoids have been reported to be localized in the appendix. Mean age of presentation is 32–43 years and females are more frequently affected.

Appendiceal carcinoids are mostly detected incidentally during appendectomy or described by pathologists in the resected appendix. They are mostly situated in the distal third of the appendix. By obstructing the lumen they can produce appendicitis. Clinicopathologic staging is summarized in Table 11. Most appendiceal carcinoids are well-differentiated tumors consisting of EC-cells but some contain glucagon-like peptides and PP/PYY-producing cells.

Most patients with appendiceal carcinoids have a favourable prognosis. Several well conducted studies demonstrate that carcinoids of less then 2 cm size confined to the appendiceal wall and not angioinvasive are completely cured by appendectomy. Invasion of the mesoappendix, a size >2 cm and angioinvasion carry an uncertain malignant potential and right sided hemicoletomy should, therefore, be performed as in patients with metastatic spread into regional lymph nodes. Also location of a carcinoid at the base of the appendix with involvement of the cecum has a more unfavourable prognosis requiring right sided hemicolectomy.

Goblet cell carcinoids are more aggressive tumors and should be treated by right sided hemicolectomy since these carcinoids frequently invade the wall of the appendix.

Endocrine Tumors of the Colon and Rectum

With an incidence of up to 0.21 cases per 100.000 population per year hindgut carcinoids (left sided colon, rectosigmoid) are less frequent then midgut carcinoids (see Fig. 7f) (jejunum, ileum, appendix). They account for 20% of all gastrointestinal carcinoids. Within the hindgut most carcinoids are situated in the rectum (54%). Average age for colonic carcinoids is 66 years and for rectal carcinoids 58 years. Histologically, colonic carcinoids consist of EC-cells or L-cells (glucagon-like peptides and PP/PYY-producing carcinoids) and rectal carcinoids mainly of L-cells. Most colonic carcinoids are found in the right colon with an average size of 4,9 cm. Rectal carcinoids represent as submucosal nodules or yellow polypoid lesions situated mostly 4 cm proximal the dentate line. Mostly, they are less then 1 cm in diameter and only in 13% greater then 2 cm (see Table 10). Carcinoids of the colon/rectum are generally non-functioning and present with abdominal pain due to bowel obstruction, bleeding or are detected incidentally during screening colonoscopy or in case of carcinoids >2 cm with liver metastases. Very few colonic carcinoids are associated with a carcinoid syndrome. Few hindgut carcinoids are poorly differentiated and aggressively growing. Their prognosis is poor. Carcinoids >2 cm have a higher malignancy rate with metastases mostly to the liver.

Established malignancy criteria of rectal carcinoids are a size >2 cm, invasion of the muscularis propria, DNA aneuploidy and the presence of 2 mitosis and more per 10 high power microscopic fields (magnification: ×400). The prognosis is in general more favourable then the prognosis of patients with carcinoids situated in the jejunum and ileum.

General Aspect of Management

Surgery

Surgery and endoscopic resection is the only available curative treatment and should always be considered. Solitary tumors (insulinomas, gastrinomas, gastrointestinal carcinoids) should be resected by laparotomy or endoscopy. Surgical management in patients with metastatic spread is not very well defined but should be an important treatment module of a multidisciplinary approach. Single and few liver metastases are exepted examples for palliative surgery. Many patients with slowly growing metastatic GEP tumors whether functionally active as some malignant insulinoma or functionally inactive have a benefit from this approach. Not well established is the place of surgery in patients with multiple, non-functioning endocrine pancreatic tumor as part of MEN-1 syndrome.

Liver transplantation should be considered in patients with resected primary tumorbut metastases only to the liver as shown by Octreoscan and other sensitive imaging methods and unresponsive to established medical and interventional treatment. However, reoccurrence of metastases in the transplanted liver has been observed as well as newly formed extra-hepatic metastases. Nevertheless, some patients have a significant benefitfrom liver transplantation with prolonged survival and quality of life.

Medical Treatment of Symptoms

The respective pharmaceutical principles have been in detail discussed elsewhere in this chapter.

Control of Tumor Growth in Malignant and Metastatic Tumors

Non-surgical control of tumor growth includes biotherapy with long-acting somatostatin analogues and α-interferon, systemic chemotherapy, ablative methods including chemoembolizaton, thermo- and alcohol treatment of liver lesions and tumor targeted radiotherapy.

Every therapeutic modality should recognize that well-differentiated endocrine GEP tumors are mostly slow growing and often exhibit phases of stable disease or such a slow growth that a significant increase in tumor size can only be substantiated with CT- or MRI scans performed in 6–12 months intervals. Therefore, non-surgical treatment options should not be considered in patients with stable disease and uncompromised life quality. Such patients should be offered regular control visits in 6 months intervals and treatment only offered in case of significant tumor growth (>20–25% increase in 3–6 months). Therefore, patients with newly-diagnosed metastatic disease from well-differentiated endocrine GEP-tumors and low mitotic activity should not be offered a specific treatment immediately.

Long Acting Somatostatin Analogs

Evidence for antiproliferative properties of somatostatin and its analogs derives from in vitro and in vivo studies. As discussed earlier, currently available somatostatin analogues bind preferentially to sst2 and sst5 receptors which mediate antimitogenic, antiproliferative and anti-apoptotic signals. Besides these receptor-dependent effects, somatostatin controls cell growth via receptor-independent effects. These include endocrine effects with inhibition of the release of circulating or paracrine tumor growth promoting factors, vascular antiangiogenetic effects and effects on the immune system.

Anecdotal reports of tumor regression in patients with metastatic endocrine tumors of the GI tract and of stable disease over a period of 4 years in two patients with carcinoid syndrome due to malignant metastatic neuroendocrine tumors of the lung are consistent with the above mentioned experimental data.

A retrospective report of the National Institute of Health on 96 patients with metastatic endocrine tumors showed a partial tumor response in 13%, stable disease in 63% and tumor progression in only 24%. However, partial tumor response was a very rare event in prospective studies and disease stabilization occurred in 36–70% of patients. However, even stable disease was short-lasting for a minimum of 2 months and a maximum of 60 months. In one study, patients were classified into those with rapidly-progressing tumors (increase >50% in 3 months) and slowly progressing tumors (increase >50% in 3 months). Inhibition of tumor growth occurred predominantly in slow-growing tumors [27]. All trials were uncontrolled. Regarding the unpredictable course of the disease and the moderate response to treatment for a relatively short period of time, it cannot be excluded that the phases of stable disease and even partial response observed in a few patients reflect the natural course of the disease. Since long-term treatment with somatostatin analogs is expensive, placebo-controlled studies are now necessary to prove or to disprove the antiproliferative potency of long-acting somatostatin analogs in patients with metastatic endocrine GEP-tumors. Unresolved issues include the therapeutic dose, the equipotency of octreotide and lanreotide versus the longer acting release formulations and the treatment effect with regard to prolongation of live.

α-Interferon

Interferons affect tumor growth by blocking the cell cycle during the G_0-G_1 phase with prolongation of the S-phase. Experimental data suggest that α-interferon induce apoptosis and that tumor cells are replaced by fibrotic tissue. α-interferon, in addition, induces increased expression of class I antigens on the tumor cell surface which renders cells as targets for cytotoxic T-lymphocytes.

Several studies in metastatic endocrine GEP-tumors demonstrate both a symptomatic effect with improvement of flushing and diarrhea in patients with carcinoid syndrome, a concomitant decrease of biochemical markers and a stabilization of tumor growth in 20–40% and a reduction in tumor size in 12–20% of patients. As shown for long-acting somatostatin analogues, these effects are transient (6–20 months). Side effects of α-interferon treatment have a much greater impact on patients well-being and include flu-like symptoms, weight loss, fatigue, anemia, leukopenia, thrombocytopenia, autoimmune manifestations and psychiatric disturbances.

Combination Treatment with Octreotide and α-Interferon

In a prospective trial inhibition of tumor growth was observed in 67% of 21 patients with metastatic endocrine tumors of the GI-tract who were unresponsive to prior octreotide monotheraphy. Responders to combined treatment had a significant survival benefit. However, these data could not be confirmed by a prospective two arm study, comparing octreotide versus octreotide plus α-interferon in 105 patients performed by the authors of this chapter demonstrating the need for well-controlled and prospective trials in well-defined subgroups of patients with endocrine GEP-tumors.

Chemotherapy

Several chemotherapeutic agents have been used as single agents and as combinations in metastatic endocrine GEP tumors. The respective original data demonstate that chemotherapy is indicated only in patients with well-differentiated endocrine carcinomas of pancreatic origin and in rapidly growing undifferentiated and small cell endocrine carcinomas [8]. According to a 20 years old prospective study from the Eastern Cooperative Oncology Group (ECOG) which enrolled 125 patients with histologically proven unresectable islet-cell carcinomas streptozotocin plus doxorubicin was found superior to streptozotocin plus 5-fluouracil (5-FU) and to chlorozotocin. Tumor regression occurred in 69% of patients treated with streptozotocin plus doxorubicin and in 45% of patients treated with the combination of streptozotocin and 5-FU. Median duration of regression was 18 months for the doxorubicin combination and 14 months for the 5-FU combination. These beneficial effects influenced also survival. These favourable effects of tumor growth are contrasted by toxic reactions to treatment as nausea, vomiting, alopecia, hematologic and kidney toxicity. Heart failure has been observed in patients receiving the doxorubicin regimen and a cumulative dose of 400–500 mg/m² should, therefore, not be exceeded. In the institution of the authors patients are treated with the streptozotocin/doxorubicin combination. In case of response, treatment is changed to streptozotocin plus 5-FU if the limiting doxorubicin dose is reached. The dosages are summarized in table 16. Unfortunately it is impossible to identify patients responding to this treatment and patients not responding. In the latter situation one should try dacarbacine (150 mg/m²) as short infusion and repeat it every 28 days. At least 3 courses of treatment should be performed to prove or disprove success.

Importantly, streptozotocin combinations and dacarbacine are only effective in tumors of pancreatic origin. There is no established chemotherapy for malignant carcinoids of the stomach, small and large intestine. In patients with exploding undifferentiated tumors the following chemotherapeutic strategy should be offered: 130 mg/m^2 and day etoposide for 3 days plus 45 mg/m^2 and day cisplatin on days 2 and 3. Each agent is given by 24 hours infusion and cycles repeated every 6 weeks. These tumors may originate from the pancreas, stomach, small and large bowel and most patients with these rare undiffentiated tumors will respond at least for 2 to 3 cycles. Drug toxicity is a significant problem of these formulations requiring dosage reduction or cessation of treatment in some patients.

Ablative Measures

Ablative measures include transarterial chemoembolization and radio-frequency tissue or alcohol ablation. Transarterial chemoembolization [8] is based on the concept that arterial blood supply of metastases (via hepatic artery) from endocrine GEP tumors is more intense then that of other malignancies except primary hepatocellular carcinoma and that local ischemia induces cell necrosis. Unproven is the concept that the combination of desarterialization vial embolization and local cytotoxic chemotherapy increases response rates. Embolization is performed by selective injection of a mixture of iodinized oil plus doxorubicin followed by injection of gelatine sponge particles. Response rates with a decrease of symptoms in patients with carcinoid syndrome of 68–100%, decreases of hormone levels in 80% and a decrease in size of liver metastases in 37–100% of patients have been described by several institutions. Mean duration of response is approximately 24 months. In the own institution it has been shown that patients with a tumor burden >75% of the liver have not benefit from chemoembolization. Increased survival has been observed in patients with a tumor burden <50% and an accumulation of lipiodol in more then 50% of the tumor mass. Side effects include abdominal pain, nausea, vomiting and fever. Fatal complications are infection and sepsis and hepatic failure.

Radiofrequency treatment [33] is a novel advice to destroy liver metastases and can be performed percutaneously and intraoperatively using a cooled-tip needly applying 50 to 90 watts over 10–12 minutes under ultrasound control. This experimental procedure as well as ablation by injection of alcohol can be considered in case of few and small liver metastases.

Table 16

Chemotherapeutic protocols for well differentiated metastatic islet cell carcinoms

Streptozotocin plus 5-fluorouracil	500 mg/m^2 streptozotocin/day as intravenous injection for 5 consecutive days; *plus* 400 mg/m^2 5-fluorouracil/day as intravenous injection for 5 consecutive days, repeated every 6 weeks
Streptozotocin plus doxorubcin	500 mg/m^2 streptozotocin/day as intravenous injection for 5 consecutive days; *plus* 50 mg/m^2 doxorubicin as intravenous injection on days 1 and 22; repeated every 6 weeks

Maximal dose of doxorubicin: 4500 mg/m^2. Reduced dosages of every drug in case of severe nausea, vomiting, stomatitis, diarrhea, leukopenia, thrombozytopenia. Reduced dosages of streptozotocin in case of elevated creatinine or proteinuria and discontinuation if abnormalities persist.

Radioligand Therapy

Tumor-targeted metabolic endo-radiotherapy using specific receptor ligands such as octreotide or lanreotide coupled to beta-emitting radionuclides is of special interest in endocrine malignancies since biotherapy is only effective in slow growing tumors and systemic chemotherapy in a subpopulation of patients with pancreatic tumors. Almost no treatment modality has been shown to affect bone metastases. Whereas radioiodinated somatostatin analogues usually show target-to-background ratios not high enough for therapeutic applications, which is mainly due to their lipophilicity and rapid intracellular degradability, radiometal-labelled analogues display excellent biodistribution properties. To bind radioisotopes such as ^{111}Indium, ^{90}Yttrium and ^{177}Lutetium tightly to somatostatin analogs, mono- and bifunctional chelators have been developed consisting of polyaminopolycarboxylic acids or their macrocyclic derivatives such as DTPA, TTHA, DFO, DOTA or TETA. To reach biofunctionality, aliphatic side chain, thiourona-tobenzyl,-, acetamidobenzyl- or succinylbenzyl linkers connect the chelators with octreotide and related peptides. ^{111}In-labelled [DTPA]-octreotide has been shown to display an appropriate biodistribution profile in man.

Although generally regarded as mainly diagnostic, [111]-Indium emits Auger and conversion electrons, which display a tissue penetration of 0.02–10 μm and 200–500 μm respectively, and which can be used therapeutically. More therapeutic experience has been gained with [90]Yttrium, which is a classical β-particle emitter. To avoid dissociation of [90]Yttrium with a maximum path length of 9 mm from the chelated somatostatin analog, a stable [DOTA°, Tyr³]-octreotide complex has been developed. Replacement of phenylalanine at the 3-position of octreotide by tyrosine has been shown to even increase the affinity of this compound for the sst2 receptors. The effect of endo-radiotherapy depends on binding to the sst2 receptor and requires internalization of the radioligand. Therefore, a sufficient number of sst2 binding sites and rapid internalization are prerequisits for successful therapy. The principal efficacy of somatostatin receptor-mediated radiotherapy has been demonstrated in animal models. Recently, several studies including a limited number of patients with malignant endocrine tumors have been published, suggesting that radiotherapy with [111]In- and [90]-Y-labelled octreotide analogs is able to control symptoms in patients with functionally active endocrine tumors and to inhibit or even significantly decrease tumor load. Whether or not [^{177}Lu-DOTA, Typ³]-Octreotate with a tissue penetration of 2 mm is superior to [111]Indium and [90]Yttrium labelled octreotide in the treatment of endocrine GEP tumors is currently under investigation.

How Should we Proceed in Patients with Metastatic Neuroendocrine GEP-Tumors?

Despite the availability of several antiproliferative strategies that can be offered to patients with metastatic disease, current recommendations how to start with non-surgical modalities are controversial and not supported by prospective and controlled studies. Therefore, therapeutic strategies for a single patient are based frequently on personal experiences of expert centers and vary, therefore, from center to center. To harmonize therapeutic ways of proceeding European experts in the field have founded the Eureopean Network for the Study of Endocrine GEP Tumors (ENET) to define the place of currently available and future diagnostic and therapeutic principles. According to the experiences of the authors of this chapter the following recommendations can be applied to patients with metastatic GEP tumors:

1. Surgery with curative resection of the primary in the absence of metastatic spread and tumor debulking in metastatic disease should be intended where ever possible.

2. Antiproliferative strategies should consider the growth characteristics and biology of a given tumor. Do not treat non-growing metastases which are stable by CT for 6 months and longer! It is questionable whether these patients have any benefit from anti-proliferative measures. Consider surgery or local ablative measures (radiofrequence ablation) in these patients.

3. In the case of moderately rapid progression chemotherapy should be offered in patients with tumors of pancreatic origin (streptozotocin combinations, dacarbacine). Chemotherapy should not be offered to patients with well-differentiated non-functional or functional tumors arising from the intestine (from stomach to rectum).

4. Offer chemotherapy (etoposid + cisplatin) in exploding tumors as small cell and undifferentiated neuroendocrine carcinomas.

5. Offer local irradiation in case of pain in patients with bone metastases since bone metastases do not respond to chemotherapy and biotherapy.

6. Offer octreotide to patients with well-differentiated slowly growing neuroendocrine tumors. In case of further growth add α-interferon.

7. Consider chemoembolization primarily in patients with liver metastases due to mid- and hindgut tumors since this group of patients does not respond to chemotherapy.

8. Consider radioligand therapy only within controlled and prospective studies since it is unsettled whether this modality should be offered to patients as first-line treatment or to patients unresponsive to other therapeutic alternatives.

References

1. Solcia E, Klöppel G, Sobin H (2000) WHO: Histological typing of endocrine tumours. Springer: Berlin-New York
2. Chandrasekharappa SC, Guru SC, Manickam O et al. (1997) Positional cloning of the gene for multiple endocrine neoplasia type I. Science 276: 404–407
3. Debelenko, LV, Zhuang Z, Emmert-Buck MR et al. (1997) Allelic deletions on chromosome 11q13 in multiple endocrine neoplasia type 1-associated and sporadic gastrinomas and pancreatic endocrine tumors. Cancer Res 57: 2238–2243
4. Jensen RT, Gardner JD (1993) Gastrinoma In Go VLW, DiMagno EP, Gardner JD et al. (eds): The Pancreas: Biology, Pathobiology, and Disease, 2nd ed. New York, Raven Press

5. Metz DC, Jensen RT, Bale AE et al. (1994) Multiple endocrine neoplasia type 1: Clinical features and management. In Bilezekian JP, Levine MA, Marcus R (eds): The Parathyroids. New York, Raven

6. Soga J, Yakuwa Y (1998) Glucagonomas/diabetico-dermatogenic syndrome (DDS): A statistical evaluation of 407 reported cases. J Hepatobiliary Pancreat Sur 5(3):312–319

7. Modlin IM, Sandor A (1997) An analysis of 8305 cases of carcinoid tumors. Cancer 79:813–829

8. Jensen RT and Norton JA (2002). Pancreatic Endocrine Tumors. In Feldman M, Friedman LS, Sleisenger MH (eds.): Gastrointestinal and Liver Disease. Vol 1, 7th ed. Philadelphia, WB Saunders, p 988–1018

9. Rindi G, Azzoni C, La-Rosa S et al. (1999) ECL cell tumor and poorly differech GD, Brandi ML, Friedman E. Allelic loss on chromosome 11 in hereditary and sporadic tumors related to familial multiple endocrine neoplasia tyntiated endocrine carcinoma of the stomach: prognostic evaluation by pathological analysis. Gastroenterology 116:532–542

10. Solcia E, Capella C, Sessa F et al. (1986) Gastric carcinoids and related endocrine growths. Digestion 35 [Suppl 1]: 3–22

11. Vinik AI, McLeod MK, Fig LM et al (1989) Clinical features, diagnosis, and localization of carcinoid tumors and their management. Gastroenterol Clin North Am 18:865–896

12. Service FJ, Mc Mahon MM, O'Brion PC (1991) Functioning insulinoma – incidence, recurrence, and long-term survival of patients: a 60 year study. Mayo Clinic Proc 66:711–719

13. W. Creutzfeldt (1975) Pancreatic endocrine tumors: the riddle of their origin and hormone secretion. Isr J Med Sci 11:762–776

14. Creutzfeldt W, Arnold R, Creutzfeldt C et al. (1973) Biochemical and morphological investigations of 30 human insulinomas. Diabetologia 9:217–231

15. Creutzfeldt W, Arnold R, Creutzfeldt C et al. (1975) Pathomorphologic, biochemical and diagnostic aspects of gastrinomas (Zollinger-Ellison syndrome). Hum Pathol 6:47–76

16. Capella C, Heitz Ph U, Hofler H et al. (1994) Revised classification of neuroendocrine tumors of the lung, pancreas and gut. Digestion 55 (suppl.3):11–23

17. Zhuang Z, Vortmeyer AO, Pack S et al. (1997). Somatic mutations of the MEN1 tumor suppressor gene in sporadic gastrinomas and insulinomas. Cancer Research 57:4682–4686

18. Hessmann O, Lindberg D, Skogseid B et al. (1998). Mutation of the multiple endocrine neoplasia type 1 gene in nonfamilial, malignant tumors of the endocrine pancres. Cancer Research 58:377–379

19. La Rosa S, Sessa F, Capella C et al. (1996). Prognostic criteria in non-functioning pancreatic endocrine tumours. Virchow Archiv: An International Journal of Pathology 429:323–333

20. Muscarella P, Melvin WS, Fisher WE et al. (1998). Genetic alterations in gastrinomas and nonfunctioning pancreatic neuroendocrine tumors: an analysis of p16/MTS1 tumor suppressor gene inactivation. Cancer Research 58:237–240

21. Bartsch D, Hahn SA, Danichevski KD et at. (1999). Mutations of the DPC4/Smad4 gene in neuroendocrine pancreatic tumors. Oncogene 18: 2367–2371

22. Agarwal SK, Guru SC, Heppner C et al. (1999). Menin interacts with the AP1 transcription factor JunD and represses JunD-activated transcription. Cell 96:143–152

23. Mulligan LM, Kwok JB, Healey CS et al. (1993). Germ-line mutations of the RET proto-oncogene in mulitple endocrine neoplasia type 2A. Nature 363:458–460

24. Hammel PR, Vilgrain V, Terris B et al. (2000). Pancreatic involvement in von Hippel-Lindau disease. The Groupe Francophone d'Etude de la Maladie de von Hippel-Lindau. Gastroenterology 115:1087–1095

25. Service FJ, McMahon MM, O'Brien PC et al (1991) Functioning insulinoma – incidence, recurrence, and long-term survival of patients: a 60-year study. Mayo Clinic Proceedings 66:711–719

26. Rothmund M, Angelini L, Brunt LM et al. (1990) Surgery for benign insulinoma: An international review. World J Surg 14:393–398

27. Arnold R, Wied M, Behr TH (2002). Somatostatin analogues in the treatment of endocrine tumours of the gastrointestinal tract. Expert Opin Pharmacother 3:643–650

28. Arnold R, Frank M, Bülchmann G (1998). Insulinoma and persistent neonatal hyperinsulinemic hypoglycemia (nesidioblastosis). In Beger HG, Warshaw AL, Buechler MW et al. (eds.): The pancres, Volume 2, Blackwell Science p 1187–1202

29. Someya T, Miki T, Sugihara S et al. (2000). Characterization of genes encoding the pancreatic beta-cell ATP-sensitive K+ channel in persistent hyperinsulinemic hypoglycemia of infancy in Japanese patients. Endcr J 47(6):715–722

30. Fibril F, Venzon DJ, Ojeaburu JV et al. (2001). Prospective Study of the Natural History of Gastrinoma in Patients with MEN-1: Definition of an Aggressive and a Nonaggressive Form. The Journal of Clinical Endocrinology & Metabolism, 86(11):5282–5293

31. Norton JA, Fraker DL, Alexander HR et al. (1999). Surgery to cure the Zollinger-Ellison syndrome. N Engl J Med 341(9):635–644

32. Debray MP, Geoffroy O, Laissy JP et al. (2001). Imaging appearances of metastases from neuroendocrine tumours of the pancreas. Br J Radiol 74(887):1065–1070

33. Wessels FJ, Schell SR (2001). Radiofrequency ablation treatment of refractory carcinoid hepatic metastases. J Surg Res 95(1):8–12

Biliary System and Papilla of Vater

16 Carcinoma of the Gallbladder and Bile Ducts

K. SCHOPPMEYER, K. CACA, J. MÖSSNER

Summary

Biliary tract cancers are rare tumors that have a poor prognosis. Predisposing conditions are characterized by chronic inflammatory and proliferative stimuli of the biliary epithelium. Despite a wealth of diagnostic tools, these cancers are often detected late due to their insidious symptomatic appearance. In patients with localized cancer, surgery is the only curative treatment option. In hilar bile duct tumors, an extended operation including partial hepatectomy may improve long-term outcome. Currently, there is no adjuvant or palliative radio- or chemotherapy available that has been shown to be effective. Treatment in patients with severe comorbidities or advanced stages of disease is directed towards palliation of symptoms. Endoscopic interventions like biliary decompression play a central role in palliative concepts. Prognosis is determined by disease stage and effective prevention of complications, prominent among them being cholangitis.

Epidemiology

Biliary tract cancers are rare tumors. Approximately 7500 cases are newly diagnosed in the United States each year, including 5000 gallbladder cancers and about 2500 patients with carcinoma of the bile ducts. These tumors result in 3600 deaths per year, or approximately 1% of cancer deaths [1].

The frequency of biliary tract cancers has a distinct geographical pattern, possibly reflecting environmental influences. The prevalence of gallbladder carcinoma varies widely among different populations, which may partially relate to variations in the prevalence of gallstones in these populations. The tumor is rare in most white populations but is frequently diagnosed in the native populations of North and South America. Cholangiocarcinomas, which can be divided into intrahepatic, perihilar and extrahepatic tumors and those of the ampulla of Vater (discussed in chapter 18), account for about 15% of liver cancers worldwide. Their prevalence is highest in parts of Southeast Asia.

Biliary tract cancer is a tumor of the elderly. Its incidence increases with age and the tumor is most often diagnosed in the seventh decade of life. In gallbladder carcinoma, the female to male ratio varies between 1.2 to 1 and 3 to 1, depending on the country and population. However, there is a slight male preponderance for carcinoma of the bile ducts.

Etiology

Various risk factors have been associated with the development of gallbladder and bile duct cancer, respectively. Gallbladder cancer is strongly associated with the presence of gallstones, especially if they are symptomatic and large. Other risk factors include obesity, female sex, and high carbohydrate intake, all of which also predispose to the development of gallstones. Patients who suffer from chronic cholecystitis, especially when calcification of the gallbladder wall is present and those with polyps also have an increased risk.

In general, chronic inflammation of the biliary tract promotes carcinogenesis. Prominent among other risk factors is primary sclerosing cholangitis. Lifetime risk of developing carcinoma in this condition has been reported to be about 10%. The time lag between diagnosis of primary sclerosing cholangitis and the development of cholangiocarinoma ranges from 1 to more than 25 years with more than one third of carcinomas occuring within the first 2 years [2]. Patients with ulcerative colitis without manifest primary sclerosing cholangitis also have an increased risk. The risk is not affected by proctocolectomy.

Other conditions predisposing to chronic bacterial infections such as Caroli's disease (cystic dilatation of intrahepatic bile ducts) or choledochal cysts also represent known risk factors. The once endemic infestation with the liver flukes Opisthorchis viverrini and Clonorchis sinensis in Southeast and East Asia, respectively, may explain the frequency of bile duct carcinoma in these regions. The prevalence of parasite infestation correlates with that of biliary tract cancers, though the mechanism of carcinogenesis is not fully understood. Bile duct adenomas and multiple biliary papillomatosis are known precancerous lesions similar to carcinogenetic mechanisms in other gastrointestinal malignancies.

Biliary carcinogens include the radiopaque contrast medium Thorotrast, a radioactive α-particle emitter. The carcinogens that lead to an increased incidence of biliary tract cancer in rubber and chemical industry workers remain unidentified as yet. The role of tobacco smoking as a risk factor is not well established, since conflicting results were found in different series.

Despite a number of established risk factors, many biliary tract cancers occur in the absence of any obvious predisposing condition.

Symptoms and Clinical Signs

Symptoms vary depending on the location of the tumor. In distal bile duct carcinoma, symptoms caused by bile duct obstruction are most common and include jaundice, clay-colored stools, brownish urine and pruritus. In hilar carcinoma, these symptoms develop later, whereas in gallbladder and intrahepatic cholangiocarcinoma they signal an advanced stage of disease. Pain in the right upper quadrant is the most common presenting symptom in gallbladder cancer. In hilar cholangiocarcinoma, nonspecific symptoms like abdominal discomfort, fatigue, anorexia and weight loss may be the earliest indicators of disease. Fever and chills do occur rarely at first presentation.

Physical examination may reveal jaundice and skin excoriations as a result of pruritus. Dependent on the stage and location of disease, hepatomegaly, a palpable gallbladder in distal obstructing cholangiocarcinoma or a mass in the right upper quadrant in advanced stages of biliary tract cancer may be apparent. Involvement of the portal vein may lead to signs of portal hyper-

tension including ascites, bloating or signs of gastrointestinal bleeding. Rarely at presentation, but more frequently in the course of disease, cholangitis may lead to fever, chills and acute painful sensation in the right upper quadrant.

Diagnostics

Synopsis

Standard imaging techniques for detection and staging of biliary tract cancer

▸ Ultrasound and Duplex sonography
▸ Cholangiography [endoscopic retrograde cholangiography (ERC), percutaneous transhepatic cholangiography (PTC)]
▸ Computed tomography
▸ Magnetic resonance imaging (MRI), MR cholangiography and MR angiography
▸ Conventional angiography
▸ Histology (surgical, transcutaneous or intraductal biopsy) and cytology (brush cytology).

Abnormal laboratory test results due to inhibition of normal bile flow or tumor invasion into the liver are frequent signs of disease. Elevated serum alkaline phosphatase, gamma glutamyltranspeptidase or bilirubin levels may lead to further evaluation of the patient. Serum transaminases are sometimes mildly elevated. As a result of longstanding cholestasis, fat- soluble vitamin uptake may be reduced and prothrombin time increased. Transformed cells secrete tumor-associated antigens, the so-called tumor markers, into the bile or serum. Unfortunately, none of them is sufficiently specific to establish a diagnosis. However, tumor markers are useful to monitor therapy once a diagnosis has been made. Of these, CA 19–9 is the most accurate.

Due to its widespread availability and lack of contraindications, ultrasound is the first diagnostic imaging procedure. It may detect mass lesions or indirect signs of biliary obstruction and thus direct further diagnostic work-up. Although ultrasound often fails to detect the tumor in perihilar or extrahepatic cholangiocarcinoma, it is useful to rule out other causes of biliary obstruction like gallstones. Monitoring of the success of therapeutic interventions like biliary drainage can be done by repeated ultrasound. In addition, duplex sonography and contrast-enhanced ultrasound may help to visualize vascular invasion of the tumor or thrombosis of the portal vein as well as hidden tumor growth.

Contrast-enhanced spiral CT scan has an improved sensitivity to detect intrahepatic or gallbladder mass lesions. It is slightly better than ultrasound to detect perihilar or extrahepatic tumors, but indirect signs are more commonly discovered. A specific finding is the dilatation of the intrahepatic bile ducts in a small hepatic lobe, often associated with hypertrophy of the contralateral lobe (Fig. 1).

This atrophy-hypertrophy-complex suggests a tumor chronically obstructing the bile duct and infiltrating the ipsilateral portal vein. The location of obstruction may also be indicated by the distribution of the dilated biliary segments, a distal location resulting in a distended gallbladder and bilobar dilatation, while more proximal tumors lead to unilobar dilatation and a normal or collapsed gallbladder.

MRI, especially when combined with MR-angiography or cholangiography yields excellent visualization of hepatic parenchymal abnormalities including vascular involvement (Fig. 2).

It may substitute for more invasive diagnostic procedures in the preoperative assessment of biliary tract cancers, although results critically depend on the compliance of the patient and do not always delineate precisely the biliary anatomy.

Mapping of the intraductal tumor extent can be achieved by cholangiography. Both ERC and PTC are performed, depending on the location of the tumor, preceding operations and the expertise of the operator. Obtaining bile samples or brush cytological or biopsy specimens can increase the diagnostic yield. The sensitivity of these techniques varies widely but may confirm the diagnosis of carcinoma in up to 70%. Frequently though, these methods fail to detect malignant cells because of the desmoplastic reaction of the tumor. Cholangiography has the further advantage that decompression of the biliary tree via placement of a biliary endoprosthesis can be achieved in the same session. Current data do not support preoperative biliary drainage solely to reduce perioperative mortality. It is obligatory though in patients with cholangitis or poor liver function due to biliary obstruction or as a palliative measure in inoperable patients. The role of intraductal ultrasound during ERC remains to be defined (Fig. 3).

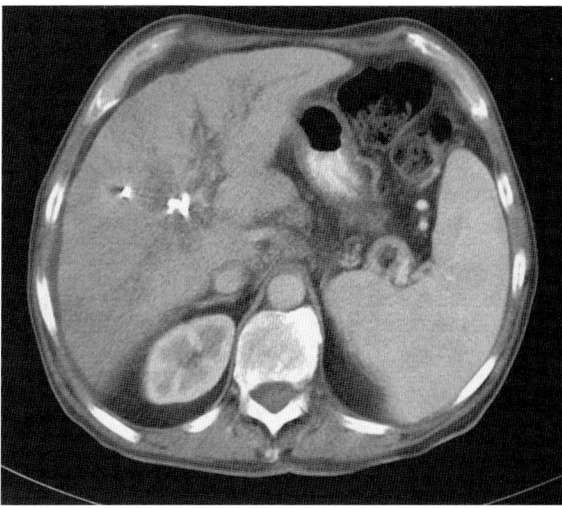

Figure 1
Atrophic appearance of the left liver lobe with crowding of the ipsilateral bile ducts as an indirect sign of a perihilar tumor invading the left portal vein and obstructing the bile duct on CT scan

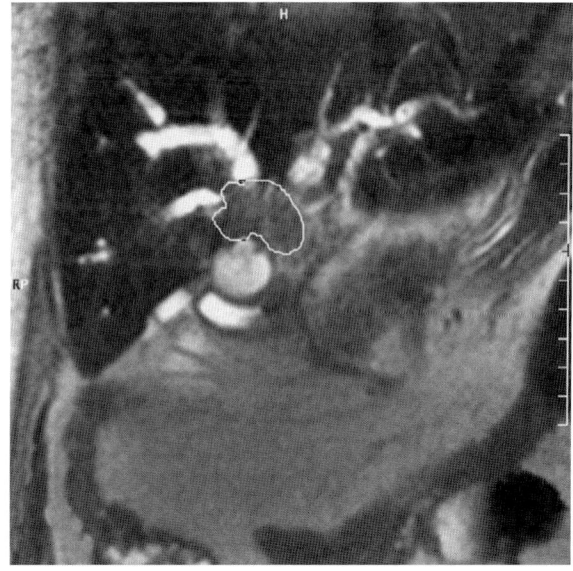

Figure 2
MRCP of a Klatskin tumor. The tumor (*encircled*) is located at the liver hilus, obstructing the bile ducts

Endoscopic ultrasound is useful in distal and periampullary tumors but not in peripheral cholangiocarcinomas.

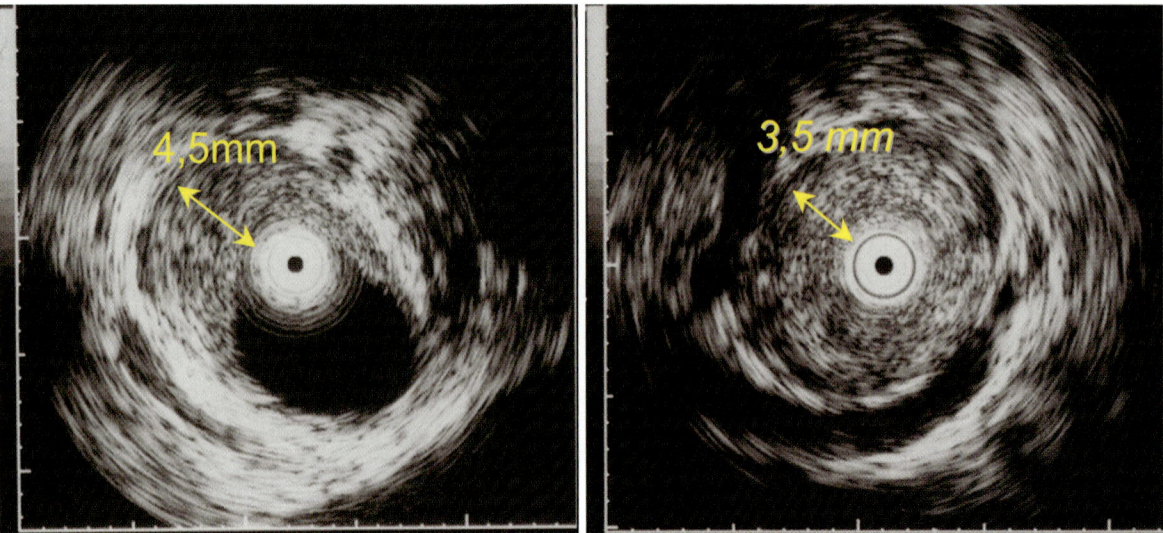

Figure 3
Intraductal ultrasound (IDUS) showing semicircular and circular growth (*arrow*) of a bile duct tumor

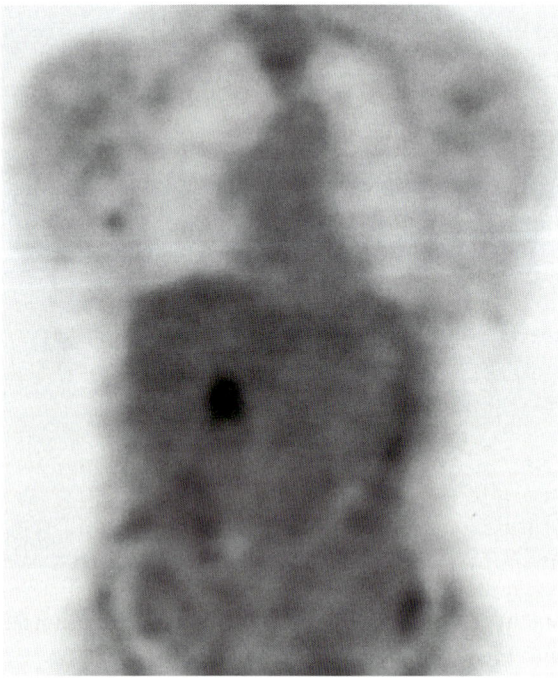

Figure 4
Positron emmission tomography demonstrates metabolic activity in a perihilar tumor that was postoperatively staged as pT3pN1M0

Angiography accurately predicts vascular involvement, thrombosis of the portal vein or vascular anomalies. It can thus help to differentiate operable from inoperable tumors. In the majority of cases, however, it can be replaced preoperatively by the above mentioned imaging techniques.

Despite considerable technical advances, radiographic evaluation often fails to detect peritoneal or nodal metastasis. The role of staging laparoscopy in the staging of cholangiocarcinoma remains to be defined. Laparoscopy, especially when combined with laparoscopic ultrasound, is able to detect radiographically-occult metastasis. The impact of laparoscopy on treatment strategies in cholangiocarcinoma needs to be determined in future trials.

A newer imaging technique is positron-emission tomography (PET) (Fig. 4).

It relies on the increased metabolism of malignant cells. Any inflammation in the body will, however, evoke conflicting results. In addition, the rather high content of fibrous tissue in cholangiocarcinoma may obscure the metabolic activity of some tumors. It has been reported that PET has a reasonable sensitivity and specificity to detect primary cholangiocarcinomas and distant metastasis, but not lymph node involvement. Chest radiography, CT or bone scanning is useful to detect distant metastases in the most common locations.

An eventual diagnosis should always be based on histology. Tissue samples can be obtained during surgery or alternatively as mentioned above by intraductal biopsy or brush cytology.

Histological Classification and Molecular Genetics

Synopsis

Most common epithelial tumors:
▸ Adenocarcinoma
▸ Papillary carcinoma
▸ Mucinous carcinoma

Molecular genetics:
Genetic alterations in various tumor suppressor genes and proto-oncogenes have been described but no carcinogenetic model can be established yet.

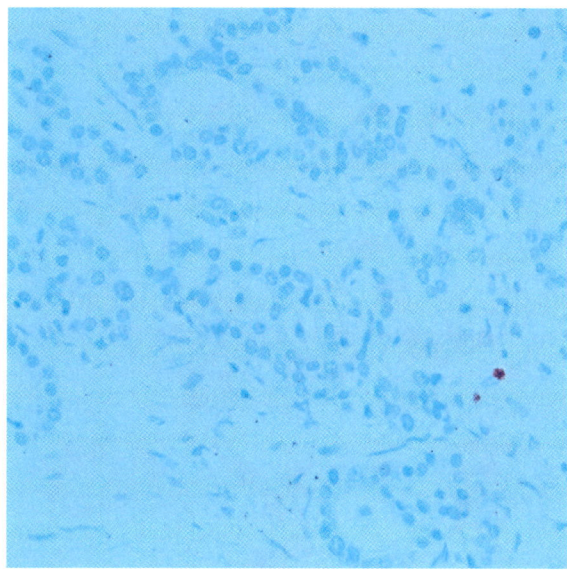

Figure 5
Histology of a bile duct carcinoma. Typical is an adenomatous tumor with a strong desmoplastic reaction

Carcinomas of the gallbladder and bile ducts are by far the most common malignant tumors of the biliary tract. The majority of carcinomas are adenocarcinoma, papillary carcinoma and mucinous carcinoma. Other tumor types occur in less than five percent of cases and include clear cell carcinoma, signet-ring cell carcinoma, adenosquamous carcinoma, squamous carcinoma and small cell carcinoma. The histologic grade varies from well differentiated to undifferentiated. Papillary carcinomas of the gallbladder have a better prognosis than other histologic types.

Clusters of cells surrounded by a sometimes extensive fibrous tissue characterize tumors (Fig. 5).

This feature often poses diagnostic problems. Immunohistochemistry can corroborate a diagnosis but is unable to establish it because there are no known proteins unique to bile duct cells or biliary tract carcinoma. Immunohistochemical stains for cytokeratins and mucins are most commonly used.

There is limited information about the molecular carcinogenesis in gallbladder carcinoma. Several studies indicate that the gene loci 17p13 and 9p21, encoding the

tumor suppressors p53 and p16INK4a, display early and frequent abnormalities. They sometimes precede the onset of histological changes and invasion. Other chromosomal alterations involve deletions at 8p21 and 18q21 (encoding DCC). Mutations of the k-ras protooncogene, however, are an infrequent event in this malignancy with the exception of carcinomas associated with congenital abnormalities of the biliary tract. However, molecular mechanisms are not yet fully understood and do not consistently correlate with histologic alterations in gallbladder carcinogenesis.

In bile duct carcinoma, several genetic alterations are known. The most common of these are oncogenic activation of k-ras, C-Myc, C-erbB2 and C-Met, as well as inactivation of tumor suppressors Bcl2, p16INK4a (Fig. 6) and p53 [3].

This may lead to phenotypic changes but not consistently. In addition, mutation and phenotypic changes also occur in nonmalignant conditions, precluding their use as diagnostic tools. How carcinogens trigger genetic alterations is a matter of speculation as is the relevance of the different genetic events in carcinogenesis.

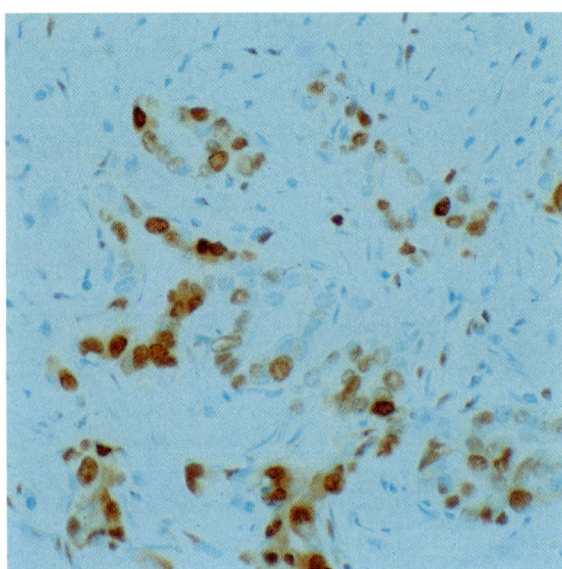

Figure 6
Immunostaining with an anti-p16INK4a antibody shows immuno-
reactivity predominantly in the nucleus in the majority of tumor cells

Staging

Synopsis

TNM classification of gallbladder carcinoma

T	Primary tumor
TX	Primary tumor cannot be assessed
T0	No evidence of primary tumor
Tis	Carcinoma in situ
T1	Tumor invades lamina propria (T1a) or muscle layer (T1b)
T2	Tumor invades the perimuscular connective tissue, no extension beyond the serosa or into the liver
T3	Tumor perforates the serosa or directly invades an adjacent organ, or both (extension 2 cm or less into the liver)
T4	Tumor extends more than 2 cm into the liver, and/or into two or more adjacent organs
N	Reginal lymph nodes
NX	Regional lymph nodes cannot be assessed
N0	No regional lymph node metastasis
N1	Metastasis in cystic duct, pericholedochal, and/or hilar lymph nodes
N2	Metastasis in peripancreatic (head only), periduodenal, periportal, celiac, and/or superior mesenteric lymph nodes
M	Distant metastasis
MX	Distant metastasis cannot be assessed
M0	Distant metastasis
M1	Distant metastasis

Stage groupings	T	N	M
Stage 0	Tis	N0	M0
Stage 1	T1	N0	M0
Stage 2	T2	N0	M0
Stage 3	T1–3	N1	M0
	T3	N0	M0
Stage 4a	T4	N0–1	M1
Stage 4b	T1–4	N2	M0
	T1–4	N0–2	M1

TNM Classification of Extrahepatic Bile Duct Carcinoma

T	Primary tumor
TX	Primary tumor cannot be assessed
T0	No evidence of primary tumor
Tis	Carcinoma in situ
T1	Tumor invades subepithelial connective tissue or fibromuscular layer
T1a	Tumor invades subepithelial connective tissue
T1b	Tumor invades fibromuscular layer
T2	Tumor invades perifibromuscular connective tissue
T3	Tumor invades adjacent structures: liver, pancreas, duodenum, gallbladder, colon, stomach
N	Regional lymph nodes
NX	Regional lymph nodes cannot be assessed
N0	No regional lymph node metastasis
N1	Metastasis in cystic duct, pericholedochal and/or hilar lymph nodes (i.e., in the hepatoduodenal ligament)
N2	Metastasis in peripancreatic (head only), periduodenal, periportal, celiac, and/or superior mesenteric and/or posterior pancreatico-duodenal lymph nodes
M	Distant metastasis
MX	Presence of distant metastasis cannot be assessed
M0	No distant metastasis
M1	Distant metastasis

Stage groupings	T	N	M
Stage 0	Tis	N0	M0
Stage I	T1	N0	M0
Stage II	T2	N0	M0
Stage III	T1–2	N1–2	M0
Stage IVa	T3	N0–2	M0
Stage IVb	T1–3	N0–2	M1

TNM Classification of Intrahepatic Cholangiocarcinoma

TX   Primary tumor cannot be assessed

T0   No evidence of primary tumor

T1   Solitary tumor 2 cm or less in greatest dimension without vascular invasion

T2   Solitary tumor 2 cm or less in greatest dimension with vascular invasion; or multiple tumors limited to one lobe, none more than 2 cm in greatest dimension without vascular invasion; or a solitary tumor more than 2 cm in greatest dimension without vascular invasion

T3   Solitary tumor more than 2 cm in greatest dimension with vascular invasion; or multiple tumors limited to one lobe, none more than 2 cm in greatest dimension, with vascular invasion; or multiple tumors limited to one lobe, any more than 2 cm in greatest dimension, with or without vascular invasion

T4   Multiple tumors in more than one lobe or tumor(s) involving a major branch of portal or hepatic vein(s) or invasion of adjacent organs other than the gallbladder or perforation of the visceral peritoneum

Note: For classification, the plane projecting between the bed of the gallbladder and the inferior vena cava divides the liver into 2 lobes.

NX   Regional lymph nodes cannot be assessed

N0   No regional lymph node metastasis

N1   Regional lymph node metastasis

Note: The regional lymph nodes are the hilar (i.e., those in the hepatoduodenal ligament, hepatic and periportal nodes). Regional lymph nodes also include those along the inferior vena cava, hepatic artery, and portal vein. Any lymph node involvement beyond these nodes is considered distant metastasis and should be coded as M1. Involvement of the inferior phrenic lymph nodes should also be considered M1.

MX   Distant metastasis cannot be assessed

M0   No distant metastasis

M1   Distant metastasis

Note: Metastases occur most frequently in bones and lungs. Tumors may extend through the capsule to the diaphragm.

Stage groupings	T	N	M
Stage I	T1	N0	M0
Stage II	T2	N0	M0
Stage IIIa	T3	N0	M0
Stage IIIb	T1–3	N1	M0
Stage IVa	T4	N0–1	M1
Stage IVb	T1–4	N0–1	M1

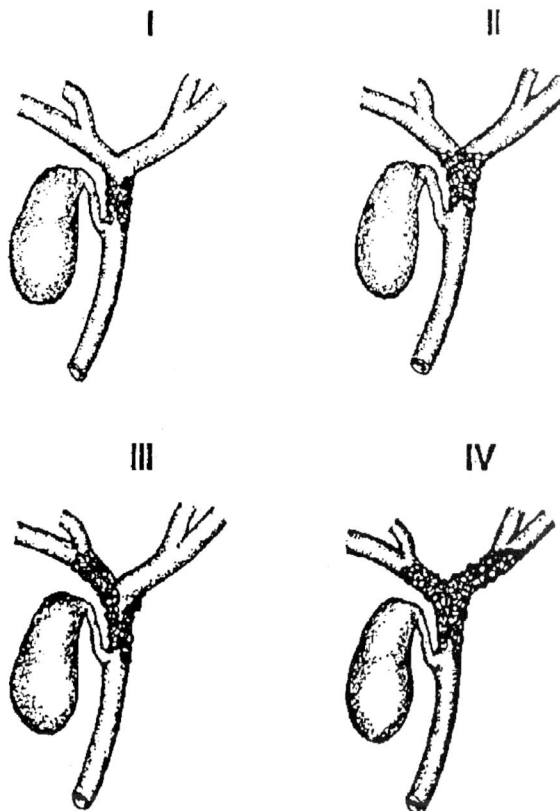

Figure 7
Bismuth classification of perihilar tumors

Gallbladder carcinoma is commonly detected at an advanced stage. In the minority of cases when the tumor is confined to the gallbladder wall (stage 1 and 2) it can be completely resected. In more advanced stages treatment is directed at palliation.

Cholangiocarcinomas are classified according to their anatomical distribution as intrahepatic, perihilar and distal extrahepatic tumors of the bile duct. Perihilar tumors have been further divided by Bismuth et al. as tumors distal to the confluence of the left and right hepatic duct (type I), tumors reaching the confluence (type II), tumors involving the common hepatic duct and either the right or the left hepatic duct (type IIIa and IIIb respectively), and tumors that are multicentric or that expand beyond the confluence into both the right and left hepatic duct (Fig. 7) [4].

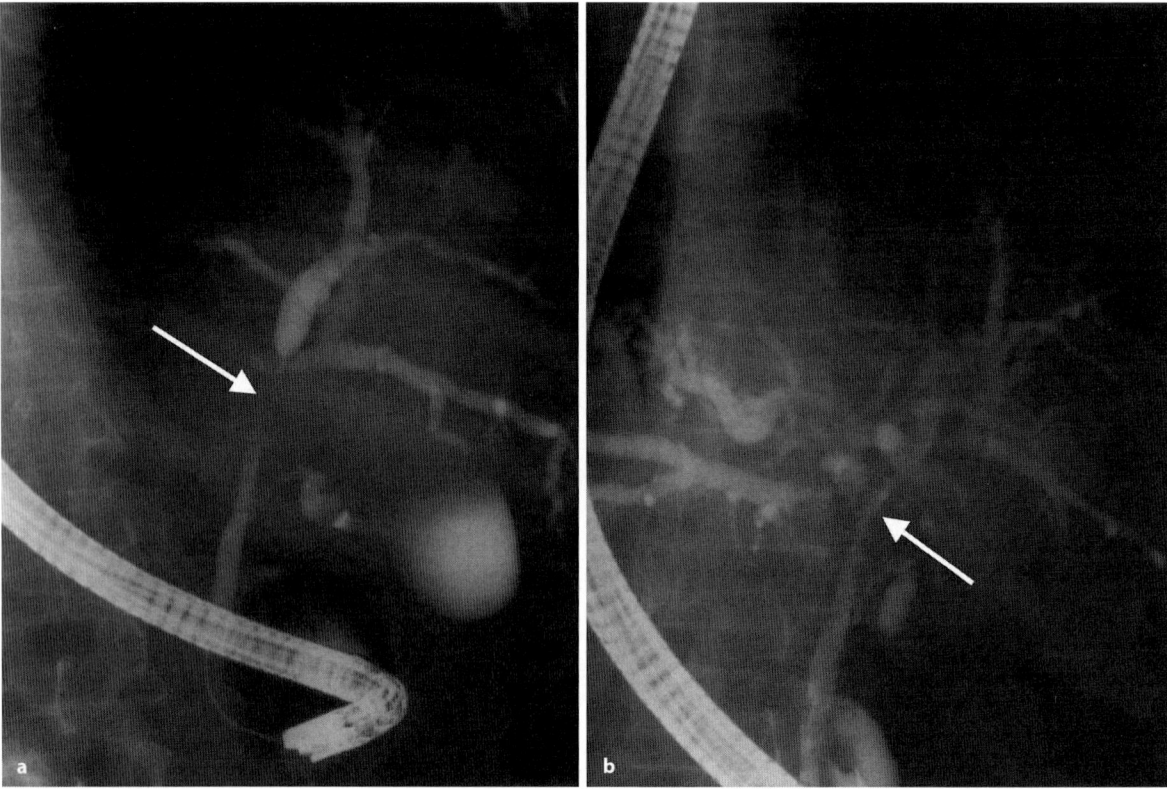

Figure 8a,b
a ERC of a bile duct carcinoma obstructing the proximal common bile duct (arrow) and bifurcation with dilatation of the intrahepatic bile ducts. **b** The stenosis has been dilated and treated by laser after intravenous application of a photosensitizing drug. Results are shown 90 days post treatment

Staging according to the TNM classification is given in tables 2 and 3. Appropriate therapy critically depends on an exact staging, which is detailed below.

Treatment

Synopsis

Surgery is the only treatment with curative intent. Palliative treatment options include maintenance of biliary or enteric passage either endoscopically or by surgical means. Radio- and chemotherapy should be further studied in clinical trials.

Endoscopy (Palliation/Resection)

Endoscopy is useful to diagnose and stage a cholangiocarcinoma and to confirm diagnosis by histology or brush cytology. In addition, endoscopy plays a crucial role in palliative treatment of inoperable malignant biliary obstruction [5]. Stents can be placed endoscopically or percutaneously to decompress obstructed bile ducts. The route of administration is usually endoscopic because external drainage is inconvenient and psychologically burdening for the patient and it may be associated with pain and bile leakage. A percutaneous approach is chosen when endoscopy has failed, as in patients with a history of partial gastrectomy or with gastric outlet obstruction. Plastic and self-expanding biliary metal stents are available. Metallic stents stay patent for longer periods but are more expensive. Plastic stents can be changed once they are occluded. However, it is prudent to do so routinely to prevent recurrent obstruction with the risk of cholangitis. Cholangitis develops in about 5% of cases in the short-term after biliary stenting and can be prevented or treated by antibiotics. Even rarer short-term complications are hemorrhage and bile leakage. The long-term complication encountered most frequently is occlusion of the stent due to tumor ingrowth or to biliary or food debris.

For palliation of multiple biliary stenosis the use of a hematoporphyrin derivative as a light sensitizer, followed 24 to 48 hours later by intraluminal photoactivation, may be a promising option. This treatment is able to improve biliary drainage and quality of life of patients (Fig. 8).

Another palliative measure is the placement of an enteric stent for gastric outlet obstruction. Although treatment of gastric outlet obstruction used to be a surgical domain, both surgical and endoscopic approaches have advantages and inconveniences. A general recommendation as to which approach is preferable cannot be given, because randomized studies do not exist.

Surgery

Only complete surgical resection is associated with an improved five-year-survival in biliary tract cancer. Staging of the tumor as well as the general health condition of the patient need to be considered when assessing resectability. Patient related factors that may preclude radical operation are poor performance status, liver cirrhosis or severe cardiopulmonary disease. In many instances the tumor leads to a deterioration in the patient's health, problems including cachexia, cholangitis with sepsis or reduced liver function due to cholestasis. Some of these may be reversible preoperatively. Obviously, tumor spread to distant sites, into blood vessels or to regional lymph nodes preclude curative surgery.

Localized gallbladder carcinoma that is confined to the gallbladder wall can be completely resected. In about 1% of cases, carcinoma is found incidentally in gallbladder specimens removed laparoscopically. Survival rates decline sharply once the cancer invades the muscle layer or beyond. Therefore, T2-tumors should always be re-

moved in an open surgical procedure that includes regional lymph nodes. Patients with stage III-IV gallbladder carcinoma (except T1–2 N1) have cancer that cannot be completely resected. Radical cholecystectomy including partial hepatectomy is sometimes performed, but with more aggressive surgery morbidity and mortality have been high.

Intrahepatic cholangiocarcinoma is best treated by partial hepatectomy. Even when macroscopic complete resection is achieved, recurrence rates approximate 50% during the first 12 months post-operation. Orthotopic liver transplantation yielded disappointing results and has been abandoned as a routine option in cholangiocarcinoma.

Independent of the tumor location, the goal of surgical intervention in perihilar and extrahepatic cholangiocarcinoma is radical resection of the tumor-bearing bile duct and complete removal of lymph nodes in the hepatoduodenal ligament and of those adjacent to the common hepatic artery. In perihilar carcinoma, treatment depends on the Klatskin type of tumor. In type II and III carcinomas an extended partial hepatectomy is usually performed with Roux-en-Y hepaticojejunostomy [6]. Type I carcinoma can be exceptionally treated by resection of the hepatic confluence and hilus followed by reconstruction of a biliodigestive anastomosis. Resection of the extrahepatic duct together with hilar resection is recommended for tumors in the mid part of the extrahepatic common bile duct. A partial duodenopancreatectomy (Whipple's procedure) is the standard operation for distal bile duct cancer.

Type IV perihilar carcinomas and/or tumors with vascular infiltration or advanced liver metastasis are considered nonresectable. In this situation a biliodigestive bypass or gastroenteric anastomosis may be indicated to palliate symptoms.

Radiotherapy

Radiotherapy has been tested in the adjuvant setting as well as a palliative treatment. A single prospective trial could not demonstrate a survival advantage for postoperative external radiotherapy [7]. In retrospective uncontrolled studies, single patients benefited from either external or intraluminal radiotherapy. Some report increases in survival compared to historical controls or in a non-randomized control group. In general, therapy was well tolerated. But due to a lack of randomized trials, no definitive conclusion can be drawn about the role of radiotherapy in multimodal therapy of biliary tract cancer [8].

Chemotherapy

Chemotherapy is not a routine option in the management of biliary tract cancer. A variety of chemotherapeutic agents have been studied either as a monotherapy or as combination chemotherapy via different routes of administration. Despite anecdotal reports of survival advantages and symptomatic relief, most clinical trials were uncontrolled and involved only small numbers of patients. Response rates did not exceed 30% and were not sustained. The most commonly used drugs were 5-fluorouracil, mitomycin C and doxorubicin both in the adjunct therapy to surgery and in palliative treatment of advanced disease. A single randomized trial could demonstrate a non-significant survival advantage for patients treated with 5-fluorouracil, leucovorin and etoposide in a small number of subjects with advanced disease. Data are also scarce for adjuvant treatment following a successful operation. Thus, patients with advanced biliary tract cancer present a difficult problem to clinicians as to whether to choose a strictly supportive approach or to expose patients to the side effects of a potentially ineffective treatment [8].

Radiochemotherapy

The rationale for radiochemotherapy is supported by preclinical trials and by the effectiveness of this treatment modality in other types of carcinoma like rectal carcinoma. Survival times in a number of non-standardized trials varied widely between 8 and 30 months. Promising results were reported for neoadjuvant radiochemotherapy of extrahepatic cholangiocarcinoma and of gallbladder carcinoma. However, prospective randomized trials are lacking to confirm these results.

Prognosis and Follow-Up

Prognosis of biliary tract cancers is poor. Only complete surgical resection of the tumor is associated with an increased five-year survival.

In gallbladder carcinoma, the mean five-year survival for all stages is between 5 and 10%. Obviously, variation is exceedingly high when comparing patients with resectable stage 0 or 1 disease to those with inoperable tumors. Patients with intrahepatic cholangiocarcinoma have a five-year survival between 10 and 45%. Median survival varies between 18 and 30 months. Even after curative resection, recurrence rates after 12 months can be as high as 60%.

Median survival for patients with perihilar cholangiocarcinoma has been reported to be from 12 to 24 months. A more aggressive surgical approach may yield better results. Prognosis is limited by the occurrence of complications like cholangitis and liver failure more than by tumor progression or metastasis. Five-year survival rates in patients with distal extrahepatic cholangiocarcinoma vary between 15 and 25%.

Due to the lack of effective therapies for recurrent disease no standardized follow-up of patients whose tumor had been resected is recommended. Individual follow-up to prevent or treat complications is necessary. This may be achieved by clinical examination, laboratory test results and transabdominal ultrasound. When a biliary stent has been placed to relieve obstructive jaundice, changing plastic stents at three month intervals is recommended, while metal stents may remain in place as long as they stay patent.

Screening patients with risk factors is not recommended. Screening of patients with gallstones is not effective because gallstones are highly prevalent, incidence of carcinoma is rather low and screening methods are not sufficiently sensitive. Patients with primary sclerosing cholangitis may be screened by repeated measurements of the tumor marker CA 19–9, although its value is disputable.

Future Perspectives

Since only early detection of disease offers a chance of cure some hope is set on the development of new diagnostic tools. This may include molecular markers or a panel of markers that offer higher accuracy in the diagnosis of early stage cancer. Imaging modalities like PET may be a valuable supplementation. Endoscopic and intraluminal ultrasound may prove helpful in preoperative staging.

Goals in optimizing therapy will include chemopreventive agents currently being studied in other types of cancer, that could be assessed in a population at risk. Adjuvant therapy after resection of high-risk cancer is imminent and prospective randomized studies should be performed. In palliative treatment, the field is wideopen for new treatment modalities. Among them angiogenesis inhibitors or immunotherapies will be tested in clinical trials. In addition, when the complex molecular carcinogenesis of biliary tract cancer becomes clearer, this may lead to the development of targeted therapies.

References

1. Landis SH, Murray T, Bolden S, Wingo PA (1998) Cancer statistics, 1998. CA Cancer J Clin 48:6–29
2. Broome U, Olsson R, Loof L et al. (1996) Natural history and prognostic factors in 305 swedish patients with primary sclerosing cholangitis. Gut 38:610–615
3. Holzinger F, Z´graggen K, Büchler MW (1999) Mechanisms of biliary carcinogenesis: a pathogenetic multi-stage cascade towards cholangiocarcinoma. Ann Oncol 10 Suppl 4:122–126
4. Bismuth H, Nakache R, Diamond T (1992) Management strategies in resection for hilar choangiocarcinoma. Ann Surg 215:31–38
5. Shah SK, Mutignani M, Costamagna G (2002) Therapeutic biliary endoscopy. Endoscopy 34:43–53
6. Jarnagin WR, Fong Y, DeMatteo RP et al. (2001) Staging, resectability, and outcome in 225 patients with hilar cholangiocarcinoma. Ann Surg 234:507–519
7. Pitt HA, Nakeeb A, Abrams RA et al. (1995) Perihilar cholangiocarcinoma: postoperative radiotherapy does not improve survival. Ann Surg 221:778–797
8. Hejna M, Pruckmayer M, Raderer M (1998) The role of chemotherapy and radiation in the management of biliary cancer: a review of the literature. Eur J Cancer 34:977–986

17 Benign Tumors of the Biliary System

K. Schoppmeyer, K. Caca, J. Mössner

Summary

Benign tumors of the bile ducts are a rarity, while tumors of the gallbladder are more frequently encountered. Benign lesions of the gallbladder are usually detected incidentally, whereas in the bile ducts they may cause obstructive jaundice. The latter should be resected whenever possible, due to the difficulty of differentiating benign lesions from early cancer.

Epidemiology

Polypoid lesions of the gallbladder of different histology affect approximately 5% of the adult population. Most of them are benign cholesterol polyps. Benign bile duct tumors are very uncommon, though their incidence might be underestimated due to their silent clinical appearance. In a series of patients with symptomatic hilar lesions, 15% were benign lesions [1]. Biliary cystadenoma is an uncommon tumor that typically occurs in adults, especially in women. But no reliable epidemiologic data are available about the frequency of these lesions in the general population.

Etiology

The etiology of benign biliary lesions is in good part a matter of speculation. Since some benign tumors are believed to be precursors of malignancy, it can be assumed that they arise due to the same conditions as carcinoma. This may apply to gallbladder polyps as well as bile duct adenomas, which may be associated with gallstones or chronic inflammation of the biliary tree. However, others believe that bile duct adenoma is a reactive process to injury rather than a true neoplasm. Developmental anomaly may be still another condition leading to bile duct adenoma or to bile duct hamartoma, also known as von Meyenburg complex. Finally, the cause of biliary cystadenoma is not known. It may represent a congenital anomaly of the biliary tree.

Symptoms and Clinical Signs

Benign tumors of the gallbladder are almost always diagnosed incidentally. Right upper quadrant discomfort or elevated transaminases caused by unrelated conditions like gallstones may lead to a diagnostic exploration discovering benign gallbladder lesions. Only in rare cases when a benign lesion is located in the gallbladder infundibulum may it cause intermittent symptomatic gallbladder distension.

Patients with biliary cystadenoma may complain about chronic abdominal pain. Biliary hamartomas and adenomas are typically discovered incidentally at imaging studies, during surgery, or at autopsy. Papillary adenomas and the rare granular cell tumors of the bile duct cause obstructive jaundice and thus pose a serious problem in the differential diagnosis to cholangiocarcinoma.

Diagnostics

Synopsis

Standard imaging techniques for biliary tract lesions

▶ Ultrasound, endoscopic ultrasound
▶ Cholangiography (endoscopic retrograde cholangiography, percutaneous transhepatic cholangiography)
▶ Computed tomography
▶ Magnetic resonance imaging (MRI), MR cholangiography and MR angiography.

Imaging studies often reveal benign lesions incidentally. Gallbladder polyps are usually detected by abdominal ultrasound. Due to their immobility they can be distinguished from gallstones. Ultrasound is also an invaluable tool to determine polyp size and number and to follow up their growth, both discriminating features between benign and malignant polyps. While adenomas of the bile duct are difficult to visualize by ultrasound, multiple hamartomas may mimic small abscesses or diffuse metastasis. These alterations must then be further differentiated by clinical and laboratory findings. Cystadenomas can be differentiated from simple cysts because they often have a visible wall and internal septations. Obstructing papillary adenomas may present with indirect signs of a mass-forming tumor, i.e. bile duct dilatation, the distribution of dilated segments giving a clue as to the location of the tumor.

Endoscopic ultrasound allows closer study of extrahepatic bile duct and gallbladder lesions. Intraluminal ultrasound of the bile duct may demonstrate a mass lesion confined to the epithelium. Any sign of infiltration precludes the assumption of a benign lesion.

Contrast enhanced CT scan supplements information gained by ultrasound. A bile duct hamartoma or adenoma usually appears as a small, well-defined mass that demonstrates little if any enhancement after administration of contrast medium. In contrast, biliary cystadenoma appears well defined and cystic but the cyst walls enhance after intravenous administration of contrast material. Solitary papillary adenomas usually occur in the common hepatic duct and less commonly arise in the right or left hepatic duct. Most papillary adenomas are small, intraductal masses that are not visualized by CT.

At MR imaging, the appearance of a bile duct hamartoma or adenoma is nonspecific. The MR imaging appearance of biliary cystadenoma varies depending on the protein content of the fluid and the presence of an intracystic soft-tissue component [2].

Cholangiography is performed in cases where a biliary mass causes bile duct obstruction. It is useful to further classify the lesions, to detect multiple locations, to take biopsy samples and to decompress a symptomatic stenosis. The preoperative determination, as to whether a biliary tumor is benign or malignant, is the ultimate goal in order to plan the therapeutic strategy.

Histological Classification and Molecular Genetics

Synopsis

Tumors derived from the epithelium are adenomas, cystadenomas and papillary adenomas. Tumors originating from nonepithelial structures are very infrequent.

Benign tumors of the gallbladder are histologically composed of various structures including cholesterol polyps, adenomyomatous hyperplasia, xanthogranulomatous cholecystitis and heterotopias. Cholesterol polyps are the most common masses in the gallbladder apart from stones. They represent cholesterol deposits in the lamina propria that may over time protrude into the gallbladder lumen. While cholesterol polyps do not degenerate into malignant tumors, true gallbladder adenomas may be transformed, in analogy with other adenomas in the gastrointestinal tract.

Biliary cystadenoma is a multilocular cystic liver mass that originates in the bile duct and usually resides in the right hepatic lobe. Histologically, the cystic mass is lined with cuboid or columnar epithelium and contains proteinaceous fluid. Intracystic soft-tissue components may be present as well as focal calcifications. Malignant transformation is not uncommon and therefore histologic examination of the whole tumor is obligatory.

Bile duct hamartoma, also known as von Meyenburg complex, is a benign tumor composed of disorganized bile ducts of various sizes surrounded by fibrocollagenous stroma. It usually occurs as a multilocular mass. Bile duct adenoma is usually a well circumscribed, subcapsular mass ranging from 1 mm to 1 cm in diameter. It is composed of small bile ducts and various amounts of inflammatory reaction and fibrosis. It is often difficult to distinguish a bile duct adenoma from a hamartoma at pathologic analysis.

Papillary adenomas most often arise in the common hepatic duct as a solitary lesion. They may sometimes spread as multiple lesions into the right and left hepatic duct. Histologically, they are composed of columnar epithelium supported by connective tissue from the lamina propria with capillary fronds extending into the lumen.

Lesions originating from nonepithelial structures are granular cell tumors, leiomyomas, neurofibromas and ganglioneuromas. They are histologically composed identically to their counterparts in other locations of the body. Manifestation in the biliary tree is a rarity.

Staging

Synopsis

By definition all benign tumors do not infiltrate their vicinity and do not metastasize. They may grow as multiple lesions, such as in biliary papillomatosis.

Treatment

Synopsis

Standard treatment: Surgery.

Surgical resection is the standard treatment for benign biliary tumors. Under certain conditions, observation of gallbladder polyps seems justifiable. However, bile duct tumors of uncertain pathology should undergo early resection in view of treatment limitations and the dismal prognosis of established cancers.

Endoscopy (Palliation/Resection)

Endoscopy is mainly diagnostic in the treatment of benign biliary lesions. Endoscopic retrograde cholangiography may be performed prior to cholecystectomy when cholangiolithiasis is a concern. In inoperable patients with biliary obstruction, biliary drainage can be achieved endoscopically. The same procedure may be chosen when septic cholangitis has complicated bile duct obstruction by a benign tumor. Definitive surgical therapy can then be performed later under safer circumstances.

Surgery

Polypoid lesions of the gallbladder are a frequent incidental finding. Although the majority of them are benign, there is a risk of malignant transformation. To distinguish benign from malignant polyps can be challenging. Discriminating features have been proposed to weigh the risk of malignant transformation and thus to proceed with surgery. Resection is recommended in symptomatic patients, patients over 50 years of age, or those with polyps greater than 10 mm in diameter, or associated with gallstones or polyp growth on serial imaging studies [3]. The standard technique is cholecystectomy, either open or laparoscopic.

Benign bile duct lesions should be resected when they are symptomatic. In addition, in the case of an incidental lesion, differential diagnosis between benign and malignant lesions will never be unequivocal without histology. Every effort should be made, however, to establish the most likely diagnosis preoperatively, so as to avoid an unnecessary extensive operation with potentially debilitating consequences [4].

Biliary cystadenoma as well as papillary adenoma carries a risk of malignant transformation. Multiple lesions can occur with both entities. When the intraoperative finding and frozen sections confirm a benign mass, the least extensive operation should be performed. Bile duct hamartomas may coalesce into larger masses and be confounded with diffuse metastasis or microabscesses. The clinical aspect may then control the decision. An incidental finding of an asymptomatic lesion makes the so-called von Meyenburg complex likely, which justifies no further therapy.

Prognosis and Follow-Up

Most gallbladder polyps are benign, although malignant transformation is a concern. Therefore, in high-risk situations cholecystectomy is the treatment of choice. When a lesion turns out to be benign histologically, no follow-up is required. If watchful waiting has been chosen at first, individual follow-up intervals depending on the risk of malignant transformation and the operability of the patient are warranted.

Bile duct adenomas tend to recur after resection and malignant transformation has been reported. Therefore, histologic confirmation is required. In biliary cystadenoma, recurrence after surgical resection is common and malignant transformation to cystadenocarcinoma can occur. There have been reports that multiple bile duct hamartomas are associated with cholangiocarcinoma. Papillary adenomas also demonstrate a high rate of recurrence and some authors report malignant transformation.

No structured follow-up is recommended after resection of a tumor despite a significant rate of recurrence, because malignant transformation is a rare event.

Future Perspectives

Elucidating the molecular pathway from benign biliary lesions to carcinoma will help to develop new tools in differential diagnosis. Novel imaging techniques including endoscopic ultrasound and MR imaging may further aid in distinguishing between benign and malignant biliary tract lesions. The role of other procedures such as positron emission tomography in the combination of diagnostic measures used to detect and stage biliary tumors has not yet been defined.

References

1. Gerhards MF, Vos P, van Gulik TM, Rauws EA, Bosma A, Gouma DJ (2001) Incidence of benign lesions in patients resected for suspicious hilar obstruction. Br J Surg 88:48–51
2. Levy AD, Murakata LA, Abbott RM, Rohrmann CA Jr. (2002) From the archives of the AFIP. Benign tumors and tumorlike lesions of the gallbladder and extrahepatic bile ducts: radiologic-pathologic correlation. Radiographics 22:387–413
3. Myers RP, Shaffer EA, Beck PL (2002) Gallbladder polyps: epidemiology, natural history and management. Can J Gastroenterol 16:187–194
4. Friess H, Holzinger F, Liao Q, Büchler MW (2001) Surveillance of premalignant disease of the pancreatico-biliary system. Best Pract Clin Gastroenterol 15:285–300

18 Malignant Tumors of the Ampulla of Vater

W. SCHEPPACH, H.-J. GASSEL, J. G. MUELLER

Summary

About half the ampullary carcinomas cause jaundice early and are thus diagnosed at a resectable stage. Ampullectomy is acceptable for stage 0-I tumors. Whipple's operation is appropriate for patients with stage II, III and IV tumors showing pancreatic but not extrapancreatic infiltration. These patients should be devoid of any other significant comorbidity. Palliative endoscopic stenting of the bile duct alleviates symptoms associated with obstructive jaundice in patients with advanced cancer (stage IV/extrapancreatic infiltration, distant metastases) or inoperability. At present there is no indication for multimodal treatments (e.g., radiotherapy, chemotherapy, radiochemotherapy). The prognosis of ampullary carcinoma is better than that of pancreatic or cholangiocellular cancer. The single most important factor predicting survival is disease stage at the time of diagnosis.

Epidemiology

Recent versions of the International Classification of Diseases classify biliary tract cancers as cancers of the gallbladder, the extrahepatic bile ducts, and of the ampulla of Vater. These three neoplasms differ in their descriptive epidemiology and should be considered separately in clinical investigations. According to limited data from nine cancer registries worldwide, cancer of the ampulla of Vater is the least common of the three entities. In Cote-d'Or, France, the incidence rates are 0.38 and 0.27 per 100.000 male and female inhabitants, respectively. Although cancer of the ampulla of Vater remains a rare tumor in both sexes, the incidence is slightly higher in men. An increase of the incidence rate over time (from 0.19 in the period of 1976–1980 to 0.59 in the period of 1991–1995) has been noted in men whereas in women, they have remained stable [1]. The incidence of this rare tumor also increases with age which limits the options for a radical resection in elderly patients.

Etiology

Environmental risk factors of ampullary cancers are poorly understood. In a case-control study conducted in Los Angeles County, California, the risk of cancer of the extrabiliary tract and of the ampulla of Vater increased with smoking cigarettes or cigars/pipes. For both men and women, risks increased twofold or more among those who had been smoking cigarettes for 50 or more pack-years [2]. A similar risk factor is found in adenocarcinomas of the pancreas although, on the basis of histology and clinical behaviour, a clear distinction has to be made between pancreatic and ampullary neoplasms.

A genetic background is found in periampullary adenomas and adenocarcinomas complicating familial adenomatous polyposis (FAP) described elsewhere.

Symptoms and Clinical Signs

Jaundice is the leading symptom of ampullary cancer often occuring early in the course of disease. Under these circumstances localized cancer is amenable to radical surgical resection. Jaundice may be accompanied by acholic stools, bilirubinuria and pruritus in severe cases. Malignant obstruction of the biliary and pancreatic ducts rarely leads to clinically manifest cholangitis or pancreatitis.

Physical examination is unrevealing in most patients as tumors are usually small at the time of diagnosis. Rarely, the gallbladder may be palpable (Courvoisier's sign) due to biliary obstruction. In lean patients suffering from advanced cancer, masses may be palpable in the right upper abdominal quadrant (primary tumor) and on the surface of the liver (metastases). Pallor and melena may indicate upper intestinal bleeding from friable tumors.

Diagnostics

Synopsis

Standard imaging techniques for detection and staging of ampullary cancer

▸ Transabdominal ultrasound
▸ Endoscopic retrograde cholangiopancreatography (ERCP)
▸ Endoscopic ultrasound (EUS)
▸ Spiral computerized tomography (CT)

Laboratory tests show varying degrees of cholestasis by increased activities of serum alkaline phosphatase (AP), gamma glutamyltranspeptidase (γGT) and glutamate dehydrogenase (GLDH), with or without hyperbilirubinemia. Serum transaminases may also be elevated, usually less than the cholestatic enzymes. Obstruction of the main pancreatic duct may be reflected by increases of serum amylase and lipase levels. There is no serum tumor marker specific for ampullary neoplasms; however, carbohydrate antigen (CA) 19–9 may be mildly elevated secondary to cholestasis. Gastrointestinal bleeding of low intensity leads to iron-deficiency anemia and a positive fecal occult blood test.

Standard imaging techniques for the diagnosis of ampullary neoplasms include transabdominal ultrasound, endoscopic retrograde cholangiopancreatography (ERCP), endoscopic ultrasound (EUS), and spiral computerized tomography (CT). The strength of conventional transabdominal ultrasound certainly lies in the detection of a uniformly dilated intra- and extrahepatic bile duct. Sonography is less reliable with regard to the detection of a duodenal mass, lymph node involvement, or portal venous infiltration, but it can visualize liver metastases from ampullary tumors greater than 0.5–1 cm.

A definite diagnosis is usually made by endoscopy using a side-viewing ERCP scope. When taking biopsies (or a brush cytology from the bile duct) the endoscopist

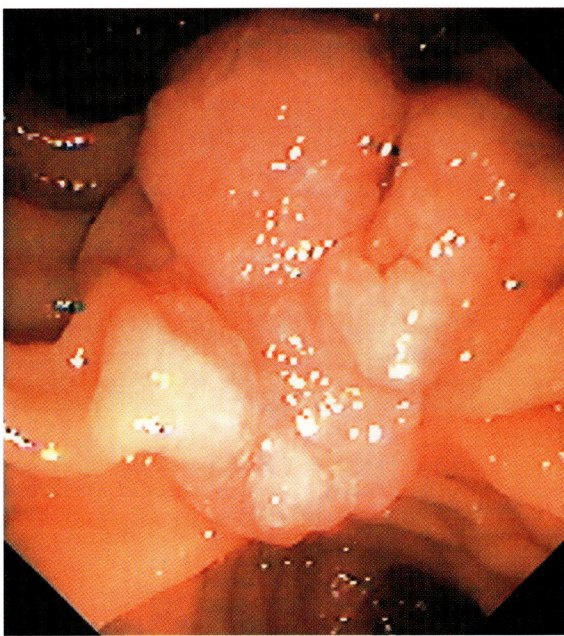

Figure 1
Adenocarcinoma of the ampulla of Vater with infiltration of the adjacent duodenal wall (endoscopic aspect)

should take the diagnosis of the pathologist into account and be aware that adenocarcinoma may be coexistent. The infiltration of the duodenal wall and the obstruction of the duodenal lumen are easily recognized during endoscopy. Usually, a small papillotomy is performed and, after radiological visualization of both ducts, a plastic stent (preferably 10 F) is endoscopically inserted into the bile duct. Thus, biliary decompression can be achieved preoperatively provided the patient is a candidate for surgery (Fig. 1).

Otherwise, biliary stenting is considered the definite procedure to alleviate obstructive jaundice. Compression of the bile or pancreatic duct by the tumor as well as the prestenotic dilatation can be visualized by magnetic resonance cholangiopancreatography (MRCP), if the major duodenal papilla cannot be cannulated at ERCP, however, without the option of therapeutic intervention.

Endoscopic ultrasound (EUS) has been found to be especially effective for local tumor staging of ampullary carcinomas [3]. It is superior to abdominal ultrasound

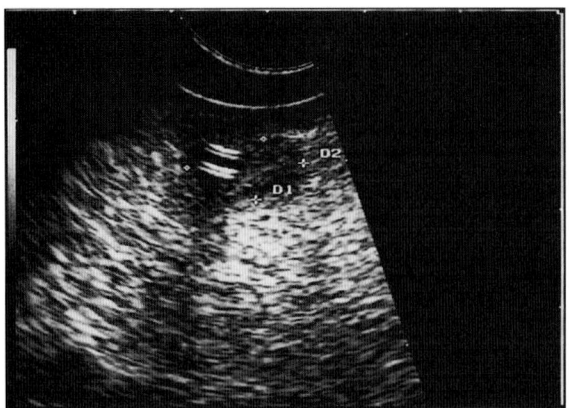

Figure 2
Endosonographic appearance of a small ampullary adenocarcinoma: A hypoechoic mass (1.2×0.6 cm) is infiltrating into the head of pancreas. A plastic stent marks the location of the common bile duct

and computerized tomography in determining tumor size (T stage) as well as infiltration into the pancreas. However, the presence of an endobiliary stent at EUS may result in understaging especially T2/T3 tumors. Hence, stent placement should follow EUS examination, if possible. Taken together, EUS is the best technique to demonstrate portal venous infiltration by the tumor. However, arterial encasement is less reliably detected by EUS. With regard to the extent of lymph node involvement (N stage), EUS and CT are complementary procedures: EUS is probably superior in identifying lymph nodes close to the head of pancreas, whereas CT has advantages in the evaluation of distant lymph nodes. The EUS technique clearly improves the assessment of tumor resectability and decreases the need for explorative laparotomy (Fig. 2).

Spiral CT scan has an established role as a staging procedure in pancreatic and ampullary malignancies. Compared with ultrasound techniques, it is less observer dependent. It clearly distinguishes duodenal masses of 1 cm or more, tumor infiltration into surrounding tissues, dilated bile ducts, lymph nodes of more than 1 cm in diameter (suspected to be metastatic), and hepatic metastases. More recently, magnetic resonance imaging (MRI) has been used with the same indications as CT. However, its definite role in the staging of ampullary tumors remains to be defined. Arterial angiography and CT arterial portography are not recommended for rou-

tine staging of ampullary carcinomas. Preoperative laparoscopy which has been suggested in T3/T4 gastric and pancreatic cancers has not been shown to give additional information concerning resectability of ampullary neoplasms.

Histological Classification and Molecular Genetics

Synopsis

Histology of Malignant Ampullary Neoplasms

Over 98% of all malignant ampullary tumors are adenocarcinomas. Carcinoid tumors, sarcomas, and malignant lymphomas together account for less than 2%. Because of their initial exophytic growth pattern, adenocarcinomas may cause early clinical signs due to obstruction of the common bile duct, giving the patient a chance for early detection of the tumor and potentially curative surgery. Chronic ulcerations with regenerative epithelial changes, and distortion of the complex epithelial-muscular anatomy by granulation tissue in papillitis stenosans may mask an underlying malignant tumor and cause considerable delay in diagnosis.

Anatomically, the ampulla of Vater joins the epithelium of the bile duct, the pancreatic duct and the duodenum. As tumors arising from these anatomically distinct epithelial cells share many morphological features and have a common clinical presentation, they are usually considered together. However, they may differ in their initial presentation. Carcinomas arising from the intra-ampullary region initially cause swelling of the Papilla of Vater. Histological diagnosis at this stage requires papillotomy and a biopsy taken from within the ampullary region. Only the extension of the tumor into the duodenal mucosa, will make it visible from the duodenum. Carcinomas arising from the periampullary duodenum, however are visible from the beginning, and may form a target-like mass around the Papilla of Vater. Histologically, most of these tumors represent the intestinal type of adenocarcinoma, with about 1/5 representing the pancreato-biliary type, and some exhibiting a mixed pattern [4].

The transition from adenoma to carcinoma in the intestinal type of periampullary tumors is a focal one, leaving one or more areas of adenoma in 42% of invasive ampullary carcinomas. Therefore, extensive sampling of the tumor is required to obtain the representative areas of the lesion. According to large statistics, only about 5% of periampullary epithelial tumors are pure adenomas and 95% of periampullary epithelial tumors are carcinomas or carcinomas with residual areas of adenoma [5]. Therefore, further sampling or local complete resection of the lesion should by initiated, if a biopsy specimen yields the diagnosis of adenoma without signs of malignancy, In difficult cases, the final diagnosis may be made only intraoperatively after open wedge biopsy following duodenotomy. With increasing T stage and degree of malignancy, the frequency of residual adenoma in a carcinoma decreases.

Ampullary adenocarcinomas may spread by local invasive growth, by intraductal growth in the common bile and/or pancreatic duct, as well as via the lymphatic and hematogenous route. The biology of peri-ampullary carcinomas may differ from that of adenocarcinomas of the pancreas, since patients with periampullary carcinomas with regional lymph node metastases have a better prognosis than patients with pancreatic adenocarcinomas without lymph node metastases. Among the pancreato-biliary type adenocarcinomas, two subgroups require special attention. One of them consists of tumors with an invasive and an intraductal spread. The intraductal component may exhibit a flat (dysplastic) or a papillary growth, and may well extend beyond the resection margins of the common bile duct or the pancreatic body. There is currently no general agreement about the optimal therapeutic procedure in these cases. The other subgroup includes well differentiated tumors, forming regular glands with or without minimal cellular atypia. These tumors can be diagnosed only in larger resection specimens.

No detailed investigation is available on the molecular differences between the intestinal and the pancreato-biliary type of periampullary carcinomas. With regard to the intestinal type, there is some evidence that ampullary carcinogenesis follows an adenoma-to-carcinoma sequence, similar to that found in cancers of the colorectum. Adenoma and adenocarcinoma of the duodenum and periampullary carcinoma occur in 60–90% of patients with FAP and may be a life-threatening complication in FAP patients even after total colectomy. Somatic APC gene mutations, 5q loss of heterozygosity and ras mutations are present at early stages, whereas p53 inactivation and 17p loss of heterozygosity occur with progression of malignancy. It has been shown that some of these molecular events are associated with a poor prognosis (e.g., p53 overexpression, microsatellite stability, chromosome 17p loss of heterozygosity) [6].

Staging

Synopsis

TNM classification of cancers of the ampulla of Vater

T	**Primary tumor**
TX	Minimum requirements to assess the primary tumor cannot be met
T0	No evidence of primary tumor
Tis	Carcinoma in situ
T1	Tumor limited to ampulla of Vater or sphincter of Oddi
T2	Tumor invades into duodenal wall
T3	Tumor invades 2 cm or less into the pancreas
T4	Tumor invades more than 2 cm into the pancreas or surrounding organs
N	**Regional lymph nodes**
NX	Minimum requirements to assess the regional lymph nodes cannot be met
N0	No metastases to regional lymph nodes
N1	Regional lymph node metastases
M	**Distant metastases**
MX	Minimum requirements to assess distant metastases cannot be met
M0	No distant metastases found
M1	Distant metastases

Stage groupings	T	N	M
Stage 0	Tis	N0	M0
Stage I	T1	N0	M0
Stage II	T2–3	N0	M0
Stage III	T1–3	N1	M0
Stage IV	T4	N0–1	M0
	T1–4	N0–1	M1

Pre-operative staging techniques (primarily transabdominal ultrasound, endoscopic retrograde cholangiopancreatography, endoscopic ultrasound, and spiral computerized tomography) have been described above. Despite considerable progress in the accuracy of imaging techniques in predicting tumor stage, a definite evaluation is made by the pathologist on the basis of the resection specimen.

Treatment

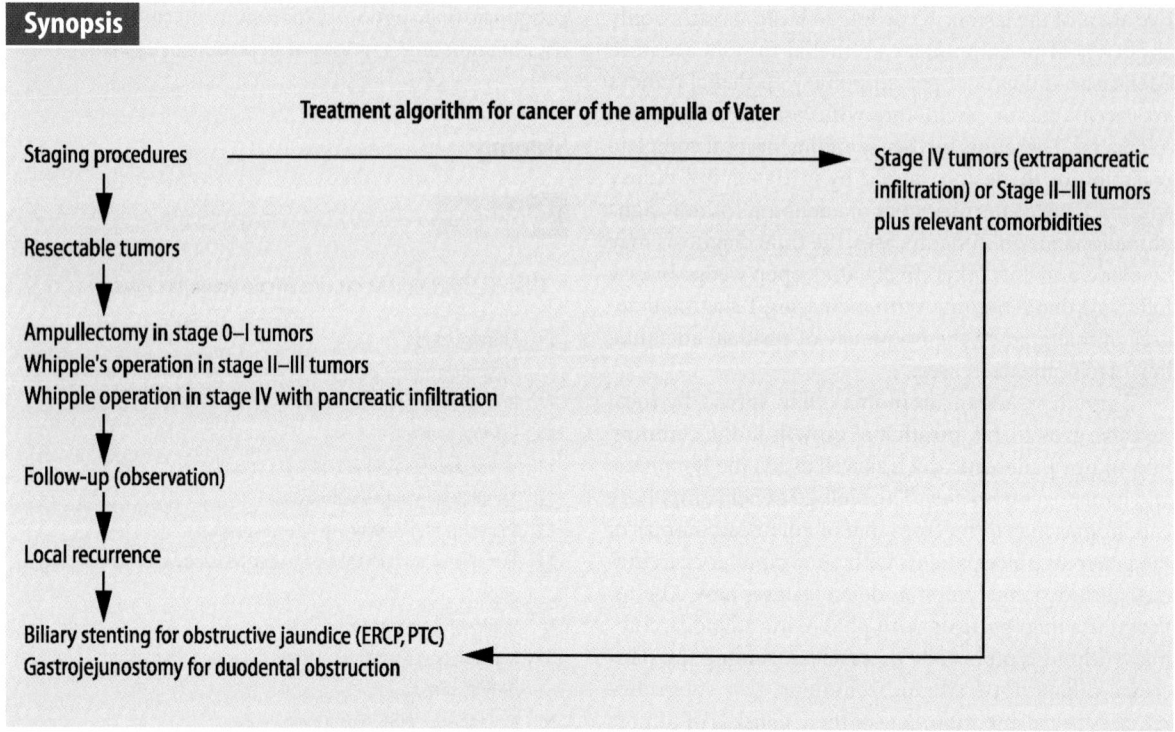

Treatment algorithm for cancer of the ampulla of Vater

Staging procedures ⟶ Stage IV tumors (extrapancreatic infiltration) or Stage II–III tumors plus relevant comorbidities

↓

Resectable tumors

↓

Ampullectomy in stage 0–I tumors
Whipple's operation in stage II–III tumors
Whipple operation in stage IV with pancreatic infiltration

↓

Follow-up (observation)

↓

Local recurrence

↓

Biliary stenting for obstructive jaundice (ERCP, PTC)
Gastrojejunostomy for duodental obstruction

Surgery

The aim of surgical treatment of cancer of the ampulla of Vater is the curative resection of the tumor. In general this can be achieved by resection of the pancreatic head performing a pancreatoduodenectomy (Whipple operation). Only in defined cases an ampullectomy may be performed as a less invasive form of treatment. The decision for surgery is dependent mainly on two factors: (a) the results of the preoperative staging, and (b) the existence of concomitant diseases (comorbid conditions). Hence, the indication for operation should be based on the results of a detailed evaluation of the preoperative tumor staging and a cardiopulmonary risk evaluation.

Patients presenting distant metastases, e.g. in the liver, lung or with peritoneal carcinosis should be excluded from resectional pancreatic surgery. Infiltration of the superior mesenteric artery, the celiac trunc or the inferior vena cava (IVC) are contraindications as well. By contrast, infiltration of the mesenteric vein or the portal vein, occasionally shown by preoperative EUS or MRI, should not lead to exclusion of the patient from pancreatic resection, since vein resection followed by either direct anastomosis or, autologous or prosthetic replacement does not increase perioperative mortality and morbidity. Hence any local tumor (T1 –T3) and tumors with more than 2 cm infiltration into the pancreas (T4) but excluding other organs are suitable for curative resection. Only patients showing either precancerous lesions or tumors limited to the ampulla of Vater or sphincter of Oddi (T1, stages 0 and I) or with an increased risk for the Whipple operation should be considered for local resection of the ampulla.

Pancreaticoduodenal resection includes cholecystectomy, transection of the common hepatic duct just below its bifurcation, transection of the pancreas left of the superior mesenteric vessels and transection of the je-junum 15 cm distal of the ligament of Treitz including complete lymphatic clearance along the superior mesenteric vessels, the portal vein, the common hepatic artery, the aorta and IVC. Despite the lack of randomized controlled studies demonstrating the necessity of such lymph dissection it is widely accepted today and recommended particularly for an exact staging. The surgical method of choice is the pylorus preserving modification of the classical Whipple operation [7]: 2–3 cm of the postpyloric duodenum are preserved in order to keep the integrity of the stomach. Several studies showed an improved motility of the stomach with better digestive function and improved quality of life without reduction of oncological radicalness. Major complications are anastomotic leakages at the hepaticojejunostomy and the development of pancreatic fistulas (5–9%) which can usually be treated without reoperation. In experienced centers the postoperative mortality rate ranges from 1.5 to 4%, the morbidity rate ranges at about 8–10% and thus justifies indication for operation in a broad sense.

Ampullary resection is a less invasive surgical procedure which includes a tumor excision after mobilization of the duodenum and duodenotomy. The procedure is finished by reimplantation of the pancreatic and bile ducts into the duodenum and closure of the duodenotomy. Duodenal leakage, biliary or pancreatic leakage, cholangitis and pancreatitis due to strictures of the ducts are rare but serious complications. Though there are no randomized trials the 5-year survival rates reported from small series are quite promising (44%) [8]. Hence, this procedure is recommendable for selected patients.

Bypass operations are recommended for patients not suitable for ampullary or pancreaticoduodenal resection. The endoscopic procedure is preferred for bilary obstructions where applicable. Otherwise a hepaticojejunal bypass operation may be indicated and combined with gastroenterostomy if gastrointestinal obstruction is diagnosed.

Endoscopy (Resection/Palliation)

In experienced centers, endoscopic snare excision of benign adenomas of the papilla of Vater has become the procedure of choice. This technique has also been applied to selected patients with small ampullary adeno-carcinomas, not considered candidates for surgery [9]. In the majority of cases, however, endoscopic intervention will be restricted to stent insertion into the bile duct after sphincterotomy; pancreatic stenting is not required. As most ampullary carcinomas grow more slowly than pancreatic carcinomas, palliative biliary stenting is associated with a prolonged clinical benefit concerning the prevention of obstructive jaundice. There is no clear evidence wether plastic or metal stents should be preferred in ampullary carcinoma. Stent insertion via percutaneous transhepatic cholangiography (PTC) remains an alternative, if access to the papilla of Vater cannot be achieved by ERCP. This more invasive two-stage procedure should be reserved only for ERCP failures.

Radiotherapy, Chemotherapy, Radiochemotherapy

Ampullary cancer is a domain for surgical and endoscopic interventions. At present, there is no clearly defined role for multimodal treatments, such as radiotherapy, chemotherapy, or radiochemotherapy. Adjuvant radiotherapy in combination with 5-fluorouracil (5-FU) has been safe and well tolerated; however, the survival benefit was small and locoregional recurrences were not prevented [10]. Preoperative chemotherapy or radiochemotherapy has been described in small series with conflicting results. Infusional 5-FU (500 mg/m^2 body surface area, day 1–5, repeated day 28) has been tried in the palliative setting with limited efficacy. To date, the use of radiotherapy, chemotherapy, or radiochemotherapy is not warranted as standard treatment of cancers of the ampulla of Vater.

Prognosis and Follow-Up

The prognosis of ampullary cancer is substantially better than that of pancreatic cancer or cholangiocarcinoma. Overall survival rates may be as high as 60% at 1 year, 30 to 55% at 3 years, and 20% at 5 years [1]. The single most important factor predicting survival is disease stage at diagnosis: The 5-year survival rate is 73% if a diagnosis was made in stage I or 7% in stage IV. Five-year survival ranges from 15% for patients with involved resection margins to 60% for those with free margins. Survival at 3 years is significantly worse for patients with positive lymph nodes (23%) than for those with free nodes (73%). The tumor biology also correlates with survival; prognosis is poor with high S-phase fraction or aneuploidy. Recently, molecular biomarkers associated with poor prognosis have been described (e.g., p53 overexpression, microsatellite stability, chromosome 17p loss of heterozygosity).

There is no well-established post-operative followup scheme with regard to ampullary carcinoma, similar to that applied in colorectal cancer. The consequences of an early detection of a local tumor recurrence are limited. In very few cases a second operation with curative intention will be successful. In young patients with a low operative risk the resection of localized hepatic metastases will be performed by most surgeons. However, there are no prospective data to support this view. Costeffective follow-up procedures will include transabdominal ultrasound and laboratory tests to detect recurrent cholestasis for the majority of patients.

Endoscopic surveillance is recommended for patients with familial adenomatous polyposis (FAP) because of the high prevalence of duodenal adenomas. Although the risk of progression from periampullary adenoma to carcinoma seems small, endoscopic surveillance with intervals of at least 3 years may be appropriate. The interval between endoscopies should be shortened to 1 year if adenomas are present.

Future Perspectives

There is an ever growing number of imaging techniques which might be useful in the detection and staging of ampullary tumors. It is not quite clear wether MRI imaging predicts tumor resectability better than spiral CT. Combining ERCP with intraductal ultrasound (IDUS) may offer advantages in the staging of small ampullary tumors. The role of positron emission tomography (PET) in the diagnosis of positive lymph nodes and distant metastases has not been established with this indication.

However, all these techniques will not be used sequentially but rather in a combination that will enable us to diagnose and stage cancer reliably and cost-effectively.

Considerable progress has been made towards the diagnosis of tumors at the pancreatico-biliary junction within the past two decades [1]. However, only a better understanding of the molecular biology of these tumors may finally lead to improved targeted systemic therapies even at inoperable stages of disease.

References

1. Benhamiche AM, Jouve JL, Manfredi S, Prost P, Isambert N, Faivre J (2000) Cancer of the ampulla of Vater: results of a 20-year population-based study. Eur J Gastroenterol Hepatol 12:75–79
2. Chow WH, McLaughlin JK, Menck HR, Menck TM (1994) Risk factors for extrahepatic bile duct cancers: Los Angeles County, California (USA). Cancer Causes Control 5:267–272
3. Cannon ME, Carpenter SL, Elta GH et al. (1999) EUS compared with CT, magnetic resonance imaging, and angiography and the influence of biliary stenting on staging accuracy of ampullary neoplasms. Gastrointest Endosc 50:27–33
4. Albores-Saavedra J, Henson DE, Klimstra DS (2000) Tumors of the Gallbladder, extrahepatic bile ducts, and ampulla of Vater. AFIP Atlas of Tumor Pathology, Third series, Fascicle 27
5. Takashima M, Ueki T, Nagai E, Yao T, Yamaguchi K, Tanaka M, Tsuneyoshi M (2000) Carcinoma of the Ampulla of Vater associated with or without adenoma: A clinico-pathologic analysis of 198 cases with reference to p53 and Ki67 immunohistochemical expressions. Mod Pathol 13:1300–1307
6. Scarpa A, DiPace C, Talamini G et al. (2000) Cancer of the ampulla of Vater: chromosome 17p allelic loss is associated with poor prognosis. Gut 46:842–848
7. Klinkenbijl JH, van der Schelling GP, Hop WC, van Pel R, Bruining HA, Jeekel J (1992) The advantages of pylorus-preserving pancreaticoduodenectomy in malignant disease of the pancreas and periampullary region. Ann Surg 216: 142–145
8. Klein P, Reingruber B, Kastl S, Dworak O, Hohenberger W (1996) Is local excision of pT1-ampullary carcinomas justified? Eur J Surg Oncol 22: 366–371
9. Park SW, Song SY, Chung JB, Lee SK, Moon YM, Kang JK, Park IS (2000) Endoscopic snare resection for tumors of the ampulla of Vater. Yonsei Med J 41:213–218
10. Kinkenbijl JH, Jeekel J, Sahmoud T et al. (1999) Adjuvant radiotherapy and 5-fluorouracil after curative resection of cancer of the pancreas and periampullary region: phase III trial of the EORTC gastrointestinal tract cancer cooperative group. Ann Surg 230:776–782

Liver

IX

19 Hepatocellular Carcinoma

M. SCHEURLEN, H.-J. BRAMBS, H.-J. GASSEL

Summary

Hepatocellular carcinoma (HCC) is one of the most frequent tumors worldwide. Its etiology is dominated by exogenous factors. Liver cirrhosis due to chronic viral hepatitis, or hereditary hemochromatosis is most frequently associated with the disease. HCC occurs in a non-cirrhotic liver only very rarely. Because the underlying disease may dominate the clinical picture, signs of an early tumor may be missed.

The most important diagnostic tools are abdominal ultrasound (US), contrast-enhanced computed tomography and magnetic resonance tomography. Alpha-fetoprotein (AFP) is elevated in up to 90% of HCC cases, but specificity is reduced because of the co-existing cirrhosis.

Surgical removal of the tumor, either by partial hepatectomy or by liver transplantation, offers the best chance for cure. However, several minimally invasive local procedures, aiming at either chemical or thermal ablation of malignant tissue under sonographic or radiological control, have also been shown to result in the complete destruction of small HCCs. Antineoplastic chemotherapy is ineffective in HCC, and no effective palliative, adjuvant or neoadjuvant strategies are available. Other therapies with tamoxifen, octreotide, megestrol or pravastatin are at present under investigation or have already been shown to be ineffective.

Epidemiology

On a global scale, HCC is one of the most frequent malignant tumors, with probably more than one million new cases per year worldwide. However, the incidence varies considerably between different countries, with the highest rates being found in East Asia (up to 36.6 per 100,000 in men) and Africa (up to 48 per 100,000 in men). In developed countries, HCC is a relatively rare tumor, but incidence rates have risen from 1.4/100,000 in the years 1976–80 to 2.4/100,000 between 1991 and 1995. In general, the incidence is higher in men than in women.

Etiology and Pathogenesis

In nearly all cases, HCC occurs in a chronically diseased liver. The main risk factors that may eventually lead to the development of HCC have been identified during the last decades. However, the exact pathogenetic mechanisms are not yet clear. As with other cancers, HCC is the result of a multistep process that includes genetic alterations in oncogenes and tumor suppressor genes as well as chromosomal deletions or translocations. The pathway to HCC may differ according to the underlying disease process. In the vast majority of cases, HCC does not develop before liver cirrhosis is present. The coexistence of chronic liver damage – characterized by hepatocellular necrosis and simultaneous liver regeneration – with a chronic inflammatory process facilitates genetic alterations and thereby HCC formation. However, the risk of an HCC differs considerably depending on the etiology of the liver cirrhosis. Cirrhoses following chronic infection with hepatitis B virus (HBV) or hepatitis C virus (HCV) bear the highest risks for HCC.

Worldwide, hepatitis B is the single most important agent leading to the development of HCC. Individuals positive for HBs antigen have a 30–100 fold risk of developing an HCC as compared to HBs antigen-negative people. Data on the global distribution of HCC show the highest prevalence in those regions of the world where hepatitis B is endemic, and where large parts of the population have acquired the infection at birth or in early childhood. In a considerable proportion of these individuals, cirrhosis develops after long-standing chronic hepatitis. Although in patients with chronic hepatitis B and concomitant liver cirrhosis the risk of HCC is about ten-fold higher than in HBV infected individuals without cirrhosis, HCC may occasionally occur without an underlying cirrhosis. Therefore, HBV itself seems to promote HCC development. However, the exact mechanisms for HBV carcinogenesis have not been elucidated so far. The virus is integrated into the genome of liver cells, and virus DNA is found in HCCs of patients with chronic hepatitis B. Direct involvement of viral genes (e.g. the x gene) or gene products into tumorigenesis has also been considered but has not been definitely proven so far.

In contrast to the developing countries of Asia and Africa, the most important cause of HCC in the industrialized regions (Japan, the USA, Western Europe) is hepatitis C infection. HCV infection becomes chronic in an estimated 80% of cases. In most infected individuals, the disease progresses very slowly over many years from chronic inflammation to fibrosis to cirrhosis. In between 10 and 20% of all hepatitis C patients, the disease will progress to liver cirrhosis, and only a minority of patients with chronic hepatitis C will die of the consequences of the infection. Among patients with HCV associated cirrhosis, 1–4% per year will develop HCC. In contrast to HBV, HCV is not integrated into the human genome, and cases of HCC without an underlying cirrhosis are very rare in patients with chronic hepatitis C. Therefore, the effect of the chronic inflammation together with the liver cirrhosis is considered to be the primary cause for cancer formation in chronic hepatitis C.

Remarkably, hepatocellular cancer is only very rarely observed in individuals with chronic autoimmune hepatitis, although this disease is also characterized by chronic inflammation and leads frequently to liver cirrhosis. A direct involvement of viral proteins in hepatic carcinogenesis in patients with chronic viral hepatitis must therefore be considered. Transgenic mice harboring either the HBx or the HCV core gene product develop HCCs frequently and at an early age. Although this observation supports the hypothesis that the hepatitis viruses and/or their gene products are directly carcinogenic, the exact mechanisms of these tumor-promoting effects are unclear. An interaction between virus gene products and tumor suppressor genes such as p53 is under discussion.

In developing countries with a warm climate, the impact of chronic viral hepatitis on the epidemiology of HCC is aggravated by the risk of an exposure to aflatoxins. These mycotoxins that are produced by the fungus

Aspergillus flavus contaminate food in hot and humid regions when grains are stored without adequate cooling. The exact pathomechanism for tumor induction by aflatoxins is not entirely clear. It has been shown that chemical reactions of host DNA with specific electrophilic derivatives of aflatoxin lead to DNA damage and mutations in tumor suppressor genes, thereby augmenting the carcinogenic effects of concomitant viral hepatitis. Molecular analysis of HCCs from South Africa and China showed an accumulation of mutations in the p53 gene. This tumor suppressor gene therefore seems to be a "hot spot" for the tumor-promoting effects of aflatoxin.

Another condition that is associated with a high risk of developing HCC is hepatic iron overload, as found particularly in hereditary hemochromatosis. Liver cirrhosis seems to be a prerequisite for tumor formation in hemochromatosis as in viral hepatitis. Only in very rare instances, has HCC been found in patients with hemochromatosis but no underlying cirrhosis. The carcinogenic mechanism of hepatic iron overload seems to be mainly the induction of oxidative stress by reactive oxygen species and free radicals due to redox cycling of iron. Other mechanisms under discussion are the facilitation of tumor growth and an immune modulation by tissue iron leading to a reduced antitumor defense.

In patients with hemochromatosis, iron depletion by repeated phlebotomy with depletion of hepatic iron does not obviate the HCC risk completely once cirrhosis has developed.

The HCC rate in alcoholic cirrhosis is considerably lower than the rates in cirrhosis induced by chronic viral hepatitis or hereditary hemochromatosis. Liver cirrhosis due to other etiologies (e.g. autoimmune hepatitis, Wilson's disease or primary biliary cirrhosis) is associated with only a low HCC risk.

Symptoms and Clinical Signs

Because the symptoms of the underlying liver disease may dominate the clinical picture, the clinical manifestation – if present at all – of a small HCC is easily missed or misinterpreted. Normally, the presence of an HCC does not become obvious until considerable tumor progression has already taken place and symptoms such as icterus, hepatomegaly and weight loss are evident. There is no typical clinical symptom of the incipient disease.

Symptoms caused by extensive tumor necrosis or spontaneous rupture of an HCC with intra-peritoneal bleeding are complications of the advanced tumor.

Metastatic spreading of the tumor occurs first within the liver, leading to multifocal growth that in up to 40% of the cases is already present at the time of diagnosis. Extrahepatic metastases are usually found in local lymph nodes, the peritoneum, the lung and the skeletal system.

As in other malignant diseases, paraneoplastic symptoms may also occur in patients with HCC (Table 1). These symptoms may precede the clinical manifestation of the actual tumor. Of special importance among these paraneoplastic symptoms are polycythemia and symptomatic hypoglycemia in 10% and 5% of the patients, respectively. Polyglobulia is thought to be the result of paraneoplastic erythropoietin production by the tumor. If observed in a patient with liver cirrhosis, this symptom should prompt the search for a hepatocellular carcinoma undetected so far.

Diagnostics

Synopsis

Diagnostic Procedures in HCC

Test	Sensitivity	Specificity
Serum AFP		
– Cutoff value 100 ng/ml	++	(+)
– Cutoff value 1000 ng/ml	(+)	++
Ultrasound		
– Conventional	++	++
– Contrast-enhanced	+++	+++
MRT	+++	+++
CT (contrast-enhanced)	+++	+++

Laboratory Parameters

No hematological or clinical chemical parameters of routine laboratory testing are specific for HCC. Transaminases, alkaline phosphatase and/or LDH may increase gradually with tumor growth. In a subgroup of cases, erythrocytosis due to extrarenal production of erythropoietin may occur, leading the attention to the underlying neoplastic process.

Table 1

Paraneoplastic symptomes in patients with HCC

Hematologic	Polycythemia (erythrocytosis)
	Hemophagocytic syndrome
	Hypereosinophilia
Endocrine system	Hypoglycemia
	Cushing syndrome
	Hyperestrogenemia
	Hyperthyroidism
	Carcinoid syndrome
Metabolic	Porphyria
	Hypercalcemia
	Hypophosphatemia
	Hypercholesterolemia
Neurologic/	Encephalomyelitis
Musculoskeletal	Chronic demyelinating
	polyradiculoneuropathy
	Polymyositis
	Multifocal necrotizing leukoencephalopathy
	Polyarthritis
Cutaneous	Dermatomyositis
	Lichen myxedematosus
	Sign of Leser-Trelat
	Pityriasis rotunda
Other	Arterial hypertension
	Thrombophlebitis migrans

Tumor Markers

To improve the prognosis of hepatocellular carcinoma, diagnosis at an early and potentially curable state is of the utmost importance. For the screening of high-risk groups, but also to facilitate the definition of suspicious focal lesions within the liver, a tumor marker with a high sensitivity and specificity for HCC is required. Unfortunately, no such tumor marker is available at present. In clinical routine, AFP is most frequently used. AFP is a glycoprotein with a molecular weight of 72 kD that is produced in large amounts until after birth, when its serum concentration drops to a maximum of 5 ng/ml for the rest of life in healthy individuals.

In 50–90% of patients with HCC, serum levels of AFP are elevated, depending on tumor size and type. In up to 46% of patients with small HCCs measuring less than 5 cm, only moderately elevated AFP levels

(<400 ng/ml) are found. Hepatoblastoma is characterized by very high serum levels, mostly above 1000 ng/ml, while in fibrolamellar HCC, AFP is within the normal range in most cases. The specificity of AFP is reduced by the fact that this marker can also be elevated in benign liver diseases. In chronic liver disease, especially in chronic viral hepatitis, fluctuating rises of AFP to moderate levels (up to 100 ng/ml) are frequently observed, and are often associated with increased inflammatory activity. During flare-ups of viral hepatitis or after liver resection, very high AFP levels are occasionally found (up to greater than 1000 ng/ml). If the cutoff value is set to 100 ng/ml, AFP has a sensitivity of 39–64% and a specificity of 76–91% for HCC.

Desgamma-carboxy-prothrombin (DCP; synonym: "protein induced by vitamin K absence") is another tumor marker that has been studied in HCC. Because this abnormal protein is produced mainly by malignant liver cells, its specificity for HCC is probably greater than that of AFP. However, as regards the sensitivity for detection of small tumors in particular, DCP seems to be inferior to AFP.

Imaging

The detection and characterization of hepatic neoplasms with imaging modalities depends on the tissue or contrast difference between the nodular lesions and the surrounding liver parenchyma. All imaging techniques are limited in the detection of HCC within a cirrhotic liver. The end-stage cirrhotic liver architecture is severely distorted, and the altered portal hemodynamics ultimately affect any diagnostic method that utilizes intravenous contrast material. Therefore, the presence of fibrosis, regenerating nodules, necrosis, and fatty alterations can influence the sensitivity of every imaging technique. HCC may be detected by only one of the available imaging modalities. Consequently, the diagnosis of HCC in the cirrhotic liver may involve several complementary imaging techniques.

There have been no randomized controlled studies to demonstrate that screening improves survival. Indirect evidence, however, suggests that screening may improve resectability and liver transplantation rate. Additionally, from a pragmatic point of view, it seems useful to screen high-risk patients at regular intervals by obtaining AFP levels and performing US or computed tomography, because a patient who has access to modern therapeutic modalities may benefit if the diagnosis is established early.

HCC may manifest as a solitary mass, a dominant mass surrounded by satellite nodules, a multifocal mass, or a diffusely infiltrating tumor.

Fibrolamellar carcinoma (see also below), a rare variant of HCC that accounts for only 2% of all hepatocellular malignancies, most frequently presents as a large solitary mass with a lobulated contour and a central fibrous scar, and may be confused with focal nodular hyperplasia (FNH). In one third of the patients, fibrolamellar carcinoma contains calcifications, whereas calcifications are never seen in FNH.

Ultrasound (US)

US is the first-line imaging study in the diagnostic work-up of patients with suspected hepatic disease, and a number of useful facts can be obtained. In patients with chronic liver disease, the combination of US and measurements of serum AFP levels are frequently used to screen for HCC.

The sonographic appearance of HCC is variable, depending on the size and histology of the tumor. The majority of small HCCs (<3 cm) are homogeneous and hypoechoic. Larger lesions are typically hyperechoic or of heterogeneous structure due to the presence of necrosis, hemorrhage, fatty change, and interstitial fibrosis. In advanced cases of HCC, portal vein thrombosis, hepatic or portal vein invasion and biliary obstruction may occur. The severely diseased cirrhotic liver may have such a heterogeneous echo pattern that the recognition of a focal lesion is difficult or impossible. Regenerating and dysplastic nodules measuring 0.5–1.5 cm in diameter are distinguishable by US. They tend to be hypoechoic relative to the surrounding liver parenchyma and can be confused with tumorous lesions.

The efficiency of US as a screening modality for the detection of liver masses in patients with advanced cirrhosis has been evaluated prospectively. The sensitivity of sonography in detecting lesions in a severely cirrhotic liver may be as low as 50%, with a specificity of 98% for any discrete lesion.

More recently, the use of tissue harmonic imaging and micro-bubble contrast agents has been investigated. These refinements offer a great potential for enhancing the detection and characterization of liver tumors, particularly in patients with cirrhosis.

Duplex and color Doppler sonography are useful for the evaluation of spontaneous portosystemic shunts due to decompensated liver cirrhosis, and in detecting vascular invasion by HCC. Tumor thrombi may be identified within the portal vein, hepatic veins, or vena cava.

In summary, the ability of transabdominal US to detect and differentiate small lesions within a cirrhotic liver remains poor, and its use as a single method for the detection of liver lesions prior to hepatic resection is therefore inappropriate. US is a useful modality for guidance of biopsy due to its real-time capabilities and the multiplanar views possible with scanning probes. Multiple recent studies have emphasized the role of US in the treatment of HCC in guiding percutaneous ablative therapies involving injection of ethanol or acetic acid.

Computed Tomography

The advent of helical CT has greatly improved the capabilities of CT scanning. Shorter scanning times combined with the rapid administration of intravenous contrast material allow sequential arterial and portal phase images of the liver to be obtained during a single bolus of contrast within a single breath-hold in each phase. Arterial phase scans are obtained 20 seconds after the start of intravenous injection of contrast material at a rate of 3–5 ml/sec, whereas portal venous phase scans are obtained 60–70 seconds after the administration of contrast material has started. Dual phase imaging is particularly necessary to differentiate small tumors within the liver parenchyma. The addition of arterial phase imaging to unenhanced and portal venous phase imaging depicts up to 30% more tumor nodules, and in approximately 10% of patients it may be the only phase to demonstrate the tumor lesion at all.

The small HCC is most frequently a vascular lesion, which enhances rapidly during the arterial phase and becomes isodense with the liver parenchyma during the portal phase. Large tumors have a heterogeneous pattern of enhancement in the arterial phase. Portal venous phase scans are helpful for detecting less vascularized tumors (Fig. 1a–c).

An encapsulated HCC is rarely seen in the non-Asian population. It is characterized by a hypodense rim on early enhanced CT. This capsule as well as septations within the tumor usually enhance in a delayed CT scan following intravenous contrast administration.

Regenerative and dysplastic nodules are difficult to differentiate because they do not enhance in the arterial phase and tend to enhance homogeneously and similarly to the surrounding parenchyma in the portal venous phase.

In a recent study, the sensitivity of contrast-enhanced helical CT for the detection of HCC in the surveillance of patients with cirrhosis had a low sensitivity of only about 30% [1]. The tumor nodules that were not detected with CT and found only at surgical-pathologic analysis ranged in size from 2 to 40 mm (mean, 13 mm).

Preoperative three-dimensional helical CT scan angiography provides an arterial and portal venous "road map" in patients undergoing evaluation for liver resection or transplantation.

The injection of a small amount of iodized oil into the hepatic artery results in the retention of this contrast material within tumor nodules. The reported sensitivity of this technique varies widely between 40 and more than 90%, probably related to tumor size and the degree of cellular differentiation. The sensitivity is low for well-differentiated carcinomas and high (90%) for small, moderately or poorly differentiated nodules.

Nuclear Magnetic Resonance (NMR)

Usually, HCC presents as a hypointense lesion on T1-weighted images, and is hyperintense on T2-weighted images. However, the NMR imaging appearance correlates with the histology, and the presence of fatty alterations, necrosis, or hemorrhage may result in increased signal intensity on T1-weighted images. Dynamic multiphase gadolinium-enhanced NMR imaging has been shown to improve detection of HCC and may be superior to dual-phase spiral CT. Following the administration of intravenous contrast material, HCC is typically depicted as a hypervascular mass, but vascularity and enhancement are variable. Therefore, any lesion in a cirrhotic liver that does not fulfill the criteria for a cyst or a hemangioma should be considered an HCC until proven otherwise.

Recent developments and refinements in NMR imaging, such as the use of liver-specific contrast materials and dynamic scanning, have underlined the role of this technique in the detection and characterization of liver

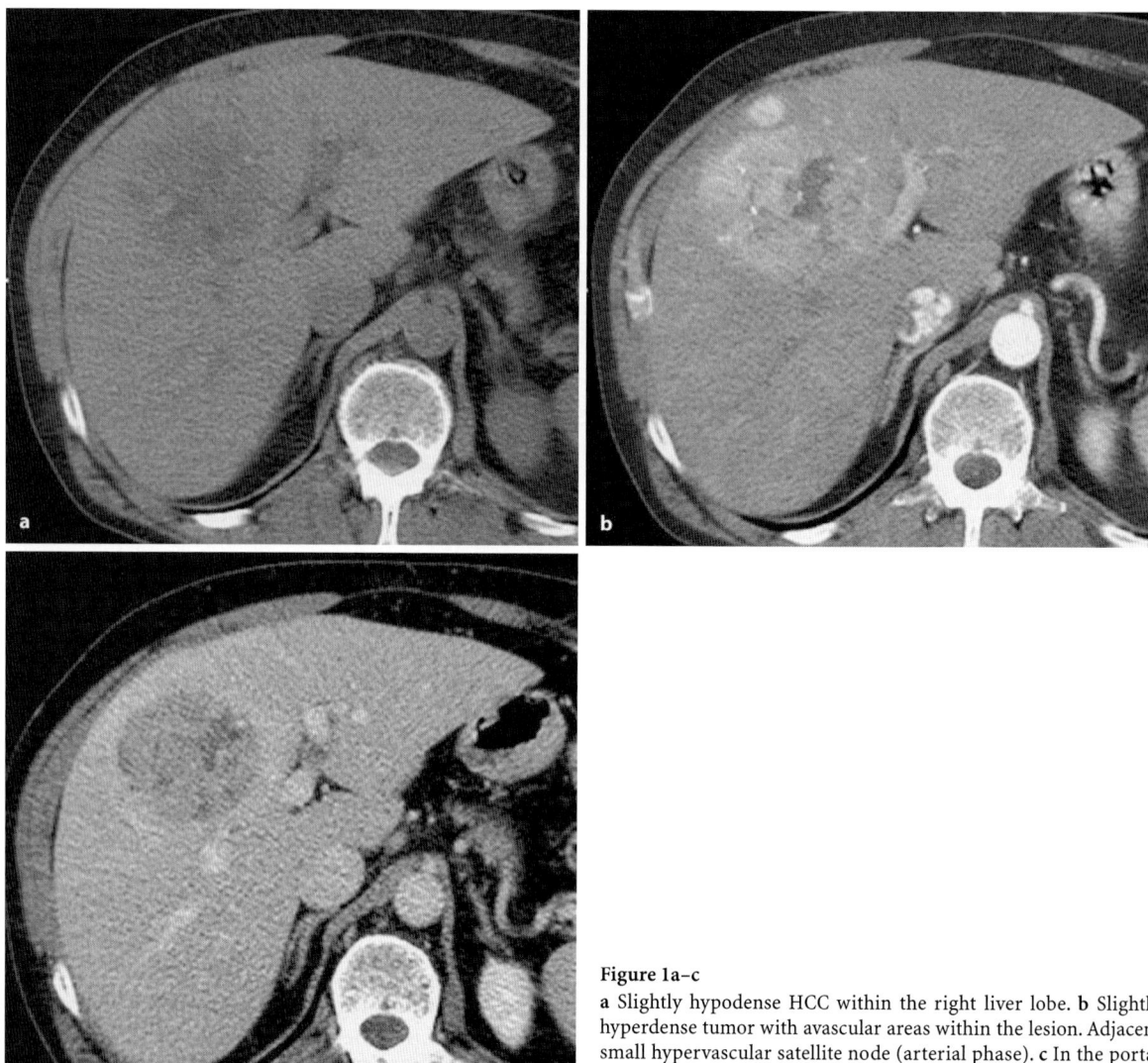

Figure 1a–c
a Slightly hypodense HCC within the right liver lobe. **b** Slightly hyperdense tumor with avascular areas within the lesion. Adjacent small hypervascular satellite node (arterial phase). **c** In the portal venous phase the tumur becomes hypodense compared to the surrounding liver tissue

lesions. Two kinds of liver-specific contrast agents have been developed for liver NMR imaging: iron oxide contrast agents and hepatobiliary contrast agents.

Ferumoxide particles are cleared from the blood by phagocytosis in the reticuloendothelial system. On T2-weighted images, signal loss caused by the uptake of ferumoxide particles maps Kupffer cell distribution. Usually, malignant tumors are devoid of Kupffer cells, and therefore an improved contrast between the liver parenchyma and malignant lesions can be observed. Scarring, inflammation, the development of regenerative nodules, and shunting within the cirrhotic parenchyma reduce hepatic uptake of ferumoxides. These drawbacks, however, affect the performance only in the most severe cirrhosis. In patients with hepatic iron overload, the intravenous administration of ferumoxides rarely increases the detection rate for tumorous lesions. On the other hand, well-differentiated HCC may posses the capacity for phagocytosis, and a HCC may remain isointense to the liver parenchyma even after administration of ferumoxides.

Hepatobiliary contrast agents comprise a heterogeneous group of soluble paramagnetic molecules that are taken up by the hepatocytes and secreted into the bile. Usually, malignant tumors do not absorb these agents in contrast to normal liver parenchyma.

In the detection of HCC, the sensitivity of ferumoxides-enhanced NMR imaging has been reported to be 80–93% [2], while that of hepatobiliary-enhanced NMR imaging was found to be 82–89%. According to a recent study, ferumoxides-enhanced NMR imaging demonstrated superior diagnostic accuracy in lesions smaller than 10 mm. In the preoperative detection of HCC, it was superior to hepatobiliary contrast-enhanced NMR imaging.

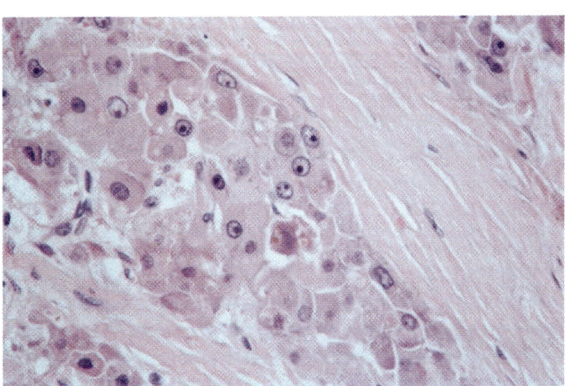

Figure 2
Histology of the fibrolamellary type of hepatocellular carcinoma: typical pleomorphic tumor cells of hepatoid morphology in a dense fibrous stroma. (H.E. stain, ×250). (This figure was kindly provided by Dr. A. Gassel, Institute of Pathology, University of Würzburg)

Positron Emission Tomography (PET)

Malignant tumors, including HCC, have increased aerobic glycolysis and glucose metabolism. Fluoro-deoxy-glucose (FDG) is a glucose analogue that competes with glucose at transport sites on the cell membrane and in the intracellular enzymatic pathways. Well-differentiated HCCs have a low detection rate in FDG PET, because their metabolic activity is low and similar to that of the surrounding liver. Large, moderately or poorly differentiated HCCs, however, are more likely to be defined with this technique because of their increased metabolic activity. The overall sensitivity of FDG PET in the diagnosis of HCC is only about 50%. FDG PET, however, is valuable for the delineation of extrahepatic disease that may escape detection at cross-sectional imaging.

PET scans have poor spatial resolution, and complementary information obtained from cross-sectional imaging studies, such as CT scans, is necessary. A new refined approach is the combination of a PET scan and a multidetector helical CT.

Histological Classification

Whether there is a direct pathway of histological changes from a benign histology in a cirrhotic liver to HCC is not clear at present. Dysplastic nodules or foci, as characterized by clustering of cells with cytoplasmic and nuclear abnormalities, are frequently found in the neighborhood of HCC. A progression of the disease from macro regenerative to dysplastic nodules of advancing grades, and from there to HCC is assumed by some authors, although this histological progression can be proven only with difficulty.

The histological features of HCC may vary considerably between cases. Generally, the cells conserve some characteristics of normal liver cells, and may form trabeculae similar to normal liver tissue. The tumor can occur in a pseudoglandular, cirrhous or solid pattern. However, the histological group does not seem to have an impact on prognosis.

Hepatoblastoma is a rare variant of HCC that occurs mostly in children and only very rarely in adults. The tumor originates from embryonic or fetal hepatocytes. Histologically, the tumor is hypervascular, and may contain other mesenchyme-derived tissue, for example osteoid. AFP is frequently elevated excessively in hepatoblastoma, and levels may be above 1 million ng/ml.

Another special form of HCC that differs from the other variants with respect to prognosis is *fibrolamellar HCC* (Fig. 2). This type of HCC is only rarely associated with cirrhosis and therefore often difficult to diagnose. It is characterized by the presence of multiple fibrous septa within the tumor. The malignant cells are large and polygonal with some resemblance to endocrine tumors. The etiology seems to be different from that of the

Table 2

TNM classification of hepatocellular carcinoma (UICC)

T0	No primary tumor
T1	Solitary tumor, diameter ≤ 2 cm, no vascular invasion
T2	Solitary tumor, diameter ≤ 2 cm, vascular invasion present, *or* Multiple tumors in the same lobe, < 2 cm, no vascular invasion, *or* Solitary tumor, > 2 cm, no vascular invasion
T3	Solitary tumor, > 2 cm, vascular invasion present, *or* Multiple tumors in the same lobe, ≤ 2 cm, vascular invasion present, *or* Multiple tumors in the same lobe, > 2 cm, with or without vascular invasion
T4	Multiple tumors in more than one lobe, *or* Invasion of portal or liver veins, *or* Invasion of neighboring organs (except gall bladder), *or* Perforation of visceral peritoneum
N1	Regional lymph node metastases

Stage groupings	T	N	M
Stage I	1	0	0
Stage II	2	0	0
Stage IIIA	3	0	0
Stage IIIB	1	1	0
	2	1	0
	3	1	0
Stage IVA	4	0–1	0
Stage IVB	1–4	0–1	1

other forms of HCC, since predisposing conditions such as viral hepatitis are not found. Fibrolamellar HCC occurs at an earlier age (20–30 years) than the other forms of primary liver cell cancer, and in an otherwise intact liver. Therefore, and because it resembles focal nodular hyperplasia on conventional imaging techniques as well as microscopically, it is often misdiagnosed at first. AFP is also frequently not helpful, since it is not elevated in most cases of fibrolamellar HCC. Because of this difficult differential diagnosis, the possibility of fibrolamellar carcinoma has to be considered in patients with FNH. In every newly diagnosed case of FNH, rapid tumor growth has to be excluded by follow-up with sequential abdominal US. In general, the prognosis of fibrolamellar HCC seems to be better than that for the other forms of HCC with later spreading and better operability because of the absence of cirrhosis.

Staging

Synopsis

Barcelona Classification of Liver Cancer (BCLC) staging system for HCC

Stage	Performance Status	Tumor stage	Liver function
Stage A (early HCC)			
A1	0	Single, <5 cm	No portal hypertension, normal bilirubin
A2	0	Single, <5 cm	Portal hypertension, normal bilirubin
A3	0	Single, <5 cm	Portal hypertension, elevated bilirubin
A4	0	3 tumors <3 cm	Child-Pugh stage A-B
Stage B (Intermediate HCC)	0	Large multi-nodular	Child-Pugh stage A-B
Stage C (Advanced HCC)	1–2	Vascular invasion/ Extrahepatic spread	Child-Pugh stage A-B
Stage D (End-stage HCC)	3–4	Any	Child-Pugh stage C

The TNM staging system is summarized in Table 2. It has been challenged insofar as it does not reliably separate the patient groups in whom the tumor may still be cured surgically. Stage IVA, for example, is not homogenous with respect to prognosis. It contains a subgroup of patients with T4N0M0 (small tumors in both liver lobes, but no metastases) whose prognosis is not worse than that of stage IIIA (one large or multiple small tumors in the same liver lobe) if these patients are treated with liver transplantation. On the other hand, patients with T4N1M0 are also classified as stage IVA, but neither liver resection nor transplantation will offer cure for this patient group, because of extrahepatic spreading of the disease. Additionally, the TNM staging system only refers to tumor size and spreading, but does not take into account the additional problems arising from the underlying liver disease. Apart from liver transplantation, all other potentially curative treatment modalities, liver resection as well as local tissue destruction or the application of chemotherapy, will require a residual liver function that is adequate to tolerate these aggressive treatments.

The Okuda staging system (Table 3) was the first to group patients not only according to their tumor spread, but also to include liver function into patient classification. However, the Okuda system classifies tumor stage very roughly, and only intrahepatic manifestations are measured. Therefore, an alternative staging system has been suggested by the Barcelona Group (BCLC staging system; see synopsis). This classification discriminates patients with HCC not only according to their tumor manifestations, but also includes their performance status and liver function. With this staging system, the patient groups that can be treated with the various modern treatment modalities (resection/transplantation, local tumor destruction, experimental or palliative therapies) are more easily discriminated from each other.

Treatment

Synopsis

Therapy of HCC according to tumor stage

Stage	Description	Aim of therapy	Treatment
Early	1 single node up to 5 cm or up to 3 nodes with up to 3 cm each *(BCLC A, Okuda 1–2, UICC I–IIIA, (IVA))*	Cure	Resection/Transplantation/Local ablation (dependent on technical and functional resectability)
Intermediate	3 nodes or at least one node >5 cm *(BCLC B, Okuda 1–2, UICC IVA)*	Palliation	Local therapy (trans-arterial chemoembolization (TACE); radiofrequency ablation (RFA); laser-induced thermotherapy (LITT); percutaneous ethanol injection (PEI))
Advanced	Major vascular invasion, extrahepatic spread *(BCLC C, Okuda 1–2, UICC IIIB, IVA, IVB)*	Palliation	Local therapy (TACE, RFA, LITT, PEI; experimental systemic therapy)
Terminal	Severely reduced performance, Child C cirrhosis, advanced tumor stage *(BCLC D, Okuda 3, UICC not classified)*	Palliation	Symptomatic treatment

Table 3
Okuda staging system

Clinical parameters	Cut-off values	Points
Tumor size (cross-sectional area on imaging)	>50%	1
	<50%	0
Ascites	Present	1
	Absent	0
Serum albumin (mg/dL)	>3	0
	<3	1
Serum total bilirubin (mg/dL)	>3	0
	<3	1

Number of points	Stage
0	1
1–2	2
3–4	3

Surgery

At present the radical removal of the tumor by surgical resection is the only form of curative treatment for HCC. Beside the different variations of liver resections, a total hepatectomy with consecutive liver transplantation may be the only therapeutic option in certain cases with a progressive form of liver cirrhosis as underlying disease [3]. Thus, in many patients the grade of liver disease, e.g. fibrosis or cirrhosis, will limit the intention to liver resection. The choice of the optimal form of treatment is based on an individual decision for each patient, finding the balance between the oncological needs mainly based on the stage of the tumor and the grade of cirrhotic liver damage limiting the functional reserves of the remaining liver. Liver resection applies only to about 20% of patients suffering from HCC. As compared to liver resections for metastases or benign lesions, liver surgery for HCC requires experienced surgeons and should be performed at centers with a close interdisciplinary collaboration between gastroenterologists, radiologists, anesthesiologists and high volume surgeons.

Due to an improved understanding of liver anatomy, rapid advances in imaging techniques such as three-dimensional computed tomography and NMR imaging and intraoperative US devices, the pre-and intra-operative planning of the resection has gained high accuracy. The surgical part of an oncological liver resection has been standardized and is facilitated by technical devices such as US or waterstream dissection devices that allow resections outside anatomical lines. Continuing improvements in anesthesiology and intensive care medicine allow major operations on elderly patients with certain comorbidities as well as on cirrhotic patients.

Liver Anatomy and Liver Resection

The liver is divided in eight segments. Each segment is perfused via a single portal vein branch, artery and bile duct. Hemihepatectomies (right side: segments 5–8, left side: segments 2–4) and extended hemihepatectomies (synonym trisectorectomies) are summarized as major liver resections; bisegmentectomies (left side: segments 2 and 3, right side: segments 7 and 8) are minor liver resections. These anatomical liver resections form the majority of liver resections, particularly in non-cirrhotic livers. However, single segmentectomies and even non-anatomical wedge resections are approved surgical procedures for the resection of HCC in order to save liver parenchyma in fibrotic or cirrhotic patients. At present no surgical guidelines concerning the extent of liver resection can be formulated from an oncological point of view. In earlier studies a margin of more than 1 cm between tumor and resection plane was proposed. At present it is accepted that, independent of the width of the surgical margin, the main prognostic factor besides the degree of liver cirrhosis is a Ro resection, e.g. no macroscopic or microscopic tumor residuals after resection [4]. The resection plane should be marked with ink for an accurate pathological examination.

Since bile ducts and blood vessel branches do not cross intersegmental barriers the anatomical resections show less surgical complications, e.g. intraoperative blood loss or postoperative bile fistulas. Therefore the anatomical surgical resection is recommended as the standard procedure for resection of HCC both in cirrhotic and non-cirrhotic livers (Fig. 3).

HCC in Non-cirrhotic Livers

In the Western hemisphere HCCs develop in a non-cirrhotic liver only in a minority of patients. Therefore the late diagnosis of the tumor often reveals large nodules. After exclusion of extrahepatic tumor spread, these tumors are best treated by liver resection. Unsuspected local infiltration of the diaphragm or stomach may require extended operations. Centrally located tumors can be treated by mobilization of the liver, clamping of the ligament and division of the suprahepatic inferior vena cava in order to perform an *ante situm* resection of the tumor. During clamping, the gut can be protected by a veno-venous porto-femoro-axillary bypass.

Tumor recurrence is the major problem after liver resection for HCCs in non-cirrhotic livers, occurring at a frequency of 30 to 60%. Depending on localization and the function of the regenerating liver, reresections are appropriate. Otherwise local ablative treatment and chemoembolization or even radiotherapy are therapeutic options for these patients.

HCC in Cirrhotic Livers

As described above liver cirrhosis, mainly induced by hepatitis B and C, is the underlying disease of HCC in more than 80% of the patients. Knowing the increased risk of cancer development in these patients, HCCs are primarily detected by routine screening methods including the assessment of AFP, US examinations and CT/MRT scans. Thus, these HCC nodules can be diagnosed at a rather small size. Two problems make treatment difficult; firstly, the impaired liver function due to the cirrhosis, and secondly the fact that HCC develops multifocally.

In order to assess the function of the liver and to estimate the possibility of resection, various liver function assays have been described and evaluated. For the decision as to whether to perform a liver resection or not, the Child Pugh Turcotte classification of liver cirrhosis is

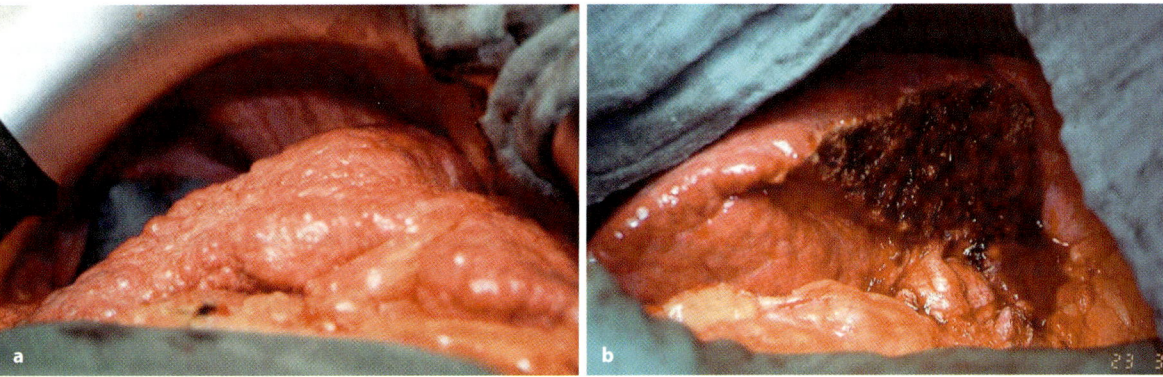

Figure 3a,b
a Intraoperative situs: Cirrhotic liver immediately prior to resection for HCC located in segments 3 and 4. Note the demarcation of the left liver lobe after dissection and ligature of the left portal vein, the left liver artery and the left hepatic vein. **b** Intraoperative situs: Liver resection plane after a left hemihepatectomy for HCC in a cirrhotic liver. Vessels and bile ducts are ligated by sutures and clips

widely accepted. Both the Okuda and the BCLC classification take into account liver function and tumor mass. However, for the clinical decision on surgery, both classifications are less frequently used at present. In Japan, the indocyanin green retention rate is used for the assessment of resectability with convincing results.

In general, major liver resections are feasible in patients with fibrosis or cirrhosis stage Child A, minor resections and atypical resections in Child B cirrhosis. In patients with cirrhosis grade Child C, a liver resection should not be performed at all. Since even an explorative laparotomy can be a serious risk for these patients, the only form of curative treatment would be liver transplantation. However, the immunosuppressive regimen after transplantation impairs the outcome, due to rapid tumor growth within the graft. Thus, this therapeutic option can be offered to selected patients only.

The perioperative mortality after liver resection for HCC in cirrhotic livers ranges from 5–20%. Postoperative morbidity is increased to 15–25% as compared to less than 5% after liver resection for metastases. The most serious complication after liver resection in cirrhotic patients is postoperative liver dysfunction. It presents with progressive jaundice and hepatorenal syndrome and is associated with a high mortality [5]. The discordant results concerning postoperative complications and long-term results can be explained by different surgical attitudes. Preoperative selection of patients with particular regard to UICC stage and liver function is mandatory in order to achieve acceptable results.

Five-year survival rates vary from 15–75% depending on the UICC stage, the selection of patients and the size of the study groups [6]. The comparison of different studies needs a critical evaluation of the patient selection, particularly concerning the grade of liver damage. In some studies, more than 80% long-term survival after resection of small tumors without vascular invasion is published. Patients with small tumors and less than 3 tumor nodules are the best candidates for resection. However, these patients are also suitable candidates for various forms of local ablative therapies, e.g. PEI, RFA and LITT. Some studies present comparable 5-year survival rates after PEI and liver resection. Hence, in patients with cirrhotic livers, particularly Child B stage, the indication for liver resection should be based on an individual benefit- risk ratio. HCCs at UICC stage IVa in cirrhotic livers cannot be treated by liver resection.

Liver Transplantation

Total hepatectomy and transplantation is an accepted form of treatment for HCCs at certain stages. The results after liver transplantation for UICC stage IV tumors were disappointing, showing 5-year-survival rates <50% even in experienced transplant centers. By contrast, small HCCs with less than 3 nodules in liver cirrhosis can be successfully treated by liver transplantation. With a postoperative mortality of less than 3% and long-term survival rates of 60–70% this procedure is recommended for selected patients. The main cause of death after liver transplantation for HCC is tumor recurrence, particularly associated with vascular invasion of the HCC.

At present liver transplantation is the treatment of choice with acceptable long-term results for patients with liver cirrhosis at stages Child C or B and HCC at stages UICC I or II with less than 3 tumor nodules. Any extrahepatic tumor spread is a contraindication for transplantation.

A serious problem for all patients bearing a HCC in a cirrhotic liver is the time on the waiting list for transplantation. Living-related liver transplantation is developing rather quickly in certain transplant centers. With increasing surgical experience the results are improving. At present the outcome is not equal to that after cadaveric liver transplantation and rare but serious complications including deaths have occurred in the otherwise healthy donor individuals. Still, living-related liver transplantation might help to partially solve the above-mentioned problems in the near future.

Fibrolamellar Type of HCC

The rare form of fibrolamellar HCC usually occurs in younger patients between the age of 18 and 40 years. Due to the long-lasting absence of clinical signs the tumors are mostly diagnosed at an UICC IV status. However, there is no association with liver cirrhosis and therefore curative liver resection is the best treatment for these rather young patients.

The reported 5-year survival rates range from 50–66% depending on the patient selection and the UICC stage. In summary, perioperative mortality and morbidity are low and the survival rates are significantly better as compared to liver resection for the common trabecular forms of HCC.

Chemotherapy

In general, results of antineoplastic chemotherapy in HCC have been disappointing. HCC is resistant to all antineoplastic drugs available so far. As yet, it has not even been possible to identify subgroups of patients with HCC, in whom antineoplastic chemotherapy might be of use. Very limited response rates (mostly below 15%) have been shown for doxorubicin, epirubicin, mi-

toxantrone, 5-FU, cisplatin, mitomycin C and gemcitabine. No combination schedule has been shown to prolong survival when used with palliative, adjuvant or neoadjuvant intention. In one study, postoperative adjuvant chemotherapy (intravenous epirubicin hydrochloride plus transarterial chemotherapy with an emulsion of iodized oil and cisplatin) was even associated with more frequent extrahepatic recurrence and a worse outcome in treated patients.

In summary, in view of the efficacy of locally ablative methods in reducing tumor size, there is no place for antineoplastic chemotherapy in the treatment of HCC, and patients should only be treated experimentally in clinical studies.

Others Medical Therapies

The anti-estrogenic drug *tamoxifen* had a beneficial effect on the duration of survival in patients with HCC in some, but not all studies. Although in a meta-analysis of these studies, the one-year survival rate of treated patients was better than that in the pooled control groups, a large prospective study in 477 patients with HCC failed to show any benefit of tamoxifen. In conclusion, tamoxifen is of no proven benefit.

Because the presence of variant liver estrogen receptors in a subset of HCCs leads to a more aggressive growth, in a single study from Italy, 45 patients with HCCs positive for these receptors were either treated with *megestrol* (160 mg daily) or served as a control group. Survival was significantly longer (18 *vs.* 7 months), and tumor growth was slowed down. Tumor regression was not observed. These results will need confirmation by further studies.

Somatostatin and its analogue *octreotide* have antineoplastic effects in several tumors originating from tissues that express somatostatin receptors. In a controlled study from Greece, in 53 patients with inoperable HCC, octreotide (250 g b.i.d. subcutaneously) was associated with a significantly increased median survival (13 *vs.* 4 months). The one-year survival rate was 37% in treated *vs* 13% in untreated patients. Additionally, AFP levels were significantly reduced after 6 months. In two uncontrolled series, these optimistic results were not confirmed. At present, other placebo-controlled studies to confirm these data are under way.

HMG-CoA reductase inhibitors (statins) have been shown to exert anti-neoplastic effects in several tumors *in vitro* and *in vivo*. The mechanisms are not entirely clear so far. One possible mode of action may be the suppression of protein isoprenylation. These drugs could then interfere with the metabolism and function of *ras*-p21 and thereby act as signal transduction inhibitors. Additionally, fast growing tissues such as malignant tumors have an enhanced demand for cholesterol, whose synthesis is inhibited by statins. In a recent controlled study from Japan, 83 patients with inoperable HCC received either *pravastatin* (dose 40 mg daily) or no treatment. The patients on pravastatin fared significantly better; the median survival was 18 months *vs.* 9 months in the control group. Although no measurable tumor regression was observed, tumor growth was slowed in the treated group, the tumor size being significantly smaller in the surviving patients at 6 and 12 months.

In conclusion, in view of the disappointing results with conventional antineoplastic chemotherapy, other forms of treatment have been developed that are directed against endocrine or metabolic characteristics of HCC. However, at present most of these treatments have only been investigated in one single study. In none of these studies, was tumor regression observed, although improvements in survival and slowing of tumor growth were observed. With tamoxifen, the only drug in which several placebo-controlled studies are available, the encouraging results of the first study could not be consistently confirmed. Therefore, further placebo-controlled studies on therapy with pravastatin, octreotide and megestrol have to be performed, before the efficacy of these drugs in the treatment of HCC can be appraised.

At present, no medical therapy whatsoever has been shown with sufficient certainty to be effective in patients with inoperable HCC. Likewise, no strategy for adjuvant therapy in operated patients exists so far.

Local Tumor Ablation

Transcatheter Arterial Embolization (TAE) and TACE - Transcatheter Arterial Chemoembolization. TAE and TACE are the techniques most commonly used to treat unresectable HCC. TACE implies localized intraarterial delivery of chemotherapeutic agents, emulsified in an oily medium, mostly combined with embolizing material. The

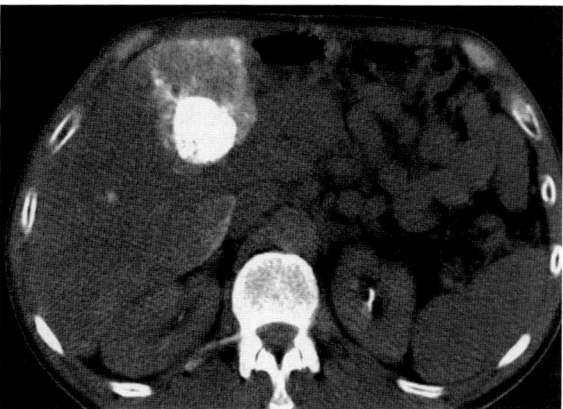

Figure 4
Following TACE the chemoembolisation agent is highly concentrated within the tumor. Small amounts of this material are seen within the surrounding parenchyma

combination of chemotherapy with a high local drug concentration and some degree of ischemia within the tumor is likely to be synergistic in achieving tumor necrosis. Embolization without chemotherapy simply implies an occlusion of the tumor's arterial blood supply. The rationale for these types of therapy comes from the observation that normal liver tissue receives most of its blood supply from the portal vein, whereas liver tumors receive the major part of their blood supply from the hepatic artery. Numerous variations of this technique are described, and there is no consensus as to what constitutes the most effective TACE technique. The common goals of TAE and TACE are to induce tumor necrosis and to control tumor growth while preserving as much functional liver tissue as possible.

A number of chemotherapeutic agents (doxorubicin, cisplatin, mitomycin C) have been proposed, but controversy persists regarding the selection of the most potent of these drugs. Poppy seed oil accumulates preferentially in HCC and has therefore become a key ingredient to the chemoembolization procedure because it is a drug-carrying, tumor-seeking, and occluding agent (Fig. 4). Several types of embolic agents that cause a temporary or a permanent occlusion of the feeding arteries have also been used for chemoembolization. However, it is generally accepted that TACE achieves maximal tumor response when repeated multiple times. Therefore, long-term arterial patency may be an essential key element to the success of this therapy. There is no consensus as to how selective chemoembolization should be, and control by more accurate imaging modalities, such as CT angiography, may be helpful.

Several predictors of survival have been studied to determine patient selection for TACE. Patients with poor baseline liver function and large tumors, diffuse tumor growth and infiltrating tumors benefit least from this kind of therapy. A relative contraindication with an increased risk of acute liver failure is the constellation of more than 50% replacement of the liver by tumor and severely increased levels of lactate dehydrogenase (>425 IU/L), aspartate aminotransferase (>100 IU/L), and total bilirubin (>34 µmol/L). TACE has been reported to be more effective in the treatment of nodular HCC than of diffuse infiltrating carcinoma. Even in patients with a tumor thrombus in the portal vein trunk or hepatofugal blood flow, TACE can be performed effectively and safely for palliation.

The issue of the efficacy of TAE and TACE in treating unresectable HCC is still controversial according to the individual study findings. A recent meta-analysis of randomized controlled trials has shown sufficient evidence to conclude that (a) chemoembolization significantly reduces overall 2-year mortality in patients with unresectable HCC and (b) TACE was not more effective than TAE, which suggests that the addition of the chemotherapeutic agents currently used does not increase the benefit of the therapy [7]. A recently published Chinese study in which patients were randomized to either chemoembolization or supportive care, could show that chemoembolization was superior to supportive care in a group of patients with unresectable HCC. Patient survival, the most relevant of the criteria for success, was found to be 57%, 31%, and 26% in the chemoembolization group versus 32%, 11%, and 3% in the group that received supportive care at 1, 2, and 3 years, respectively [1].

Percutaneous Chemical Ablation. Percutaneous chemical ablation with absolute ethanol is another established technique of imaging-guided regional therapy for HCC, with long-term survivals that compete with those after surgical resection. PEI (percutaneous ethanol injection) is generally performed for HCCs up to 3–5 cm in diameter, although acceptable results have been attained in larger tumors.

For agents with a low molecular weight, such as ethanol, acetic acid or saline, diffusion is the dominant form of interstitial transport. In contrast to the interstitium of normal tissue, tumor interstitium is characterized by several factors that result in a high interstitial fluid pressure, an elevated interstitial diffusion coefficient, and an increased tissue convection. To destroy medium-sized tumors by using PEI, multiple needle insertions must be planned to ensure that ethanol distributes throughout the entire volume of tumor to be treated.

PEI has been reported to lead to complete necrosis in 70–75% of HCC tumors 3–5 cm in diameter. However, treatment with this technique generally requires multiple sessions.

Thermal Ablation. Thermal ablation techniques, including the use of radiofrequency, lasers, microwaves, and high-intensity focused ultrasound, are gaining increasing attention as an alternative therapeutic approach in the treatment of HCC.

RFA. RFA (radiofrequency ablation) is probably the most promising of theses techniques. With this method, high-frequency alternating current is delivered to the tumorous tissue via a needle electrode. The created heat leads to localized coagulation necrosis. The essential objective of ablative therapy is achievement and maintenance of a 50–100°C temperature throughout the entire target volume for at least 4–6 minutes. However, the relatively slow thermal conduction through the tissues increases the duration of application to 10–30 minutes. Key culprits implicated in reduced coagulation include heterogeneity of tissue composition influencing electrical and thermal conductance, and blood flow, which by perfusion-mediated tissue cooling reduces the extent of thermally induced effects.

With currently available devices, the largest area of necrosis that can be induced with a single application is approximately 4–5 cm in greatest diameter. Therefore, radiofrequency ablation is limited to lesions less than 3–4 cm in diameter, because the success of this method is dependant on the ability to destroy all viable tumor tissue and an adequate (at least 1 cm-wide) tumor-free margin. Lesion size is the most important factor in determining local recurrence of disease. Strategies are being pursued to improve RFA efficacy by occluding blood flow to the liver during ablation procedures.

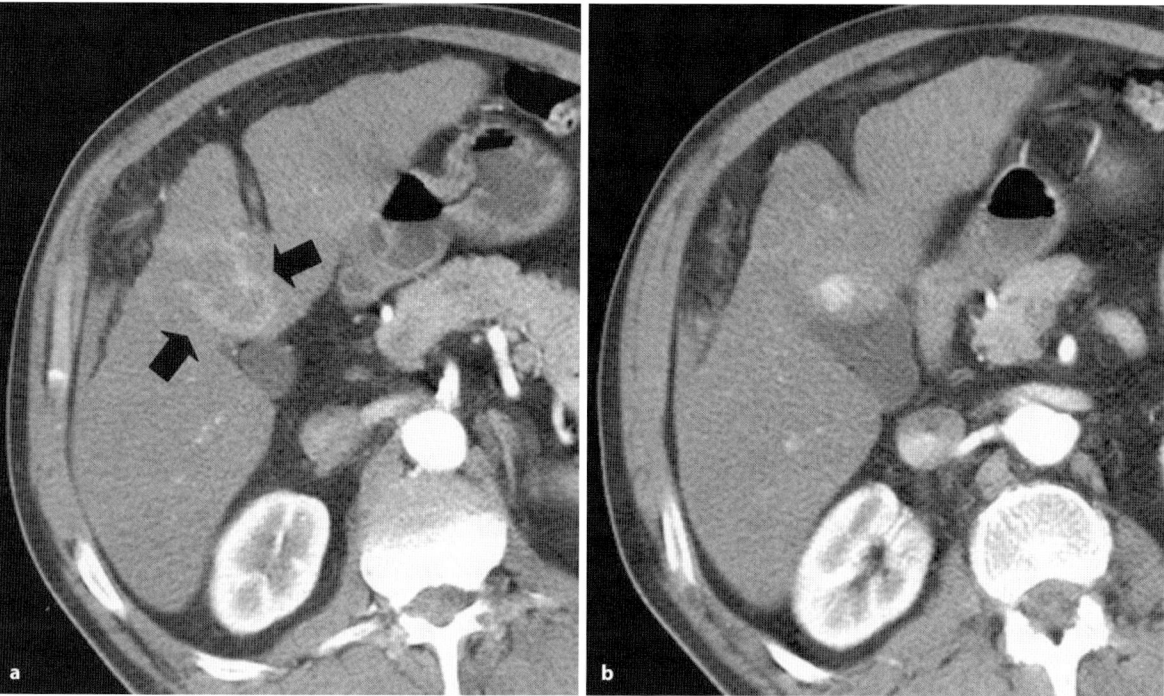

Figure 5a,b
a Hypervascular rim surrounding tissue necrosis immediately after radiofrequency ablation (*arrows*). b Incomplete tumor ablation: hypervascular tumorous nodule adjacent the gallbladder

The radiofrequency needle may either be placed percutaneously with US, CT, or MRI guidance, or by a more invasive procedure (laparoscopy or laparotomy). The guidance system is chosen largely on the basis of operator preference and local experience.

Imaging after the therapy is essential to assess the completeness of the ablation and later on to detect early recurrences (Fig. 5b), which may be amenable to repeated ablation. Posttreatment imaging is usually performed with CT and, less frequently with MRI. Peripheral enhancement at CT or NMR imaging is observed immediately after the session (Fig. 5a) and disappears over time when contrast material is given intravenously. Whereas US is valuable for guiding the ablation procedure, sonographic findings may under-or over-estimate size and completeness of necrosis, because the hyperechogenic focus that appears around the probe during the application of energy represents formation of gas bubbles and not the coagulated tissue *per se*.

The complication rate is low and makes this method a relatively safe procedure. The most commonly reported complications in liver tumor ablation are focal pain, pleural effusion, and regional hemorrhage, with most requiring no surgical intervention.

Results from a recent prospective study comparing PEI and RFA in patients with small HCC showed that RFA resulted in a 10% higher number of completely destroyed tumor nodules. RFA treatment also requires fewer sessions than PEI, and the latter has the additional disadvantage of a relatively high procedural complexity with multiple needle insertions [8].

In comparison with the other currently available percutaneous thermal therapies for HCC, RFA appears to have several advantages; RFA creates larger volumes of tumor necrosis in a shorter period of time than either laser or microwave therapy. Additionally, the equipment used for RFA is less expensive than either laser or microwave equipment.

RFA therapy appears to be more effective than TACE, in which complete necrosis can be achieved in only 15–35% of cases. In particular, the side effects and the long-term impairment of liver function associated with TACE support the use of RFA. On the other hand, TACE can be performed in multinodular disease.

Laser Ablation. For laser thermal ablation (LTA), flexible thin optic fibers are inserted into the tumor via percutaneously placed needles. The laser provides sufficient energy to allow for substantial heat deposition, thereby inducing protein denaturation and cellular death.

The use of thin fibers and fine needles with LTA makes it possible to reach a lesion safely, even if it is very deep, difficult to get at, near the gallbladder or the hepatic hilum or superficial. However, one of the major disadvantages of LTA is the inability to achieve large volumes of tumor destruction with a single fiber application. Efforts to overcome this limitation include simultaneous multiple fiber applications and other technical refinements.

Cryotherapy. Another form of local ablative therapy is cryosurgery. Although the successful local destruction of HCCs with a diameter of up to 5–6 cm is technically proven, two major disadvantages are responsible for the declining number of clinical applications. Firstly cryoablation of liver tumors requires either a laparotomy or a laparoscopy and thus is more invasive as compared to PEI, RFA or LTA. Secondly the observation of rare but life-threatening complications, such as tumor cracking with consecutive bleeding during the thawing process and the so-called cryosyndrome with hypotension and consecutive multiorgan dysfunction eventually resulting in a lethal multiorgan failure, have reduced the use of this therapy.

Prognosis

The natural history of HCC is influenced by several factors:
1. Presence or absence of cirrhosis
   Patients with advanced liver disease (Child's stage C) have the worst prognosis because of early hepatic decompensation. In spite of the fact that it occurs more frequently in a non-cirrhotic liver, HCC of non-viral origin grows particularly fast. In epidemiological studies from Africa, median survival times of no more than 1 month after diagnosis have been described.
2. Etiology of the liver disease
   In countries where aflatoxin is a major contributing factor in the etiology of HCC, an underlying liver disease may not primarily affect liver function. Therefore, the tumor grows to a considerable size without impairing liver function. On the other hand, in regions where the tumor frequently develops in advanced cirrhosis, it causes liver failure at an earlier stage.
3. Gender
   Men have a higher risk for HCC as compared to women. Additionally, survival in women seems to be somewhat better than in men, possibly due to a more benign course of the underlying cirrhosis.
4. Tumor properties
   The prognosis of HCC depends largely on the resectability of the tumor, and indirectly on the properties of the tumor itself and on patient characteristics. Chances for cure are best if there is only one single tumor and no microvascular invasion present. Patients with one single tumor and microvascular invasion or with multiple tumors have an intermediate prognosis, if none of these has a diameter of more than 5 cm. Patients with either multiple tumors any of which have a diameter greater than 5 cm, or one tumor with major vascular invasion and/or lymph node involvement have the worst prognosis. Severe fibrosis or cirrhosis reduce survival within all categories.
5. AFP level
   Survival has been shown to correlate positively with AFP level, and especially with lectin-binding AFP (AFP L3).
6. Histological type
   Since fibrolamellar HCC occurs mostly in a non-cirrhotic liver and in people of younger age, its prognosis is better as compared with other forms of HCC. Additionally, because of an expanding and less invasive growth, resectability is improved. In several small series, 5-year survival has been reported to be between 63 and 100%.

Follow-Up

Recurrence rates after curatively intended resection of HCC vary considerably between different groups and have been reported to be as high as 61.5%, mostly due to unrecognized intrahepatic spreading of the primary tumor. In patients with still adequate liver function, resection of the recurring nodule by repeated partial hepatectomy may be tried. Since no effective therapy is available for extrahepatic metastases after hepatectomy, follow-up concentrates on the recurrence of intrahepatic tumor manifestations. In tumors producing AFP, HCC recurrence may be detected by repeated measurements of this tumor marker starting early post-operatively. Tumor visualization is performed by repeated US, possibly enhanced by contrast medium, and may be confirmed by NMR. Although no systematic data are available, intervals of three months for follow-up investigations during the first 2 years, and of six months thereafter are reasonable. If not surgically resectable, small recurring tumors within the residual liver may still be treated curatively by local therapy (thermocoagulation or ethanol injection).

After resection of an HCC, every effort has to be undertaken to treat the underlying liver disease. This includes:

1. Repeated phlebotomy in patients with hereditary hemochromatosis, aiming at depletion of intrahepatic iron.
2. In patients with chronic hepatitis C treatment with alpha-interferon and ribavirin should be started, if this therapy has not been tried and proven ineffective at an earlier time.

In patients with chronic hepatitis B, therapy with a virostatic drug such as lamivudine, famciclovir or one of the newer drugs still under investigation (e.g. adefovir) has to be started. This therapy is not primarily intended as a definite cure for the hepatitis, since HbsAg seroconversion will be achieved only in rare cases, but rather to reduce viral load and thereby the mutagenic potential of the HBV, and to treat the chronic inflammation of the liver.

Screening, Surveillance, Prevention

Because of the discouraging results of conservative treatment modalities and because of the dismal prognosis of advanced HCC, mortality can only be reduced by strategies either to diagnose the disease at an early stage or to prevent tumor development by treating chronic liver disease.

In view of the bad prognosis of advanced HCC, surveillance of risk groups (patients with cirrhosis due to chronic viral hepatitis, hemochromatosis or chronic alcohol abuse) is necessary in order to detect the tumor at a still resectable stage. At present, it is recommended that measurement of serum AFP and an US of the liver are performed once every six months in these patients. Although the results of systematic screening programs for the detection of small and surgically curative tumors have not been very encouraging, mostly due to the relatively low sensitivity of conventional US to detect a small tumor within the cirrhotic liver, such studies have not yet been performed with new technical developments in US (contrast-enhancement, contrast media, power Doppler) or radiology (high-resolution CT, NMR with the use of contrast media).

The most effective strategy to reduce global HCC mortality is to reduce the high infection rate of the population in endemic areas with the HBV and HCV. In those regions, vaccination against hepatitis B will decrease the number of chronic carriers. However, because of the long time between hepatitis B infection and HCC development, it will take about 40 years before the full impact of such a vaccination program will become evident.

Because at present no vaccination for hepatitis C is available, prevention strategies have to aim at the reduction of the infection rate by preventing transfer of viruses. Injection of drugs by contaminated needles has to be avoided. Since the discovery of the HCV in 1989, testing of blood products is possible, and the risk of infection *via* transfusion has declined drastically. In patients with established HCV infection, there is a realistic chance that combination therapy with interferon and ribavirin will result in complete virus elimination and thereby stop the progression to liver cirrhosis. At present, the best results are obtained by pegylated alpha-interferon in a dose of 80–180 g once weekly in combination with 800–1200 mg ribavirin daily (adjusted to body weight). With this treatment, sustained virus elimination can be obtained in more than 40% of patients with virus genotype 1 after treatment for one year, and in up to 90% with genotype non-1 after treatment for 6 months, respectively. In several studies it has been shown, that responders to the antiviral combination therapy have a markedly reduced risk for HCC as compared to nonresponders. However, in patients where the antiviral combination therapy has not been successful, there is no effective strategy for the prevention of HCC. It has been suggested that fibrosis progresses more slowly and the incidence of liver cell cancer is reduced even in non-responders after interferon therapy. However, this result of one large Japanese study has not been confirmed by others. Theoretically, because of its anti-fibrotic effect, which is independent of the antiviral action, prolonged therapy with alpha-interferon – possibly in a reduced dose – might reduce HCC incidence.

Because of the considerable risk of developing HCC, individuals with hereditary hemochromatosis must be identified before cirrhosis is present. Genotyping offers the possibility of detecting affected persons among first-degree relatives of patients with hemochromatosis. The high frequency of hemochromatosis-associated mutations in the HFE gene makes screening of the total population in countries with a high incidence of the disease reasonable. Among conventional laboratory tests, serum iron content and transferrin saturation have the highest sensitivity and specificity. If hemochromatosis is diagnosed, iron depletion by repeated phlebotomy must be started and be continued throughout life. Serum ferritin has to be kept in the lower normal range.

In all patients with chronic liver disease irrespective of the etiology, alcohol consumption has to be stopped.

Future Perspectives

As pointed out above, the successes in the worldwide fight against HCC will be achieved mainly by strategies aiming at tumor prevention. HCC is a tumor whose genesis is dominated by exogenous factors, and therefore prevention and treatment of chronic viral hepatitis in the general population is of special importance. These strategies must include the following measures:

1. Vaccination programs against hepatitis B have to be launched on a nationwide basis in order to eliminate this infection worldwide.
2. Efforts to develop antiviral therapies against hepatitis B and C have to continue. While hepatitis C can be cured in about 50% of the patients, this is not the case for hepatitis B. A major problem with all drug therapies against viral hepatitis developed so far is the high cost of the drugs and the long duration of therapy. Additionally, interferon therapy against hepatitis C is associated with considerable side effects that reduce patient compliance and require continuous surveillance of the patients. As a consequence, the actual therapeutic strategies are either not affordable or not practicable for many of the countries with a high prevalence of chronic viral hepatitis.

Since the bad prognosis of HCC is mainly the consequence of the fact that only surgical resection, but no form of conservative therapy that has been tested so far, offers any hope for cure, the main efforts have to be undertaken in this field. The following strategies are under investigation:

1. Gene therapy aiming at prodrug activation by transfer of suicide genes, tumor cell phenotype correction by inhibition of oncogenes or transfer of either tumor suppressor genes or oncolytic viruses. However, gene therapy in HCC is still hampered by several unsolved problems such as the need to develop methods for selective gene transfer or to select the most appropriate therapeutic target.
2. Biologic or pharmacological strategies aiming at the inhibition of angiogenesis. This might be achieved either pharmacologically (e.g. by drugs such as thalidomide) or by an approach using gene transfer.
3. Although the results in this field have been disappointing so far, efforts have to go on to develop antineoplastic chemotherapeutic agents that are effective against HCC either alone or in combination and that at the same time are tolerable for patients with advanced liver disease.

References

1. Lo CM, Ngan H, Tso WK, et al: Randomized controlled trial of trans-arterial lipiodol chemoembolisation for unresectable hepatocellular carcinoma. Hepatology 35:1164–1171

2. Mori K, Scheidler J, Helmberger T, Holzknecht N, Schauer R, Schirren CA, Bittmann I, Dugas M, Reiser M: Detection of malignant hepatic lesions before orthotopic liver transplantation: accuracy of ferumoxides-enhanced MR imaging. Am J Roentgenol 179:1045–1051, 2002

3. Bismuth H, Chiche L, Adam R, Castaing D, Diamond T, Dennison A (1993) Liver resection versus transplantation for hepatocellular carcinoma in cirrhotic patients. Ann Surg 218: 145–151

4. Poon RTP, Fan ST, Lin IO, Wong J (2000) Significance of resection margin in hepatectomy for hepatocellular carcinoma. Ann Surg 231: 544–551

5. Shirabe K, Shimada M, Gion T, Hasegawa H, Takenaka K, Utsunomiya T, Sugimachi K (1999) Postoperative liver failure after major hepatic resection for hepatocellular carcinoma in the modern era with special reference to remnant liver volume. J Am Coll Surg 188:304–307

6. Neuhaus P, Jonas S, Bechstein WO (2000) Hepatoma of the liver- resection or transplantation? Langenbeck's Arch Surg 385: 171–178

7. Cammà C, Schepis F, Orlando A, Albanese m, Shahied l, Trevisani F, Androne P, Craxi, Cottone M: Transarterial chemoembolisation for unresectable hepatocellular carcinoma: meta-analysis of randomized controlled trials. Radiology 224:47–54,2002

8. Livraghi T, Goldberg SN, Lazzaroni S, Meloni F, Solbiati L, Gazelle GS: Small hepatocellular carcinoma. Treatment with radio-frequency ablation versus ethanol injection. Radiology 210:655–661, 1999

9. Befeler AS, di Bisceglie A (2002) Hepatocellular Carcinoma: Diagnosis and Treatment. Gastroenterology 122:1609–1619

10. Bruix J, Llovet JM (2002) Prognostic prediction and treatment strategy in hepatocellular carcinoma. Hepatology 35:519–524

11. Fujiyama S, Tanaka M, Maeda S, Ashihara H, Hirata R, Tomita K (2002) Tumor markers in early diagnosis, follow-up and management of patients with hepatocellular carcinoma. Oncology 62 Suppl 1:57–63.

12. Okuda K (2002) Natural history of hepatocellular carcinoma including fibrolamellar and hepato-cholangiocarcinoma variants. J Gastroenterol Hepatol 17:401–405.

13. Peterson MS, Baron RL, Marsh JW, Oliver JH, Confer SR, Hunt LE: Pretransplantation surveillance for possible hepatocellular carcinoma in patients with cirrhosis: epidemiology and CT-based tumor detection rate in 430 cases with surgical pathologic correlation. Radiology 217:743–749, 2000.

20 Colorectal Liver Metastases

H.-J. GASSEL, M. GASSER, A.M. WAAGA-GASSER, W. TIMMERMANN

Summary

The liver is the main site of manifestation of metastases of colorectal neoplasms. Diagnostic examination must address the primary tumor site, the extent of liver involvement and the presence of extrahepatic disease by endoscopy, ultrasound, computed tomography, chest x-ray and carcinogenic antigen (CEA) level assessment. Surgical resection represents the treatment of choice and is the only curative therapy at present. It should be performed for resectable metastases after exclusion of extrahepatic tumor (except pulmonary metastases), if the patient's general health status and the remaining liver parenchyma are functionally sufficient. The achievement of a R0 status is the main prognostic factor. Adjuvant and neoadjuvant treatment protocols are under current investigation and cannot be recommended unless in clinical trials. Palliative options include chemotherapy (at present gold standard) and local ablative procedures, e.g. by radiofrequency or laser induced thermoablation and cryoablation. A close follow-up of the patients is necessary since secondary treatment can prolong survival.

Epidemiology

In Europe and the U.S. the incidence rate of colorectal cancer is 15 to 30 per 100,000 inhabitants per year. It is the third most common malignancy in the developed world and accounts, for instance, for 20% of cancer-related deaths in the U.S. The incidence increases dramatically above age 50, approximately equally in men and women. The liver is the main site for manifestation of metastases of colorectal neoplasms. Thus, colorectal metastases form the largest group of secondary malignancies in the liver. About 15 to 25% of patients with colorectal cancer present with synchronous liver metastases [1] and an additional 20% develop metachronous hepatic secondaries, usually within the following 3 years. About a quarter of these patients are candidates for liver resection. Twelve to fifteen percent of patients with colorectal cancer may become at least candidates for curative resection of liver metastases. If neoadjuvant chemotherapy and increasingly aggressive surgical procedures are utilized, this number may approach nearly 20%. Moreover, without any treatment, long-term survival of patients bearing colorectal metastases will not occur.

Etiology and Pathogenesis

The pathogenesis of colorectal cancer involves genetic and environmental factors. The most important one is probably diet. Beyond regional lymph nodes, metastases for colorectal cancer are manifested first in the liver. In the case of synchronous metastasis, the hepatic neoplasm is detected at the same time as the primary lesion, whereas in the case of metachronous metastasis, its appearance is delayed, following the successful removal of the primary tumor. Colorectal metastases reach the liver by different routes:

▸ portal venous circulation,
▸ lymphatic spread, and
▸ via the hepatic arterial system.

Beside hemodynamic factors, several other parameters have been reported to be essential for the formation of colorectal liver metastases [2]. Metachronous cancer cells are migrating step-wise from the site of the primary tumor into the liver, resulting in a mechanical entrapment of tumor cells within the sinusoids. Several adhesion molecules seem to play a crucial role in the settlement of colorectal cancer cells. Subsequently these cells build a metastatic lesion within the liver. Recent data have shown that metastatic tumor growth is often correlated with defective function of cell-cycle regulatory proteins, such as apoptosis-inducing proteins or tyrosine kinases. To facilitate further growth and spreading of a metastatic lesion in the liver, tumor cells seem to have the potential to produce and release factors inducing apoptosis in the local environment of surrounding liver tissue. Furthermore, these cells have the ability to induce adequate vascularization, known as angiogenesis, which is necessary for the expansion of metastases. In this process, angiogenic factors mediate the acceleration of migration of endothelial cells and formation of new blood vessels derived from preexisting ones. Since the capillaries of liver metastases are lined with endothelial cells derived from the sinusoids of the liver, fatty livers or those with cirrhosis have been observed to form fewer metastases. This may be explained by a reduced rate of angiogenesis.

The growth rate of metastatic hepatic neoplasms is often more rapid than that of the original lesion, and the mitotic count of these tumors has been shown to be up to five times greater than that of the extrahepatic primary lesion. These morphological alterations in liver metastases correspond with histopathological and molecular changes within the primary tumor. However, precise understanding of the molecular pathological basis of the formation and further tumor growth of a metastatic lesion in the liver requires further investigations.

Symptoms and Clinical Signs

Symptoms referable to the liver are present in 67% of patients with proven metastases, including hepatic pain, ascites, jaundice, anorexia, and weight loss. In half of these patients, hepatic nodularity becomes apparent and jaundice, ascites, and signs of portal hypertension are present in approximately 25 to 33%. Moreover, the alkaline phosphatase level is increased in over 80% of these patients and in approximately two-thirds of them an elevated serum glutamic oxalacetic transaminase level is usually observed. Whereas in these patients the serum alpha-fetoprotein determination is negative, the CEA and CA 19–9 are often positive. Therefore they may be used as markers for metastatic colon carcinoma and thus are recommended for both diagnostic purposes and for evaluation of the success of therapeutic strategies.

Diagnostics

Synopsis

▶ CEA level
▶ Endoscopy
▶ Ultrasound
▶ CT scan (3-phase contrast enhanced) or MRI (contrast enhanced by Resovist or Endorem)
▶ Chest x-ray

Preoperative diagnostic examination must address the primary tumor site, the extent of liver involvement, and the presence of extrahepatic disease. The basic methods to achieve these goals are:

▶ Endoscopy of the colon, digital examination of the anastomotic site after low anterior resection accompanied by endoluminal ultrasonography;

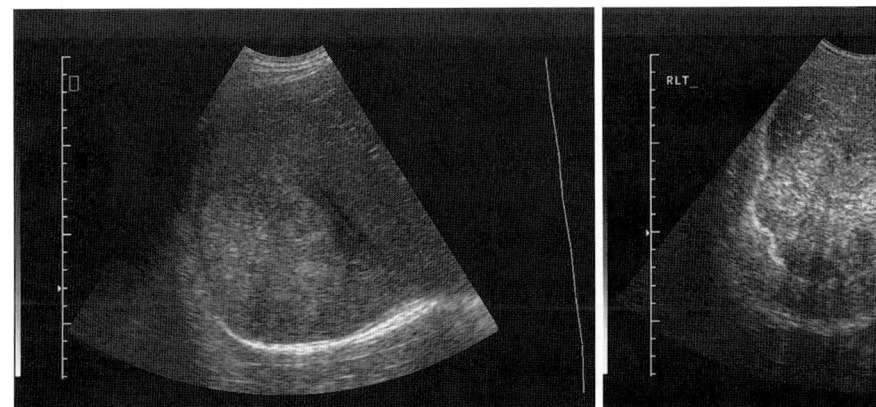

Figure 1
Detection of colorectal metastases by ultrasound examination. *Left:* conventional B-mode; *right:* enhanced presentation by contrast harmonic imaging, late phase. (Courtesy of M. Jenett, MD, Institute of Radiology, University of Würzburg)

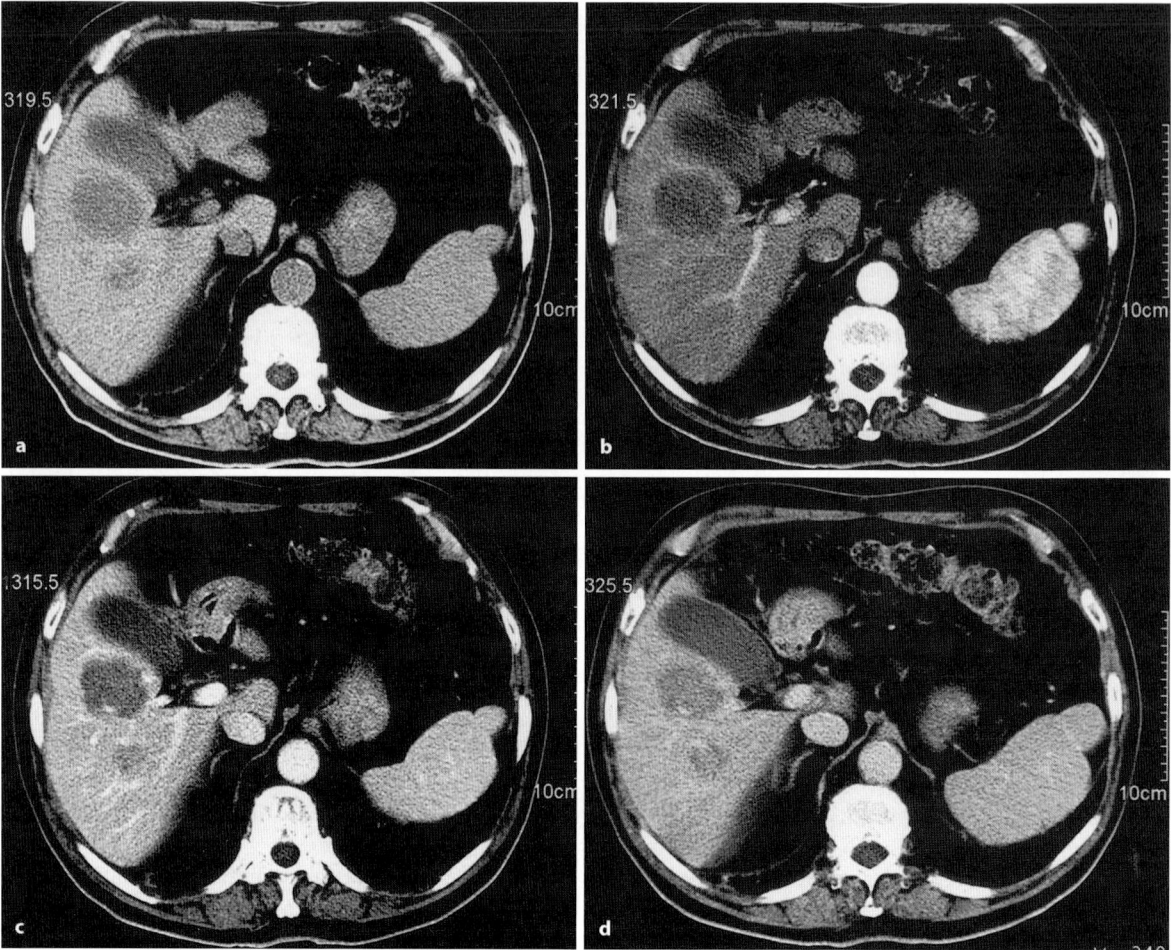

Figure 2a–d
Detection of colorectal metastases by 3-phase computed tomography. a native; **b** i.v. contrast medium, arterial phase; **c** i.v. contrast medium, portal venous phase; **d** i.v. contrast medium, venous phase. (Courtesy of G. Schindler, M.D. and R.Moll, M.D., Institute of Radiology, University of Würzburg)

▸ Ultrasound and CT scan or MRI of the pelvis after abdomino-perineal resection;
▸ Bi-directional chest x-ray, supplemented by spiral CT-scan of the lungs in cases with suspicious results;
▸ CEA and CA 19–9 determinations to provide a baseline for follow-up;
▸ Ultrasound of the liver, occasionally with harmonic imaging and contrast medium (Fig. 1);
▸ spiral CT-scan (Fig. 2) (5 mm collimation, reconstruction interval 5 mm, acquisition beginning at 60–70 s), occasionally CT arterial portography, and, increasingly, MRI of the liver (Fig. 3).

Endorem or Resovist MRI may provide a supplementary diagnostic tool for further examination of the liver. When more than half of the functional hepatic parenchyma needs to be resected, CT volumetry may optimize the choice of further therapy.

The value of immune-scintiscan, and even of single positron emission computed tomography, is not yet defined. Nevertheless, generation of more specific antibodies may have some future value, particularly in detection of disease in the extrahepatic abdomen and pelvis. Furthermore, whole-body positron emission tomography (PET) with [18F] fluorodeoxyglucose (FDG) may further

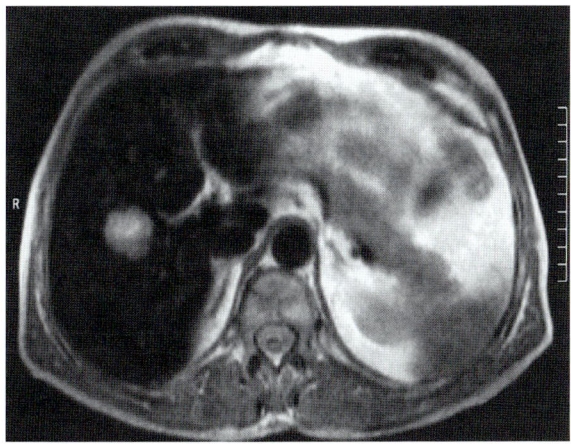

Figure 3
Visualization of colorectal metastases by magnetic resonance imaging enhancement by Endorem contrast medium. (Courtesy of D. Hahn, M.D. and W. Kenn, M.D., Institute of Radiology, University of Würzburg)

enhance diagnostic accuracy, particularly in distinguishing between metastases and benign liver lesions, as well as in the detection of extra-hepatic disease.

In summary, preoperative ultrasound and CT scan are sufficient to detect and localize colorectal metastases to the liver in patients with a medical history of colorec-

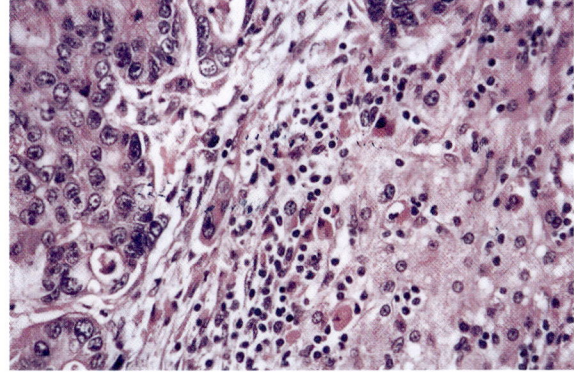

Figure 4
Histology of a typical liver metastasis of a colonic adenocarcinoma. The carcinoma in the *left third of the figure* corresponds to a moderately differentiated adenocarcinoma of the colon. Adjacent to the *right* is a wall of fibrous tissue, lymphocytes and darkly stained apoptotic liver cells. H&E, ×250. (Courtesy of A.M. Gassel, M.D., Institute of Pathology, University of Würzburg)

tal carcinoma. If the results of both procedures are similar and the metastases appear to be resectable, an operation should be performed without further diagnostic procedures. If results between ultrasound and CT scan are discordant, MRI with Endorem or Resovist may be helpful in making the decision concerning an operation. Using this protocol, the rate of negative laparotomies is reduced to less than 10%. Moreover, percutaneous biopsies should not be performed if surgery is planned, in order to avoid tumor cell dissemination and hemorrhage from the biopsy site. However, if palliative nonsurgical therapy is considered, percutaneous biopsy is recommendable for a definitive histological diagnosis. The preoperative diagnostic work-up must be supplemented by thorough intraoperative assessment. Besides clinical evaluation of the abdominal cavity including inspection and palpation of the liver, the most important method is intraoperative ultrasound. Although the latter helps to determine the anatomic location of metastases thus facilitating surgical resection, its adjunctive use in patients screened preoperatively by FDG PET has limited impact on treatment selection.

Histological Classification and Molecular Genetics

Colorectal liver metastases are the most frequent malignant liver tumors, with histological morphology which can be compared to that of the primary colorectal tumor (Fig. 4).

Histological evaluation is usually performed as follows:

▸ preoperatively, a biopsy may be taken to differentiate between a primary liver tumor and a metastatic lesion of an unknown primary tumor, or

▸ postoperatively, the size and number of metastases are examined in the resected liver.

With standard hematoxylin & eosin staining of a core biopsy, it is possible to differentiate between a primary liver tumor and a metastatic lesion. However, it may be difficult in some cases to define a lesion as a secondary tumor derived from a colorectal cancer, since cholangiocellular carcinoma may show a comparable histological pattern. In these patients, additional immunocytochemical tests may be performed. In 92% of patients with colorectal carcinoma, cytokeratin (CK) 8/18 and 20 are positive whereas CK 7 remains negative. In contrast, in cholangiocellular carcinomas of the liver, CK 20 is negative whereas CK 7 is positive.

The histopathological assessment of the resected liver has to be determined by its size and the number of metastases. It is particularly important to determine the distance between the metastasis and the resection margin within the resected part of the liver. Staining the liver parenchyma within this margin with tissue ink is increasingly accepted. It has to be remembered that the intraoperative use of thermocoagulation and ultrasound dissection devices, as well as postoperative tissue processing for histology may result in a shrinking of the solid tissue between 12–30%. Therefore, the surgeon should document the resection margin before the resected liver is fixed in formalin.

Treatment

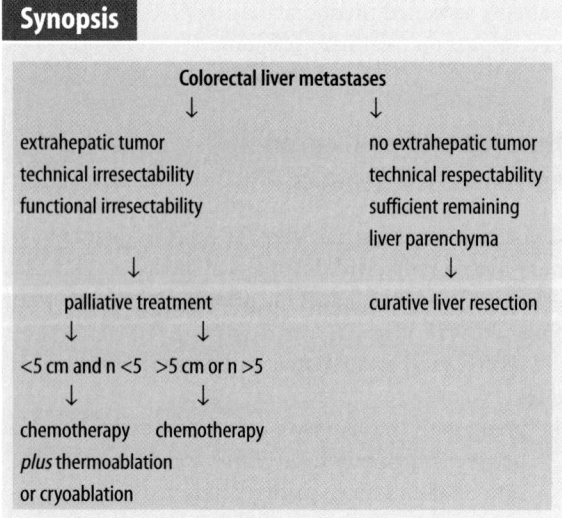

Synopsis

Colorectal liver metastases

↓   ↓

extrahepatic tumor   no extrahepatic tumor
technical irresectability   technical respectability
functional irresectability   sufficient remaining
                                     liver parenchyma

↓   ↓

palliative treatment   curative liver resection
↓   ↓
<5 cm and n <5   >5 cm or n >5
↓   ↓
chemotherapy   chemotherapy
plus thermoablation
or cryoablation

Liver Resection

Resection of liver metastases from colorectal cancer is accepted as a safe and curative treatment. The major goal of surgery is the radical removal of tumor and the achievement of long-term tumor-free survival. Surgical strategy is not uniform, particularly in those patients with resectable synchronous hepatic metastases of colorectal cancer. For the actual decision on liver resection,

given the possibility of achieving an R0 situation, safety aspects as to comorbidity and acceptable extent of parenchyma loss are the prime limitations (Fig. 5a,b).

In general, an anatomical liver resection is considered the treatment of choice, including segmentectomies and hemihepatectomies (Fig. 6).

If the liver is morphologically normal and functionally intact, resection of up to 50% of parenchyma can be performed and resections of up to 75% of the parenchyma are possible, without substantially increasing postoperative morbidity. In some cases, preoperative liver function assays like indocyanine green or monethylglycinexylidide tests may be useful for operative decision. Major complications like hemorrhage or persisting bile fistulas after liver resection occur in 1 to 6%, in noncirrhotic patients the 30-day mortality of elective liver resection ranges between 0% and 5% [3]. Liver transplantation as a treatment option for colorectal metastases is generally not accepted, first because of a dramatic shortage of donor organs and second because of the poor prognosis after liver transplantation for colorectal metastases (long-term survival lesser than 20%).

However, patients who have complex hepatic metastases at the time of diagnosis of the primary colorectal cancer and who would require extended hepatic lobectomy should have hepatic resection delayed for at least 6 to 12 weeks after colon resection. In addition, repeat hepatectomy for recurrent liver metastases has been reported to be an effective treatment to improve survival time for selected patients. In those with isolated second liver metastasis, unilateral spread of first liver metastases, and a disease-free interval between the first and second hepatectomies of more than 12 months, long-term survival or cure can be expected after repeat hepatectomy. In patients with recurrent disease, a re-resection is possible in roughly 20% and survival from the time of re-intervention ranges from 21 to 57% after 5 years (Tab. 1).

Table 1

Indication for surgery	Contraindications
technically resectable metastases	extrahepatic tumor
remnant liver parenchyma	positive lymph nodes in
sufficient	hepatoduodenal ligament
no extrahepatic tumor (except lung)	R0 status not achievable
fair general health status	

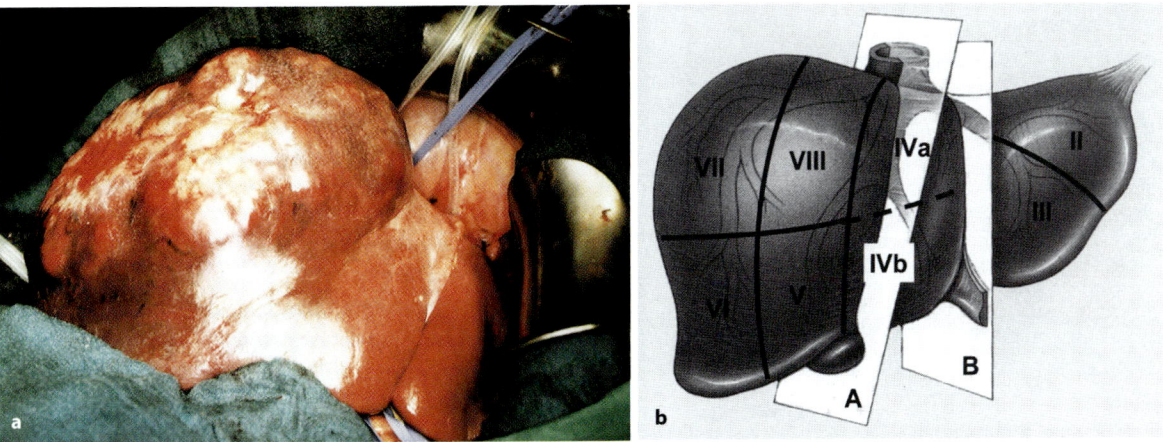

Figure 5a,b
a Intraoperative situs presenting a large liver metastatasis of colorectal cancer located in segment 5–8 (right lobe of the liver). **b** Segmental classification of the liver according to Couinaud. A: Resection phase for hemihepatectomy; B: Resection phase for left lobectomy

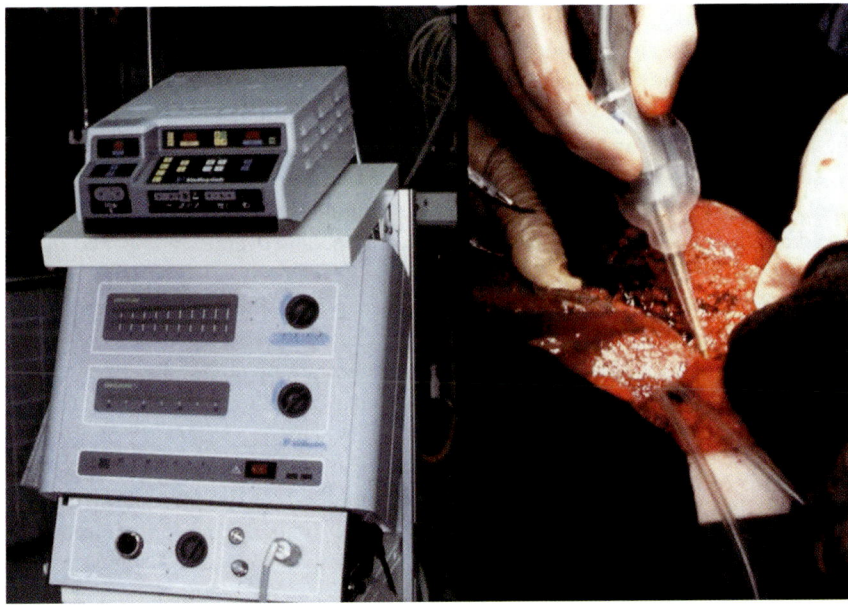

Figure 6
Anatomical liver resection. *Left*: Ultrasound device for dissection of parenchyma (CUSA); *right*: intra-operative view of hemihepat-ectomy

With respect to the operative approach, a clear margin of 1 cm or more should be the aim. However, if the size or location of metastases does not allow a 1 cm margin, resection should still be performed, making every surgical effort to ensure a complete rim of unaffected tissue (Fig. 7).

Adjuvant chemotherapy or radiotherapy after Ro resection is unlikely to improve results as no convincing data exist yet. However, there is an increasing tendency to offer resectional treatment to aged patients with concomitant disease, and far more advanced tumor burden.

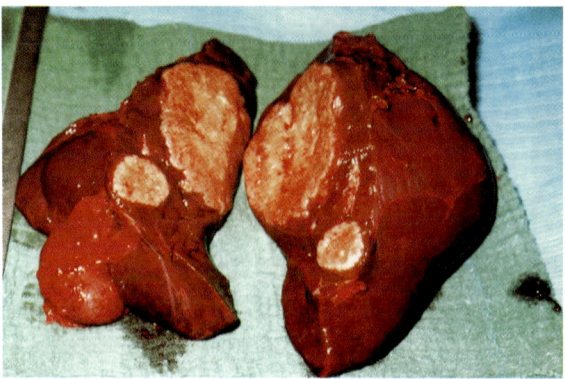

Figure 7
Resected colorectal metastases after right side hemihepatectomy:
Large metastasis with satellite nodule

The technique of unilateral portal venous embolization was first described in 1990 and is now increasingly used in order to induce increase of the remaining parenchyma after complex resections, e.g. extended right hemihepatectomies. Mortality and morbidity and the 5-year survival rates are not significantly affected.

Another approach towards the improvement of surgical strategies is a sequential two stage resection in cases with large and/or multiple metastases. In the first operation the tumor mass is reduced by a non-formally anatomical resection. After liver regeneration, the residual tumor is removed. This procedure, however, is associated with increased morbidity and mortality. Therefore, sequential resections are restricted to patients with a low individual risk profile [4].

Non-Resecting Treatment Options

Local Ablative Treatment

New methods of ablation of liver metastases have been developed in recent years, such as cryotherapy, radio frequency ablation, and laser hyperthermia. In particular, the technical devices for radio frequency ablation have proved to be rather convenient. The application procedure is safe and simple and the success rate can be monitored with ultrasound and CT scan. This method seems to be promising for combined therapy with surgical intervention. However, all of these techniques are efficient in local destruction of liver tumors and despite continu-

ing technical development and improvement, they are limited by the size of the tumor (maximum 4–5 cm in diameter). Whereas cryosurgery [5] can be applied via laparotomy or laparoscopy, radiofrequency [6] as well as laser-induced thermoablation [7] are mainly used percutaneously. Complications such as postinterventional bile fistulas, hemorrhage, abscess formation and perforation of the gut are reported at frequencies ranging from 0.5 to 1.8%. The mortality of the procedures is less than 1% [7]. In summary, although local ablative treatment of colorectal liver metastases seems to be an effective therapeutic option, it is still only used under palliative conditions. Comparison of these new techniques with the gold standard, (i.e., surgical resection) and multimodal therapies (e.g., local ablation methods combined with chemotherapy) deserves further evaluation in well-designed randomized multicentre trials.

Chemotherapy

In the past, clinical trials have shown that chemotherapy with improvement in survival and quality of life is better than symptomatic treatment alone, if administered before symptoms occur. Thus, chemotherapy became the standard treatment for most patients with colorectal liver metastases. Although patients cannot be cured with chemotherapy alone, median overall survival has increased from less than 1 year in untreated patients to more than 1 year, and even to 18 months or more, in recent trials with multidrug chemotherapy. The protocols for systemic palliative chemotherapy do not differ from those described for colorectal carcinomas (see chapter on sporadic CRC by Bresalier). They are based on 5-fluorouracil (5-FU) and leucovorin as first line therapy and combined with either irinotecan or oxaliplatin.

Probably the most promising concept to improve the outcome after surgical resection of liver metastases of colorectal origin and to cure more patients is to combine surgery with chemotherapy. Kemeny et al. [8] determined the efficacy and safety of the combination of hepatic arterial infusion (HAI) of floxuridine (FUDR) with intravenous continuous infusion of 5-FU after resection of liver metastases. The rationale for intraarterial chemotherapy relies on the dual blood supply of the liver and on the fact that liver metastases larger than one millimeter are supplied mainly by the hepatic artery. In addition, fluoropyrimidine analogs such as FUDR are extracted in the liver, resulting in decreased extrahepatic concentration of the drug. However, HAI has limitations. The first is the risk of extrahepatic progression because only the liver receives a sufficient concentration of the drug. This is observed in 50% to 70% of patients after a year of treatment and may occur in unusual sites such as the brain, bones, or adrenal glands. This pattern suggests that HAI should be combined with systemic chemotherapy to treat liver metastases and to prevent occurrence of extrahepatic metastases. In the study by Lorenz et al. [9], HAI with FUDR combined with intravenous 5-FU and folinic acid was superior to HAI with FUDR alone in time-to-progression and overall survival. The second main limit of HAI is the risk of severe side effects. Biliary toxicity depends on the protocol used and is almost exclusively observed with FUDR. The risk increases with the dose and the duration of administration. After 1 year of HAI with FUDR, hepatitis has been observed in 35% of patients and biliary sclerosis in 25%. A phase I/II study of HAI with FUDR combined with systemic irinotecan administered after resection of liver metastases demonstrated that tolerance was acceptable when irinotecan was administered every other week.

Two other recently published studies have evaluated the potential benefit of HAI as adjuvant treatment after resection of colorectal liver metastases. Lorenz et al. used HAI with 5-FU and folinic acid without systemic treatment and showed no benefit over surgery alone, with significant toxicity in the patients receiving chemotherapy. The study from the Memorial Sloan-Kettering Cancer Center compared HAI plus systemic 5-FU and folinic acid with systemic 5-FU and folinic acid only and concluded that combined treatment resulted in a decrease in the hepatic recurrence rate and an improved overall survival only at 2 years.

In summary, HAI alone is not sufficient as adjuvant treatment for liver metastases. HAI combined with systemic chemotherapy can reduce the risk of recurrences after surgery for liver metastases, but this potential benefit is counterbalanced by a significant increase in side effects. Whether the best timing for the administration of chemotherapy is before or after surgery or both and whether the best regimen should contain FUDR, 5-FU, oxaliplatin, irinotecan, or other new drugs are under current investigation. Another critical point is whether administration should be by the systemic or the intra-arterial route. As any adjuvant therapy (systemic or HAI) cannot be recommended as a standard therapy, patients should be enrolled in randomized clinical trials. The same can be applied to neoadjuvant protocols that have been shown to effectively reduce tumor size and may lead to resectability of primarily irresectable metastases.

At present surgical resection represents the treatment of choice and the standard for assessment of any competitive therapeutic approach, since no equally effective therapeutic alternative exists.

Prognosis

Surgical treatment for liver metastases from colorectal cancer is safe and potentially curative, with a 5-year survival rate of 25% to 40%. After resection, however, it is estimated that the disease recurs in 60% to 85% of the patients; and in approximately 40% of these cases, the disease occurs in the form of isolated liver metastases. The predictive factors for recurrence following first resection of liver metastases have not yet been fully clarified. Dukes' staging influenced the disease-free survival after hepatectomy. Wall invasion, mesenteric lymph node metastases, lymphatic invasion, and venous invasion in the primary tumor seem to be predictive factors for recurrence after hepatectomy. There is contradictory data regarding a positive surgical margin. In many series it was a predictive factor after hepatectomy, however, other studies showed no independent impact on outcome or suggested that the importance of a positive resected margin should not be overestimated [10].

The stage of the primary tumor and lymph node metastases are significantly associated with a poor prognosis in both univariate and multivariate analyses. Disease-free survival is significantly influenced by lymph node metastasis, a short interval between treatment of the primary and metastatic tumors and a high preoperative level of CEA.

The overwhelming indicator of prognosis is the completeness of tumor removal according to the R-classification. With respect to the liver involvement, multiplicity of metastases and bilateral disease both seem to be of minor importance after R0-resection, while satellite lesions are significant in many series. The actual number of metastases is of minor importance, with a slight superiority in 5-year survival for patients with one to three nodules relative to patients with four nodules or more in most series. Lymph node metastases at the liver hilum predict a poor outcome. They are likely to prove a clear contraindication to surgery. Whether operative blood loss, need for blood transfusion, and intra-operative hypotension have independent effects on prognosis is still unclear.

Since 1980, single institution series exceeding 100 patients have reported actuarial 5-year survival figures ranging from 18 to 46%, while collected series have reported figures of 21 to 33%. In a recent Japanese series, a 51% survival rate was reported. In a large study with 597 patients who underwent resection of initial colorectal liver metastases with curative intent, the overall 5-year survival was 33%. Ten-year survival figures, if recorded at all, were rarely based on a large enough sample of patients. However, in that large study, a 24% survival at 10 years based on 60 surviving patients with 57 remaining free of recurrent disease was reported.

In summary, the Ro status (Ro resection, no extrahepatic tumor) but not the size of the surgical margin is the main prognostic factor. Localization of the metastases, e.g. bilobar lesions, the number of metastases and the size of the lesion are of minor or even no prognostic value. The importance of tumor biology, e.g. grading and growth pattern, is increasingly recognized.

Follow-Up

Due to the regenerative capacity of the parenchyma, liver re-resections can be performed safely and with oncological benefit. Thus, the follow-up of patients should aim at the liver, the lung, and the primary tumor state. In the first year after liver resection, ultrasound, CT scans, chest x-rays, and CEA estimations should be performed every 3 months, in the second year every 6 months, followed by every 12 months. This should be supported by MRI, endoscopy, and endoscopic ultrasound examinations.

Future Perspectives

Improved results in recent years may have been supported by better preoperative imaging techniques, refinements in surgical technology, and better tailoring of the procedure to the patient's individual need. An increase in the rate of resectable metastases to more than 20% may be achieved by combination of local ablative therapies with neoadjuvant chemotherapy, portal vein embolization and sequential resections.

References

1. Scheele J, Stang R, Altendorf-Hofmann A, Paul M (1995) Resection of colorectal liver metastases. World J Surg 19(1): 59–71
2. Berman RS, Portera CA Jr, Ellis LM. (2001) Biology of liver metastases. Cancer Treat Res 109: 183–206
3. Nordlinger B, Guiguet M, Vaillant JC, et al. (1996) Surgical resection of colorectal carcinoma metastases to the liver. A prognostic scoring system to improve case selection, based on 1568 patients. Association Francaise de Chirurgie. Cancer 77(7):1254–1262
4. Adam R, Laurent A, Azoulay D, et al. (2000) Two-stage hepatectomy: A planned strategy to treat irresectable liver tumors. Ann Surg 232:777–785
5. Seifert JK, Achenbach T, Heintz A et al. (2000) Cryotherapy for liver metastases. Int J Colorectal Dis 15:161–166
6. Curley SA, Izzo F, Delrio P et al. (1999) Radiofrequency ablation of unresectable primary and metastatic hepatic malignancies: results in 123 patients. Ann Surg 230:1–8
7. Vogl TJ, Muller PK, Mack MG et al. (1999) Liver metastases: interventional therapeutic techniques and results, state of the art. Eur Radiol 9:675–684
8. Kemeny N, Fata F (2001) Hepatic-arterial chemotherapy. Lancet Oncol 2:418–428
9. Lorenz M, Mueller HH, Mattes F et al. (2001) Phase II study of weekly 24-hour intraarterial high-dose infusion of 5-fluorouracil and folinic acid for liver metastases from colorectal carcinomas. Ann Oncol 12:321–325
10. Elias D, Cavalcanti A, Sabourin JC, et al. (1998) Results of 136 curative hepatectomies with a safety margin of less than 10 mm for colorectal metastases. J Surg Oncol 69(2):88–93

21 Liver Metastases of Noncolorectal Cancer

W. Timmermann, R. Kellersmann, H.-J. Gassel

Summary

Liver metastases of noncolorectal nonneuroendocrine (NCNN) carcinoma should only be resected, if radical removal can be achieved. The surgical procedure does not differ from that of colorectal metastases. The perioperative lethality ranges from 0 to 8.3%, the morbidity from 6 to 47%. There are no defined standard prognostic factors for patients with metastases of noncolorectal (NC) carcinoma. Patients with metastases of neuroendocrine (NE) carcinoma have a superior prognosis due to the slow progression of the underlying disease. 5 year survival rates of up to 70% have been reported after resection of those metastases. For resections of NCNN metastases 5 year survival rates up to 46% have been documented in smaller series. The value of adjuvant or neoadjuvant therapies as well as local ablative procedures has yet to be defined. The indication to resection of metastases of NC carcinoma requires careful and always individual decision.

Epidemiology

Liver metastases of NC cancer mainly originate from other gastrointestinal primaries due to their portal venous drainage. However, postmortem studies have revealed hepatic involvement in 40% of patients who died of lymphatic, breast, kidney, endometrial, sarcomatous, and bone tumors as a result of generalized hematogeneous dissemination (Fig. 1). The incidence of isolated hepatic metastases of NCNN malignancies is substantially lower compared to cancers of colon and rectum. For example, more than 50% of patients with metastasizing breast cancer show at some stage tumor spread to the liver, but isolated hepatic metastases were observed in only 2–12% of patients [1–3]. In melanoma, renal cell carcinoma, and sarcomas approximately 1% of patients have isolated hepatic metastases [4]. Risk of liver metastases from NE tumors correlates with the size of the primary lesion. In most studies, more than 50% of patients with NE carcinoma showed involvement of the liver at the time of first diagnosis and up to 90% of liver metastases were already found to be bilobular.

Symptoms and Clinical Signs

Symptoms and clinical signs of liver metastases of NCNN tumors are usually caused by their local infiltrative and destructive growth. Clinical findings such as jaundice, anemia, pain of the right upper quarter, or palpable masses are unspecific, often an indication of an advanced stage of the disease, and present in only 40–65% of patients [2, 5, 6]. By contrast, the majority of NE tumors produce hormones that may result in systemic endocrine symptoms such as flush, hyper-/hypoglycemia, Cushing's syndrome, diarrhea, gastric hyperacidemia or acromegaly. Particularly in gastrointestinal carcinoids, the onset of clinical signs is often associated with liver involvement. The size of NE liver metastases does not correlate with clinical presentation, as small hepatic lesions may produce bizarre endocrine syndromes, while large liver masses remain asymptomatic. Since NE malignancies grow slowly, patients may present with large liver tumors without disturbance of hepatic functions.

Diagnostics

Synopsis

The best screening method to detect liver tumors is sonography. The standard diagnostic procedures for liver metastases are computed tomography (CT) scan and MRI with/without contrast enhancement.

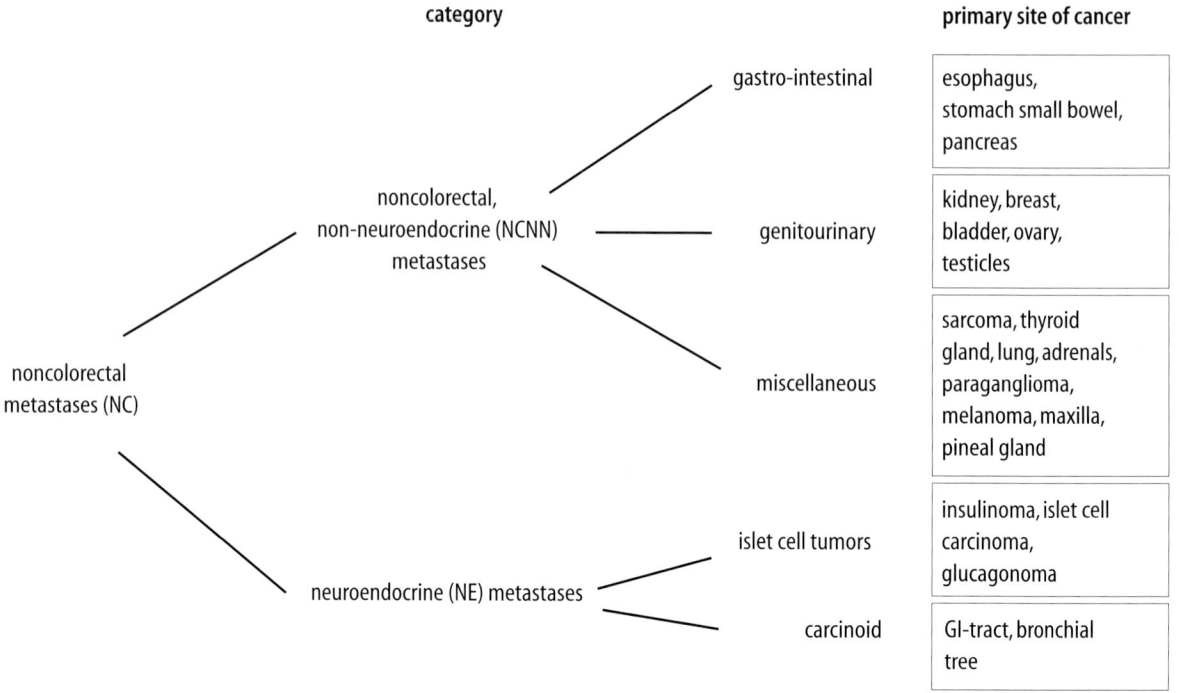

Figure 1
Categories of sites of primary tumors of noncolorectal liver metastases which have been treated by liver resection

Liver metastases of NC carcinoma are found incidentally, during staging of a newly diagnosed primary malignoma or during routine follow-up after treatment of the primary cancer. Diagnostics should pursue two major principles:

1. characterization of the liver lesion (benign vs. malignant, primary vs. secondary) and
2. description of the local, intrahepatic extent of the disease (number, size and localization of liver nodules) and presence of extrahepatic, systemic manifestations.

Abdominal ultrasound represents the screening method for detection of liver metastases of NC cancer. Further diagnostic imaging includes CT and MRI as standard tools to assess precisely liver involvement and to search for extrahepatic metastasis or local recurrence for most primary cancers. However, depending on the tumor type, endoscopy, scintigraphy of the skeleton, or positron emission tomography (PET) may be necessary for a comprehensive preoperative staging. PET, in particular, has recently set a new standard in the detection of intra- and extrahepatic tumor dissemination. In selected cases, laparoscopy may be warranted to enhance diagnostic accuracy prior to a potential liver resection. This technique may be particularly suitable for the discrimination of benign and malignant lesions allowing for direct liver ultrasound and multiple biopsies. It also provides a very sensitive method for the search for intra-abdominal tumor spread. In NCNN liver metastases, octreotide scan represents an additional technique to identify NE tissue with a sensitivity of 80–90%. Serum analysis of hormone levels and measurement of urine 5-hydroxytryptophan excretion may be used as screening methods especially during follow-up of patients who have previously been positive for these markers.

Histological Classification and Molecular Genetics

Metastases of NC cancer are usually characterized by the typical histological picture of their primaries. In some cases, the result of a liver biopsy helps to diagnose the underlying tumor. There are no staging systems for classification of NC liver metastases.

Treatment

Synopsis

The major therapeutic goal is the radical resection of NC liver metastases. All techniques of liver resection including reresection and liver transplantation have been successfully used in selected groups of patients. All kinds of local ablative therapies have been used as well, mainly if surgical resection of metastases was impossible.

Therapeutic efforts in patients with NC liver metastases aim at a radical resection of the entire malignant lesion (Ro situation). The surgical principles do not differ from those applied to colorectal liver metastases. The whole spectrum of established techniques for liver resection of colorectal metastases including atypical, anatomical, *ante-situ* resection or even liver transplantation have also been used for NC hepatic filial tumors. The mortality in these procedures ranges from o to 8.3% [8], morbidity from 6 [1] to 47% [4]. Additional removal of extrahepatic metastatic tissue has been considered an appropriate treatment as long as radical resection (Ro) can be accomplished [2–4]. Repeated resection of NC liver metastases may also be performed in selected cases [3]. Apart from surgical resection of liver metastases, local ablative methods such as chemoembolization, radiofrequency ablation, cryoablation, and laser therapy have recently been introduced as further therapeutic options.

Due to the slow growth of NE malignant tissue, incomplete hepatic resection is accepted as a useful palliative strategy in patients with NE liver metastases. Relief of tumor-related symptoms is anticipated if 90% of the tumor mass can be removed by surgical means [9, 10]. Furthermore, after careful patient selection including those who received radical resection of the primary tumor and had failure of other treatments, liver transplantation is considered an indication to treat hepatomegaly and endocrine symptoms and may offer potential cure (Fig. 2) [11]. Administration of somatostatin analoga can provide rapid and effective reduction of endocrine symptoms in liver metastases of tumors that are positive for somatostatin-receptor expression.

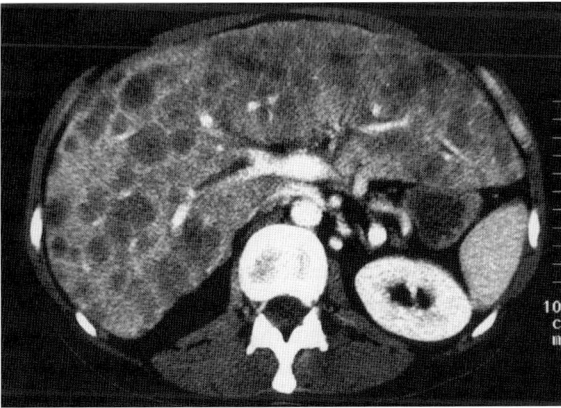

Figure 2
CT scan of a 44 year old male patient with multiple metastases of a neuroendocrine carcinoma. Because of therapy-resistant abdominal pain the patient was listed for liver transplantation. (Courtesy of G. Schindler, M.D. and R. Moll, MD, Institute of Radiology, University of Würzburg)

Prognosis and Follow-Up

Although the natural history of liver metastases of NCNN malignancies is less well defined than that of colorectal cancer, it has been reported that untreated patients with these tumors have a median survival of 2–8 month [7, 12].

There is no clear consensus about prognostic factors in NCNN liver metastases. Controversial data exist regarding primary site, time of diagnosis (synchronous vs. metachronous), presence of extrahepatic metastases, or number of hepatic metastases [5–7, 9]. A significant influence on the disease-free survival after radical resection of the primary tumor was described in 2 publications if this interval was longer than 24 or 36 month [2, 12]. In larger series, radical resection, irrespectively of the primary tumor, correlated with improved prognosis [1–3, 5].

In larger studies, overall 5 years survival rates for patients who underwent liver resection for NCNN liver metastases range from 10 to 37% with a median survival time of 12 to 32 months (Table 1). The resection of liver metastases from breast cancer is associated with survival rates of 9–51%, depending on patient selection. Patients who respond to systemic treatment or those with initially negative lymph node status may have a more beneficial outcome. The majority of patients resected for hepatic metastases of breast cancer had recurrence to the liver which suggests the usefulness of some kind of local adjuvant therapy [2]. Resection of isolated liver metastases from gastric adenocarcinoma is controversial unless liver involvement is due to direct tumor invasion of the left hepatic lobe. 5-years survival rates range from 5 to 30%, however the group of these patients is usually small and very heterogeneous. Few long-term survivors have been documented. Only patients with metachronous liver metastases may benefit from surgical resection [8]. Despite anecdotal reports of long-term survival, hepatic metastasectomy of gallbladder or pancreas carcinoma has not been recommended because the overall prognosis is very poor. Hepatic resection of liver metastases from renal and genito-urethral carcinoma as well as from melanoma and sarcoma may provide reasonable outcomes after individual, careful patient selection. Some studies demonstrated high survival rates in subgroups that were defined according to their primary tumor (Table 2); however, they again do not indicate exact treatment recommendations due to their heterogeneous character and relatively low number of patients. Similarly, results of additive treatments using systemic or loco-regional chemotherapy before and/or after liver resection for NCNN liver metastases do not allow clear assessment of their influence on patients' prognosis [1, 9].

The natural course of NE liver metastases is less aggressive compared to other malignancies. Without treatment, a 5-year survival rate of approximately 30–40% has been demonstrated. There are reports of sporadic long-term survival of more than 10 years in patients with untreated carcinoid liver metastases. If curative liver resection is possible, a 5-year survival rate of more than 60% can be achieved. After palliative resection, 5-year survival rates of 39–65% and postoperative response to tumor-related symptoms of approximately 90% with a mean duration of 19 months have been shown. Survival of patients receiving a liver transplant for metastatic disease of NE tumors was around 35% after 5 years [11]. Arterial chemoembolization may lead to significant alleviation of symptoms and control of tumor size in approximately 90% of patients. However, this non-surgical procedure is hampered by a mortality rate of up to 5%. Administration of somatostatin analogues (e.g. octreotide) also reduces clinical symptoms in nearly 80% of patients and improves quality of life, but its influence on patient survival still appears to be controversial. Partial resistance to somatostatin analogues after 3–12 months may limit their clinical use. Further palliative approaches such as systemic chemotherapy, interferon-α, cryoablation, and alcohol instillation have also shown to exert beneficial effects, but their therapeutic relevance has yet to be determined [9, 10].

Table 1

Overall survival after resection of NCNE liver metastases

Reference	n	5 years survival
Laurent et al. [12]	39	35%
Hemming et al. [5]	37	45%
van Ruth et al. [7]*	28	35%
Lindell et al. [6]	20	25%
Elias et al. [9]**	147	36%
Harrison et al. [2]	96	37%
Lang et al. [3]	127	26%
Zacherl et al. [4]	72	10%

*One patient with NE liver metastases, **27 patients with NE liver metastases (5 years survival 74%)

Table 2

Studies that define subgroups of primary tumors with beneficial outcome after resection of NCNE liver metastases

Reference	Subgroups	n	5 years survival [%]
Hemming et al. [5]	non-gastrointestinal	30	60
Elias et al. [9]	testicular	20	46
Harrison et al. [2]	genito-urethral	34	60

Future Perspectives

Future diagnostic efforts will have to focus on a better selection of patients particularly of those with NCNE hepatic involvement. Improvement of diagnostic tools will help to improve the identification of those patients who have tumor cell dissemination outside the liver and may therefore not be good candidates for an exclusively local therapy. For example, detection and characterisation of tumor cells in blood or bone marrow by immunohistochemistry or molecular biological methods may become promising diagnostic standards for a better patient selection prior to an intended liver resection. To date, there is very little consensus about prognostic factors that may influence the outcome for these patients and allow for a more tailored concept for the individual patient, since most studies only report single center experiences and often rely on low patient numbers. However, current concepts in the treatment of NCNE liver metastases agree that surgical resection is only useful if radical removal (Ro situation) can be achieved. Local ablative techniques such as cryoablation and radiofrequency ablation will expand the spectrum of surgical options for patients with NC liver metastases, but solid therapeutic guidelines for their efficient use are still required. Additionally, the rapid progress in systemic treatment strategies, e.g. polychemotherapy, will further generate effective adjuvant and neo-adjuvant approaches that will increase the number of patients who may benefit from surgical resection of NC liver metastases.

References

1. Raab R, Nussbaum KT, Behrend M, Weimann A (1998) Liver metastases of breast cancer: results of liver resection. Anticancer Res 18: 2231–2233
2. Harrison LE, Brennan MF, Newman E, Fortner JG, Picardo A, Blumgart LH, Fong Y (1997) Hepatic resection for noncolorectal, nonneuroendocrine metastases: a fifteen-year experience with ninety-six patients. Surgery 121: 625–632
3. Lang H, Nussbaum KT, Weimann A, Raab R (1999) Ergebnisse der Resektion nichtcolorectaler nichtneuroendokriner Lebermetastasen. Chirurg 70: 439–446
4. Zacherl M, Längle F, Steininger R, Scheuba C, Wenzl E, Jakesz R, Zacherl J (2001) Die chirurgische Therapie von nicht-kolorektalen und nicht-neuroendokrinen Lebermetastasen. Wien Klin Wochenschr 113: 681–687
5. Hemming AW, Sielaff TD, Gallinger S, Cattral MS, Taylor BR, Greig PD, Langer B (2000) Hepatic resection of noncolorectal nonneuroendocrine metastases. Liver Transpl 6: 97–101
6. Lindell G, Ohlsson B, Saarela A, Andersson R, Tranberg KG (1998) Liver resection of noncolorectal secondaries. J Surg Oncol 69: 66–70
7. van Ruth S, Mutsaerts E, Zoetmulder FA, van Coevorden F (2001) Metastasectomy for liver metastases of non-colorectal primaries. Eur J Surg Oncol 27: 662–667
8. Bines SD, England G, Deziel DJ, Witt TR, Doolas A, Roseman DL (1993) Synchronous, metachronous, and multiple hepatic resections of liver tumors originating from primary gastric tumors. Surgery 114: 799–805
9. Elias D, Cavalcanti dA, Eggenspieler P et al. (1998) Resection of liver metastases from a noncolorectal primary: indications and results based on 147 monocentric patients. J Am Coll Surg 187: 487–493
10. Que FG, Nagorney DM, Batts KP, Linz LJ, Kvols LK (1995) Hepatic resection for metastatic neuroendocrine carcinomas. Am J Surg 169: 36–42
11. Lehnert T (1998) Liver transplantation for metastatic neuroendocrine carcinoma: an analysis of 103 patients. Transplantation 66: 1307–1312
12. Laurent C, Rullier E, Feyler A, Masson B, Saric J (2001) Resection of noncolorectal and nonneuroendocrine liver metastases: late metastases are the only chance of cure. World J Surg 25: 1532–1536

Appendix

Metastases from an Unknown Primary Adenocarcinoma

W. Scheppach

In approximately 5% of cancer patients metastases are detected by imaging techniques but a primary tumor is missed. This situation if referred to as "cancer of unknown primary" or CUP syndrome. The gastroenterologist's problem in a subgroup of these patients is how to deal with liver metastases from an unknown primary adenocarcinoma (1, 2).

Histological Classification

Liver metastases from adenocarcinomas have to be differentiated from other entities such as squamous, hepatocellular, or neuroendocrine carcinomas. In contrast to adenocarcinomas, squamous carcinomas stain positive for cytokeratin (CK) 5 and 6. Hepatocellular carcinomas are not desmoplastic (contrary to adenocarcinomas) and are recognized by the heppar antibody. Neuroendocrine tumors are diagnosed on the basis of a typical morphology and distinctive immunohistochemistry (chromogranins, synaptophysin, neuron-specific enolase). Liver metastases from adenocarcinomas may have their origin in the intestine (stomach, pancreas, colorectum) as well as in extraintestinal organs (e.g., lung, breast, ovary). The cytokeratin pattern can be helpful to identify the primary sites in this situation. Metastases from colorectal cancers are CK 7 negative whereas adenocarcinomas from various other sites (stomach, pancreas, ductal breast, ovary, endometrium) are CK 7 positive. On the contrary, CK 20 is expressed in colorectal cancer but not in cancers of the breast, lung, ovary and endometrium; gastric and pancreatic cancers may be positive or negative for CK 20. In the differential diagnosis of CK 7 positive/CK 20 negative tumors local growth of cholangiocellular carcinoma must be considered.

Treatment

There is no well-established polychemotherapy regimen for unresectable liver metastases from an unknown primary adenocarcinoma. Historically, combinations of cisplatin/carboplatin with etoposide have shown an overall response of 20 percent. Most gastrointestinal adenocarcinomas are moderately affected by 5-fluorouracil/folinic acid (FUFA) which has been combined with paclitaxel or cisplatin. Recently oxaliplatin and irinotecan which are established in the first line treatment of metastatic colorectal cancer have both shown effectiveness in other gastrointestinal malignancies (e.g., gastric and pancreatic cancer). These newer compounds (combined with FUFA) are thus candidates for the treatment of liver metastases of unknown primary adenocarcinoma. Another combination partner is gemcitabine which has a role in the treatment of pancreatic adenocarcinomas, non small cell lung cancer, and possibly adenocarcinomas of the bile ducts. With these uncertainties in mind, we prefer combinations of oxaliplatin/FUFA or oxaliplatin/capecitabine (orally administered 5-fluorouracil prodrug) for treatment of liver metastases from an unknown primary adenocarcinoma.

Prognosis

Adenocarcinoma metastases carry a dismal prognosis with survival ranging between 2 and 6 months from diagnosis. The choice between supportive care and empirical palliative chemotherapy will be an individual decision of the patient after close consultation with his physician.

References

1. Hogan BA, Thornton FJ, Brannigan M, Browne TJ, Pender S, O'Kelly P, Lyon SM, Lee MJ (2002) Hepatic metastases from an unknwon primary neoplasm (UPN): survival, prognostic indicators and value of extensive investigations. Clin Radiol 57:1073–1077
2. Kliche KO, Kubsch K, Raida M, Masri-Zada R, Hoffken K (2002) Chronomodulated chemotherapy in metastatic gastrointestinal cancer combining 5-FU and sodium folinate with oxaliplatin, irinotecan or gemcitabine; The Jena experience in 79 patients. J Cancer Res Clin Oncol 128:516–524

22 Benign Liver Tumors

E. Biecker, H.P. Fischer, H. Strunk, T. Sauerbruch

Summary

In contrast to primary and secondary malignant hepatic tumors, benign liver tumors are relatively rare. Cavernous hemangioma is the most common, followed by focal nodular hyperplasia that is often solitary and nodular regenerative hyperplasia that involves the entire organ. Hepatic adenoma is rare but has displayed a marked increase over recent years, most likely due to the widespread use of oral contraceptives. Accurate diagnosis is crucial, since hepatic adenoma carries the risk of rupture and bleeding and, rarely, progression to hepatocellular carcinoma. Benign hemangioendothelioma of the liver is a rare entity in infants but could cause life-threatening complications. Angiomyolipoma, like inflammatory pseudotumor sometimes difficult to distinguish from a malignant process, is a very exceptional finding in the liver.

Due to advances in imaging procedures like magnetic resonance imaging, computed tomography-scan and ultrasound as well as progress in immunohistochemistry, it is possible to make the appropriate diagnosis in a high percentage of patients without laparotomy and resection.

Once the diagnosis is established and a malignant process is ruled out, most of the benign liver tumors do not need treatment. Exceptions are lesions that cause local problems or pain due to their size, hepatic adenoma because of the risk of rupture and bleeding as well as the low risk of progression to carcinoma, benign hemangioendothelioma of the infant, when it is associated with disseminated intravascular coagulation or heart failure and inflammatory pseudotumor.

Epidemiology

Cavernous Hemangioma

The most common benign tumor of the liver is cavernous hemangioma. The prevalence in large autopsy series ranges from 3% up to 20%. In contrast, an ultrasound screening survey in an otherwise healthy population revealed a prevalence of only 1.4%.

All age groups are affected but most lesions are detected in middle-aged adults. There is a preponderance of females (2–6:1).

Focal Nodular Hyperplasia

The second most frequent benign tumor of the liver is focal nodular hyperplasia (FNH). It is detected in about 3% of the population, mostly between the age of 30 and 50 years. As in cavernous hemangioma, mainly women are affected (6–8:1).

Hepatic Adenoma

Hepatocellular adenoma (HA) was a very rare entity before the introduction of the oral contraceptive (OC) agents. Nowadays, the vast majority of affected patients are premenopausal women with a long-term history of OC drug intake [1]. Long-term treatment with anabolic androgens is also known to induce HA, but only a small number of patients has been reported in the literature. In a few patients, HA are related to glycogen storage diseases. A French series of 43 patients revealed that 52% of patients with type I and 25% of patients with type III glycogen storage disease had HA at the time of the initial screening.

Nodular Regenerative Hyperplasia

Nodular regenerative hyperplasia (NRH) of the liver is relatively common. Two large series of 2535 and 577 consecutive adult autopsies have reported a prevalence of 2.6% [2] and 2.1%, respectively. The gender distribution is almost equal with a slight female predominance. Most of the patients are 50 to 70 years old; some of them are affected by rheumatologic and lymphoproliferative disorders.

Benign Hemangioendothelioma

Benign hepatic hemangioendothelioma is the most common mesenchymal hepatic tumor of infancy; most tumors are diagnosed before the age of six months. A slight female preponderance (around 2:1) has been reported. The lesion is very rare in adults. Only a few adult patients have been described so far.

Angiomyolipoma

Angiomyolipoma (AML) of the liver is a very rare condition. To date, less then 100 patients have been reported, most often women aged between 30 and 60 years.

Inflammatory Pseudotumor

Hepatic inflammatory pseudotumor (IPT) accounts for approximately 1% of all benign tumors of the liver and is found primarily in middle-aged men [3] (male:female ratio 3.5:1).

Etiology

Cavernous Hemangioma

Female preponderance has been reported in most series of cavernous hemangiomas of the liver. An increase in size has been observed during pregnancy and is associated with intake of OC and treatment with glucocorticoids. Estrogen receptors are expressed in a high percentage of cavernous hemangiomas but not in all. Growth of estrogen receptor negative hemangiomas during puberty has been shown. Sex hormones may therefore contribute to the enlargement of cavernous hemangioma.

Focal Nodular Hyperplasia

Like HA, the prevalence of FNH is predominant in women of childbearing age. This has led to the conclusion that – as in HA – endogenous estrogens or intake of OC drugs are associated with the growth and development of FNH. However, a recent study involving 136 women, who were taking either no OC, low dose OC, high-dose OC or progesterones found no relation between number or size of FNH lesions and the intake of OC during a

follow-up period of nine years [4]. In none of the 12 patients who had a pregnancy after the diagnosis of FNH, did an increase in size of the FNH occur. Similar results were shown in another series of ten pregnant women with FNH. These observations suggest that there is no clear-cut influence of exogenous or endogenous sex hormones on the growth of FNH lesions.

Hepatic Adenoma

The association of the use of OC drugs and HA is well described. First reports of increased risk of developing hepatocellular adenoma for women taking contraceptive steroids came in the early 1970s. The longer the intake of the drug, the higher is the risk of developing HA; the risk for women who have been taking the "pill" for five to seven years is increased five times. For women who have been taking the drug for more than nine years, the risk is increased 25 times. Other risk factors are an age over 30 years and OC with higher hormonal potency. This association of HA and the increased risk of development or growth of HA during pregnancy and in the postpartum period imply that estrogens are the more relevant hormonal compound. HA in glycogenosis types I and III and in patients taking androgenic steroids have also been described.

The mechanisms of sex hormone initiation or regulation of the growth of HA are the subject of speculation. Estrogen and progesterone receptors have been shown in only one third of HA. Estrogens promote hepatic regeneration in rat but it is not known if this is true in human liver. The mild cholestatic effect of contraceptive steroids might aggravate the toxicity of substances that are excreted in the bile. However, none of these theories has been proven.

Nodular Regenerative Hyperplasia

NRH is often associated with other diseases. Most cases have been reported to be associated with conditions that belong to lymphoproliferative or rheumatologic disorders [2]. Drug-related (i.e. azathioprine, busulfan, thioguanine) and familial forms are also known. The underlying cause of NRH is thought to be secondary to a microcirculatory impairment of the liver, causing atrophy and compensatory regeneration. In several patients with NRH, occlusion of small branches of the portal vein has been shown. These findings, and the observation that some patients with NRH suffered from nephrosclerosis or Raynaud's disease, support the hypothesis that an impaired microcirculation might be involved in the pathogenesis of the disease.

Benign Hemangioendothelioma

Benign hemangioendothelioma of the infant is a rare liver tumor of embryonic origin and should not be confused with the malignant epithelioid hemangioendothelioma of the adult. Hemangiomas of other organs, primarily of the skin, which are found in up to 50% of patients, are frequently associated with hepatic hemangioendothelioma.

Angiomyolipoma

The extremely rare AML of the liver is composed of three heterogeneous tissue components that include blood vessels, smooth muscle cells and fat cells. The proportions and distributions are quite variable from tumor to tumor. The exact etiopathogenesis is unknown, although it is suggested that the different cells types within the tumor might represent different development stages of one precursor cell, the so called pericyte [5].

Inflammatory Pseudotumor

IPT has been described for virtually every site in the body. Most often lungs and eyes are affected, but IPT occurs also – although rarely – in the liver. The etiopathogenesis is poorly understood. Several theories are under discussion. Different authors have described an association with a preceding fungal, bacterial or viral infection like hepatitis C, HIV or Epstein-Barr virus. Some studies, however, doubt its purely inflammatory nature. Several groups showed genomic Epstein-Barr virus material and immunoreactivity for follicular dendritic cells in the lesions and thus speculated that some IPT might be of follicular dendritic cell origin. In contrast to conventional follicular dendritic cell tumors, these IPT-like tumors have only been described for intra-abdominal sites like liver and spleen. It has been shown that some of the IPT exhibit local infiltrative growth, vascular invasion and malignant transformation and that some of the IPT have clonal characteristics. The authors referred to these lesions as a soft-tissue mesenchymal tumor with an indeterminate or low malignant potential.

Symptoms and Clinical Signs

Symptoms and clinical signs for almost all of the benign hepatic tumors are often unspecific and most often caused by a mass effect, but can be dramatic in few patients.

Cavernous Hemangioma

Cavernous hemangiomas are often found incidentally on ultrasound examinations for unspecific upper abdominal pain. Most of the lesions are less than 5 cm in diameter and do not cause any symptoms. If pain in the right upper quadrant occurs, the lesions frequently surpass 5 cm in size and may show intralesional hemorrhage, localized thrombosis or inflammation. Hemangiomas in other sites of the body like lung, skin and brain are found in some of the patients. These patients often present with multiple liver hemangiomas.

Giant cavernous hemangiomas may cause disseminated intravascular coagulation, termed Kasabach-Merritt syndrome. Affected patients commonly present with upper abdominal pain and signs of bleeding, which is often triggered by a surgical procedure. However, Kasabach-Merritt syndrome is a very rare finding in adults and appears more often in infants with benign hemangioendothelioma.

Focal Nodular Hyperplasia

FNH is an incidental finding in more than 75% of the patients [6]. If patients are symptomatic, they usually complain of mild epigastric pain or discomfort. In patients with large tumors, an abdominal mass might be palpable. Rarely, hemorrhage into the tumor occurs and may cause more pronounced pain. The latter has been shown to be more frequent in women taking oral contraceptives in some early studies, but has not been proven in more recent surveys.

Hepatic Adenoma

More than half of the patients with HA have no symptoms at all and the diagnosis is made as an incidental finding during diagnostic workup for some other reason. Approximately one third of the patients complain of mild to moderate pain in the hypochondrium or epigastrium. Some of the patients recognize a palpable mass by themselves or their physician finds it. Rarely, the first presentation of HA can be rather dramatic, as it is the case in tumor infarction with symptoms like pain, nausea and fever. Even life threatening complications like rupture and intraabdominal bleeding may occur. Bleeding and rupture as initial presentation of HA have been reported to be as frequent as 30% by some authors. Rupture and intra-abdominal hemorrhage are more frequent in large and solitary tumors and in women taking oral contraceptives.

Adenomatosis of the liver is defined by more than three adenomas in the same liver. A review of eight patients, all of them women, with adenomatosis treated in the Mayo Clinic showed that abdominal pain (87.5%) and bleeding (62.5%) were more common in these individuals with adenomatosis than in patients with only one or two lesions. All these patients underwent surgery and resection and showed an improvement of symptoms. Interestingly, immunohistochemistry for estrogen receptors showed both, receptor- positive and receptor-negative adenomas in the same liver, in eight patients [7].

Nodular Regenerative Hyperplasia

As outlined above, NRH is frequently associated with a rheumatologic or lymphoproliferative disorder that dominates the clinical picture. Therefore, NRH is often an incidental finding and many cases are not detected before autopsy [2]. The most common findings at physical examination are hepatomegaly and splenomegaly. Some patients develop portal hypertension and present with the typical clinical signs like esophageal varices and ascites [2]. Liver failure has been documented as a consequence of NRH in a few patients.

Benign Hemangioendothelioma

About half of the infants with benign hemangioendothelioma present with an abdominal mass and associated symptoms that include anorexia, vomiting, poor weight gain, and lethargy. Skin hemangiomas are present in approximately ten percent of the patients, less often hemangiomas in other organs are found. The most important and outcome-defining clinical feature is high output congestive heart failure due to massive arteriovenous shunting. The clinical triad of hepatomegaly, congestive cardiac failure and skin hemangiomas is found only in patients with large lesions. Jaundice is present in 20% of patients, anemia indicated by hemoglobin <10 g/dl in 50% of patients. Rarely, an arterial bruit may be auscultated over the liver. Infrequent but important associated conditions are disseminated vascular coagulation (Kasabach-Merritt syndrome) and liver failure.

Angiomyolipoma

Women in the age range of 30 to 60 years are the typical individuals in which AML are found. Clinical symptoms are determined almost exclusively by the tumor size. Small tumors are only found incidentally, whereas patients with large lesions – diameters up to 36 cm have been reported – present with abdominal discomfort, pain and/or a palpable abdominal mass. In contrast to AML of the kidney, less then 10% of the hepatic AML are associated with tuberous sclerosis.

Inflammatory Pseudotumor

Patients with IPT are commonly symptomatic. They present with fever, malaise, weight loss and often with unspecific right upper quadrant pain and tenderness, which makes it difficult to distinguish it from liver abscess.

Diagnostics

Synopsis

Standard techniques in the diagnostic of benign hepatic lesions

▸ Abdominal ultrasound (US) and color Doppler ultrasound
▸ Computerized tomographic (CT) scan
▸ Magnetic resonance imaging (MRI)
▸ Nuclear imaging (^{99m}Tc-labeled red blood single emission computed tomographic (SPECT) scanning, ^{99m}Tc-sulfur colloid scintigraphy, hepatobiliary scanning using trimethylbromoiminodiacetic acid (TBIDA)
▸ Hepatic arteriography
▸ Needle biopsy or open biopsy.

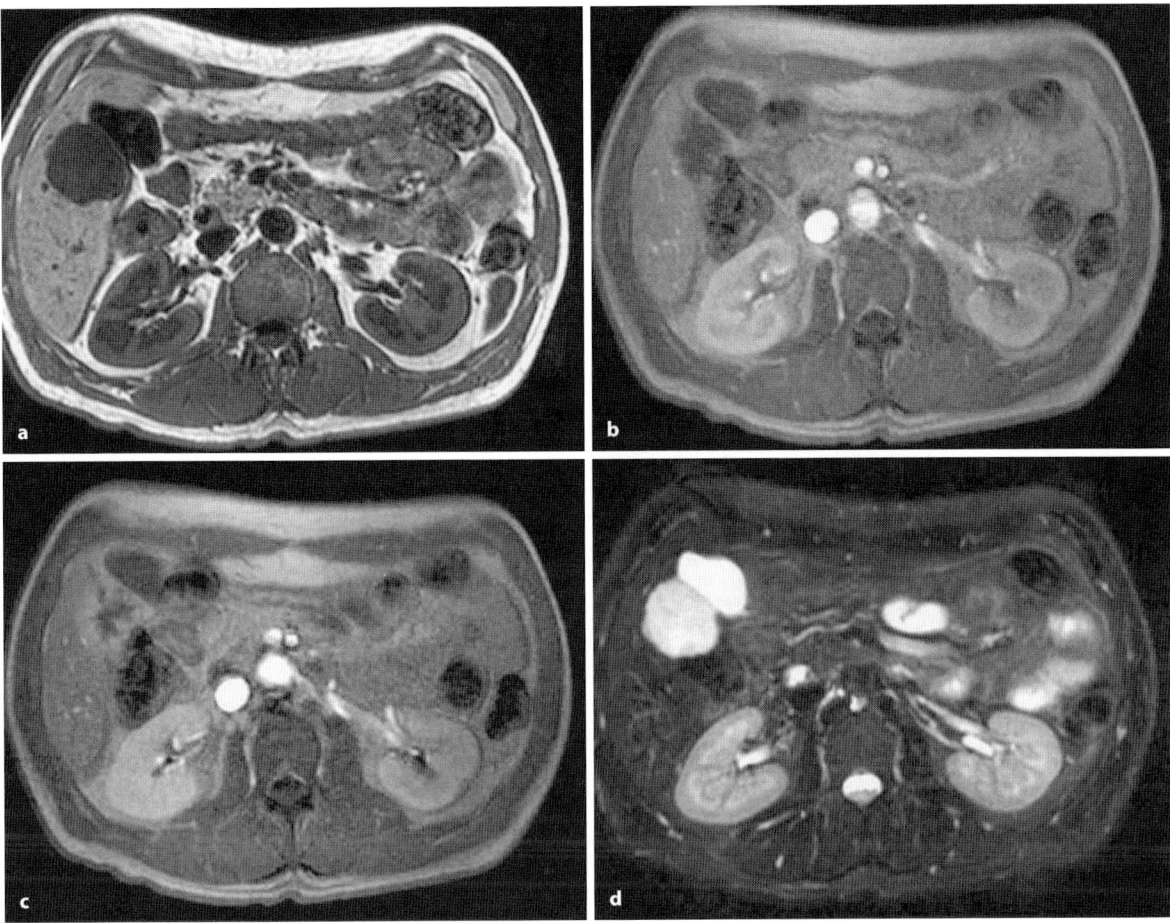

Figure 1a–d
Solitary hemangioma. **a** T-1 weighted MR image with a hypointense well demarcated, rounded lesion in the right liver lobe close to the gall-bladder. **b** Early after intravenous contrast injection there is only peripheral enhancement. Shown is also arterial as well as renal cortical enhancement. **c** In the late phase after intravenous contrast injection, contrast fills in from peripheral to central with globular enhancement. **d** T-2 weighted MR image with fat saturation (SPIR) shows a strong hyperintense lesion

Physical examination is of very limited use. A palpable mass in the right upper quadrant is found only in patients with relatively large lesions and a more detailed diagnosis is usually not possible. Similarly, liver function tests are neither sensitive nor specific in benign liver tumors. Even slight abnormalities in ALT/AST (alanine aminotransferase/aspartate aminotransferase), γ-GT (gamma glutamyltransferase) or alkaline phosphatase levels are often not present and, if they are, they are non-specific [3, 4, 8]. As is the case for other benign tumors, liver function tests in inflammatory pseudotumors may be abnormal, but are not specific. Laboratory indicators of inflammation like leucocytosis, erythrocyte sedimentation rate and C-reactive protein are frequently elevated.

Today, imaging procedures like US, CT, MRI and, with declining relevance, nuclear imaging, play the key role in the diagnosis of benign tumors of the liver.

Since US is widely available, relatively easy to perform and often used as an initial screening method, many liver lesions are detected incidentally during diagnostic work-up for some other reason.

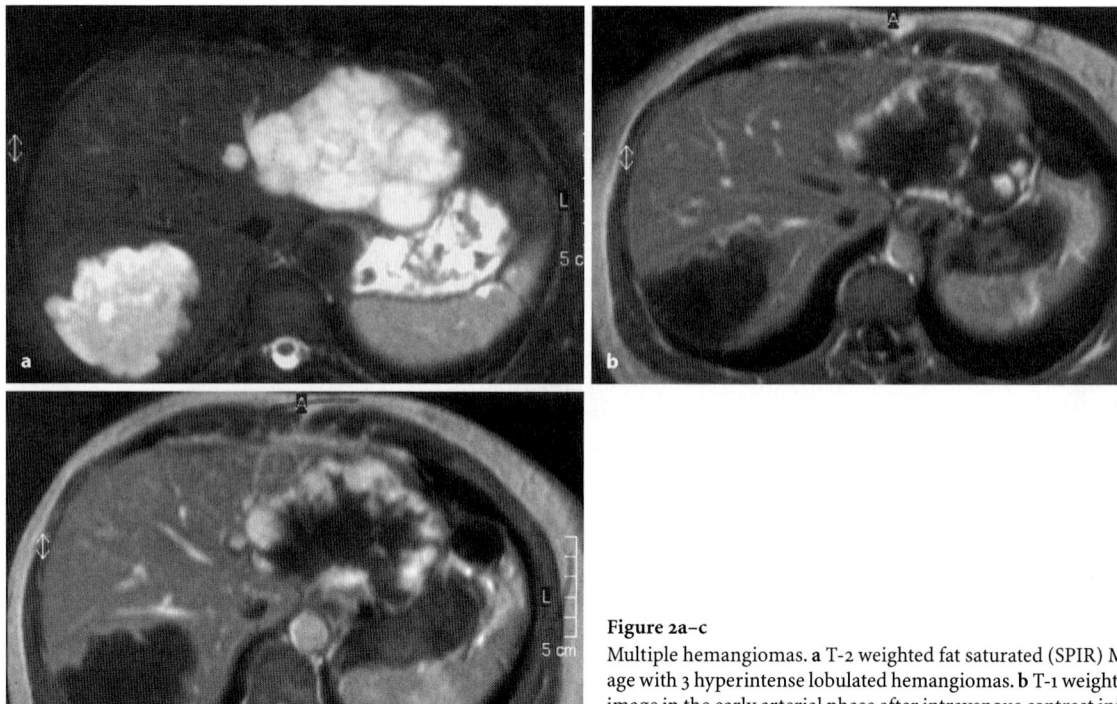

Figure 2a–c

Multiple hemangiomas. **a** T-2 weighted fat saturated (SPIR) MR image with 3 hyperintense lobulated hemangiomas. **b** T-1 weighted MR image in the early arterial phase after intravenous contrast injection with minimal peripheral, globular enhancement. **c** In the venous phase more pronounced peripheral enhancement is seen

Cavernous Hemangioma

Most of the cavernous hemangiomas have the typical appearance of a round, well-demarcated, homogenous hyperechoic mass on conventional ultrasound. However, the sensitivity (60% to 75%) and specificity (60% to 80%) of these signs are not sufficient to allow a definite diagnosis in many cases. Because of the slow blood flow in the lesion, neither color nor power Doppler imaging improve the capability of ultrasound for making a specific diagnosis of benign hepatic cavernous hemangioma. However, US contrast agents, which are more and more used in clinical routine, improve the diagnostic accuracy of US since they allow the visualization of the peripheral nodular arterial enhancement and the consecutive delayed centripetal filling [9]. On standard CT scans, hemangiomas are often missed. Good diagnostic accuracy is obtained by triple-phase (dynamic) CT scanning. Hemangiomas typically exhibit a focal globular enhancement by puddling the contrast agent in the dilated vascular spaces. More than 90% of the hemangiomas fulfill these criteria. Both, highest sensitivity (85% to 95%) and specificity (85% to 95%) are obtained with MRI (Figs. 1 and 2). Characteristic findings are a strong hyperintense signal in T2-weighted images and multiple intratumoral lobulations. Cavernous hemangiomas with a diameter >3 cm which are not located too deep in the liver parenchyma could be identified with a sensitivity and specificity that are close to MRI by ^{99m}Tc-labeled red blood cell SPECT scanning. Because of the limitations in size and localization, the procedure should be mainly used as a confirmation method. If the diagnosis is safely established and one follow-up imaging study after six months shows a stable lesion without an increase in size, no further follow-ups are necessary.

With the outlined imaging procedures, it should be possible to establish the correct diagnosis in the vast majority of cases and biopsy is rarely indicated.

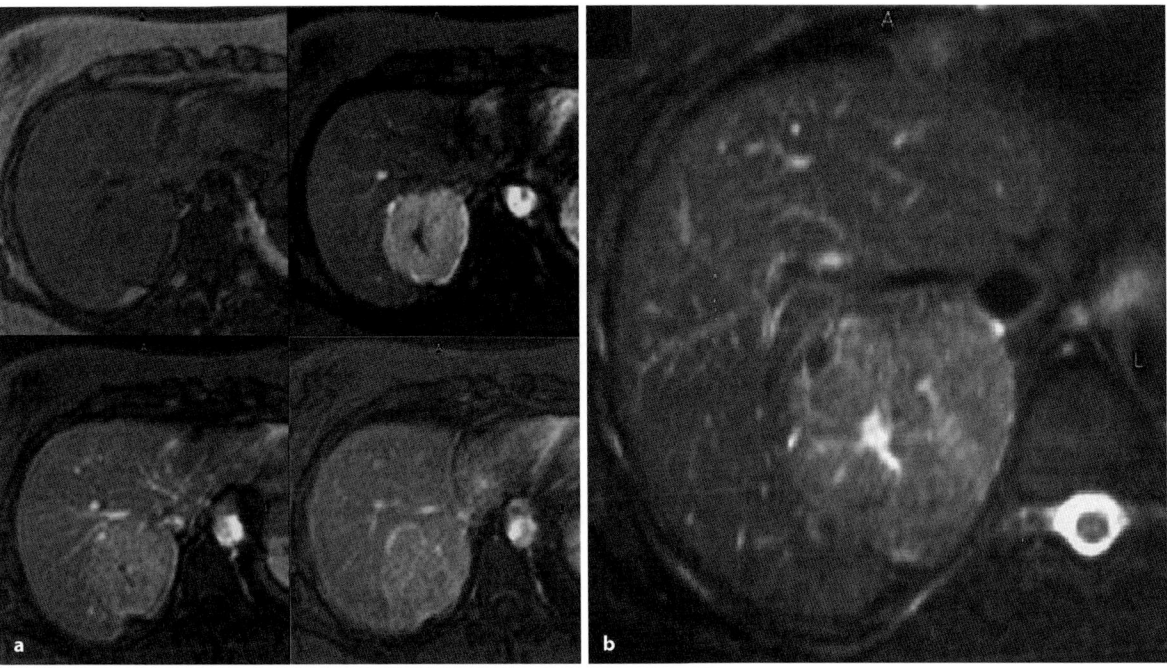

Figure 3a,b
Focal nodular hyperplasia (FNH). **a** On the T-1 weighted MR image without i.v. contrast (*upper left image*) the FNH is almost isointense to normal liver parenchyma. In the early arterial phase (*upper right image*) there is marked enhancement which is most pronounced peripherally. Central in the lesion, a hypointense scar is visible. In the venous phase (*lower left image*) the FNH again is almost isointense; the scar is still visible. In the late phase (*lower right image*) the lesion as well as the scar are isointense to normal liver. **b** On T-2 weighted fat saturated (SPIR) MR image the FNH characteristically has a hyperintense central scar

It is a subject of discussion if needle biopsy of this hypervascular tumor can safely be performed or should be considered as contraindicated because of the bleeding risk. Two recent studies have shown that US or CT guided needle biopsy with a 20 to 22-gauge needle is safe and produces tissue that is suitable for histological examination. However, more data is required before guided needle biopsy of cavernous hemangioma could be recommended as a routine procedure.

Hepatic Adenoma and Focal Nodular Hyperplasia

Because of the far-reaching implications on follow-up and treatment, the accurate differential diagnosis of FNH and HA is essential. FNH is mostly isoechoic on ultrasound but might be also hyper- or hypoechoic. The characteristic hyperechoic central scar is only present in about 25% to 45% of cases. The B-mode appearance of

HA is often mixed hyper- and hypoechoic and therefore rather unspecific. Some efforts have been made to increase the specificity of ultrasound by the use of color Doppler US. With this technique HA has been shown to exhibit a triphasic venous flow pattern, whereas in FNH the arterial flow component is predominant and reveals a spoke-wheel pattern, that is caused by arteries radiating from the center to the periphery [9].

In FNH, CT scanning with a triple-phase protocol (noncontrasted, arterial and portal venous phase) shows a hypo- to isodense lesion in the noncontrasted phase. In the early arterial phase, a peripheral and subsequent centripetal filling appears. The lesion becomes isodense again in the portal venous phase, whereas the central hypervascular scar may remain hyperdense. Similar observations are made using MRI with a contrast agent (Fig. 3).

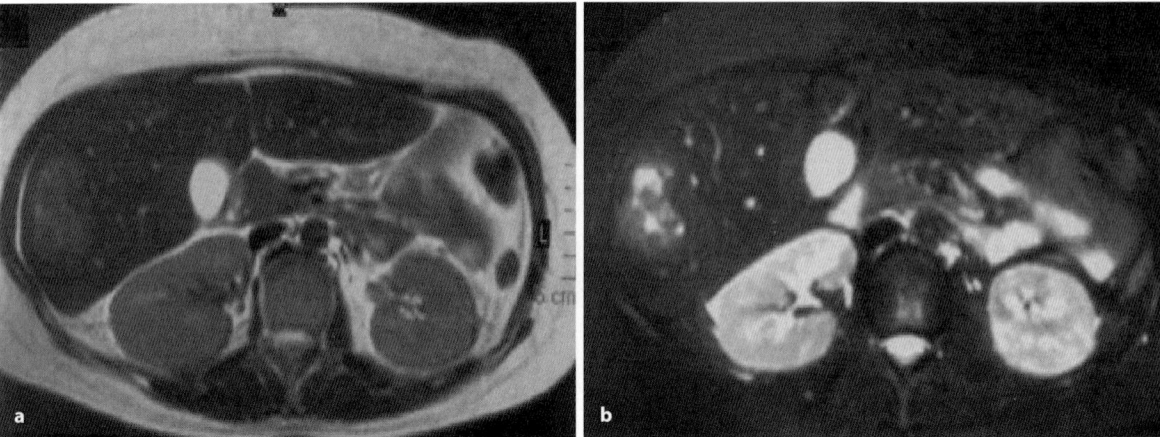

Figure 4a,b
Hepatic adenoma. **a** On this T-2 weighted MR image the adenoma is only slightly hyperintense. **b** After i.v. infusion of a Kupffer cells specific contrast agent, the liver on this T-2 weighted MR image shows a marked signal intensity decrease. Since adenomas contain only very few Kupffer cells, the lesion stays bright. Bleeding into the adenoma caused areas of high intrinsic signal

Like in sonography, CT scan findings for HA are rather unspecific. HA are hypodense on non-enhanced CT scans and might be hypo-, iso-, or hyperdense on contrast-enhanced CT. In a series of 51 pathologically proven hepatic adenomas, hyperintensity on T1-weighted MR images was observed in 59%, a peripheral rim, which corresponds to a pseudocapsule, in 31% and tumor heterogeneity, which corresponds to hemorrhagic necrosis, in 51% of the adenomas. Additionally, 67% were hyperintense on contrast-enhanced images. Differentiation of FNH and HA is also possible by ^{99m}Tc-sulfur colloid liver scintigraphy or MRI using a Kupffer cell specific contrast agent (Fig. 4). In contrast to FNH, HA contain only very few Kupffer cells. Since Kupffer cells take up ^{99m}Tc-sulfur colloid, the characteristic finding for HA in scintigraphic studies and MRI using a Kupffer cell-specific contrast agent is a focal defect in the liver. Due to hepatobiliary retention, hepatobiliary scanning of FNH with TBIDA typically reveals a "hot spot" of radioactivity in the clearing phase, usually present 60 min after application of the substance. The detectability of FNH with TBIDA is reported to be as high as 92%. If uncertainty about the diagnosis remains and a histological examination is necessary, the patient should undergo open biopsy or open needle biopsy because of the hypervascular nature of these lesions and the associated bleeding risk.

Nodular Regenerative Hyperplasia

The diagnosis of NRH is often missed by ultrasound or misjudged as micronodular cirrhosis. Findings on CT scan are normal in about half of the patients. In a few cases, well-delineated hypoechoic or isoechoic nodules can be seen. However, hyperechoic nodules have also been described. Like CT and US, MRI does not provide essential information in the diagnosis of NRH. Findings are often normal or resemble those in cirrhosis. Diagnosis of NRH may be missed even on a routine needle biopsy. In patients with clinical signs of portal hypertension – which cannot be explained by other pathological conditions like portal vein thrombosis – normal liver function tests and no abnormal findings in biopsy specimens taken by routine needle biopsy, one should consider NRH. In some patients, diagnosis can only be proven by examination of a large liver sample, which has to be taken by open biopsy.

Benign Hemangioendothelioma

B-mode US of benign hemangioendothelioma of the infant is characterized by a mostly inhomogeneous, isoechoic mass that might reveal cystic areas. Color Doppler US often shows multiple arteriovenous shunts

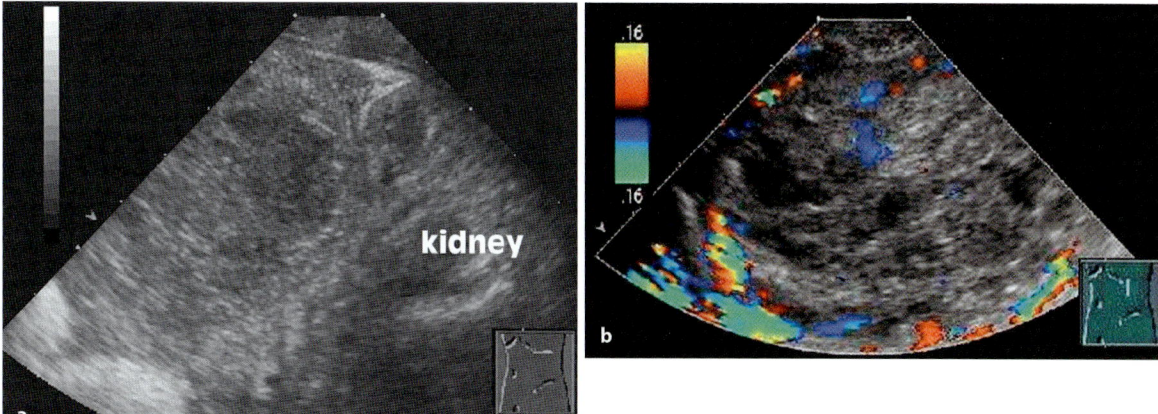

Figure 5a,b
Hemangioendothelioma in the right liver lobe. **a** B-mode sonogram with a mostly inhomogeneous, isoechoic mass with central echopoor areas. **b** Color Doppler US shows multiple arteriovenous shunts

(Fig. 5). As with US, the appearance of hemangioendothelioma on CT scan and MRI is inhomogeneous due to infarction, hemorrhage, fibrosis and calcified foci. Because of the advances in color Doppler US and visualization and reconstruction of the vessels with MRI, hepatic angiography is nowadays only rarely indicated, but provides good diagnostic accuracy. Percutaneous biopsy is contraindicated because of the risk of bleeding.

Angiomyolipoma

AML has a rather heterogeneous appearance on US, since the composition of the tissue components varies considerably. US examination mostly reveals an irregularly shaped mass but well-defined lesions have also been described. The echo-pattern might be homogenous or inhomogenous and is mostly hyperechogenic. On triple-phase CT scan, the majority of AMLs appear as hypoattenuating areas that show an early enhancement in the arterial phase. The appearance in the portal phase is more variable; hypo-, iso- and hyperattenuation have been described (Fig. 6). Using special MRI techniques like fat-suppression and dynamic MRI, the specificity could be further increased. If imaging procedures do not allow a definite diagnosis, needle biopsy should be performed.

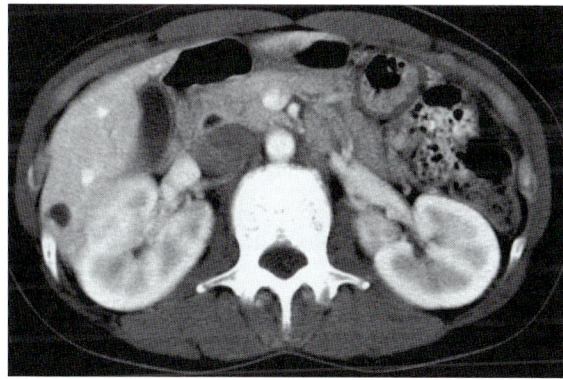

Figure 6
CT scan after i.v. contrast injection shows a 1 cm fatty lesion in the right liver lobe

Inflammatory Pseudotumor

The appearance of IPT on US (Fig. 7a) is mostly that of a homogenous, hypoechoic mass. On contrast-enhanced CT-scan, the lesion is hypodense with a slight enhancement after application of contrast medium (Fig. 7b-d). MRI findings are described as hepatic mass lesions with increased signal intensity on both T1- and T2-weight sequences. If IPT is suspected, the diagnosis has to be made histopathologically.

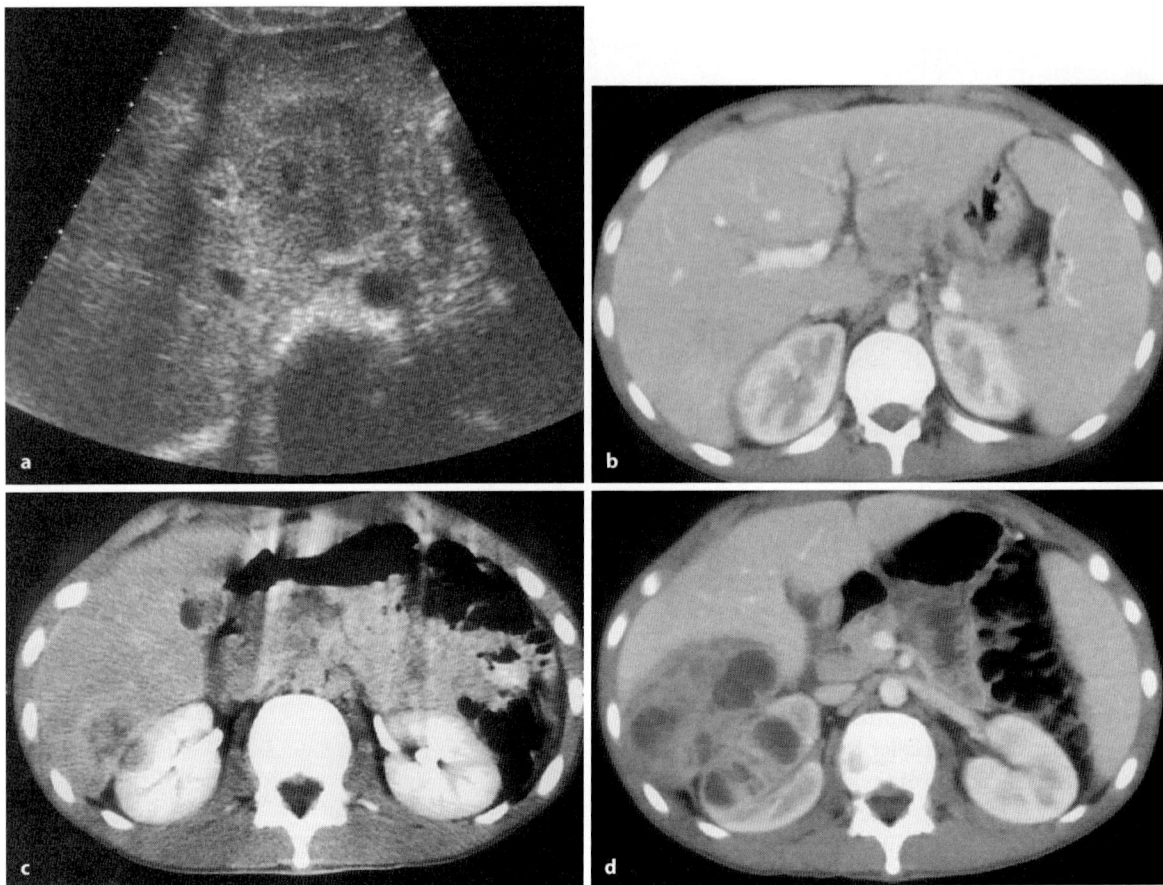

Figure 7a–d
Inflammatory pseudotumor. **a** B-mode sonogramm at presentation showed only a faintly visible, echopoor lesion between the left liver lobe and the stomach. **b** Corresponding CT scan after i.v. contrast injection with a hypodense lesion. **c** In addition there is a second lesion between the right liver lobe and the right kidney with central hypodensity and a ring enhancement. **d** This second lesion is rapidly progressive in only a few days, involving liver and kidney

Histological Classification and Molecular Genetics

Cavernous Hemangioma

Cavernous hemangiomas are solitary in about 90% of patients; in the remaining patients two or more lesions are found. The gross appearance is spongy reddish-purple or bluish (Fig. 8a). The lesions vary in size from a few millimeters up to several centimeters and are localized deep in the liver parenchyma or more frequent underneath the liver capsule. Microscopically, the lesion is

clearly demarcated from normal liver tissue (Fig. 8b). Hemangiomas consist of vascular channels of varying size that are lined by a single layer of endothelial cells and supported by collagenous walls. Thrombosis may be present. Local fibrosis and calcifications are the results of remote thrombosis.

Focal Nodular Hyperplasia

In most patients the lesions are solitary, but about 20% of patients have 2 to 5 lesions. The typical FNH is a firm, unencapsulated, nodular mass with a light-brown or yel-

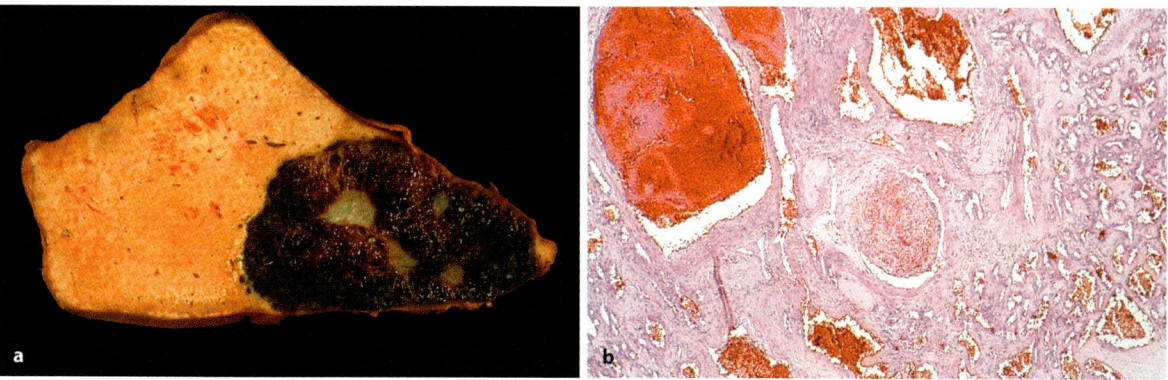

Figure 8a,b
a Cavernous hemangioma. **b** The tumor is composed of cavernous and capillary blood spaces. Some of them are occluded by organized thrombotic material (H&E)

lowish-grey color and a diameter usually smaller than 5 cm, but lesions as large as 15 cm have been described (Fig. 9a). It is frequently found in a superficial position, but like HA, it may be located deeper in the parenchyma or can be pedunculated. Necrosis and hemorrhage may be present but are not as frequent as in HA. A dense, central stellate scar is often found in FNH, but it is not pathognomonic since it may also be found in other lesions like fibrolamellar HCC (hepatocellular carcinoma). Within the scar are chronic inflammatory infiltrates and abnormal vascular structures, which include venous and capillary channels, arterial structures with muscular and intimal hyperplasia and structures that cannot be exactly classified. Immunohistochemical studies of the extracellular matrix and the distribution of endothelial cell-cell adhesion molecules and integrin receptors reinforced the hypothesis that FNH is a hyperplastic response of the liver to local vascular abnormalities. The ductular structures that are found in close approximation to the fibrous scar and its radiating bands have been studied immunohistochemically. Immunohistochemical and immunoelectronmicroscopic findings support the

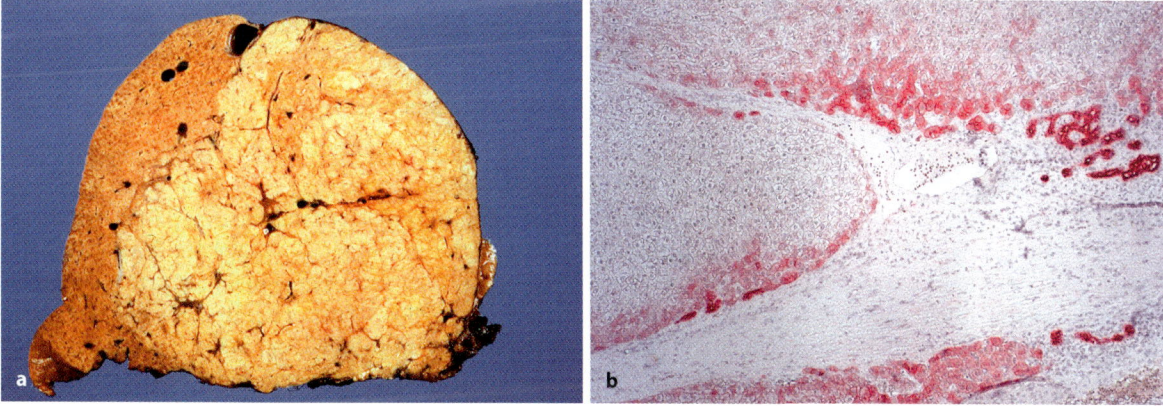

Figure 9a,b
Focal nodular hyperplasia (FNH). **a** Unencapsulated tumor in non-cirrhotic liver tissue composed of parenchymal nodules surrounded by radiating fibrous septa. **b** Characteristically these septa are lacking preformed bile ducts, but are surrounded by neoductules which are merging continuously with liver cell plates of the nodules (APAAP, anti-Keratin 7)

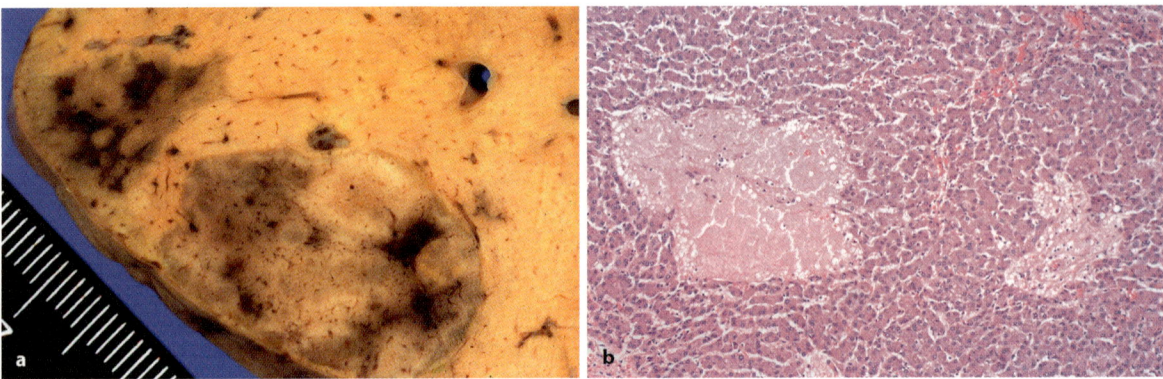

Figure 10

Liver cell adenoma. **a** Two well demarcated unencapsulated liver cell adenomas in non-cirrhotic liver tissue. **b** The tumors consist of regular hepatocytes which are arranged in two layers of liver cell plates. The adenomatous tissue contains normally appearing sinusoids and some peliotic areas (H&E)

idea that the neoductules develop from immature progenitor cells or by transdifferentiation from hepatocytes of the FNH. These findings suggest that the ductular reaction in the lesions might result from activation of these progenitor cells. The cellular composition of the nodules in FNH resembles that of cirrhotic nodules, with cords of almost normal appearing hepatocytes and sinusoidal lining cells like Ito, Kupffer and endothelial cells. Terminal hepatic venules, portal tracts and functional bile ducts are lacking (Fig. 9b). Signs of cholestasis and cholate stasis like bile plugs, cholestatic rosettes and Mallory's bodies are therefore typical findings.

Hepatic Adenoma

HA are usually located in a subcapsular position and are round with a diameter in the range of 5 to 15 cm, but may even reach 30 cm. Pedunculated adenomas and adenomas deep in the liver parenchyma have been described. On macroscopic examination, the tumor is usually light brown to yellow, relatively soft and not encapsulated (Fig. 10a). Intratumoral hemorrhage and necrosis are frequently present. Microscopically, HA closely resembles normal liver tissue but it lacks an acinar architecture. Hepatocytes are of normal apperance or only slightly atypical with a pale appearance and a finely vacuolated cytoplasm. There are few if any mitoses and no signs of malignancy. The hepatocytes are arranged in a sheetlike

fashion (Fig. 10b). Sinusoids of HA contain Ito cells and endothelial cells but virtually no Kupffer cells. Sinusoidal dilatation and blood-filled spaces are often found and could be confused with peliosis hepatis. In contrast to normal liver tissue, only very few preexisting and incorporated portal tracts or bile ducts are found in the adenomatous tissue. Small arterial branches are found within the lesion, whereas larger arteries are located in the periphery. Bile stasis is often present; lipofuscin pigment and Mallory's hyaline as well as fatty change and steatohepatitis have been described.

It is still under discussion as to whether malignant transformation to hepatocellular carcinoma occurs; there are at least two documented cases.

Nodular Regenerative Hyperplasia

Macroscopically, NRH is similar to micronodular cirrhosis. Nodules in varying sizes from 0.1 to 4 cm that have completely replaced normal liver parenchyma characterize the pathological changes in NRH (Fig. 11a). Suffilogical diagnosis. Three main features distinguish NRH from cirrhosis. First of all, fibrosis and fibrotic scar tissue are absent in uniacinar NRH, but can be found in multiacinar NRH with large nodules. Second, nodules of regenerating hepatocytes are separated by atrophic parenchyma. Regeneration is mainly present in the periportal areas with centrilobular atrophy. Third, on a reti-

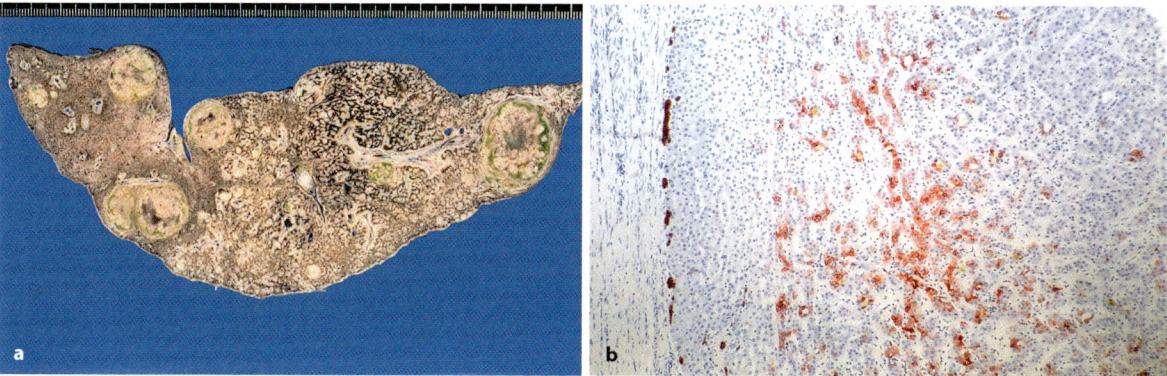

Figure 11
a Nodular (makro)regenerative hyperplasia (NRH) in a case of Budd-Chiari-Syndrome and underlying essential thrombocythemia. The liver (after liver transplantation) contains areas of acinar atrophy, a completely scarred right liver lobe as well as multiple FNH-like nodules. The caudal lobe is hyperplastic due to a separate blood drainage to the inferior caval vein. **b** This FNH-like nodule contains Keratin 7-positive canalicular and neoductular structures for bile drainage (ABC, anti-Keratin 7)

culin stain, curvilinear compression of the central veins by the regenerating nodules may be seen. These findings support the vascular hypothesis of the pathogenesis of NRH. The diminished blood flow due to occlusion of the portal venous system or of the draining hepatic veins causes an atrophy of the hepatocytes in the central areas, which is compensated by a proliferation of the hepatocytes in the periportal region [2] (Fig. 11b). However, other studies show an obliteration of portal vein branches in only the minority of cases, which refutes the vascular hypothesis.

The alternative theory hypothesizes that NRH is a proliferative disorder of the liver, because proliferative nodules are present throughout the liver. Some authors consider NRH as a premalignant condition, since hepatocyte dysplasia has been shown in 20% and 42% of cases. Hepatocellular carcinoma developing in NRH has been reported. On the other hand, the authors discuss the possibility that a preexisting HCC may have caused portal vein thrombosis that led then to NRH (vascular hypothesis).

Infantile Hemangioendothelioma

About half of the patients have a single lesion, whereas the other half present with multiple tumors. The size varies from a few millimeters to more than 15 cm. On section, the tumor is usually well demarcated and has no capsule. Small lesions are red-brown and soft, whereas the large tumors are gray to tan and may be soft or firm. Hemorrhage, fibrosis and/or calcifications may be present.

Microscopically, the tumor consists of vascular channels that may be small and capillary-like or slightly dilated in type 1 infantile hemangioendothelioma according to Dehner and Ishak [10] or may exhibit only scantily formed vascular spaces and budding of endothelial cells with larger, pleomorphic and hyperchromatic cells in type 2 hemangioendothelioma. About two thirds of the tumors present with extramedullary hematopoiesis in the tumor stroma, in tumor vessels or in both. Involutionary changes like thrombosis, fibrosis and calcifications are more likely to occur in larger tumors. Bile ducts are present in most of the tumors.

Angiomyolipoma

Macroscopically, AMLs are red to yellow soft masses that are demarcated from the liver parenchyma. Necrosis may be present. Size ranges from a few millimeters up to more than 30 cm have been reported.

Microscopically, AML is characterized by varying amounts of adipose tissue, smooth muscle cells, blood vessels and eosinophilic epithelioid cells that are arrang-

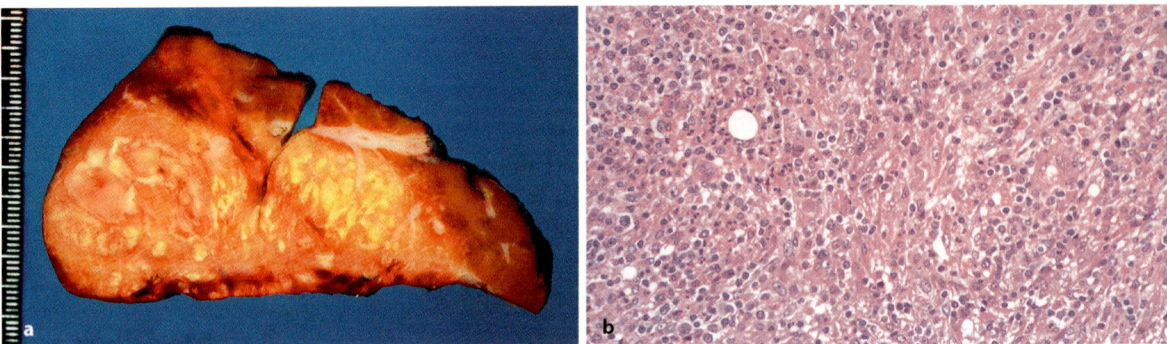

Figure 12a,b
Inflammatory pseudotumor of the liver. The lesion consists of sclerotic, myofibroblastic, xanthous and mixed inflammatory areas as shown in **b** with activated lymphoid cells, plasma cells, histocytes, neutrophilic and eosinophilic granulocytes (H&E)

ed around blood vessels. Some AML closely resemble epithelial tumors, especially the clear cell type of HCC or metastases of clear cell carcinomas, e.g. renal cell carcinoma. On immunohistochemistry, AML is the only primary liver tumor, which is immunopositive for HMB-45. HMB-45 is a marker of melanocytic differentiation and found in the myoid component. Its role in AML is not understood, but the demonstration of HMB-45 positive cells is a valuable diagnostic hint in the differential diagnosis of liver masses [5].

Inflammatory Pseudotumor

On gross examination, the tan lesion is usually only vaguely demarcated from the intact liver tissue and may infiltrate portal and hepatic veins as well as bile ducts (Fig. 12a). Histologically, IPT consists of a fibrous stroma with varying amounts of lymphocytes, macrophages, spindled cells and plasma cells (Fig. 12b). Plasma cells and lymphocytes have been shown to be of polyclonal origin. It is suggested that inflammatory pseudotumor is not a single entity, since the immunohistochemical markers for smooth muscle of the spindled cells are reported as variably positive or negative. Also, it has been shown that inflammatory pseudotumor is not purely inflammatory but may have an indeterminate or low malignant potential. Arguments include the potential for local recurrence, infiltrative local growth, vascular invasion, malignant transformation and the association with Epstein-Barr virus infection, which might be involved in the pathogenesis.

Treatment

Synopsis

Treatment options in benign hepatic tumors

1. Surgical treatment options:
  ▸ Hepatic artery ligation
  ▸ enucleation
  ▸ resection
  ▸ partial hepatectomy
  ▸ transplantation
2. Hepatic artery embolisation
3. Symptomatic medical treatment
4. Radiation therapy.

Cavernous Hemangioma

Indications for treatment of cavernous hemangioma include rupture and hemorrhage, abdominal symptoms caused by a mass effect of the hemangioma, Kasabach-Merritt syndrome and a diagnostic inconsistency that could otherwise not be solved. The risk of rupture for cavernous hemangiomas smaller than 5 cm is extremely low and even rupture of giant hemangiomas is a rare event.

Treatment modalities include resection, hepatic artery embolization and, in the exceptional case of unresectable giant hemangioma with disseminated intravascular coagulation, liver transplantation. Whether patients with upper abdominal symptoms and cavernous hemangioma should undergo treatment is under discussion. Half of the patients with symptoms who have undergone resection or embolization remained symptomatic, showing that the tumor was not responsible for the symptoms.

Focal Nodular Hyperplasia

Treatment of FNH is rarely indicated. There are several follow-up studies that show that only in the minority of patients does FNH show a progression in size or cause other problems like hemorrhage. In female patients, who are taking oral contraceptive drugs, discontinuation is not necessary since a relation of exogenous sexual hormones to the development and growth of FNH has not been shown [4].

Hepatic Adenoma

Because of the potential risk of rupture and intra-abdominal hemorrhage as well as the equivocal risk of progression to hepatocellular carcinoma, each HA larger than 5 cm should be considered for resection. In patients who are taking oral contraceptive drugs, the medication may be discontinued and the adenoma followed. In the case of regression, a resection is not mandatory.

The mortality rate for elective resection of HA is less than 1% and is reported to be 5% to 10% in cases of rupture and hemorrhage. The appropriate treatment of the patient with ruptured HA is still under discussion. Emergency resection is considered the treatment of choice by most authors. However, mortality rates in emergency resection are quite high. Alternative treatment strategies include hepatic arterial embolization and a conservative approach with hemodynamic stabilization alone. Even if laparotomy is necessary, control of bleeding could be achieved with gauze packing without immediate resection. If the patient remains stable after hemodynamic stabilization, resection of tumors larger than 5 cm could be performed on an elective basis or if rebleeding occurs. Tumors smaller than 5 cm are considered less likely to rupture and less likely to progress to hepatic carcinoma. Nevertheless, observation on a regular basis is necessary. If parallel hepatitis C or B virus infection exists, the HA should be resected, since the pathological discrimination between HA and highly differentiated hepatocellular carcinoma is extremely difficult. Figure 13 gives an overview of the treatment options of uncomplicated hepatic adenoma.

Nodular Regenerative Hyperplasia

Only a minority of patients present with signs of portal hypertension such as bleeding from esophageal varices or ascites. Liver failure is very rare. Since there is no proven treatment for NRH, the major purpose is the management of portal hypertension and its complications. This includes endoscopic treatment of varices, drug therapy to lower portal pressure and drug therapy of ascites and, if necessary, more invasive measures like porto-systemic shunt procedures. Liver transplantation in patients progressing to hepatic failure has been successfully performed.

Benign Hemangioendothelioma of the Infant

More than 85% of hepatic hemangioendotheliomas become clinically apparent before 6 months of age. According to the histological subclassification into two subtypes, type 1 shows a more benign course, whereas type 2 tends to be clinically more aggressive [10].

Uncomplicated infantile hepatic hemangioendothelioma does not require treatment, since the lesion usually involutes over the ensuing five to eight years. However, well known complications of hemangioendothelioma include congestive heart failure due to massive arteriovenous shunting, disseminated intravascular coagulation (DIC), rupture and bleeding, biliary obstruction and portal hypertension and make treatment mandatory. Mortality rates are reported to be as high as 54%. In children with mild forms of congestive heart failure, supportive treatment might be sufficient. Conservative treatment options for patients with more severe heart failure and DIC include medical treatment with corticosteroids, interferon alpha and, as a salvage therapy in life-threatening cases, cyclophosphamide. Treatment with corticosteroids is effective in 30% to 60% and interferon alpha seems to induce early regression of hemangioendothelioma in 50%. Surgical resection has the highest success rate but is problematic to perform in patients with giant hemangioendothelioma or multiple lesions. Alternative treatment modalities include radiation therapy and hepatic artery embolization or ligation,

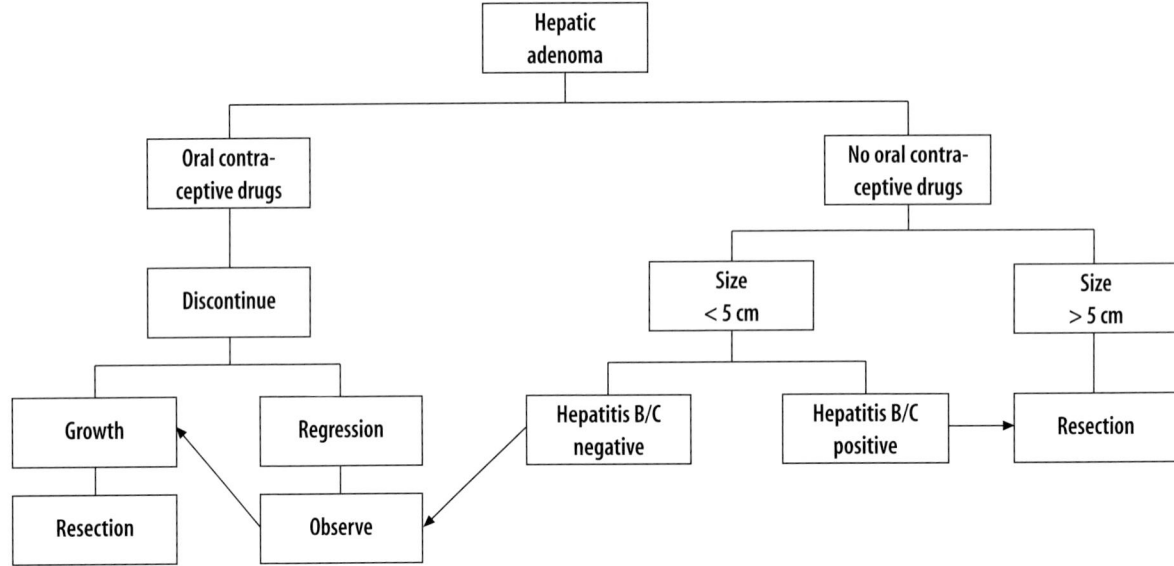

Figure 13
Suggested management of uncomplicated hepatic adenoma. Patients taking oral contraceptive drugs should discontinue the intake and have to be monitored for years. Resection is mandatory in adenomas that continue to grow after cessation of the medication. Adenomas in patients taking no oral contraceptives that a larger than 5 cm have to be resected. Also, resection should be considered for lesions smaller than 5 cm in patients which are hepatitis B or C positive

alone, or in combination with medical treatment. As an *ultima ratio*, liver transplantation has been performed in patients, who did not respond or were not eligible for the mentioned treatment modalities.

Angiomyolipoma

Any patient in whom the diagnosis of AML could not be unerringly established should undergo resection of the tumor to rule out a malignant process. Since about half of the patients present with abdominal pain, resection might be required to alleviate symptoms. Patients with lesions that cause no problems and in whom the diagnosis is safely established may be managed conservatively and monitored on a regular basis.

Inflammatory Pseudotumor

There is no consensus about the treatment of IPT. Because of its unusual clinical presentation and confusing histological picture, the accurate diagnosis is often missed and patients undergo laparotomy and resection. A review of Japanese patients involving 101 individuals

with IPT of the liver reported surgery in 66 patients and conservative treatment – either with antibiotic therapy, steroids (only one patient) or follow-up without drugs – in 34 patients. All but one patient, in whom the diagnosis was made at autopsy, survived. Several case reports of conservatively treated patients showed a favorable outcome, however, several authors consider resection as the treatment of choice.

A pragmatic approach to the treatment of patients with IPT is to treat patients in whom the diagnosis of IPT is established by imaging procedures and needle biopsy conservatively. If the diagnosis cannot be established by imaging and needle biopsy or if the condition of a conservatively treated patient worsens, a surgical resection is indicated.

References

1. Rooks JB, Ory HW, Ishak KG, et al. Epidemiology of hepatocellular adenoma. The role of oral contraceptive use. Jama 1979; 242:644–8.
2. Wanless IR. Micronodular transformation (nodular regenerative hyperplasia) of the liver: a report of 64 cases among 2,500 autopsies and a new classification of benign hepatocellular nodules. Hepatology 1990; 11: 787–97.

3. Trotter JF, Everson GT. Benign focal lesions of the liver. Clin Liver Dis 2001; 5:17–42, v.

4. Mathieu D, Kobeiter H, Maison P, et al. Oral contraceptive use and focal nodular hyperplasia of the liver. Gastroenterology 2000; 118:560–4.

5. Barnard M, Lajoie G. Angiomyolipoma: immunohistochemical and ultrastructural study of 14 cases. Ultrastruct Pathol 2001; 25:21–9.

6. Cherqui D, Rahmouni A, Charlotte F, et al. Management of focal nodular hyperplasia and hepatocellular adenoma in young women: a series of 41 patients with clinical, radiological, and pathological correlations. Hepatology 1995; 22:1674–81.

7. Ribeiro A, Burgart LJ, Nagorney DM, Gores GJ. Management of liver adenomatosis: results with a conservative surgical approach. Liver Transpl Surg 1998; 4:388–98.

8. Mathieu D, Vilgrain V, Mahfouz AE, Anglade MC, Vullierme MP, Denys A. Benign liver tumors. Magn Reson Imaging Clin N Am 1997; 5:255–88.

9. Harvey CJ, Albrecht T. Ultrasound of focal liver lesions. Eur Radiol 2001; 11:1578–93.

10. Dehner LP, Ishak KG. Vascular tumors of the liver in infants and children. A study of 30 cases and review of the literature. Arch Pathol 1971; 92: 101–11.

Appendix

X

23 Supportive Care of Patients with Gastrointestinal and Liver Tumors

W. SCHEPPACH

Summary

The preceding chapters have laid their emphasis on state-of-the-art diagnosis and therapy of tumors at various sites of the gastrointestinal tract. However, specific anti-cancer treatment modalities can only be applied if the patient is in a fair physical and emotional condition. Supportive care aimed at maintaining or improving the patient's general well-being should not be neglected. At a stage of disease when specific anti-tumor strategies have failed, the patient should be reassured that supportive treatment will continue in a meaningful way. At the end of life, compassionate comfort care can reduce suffering significantly. Health care providers should see themselves not as medical technicians but compassionate human beings, who are willing to accompany their patients through all stages of disease.

Evidence-based data concerning supportive care of cancer patients are very limited. There is a clear need to know more of the principles of palliative medicine as so many of our patients, despite all efforts, will die in the end from their gastrointestinal malignancy. Supportive care is defined as the sum of measures directed at improving the patient's physical and emotional condition, in the presence or absence of a specific anti-tumor therapy. It includes nutritional support, analgesia, antiemetic therapy, and end-of-life care. Symptomatic treatment of malignant aszites was added because it is a frequent terminal problem in patients with gastrointestinal and liver tumors.

Nutritional Support

Synopsis

Adequate nutrition is an important but often neglected component of supportive care for cancer patients. The first step is dietary counseling which takes the patient's individual food preferences into account; spontaneous intake may be supplemented by high-energy liquid formula diets. If total artificial nutrition is considered, the enteral route should be preferred. As most cancer patients have a basically functional gastrointestinal tract, polymeric diets are sufficient; oligomeric diets may be needed if the infusion site is deep in the jejunum. The choice of the appropriate application system (nasoenteral tube, PEG, PEJ, surgical jejunostomy) depends on the conceivable length of the feeding period and the risk of gastroesophageal reflux. If the gut cannot be used, total parenteral nutrition can be established after carefully balancing the advantages and procedure-related complications. Artificial nutrition can be used as an adjunct to invasive anti-cancer stategies or, when all treatment modalities have failed, can stand alone as a modality of supportive care. Research efforts are necessary to better define the potential of artificial nutrition in cancer patients, especially in longitudinal observations.

Spontaneous Oral Intake

Loss of appetite in patients with cancers at various sites occurs as a consequence of the tumor burden, but also of infection, surgery, radiation, or chemotherapy. It is often intensified by psychological factors (depression). As the extent of weight loss is a major determinant of overall prognosis, measures aimed at improving spontaneous oral intake should be taken early in the course. A weight loss of more than 10% of the pre-illness body weight within 6 months is considered clinically relevant and should prompt counter-measures. In addition to body weight, the analysis of visceral protein loss and body composition by BIA (body impedance analysis) can help to evaluate the degree of malnutrition. Early nutritional assessment and serial follow-up are indicated for patients who are at risk of developing or who have already developed nutritional deficits as a consequence of the tumor or therapy.

The first step of nutritional intervention is dietary counseling. In the absence of specific problems (e.g. swallowing disorders in esophageal cancer) a mixed diet is advised which does not differ from that of healthy individuals. As heavy meals are often not tolerated by cancer patients, smaller portions at higher frequency may be beneficial. Changes in the sensation of taste have to be considered; significant numbers of cancer patients have a higher threshold for the recognition of sweet and a lower threshold for bitter. Patients can also develop learned aversions to specific foods when they are consumed before chemotherapeutic drugs that produce nausea and vomiting. A careful selection of food preferences and provision of attractive foods, properly timed, may make the difference between weight maintenance and weight loss. At present there are no solid data in humans concerning the impact of diet on tumor growth. "Alternative" diets aimed at starving the tumor usually starve the patient instead. An evidence-based "anti-cancer" diet does not exist!

Appetite may increase following stimulants such as megesterol acetate, a gestagen also used to treat metastatic endometrial and breast cancers. At daily doses between 160 and 1600 mg this drug has shown promise in improving appetite and diminish weight loss. Following the administration of this drug, adrenal suppression, exacerbation of preexisting diabetes and thromboses have been observed. Recently, cannabinoids have been decriminalized for use in cancer patients. Dronabinol, a derivative of marijuana, reduces anorexia and weight loss, paralleled by beneficial effects on chemotherapy-induced nausea and vomiting. In a recent study in patients with advanced pancreatic cancer, eicosapentaensic acid (derived from fish oil) has shown promise as an anticachectic agent.

If dietary counseling and the prescription of appetite stimulants are insufficient, high-energy dietary supplements should be considered. Nutritionally balanced formula diets in 200 ml packages are available in a wide variety of flavors which can be offered to patients between regular meals. From there it is a small step to total enteral nutrition which may be indicated as an adjunct to invasive anti-cancer stagies or, when all treatment modalities have failed, as an integral part of supportive care.

Artificial Nutrition as an Adjunct to Anti-Cancer Therapies

There is a dilemma in malnourished patients with newly diagnosed cancer. These patients would benefit from undelayed nutritional support. On the other hand, a reversal of the nutritional changes secondary to systemic and localized effects of cancer depends on its immediate and complete eradication or significant palliation. Therefore, aggressive anti-tumor strategies (surgery, radiotherapy, chemotherapy, or multimodal treatment) should be instituted without delay, although they may further deteriorate the overall nutritional status. In such a situation, supportive care has to focus on rapid compensation of blood loss, fluid imbalances, and electrolyte disturbances. However, nutritional considerations should be incorporated early in the overall treatment program if malnutrition is present or threatening [1].

Little information is available concerning the role of enteral nutrition in the perioperative period. Randomized studies in patients who have had surgery for gastrointestinal cancer included small numbers and encountered major difficulties in providing the nutritional regimens due to nausea, distension and vomiting. Currently, there is no convincing evidence to support the routine use of artificial enteral nutrition in the postoperative period. However, seriously malnourished patients may benefit from the preoerative provision of enteral formula diets. In patients receiving chemotherapy for a variety of cancers, a clear advantage from enteral nutrition with regard to treatment toxicity, tumor response, or survival has not been demonstrated. On the contrary, malnourished patients undergoing aggressive therapies for esophageal cancer (resection, radiochemotherapy, or both) should be fed enterally (via percutaneous endoscopic gastrostomy or surgically placed jejunostomy). Severe weight loss can either be prevented or reversed in these patients as they have functional gastrointestinal tracts distally.

Numerous studies in surgical cancer patients have examined whether total parenteral nutrition (TPN) would be associated with a reduction of complications and mortality. Contradictory results have been obtained because many studies were not stratified for the degree of malnutrition. While two early metaanalyses showed a postoperative benefit from perioperative TPN, a more recent analysis concluded that routine TPN did not improve the complication rate and mortality following surgery in cancer patients. It seems that the indiscriminate use of TPN in surgical cancer patients, irrespective of their nutritional status, offers no advantage. Mal nourished patients may benefit from perioperative TPN because of improved nutritional status prior to the interference of the surgical trauma with nutrient utilization [2]. The role of TPN in patients with severe postoperative complications (abdominal abscess, anastomotic leakage) is not quite clear. These patients are usually given TPN after the operation if gastrointestinal dysfunction persists. Similarly, the nondiscriminatory use of TPN in patients treated with chemotherapy offered no outcome advantage and no decrease in complications. TPN led to some weight gain due to accumulation of water and fat, but this was not accompanied by an improvement of clinical outcome parameters. Prospective controlled trials have shown a clinical benefit from TPN only in the setting of bone marrow transplantation, but not in non-surgical treatment modalities commonly applied to patients with gastrointestinal and liver tumors.

Despite the uncertainties of clinical studies, physicians will have to make decisions concerning the initiation of nutritional intervention. The following statements are offered as a help in decision making:

1. Early nutritional support is indicated for patients who have developed or are at risk of developing nutritional deficits as a consequence of the underlying malignancy or aggressive anti-tumor therapies.

2. In patients with mild weight loss and taste changes, the evaluation of food preferences and provision of attractive natural foods and supplements may be sufficient.

3. Artificial nutrition should be instituted in the presence or likelihood of significant weight loss. Whenever feasible, the enteral route should be preferred. For example, patients with head-and-neck or esophageal tumors and dysphagia due to radiation and chemotherapy may benefit most from early enteral feeding via percutaneous endoscopic gastrostomy.

4. If the gut cannot be used for nutrient supply, parenteral nutrition via a central venous catheter is indicated in malnourished patients requiring major surgery or invasive non-surgical treatments. Patients undergoing Whipple's resection or patients suffering from 5-fluorouracil-associated mucositis may fall in this category. In surgical patients without weight loss, routine fluid and electrolyte support is indicated perioperatively, followed by early postoperative oral intake.

Artificial Nutrition After Discontinuation of Specific Anti-Cancer Treatments

Physicians taking care of oncologic patients are often confronted with a situation in which all anti-cancer treatment modalities have failed. It is important to as-

sure the patient that treatment will not stop at this stage but the objectives need to be redefined. It should then be a primary task to provide comfort care preferably on an outpatient basis and avoid unnecessary hospitalizations.

During the preceding hospital stay, the question as to whether the nutrient intake of the incurable patient is expected to be adequate should be addressed. If oral intake is sufficient, dietary advice and careful observation of body weight may be sufficient. However, if spontaneous nutrient intake is inadequate, artificial nutrition should be offered and informed consent obtained after thorough discussions with the patient and family. The PEG (percutaneous endoscopic gastrostomy) procedure has gained broad acceptance as the method of choice for patients requiring long-term enteral feeding. The physician must determine whether PEG insertion will improve the patient's subjective and objective condition in a meaningful way. The decision in favor of the PEG cannot be based solely on clinical data but must consider the impact of the procedure on the patient's quality of life and the desires of the patient and family.

If artificial nutrition (e.g. via PEG) has been initiated, patients and families need continued advice concerning the handling of the catheter and the delivery of formula diets. Ambulatory nutrition support teams have been installed to close the gap between hospital and outpatient care. The nutritional oncology service at Fox Chase Cancer Center (Philadelphia, PA) has reported a 50–80 percent success rate in getting patients to maintain or gain weight under these circumstances. It is likely that unplanned hospitalizations and tumor-related disabilities can be diminished by nutritional therapy alone, although long-term prospective data are missing. It will be important in future trials to focus not only on the objective assessment of the nutritional status but also on the subjective evaluation by the patient. The patient-generated Subjective Global Assessment may be a valuable tool to measure the quality of life of incurable cancer patients and will tell us if the medical efforts described above are justified.

Parenteral nutrition in patients with uncontrolled malignancy is not an equivalent alternative to enteral nutrition because of high complication rates and high expenses. A difficult medical and emotional problem arises when a patient with persistent intestinal obstruction due to progressive cancer is to be discharged home. The physician is then under pressure from the patient and family to institute parenteral nutrition, e.g. via ve-

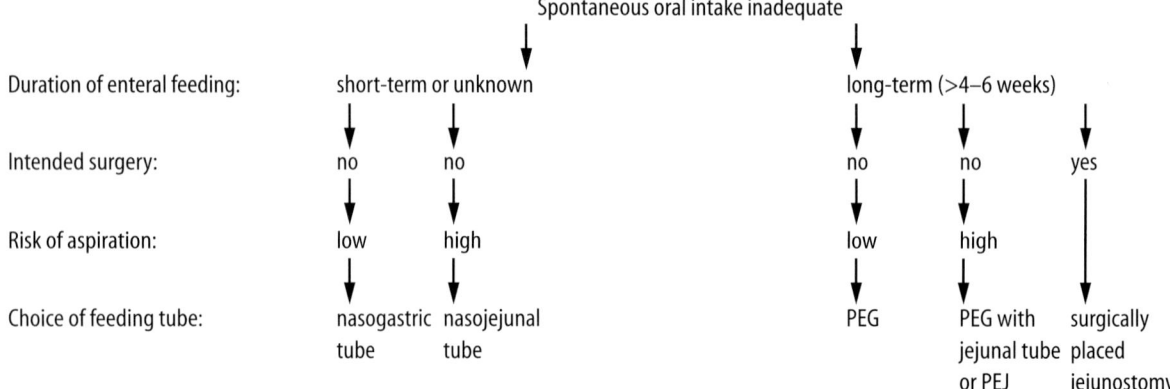

Figure 1
Choice of the appropriate feeding system for the initiation of artificial enteral nutrition (PEG, percutaneous endoscopic gastrostomy; PEJ, percutaneous endoscopic jejunostomy)

nous port systems used before for chemotherapy. Hickman or Broviac tunneled intravenous catheters can be used as an alternative. TPN can be combined with the insertion of a PEG tube used for intestinal decompression; the discomfort of a nasogastric tube is thus avoided. As these patients have usually a short life expectancy, the advantages and possible procedure-related complications need to be carefully balanced.

The situation is different in patients with a chronic dysfunctional gastrointestinal tract (due to surgery, radiation, chemotherapy) but without residual malignancy. Prolonged survival with acceptable quality of life has been reported for these rare patients on permanent TPN.

Technical Aspects of Artificial Enteral Nutrition

When the indication for artificial enteral nutrition is given, a choice has to be made concerning the route of administration. The decision may be guided by the algorithm outlined in Fig. 1.

For feeding periods of less than 4–6 weeks, nasoenteral tubes appear adequate. In most patients, nasogastric tubes which are easy to place will be sufficient. Radiographic imaging to confirm the correct position of the tube is strongly recommended before it is used for enteral feeding or the instillation of drugs. Clinical maneuvers (aspiration of gastric juice, auscultation of the abdomen during the insufflation of air) are poor predictors of tube malposition. In some patients with

gastroesophageal reflux and aspiration, jejunal placement of the tip, either fluoroscopically or endoscopically, may be required. PEG placement is not advised for short-term enteral feeding due to a small but clinically relevant morbidity and mortality.

If the feeding period is likely to exceed 4–6 weeks, permanent feeding systems should be considered. If a laparotomy is planned anyway, the surgical placement of a catheter into the first jejunal loop is the procedure of choice. This is especially beneficial in patients with esophageal resections who have a functional gastrointestinal tract distally. If surgery is not indicated, the endoscopic placement of gastrostomy tubes (PEG, percutaneous gastrostomy or PEJ, percutaneous endoscopic jejunostomy) has advanced enteral feeding technologies significantly. In most instances a 15F PEG will allow total enteral nutrition and administration of drugs; a minority of patients will need a jejunostomy tube through the PEG or a direct puncture PEJ. The placement of a PEG tube is shown in Fig. 2. A single-shot antibiotic pro-

Figure 2a–f
Endoscopic aspect during PEG placement. a Determination of the puncture site by abdominal transillumination and external application of pressure. **b** Local anesthesia. **c** Trochar entering gastric lumen. **d** Trochar after removal of metal cannula. **e** Thread passing trochar, thread grasped with biopsy forceps. **f** Internal bumper flush with gastric wall after advancement of PEG tube by the pull-through technique   ▶

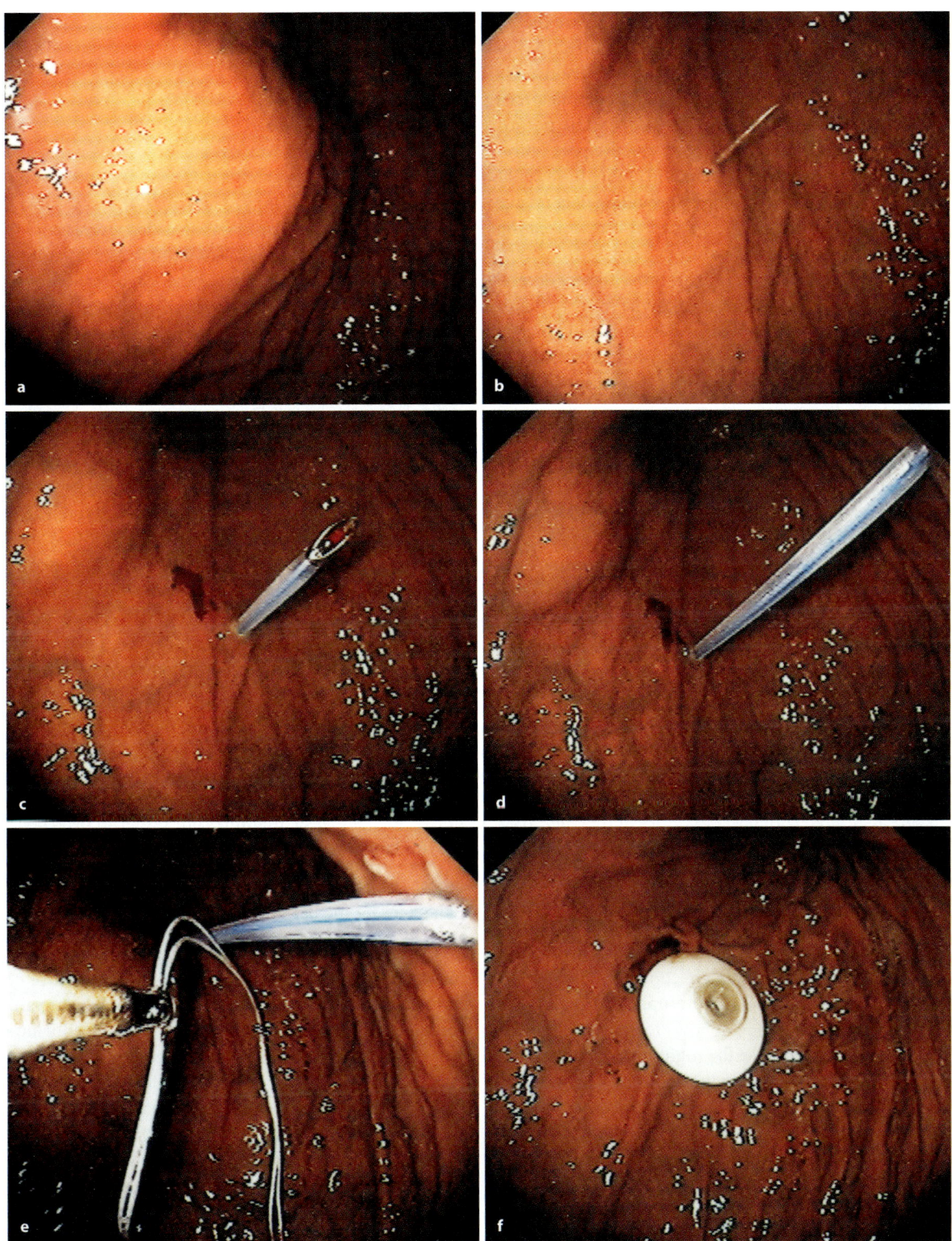

phylaxis (e.g. cefotaxim 2 g iv) 30 minutes before the intervention is recommended in Germany. Infections at the PEG puncture site (5–10% of patients) are usually treatable with local disinfectants. Major complications (abdominal abscess, peritonitis, sepsis, gastric perforation, bleeding) occur in less than 1%, the procedure-related mortality is 0–0.3%. Thus, PEG tubes have facilitated the use of enteral feeding by providing dependable access to the intestine with an acceptable complication rate and a success rate of >90%.

Although there are more than 100 different enteral formula diets on the market, they can be roughly classified as polymeric or oligomeric diets. If liquid formula diets are consumed exclusively, care should be taken to use diets fully balanced with regard to macro- and micronutrients. Polymeric diets contain polypeptides and polysaccharides and require for their digestion and absorption a functional gastrointestinal tract. These diets are suitable for routine use in cancer patients because signs of malassimilation are usually absent. Infrequently oligomeric diets may be required; these contain pre-digested oligopeptides and oligosaccharides which are easily absorbed even if not enough pancreatic and intestinal enzymes are available. A possible indication for oligomeric diets in cancer patients is enteral feeding via surgical jejunostomies placed into the second or third jejunal loops. The question as to whether dietary fiber should be integrated in formula diets has not yet been finally answered. Fiber is an integral part of normal nutrition and has pronounced effects especially in the distal gastrointestinal tract. Fiber containing formulas may be associated with fewer episodes of diarrhea; data from clinical trials are however equivocal [3]. To date it is unclear if "signal substrates" (e.g., glutamine, arginine, nucleotides, Ω-3 fatty acids, selenium) could play a role in oncologic nutrition.

Formula diets should be infused continuously (pump-assisted) because side-effects associated with enteral nutrition (diarrhea, gastroesophageal reflux) are less frequent, compared with bolus feeding. For the patient it is attractive to use the night hours for artificial feeding and to be free during the day. Total enteral nutrition is feasible at the patient's home and helps to prevent unnecessary hospitalizations.

Analgesic Therapy

Synopsis

The World Health Organization (WHO) has proposed a three-step analgesic ladder for the relief of cancer-related pain. The treatment objective is the relief and prevention of pain. It includes the use of a nonopioid (step 1), a nonopioid combined with a weak opioid (step 2), and a nonopioid combined with a strong opioid (step 3) drug. The oral route of administration should be used in the first place; transdermal administration of opioids may be considered in patients who do not tolerate oral medication. Upward dose titration should be rapid to achieve optimum analgesia. Side effects of analgesics should be treated early in the course. The principles of the WHO analgesic ladder have been found adequate to relieve pain in 70–100 percent of patients. In refractory cases the help of experts from outpatient pain clinics should be sought.

In 1986 the World Health Organization (WHO) released a monograph under the title "Cancer Pain Relief" [4]. It comprises a set of guidelines on the use of analgesic drugs with a focus on a three-step ladder of treatment escalation (see Fig. 1). Although not perfect, the principles of the WHO analgesic ladder have been found adequate to relieve pain in 70–100 percent of patients under investigation. However, pain relief in cancer patients is often not given priority because of inappropriate attitudes towards opioid therapy among health care providers, patients and their families. The following lines are not intended to give an in-depth survey of sophisticated analgesic therapies but rather to propagate the fundamental principles of the WHO scheme.

Guidelines for the Use of Analgesic Drugs

The goal of treating cancer pain is pain relief and, most importantly, pain prevention. The appropriate dose of an analgesic drug is one that relieves (or prevents) pain throughout its dosing interval; delayed release formulations are therefore given preferentially. However, a rapidly acting drug as a rescue medication for breakthrough pain should be available. Upward dose titration should be rapid to achieve optimum analgesia. The oral route of administration should be used in the first place because it is easier and less expensive than parenteral therapy. Transdermal administration of opioids may be

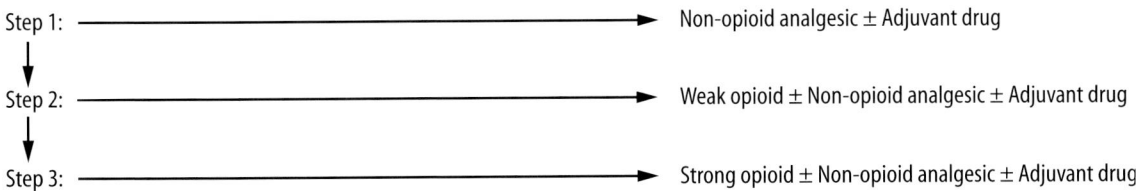

Figure 3
The World Health Organization analgesic ladder for the management of cancer pain

considered in patients who do not tolerate oral medication. Side effects of analgesics should be treated early in the course, even prophylactic treatment is considered by some authors. Typical co-medications are NSAID/proton pump inhibitor, opioid/laxative, opioid/metoclopramide [5].

Selection of the Appropriate Analgesic Drug

Drug selection is dependent on current analgesic therapy and intensity of pain (best rated semi-quantitatively on a numerical rating scale: 1–4 mild pain, 5–6 moderate pain, 7–10 severe pain). Patients under no analgesic therapy who have mild-to-moderate pain should be treated with a nonopioid drug (step 1). In patients with mild-to-moderate pain despite administration of a nonopioid drug at the maximum tolerated dose, a weak opioid analgesic should be added (step 2). Patients on a high-dose of a step 2 opioid who still suffer moderate-to-severe pain should be put on a step 3 opioid drug (Fig. 3).

Non-Opioid Drugs

Non-opioid step 1 analgesics include non-steroidal anti-inflammatory drugs (NSAIDs, e.g. diclofenac, ibuprofen), paracetamol and metamizol (Table 1). NSAIDs are effective in the treatment of somatic pain from bone metastases, soft-tissue infiltration, and recent surgery. Patients on NSAIDs should be monitored for gastropathy, gastrointestinal bleeding, and renal failure. In patients with previous gastric or duodenal ulcers, a co-medication with a proton pump inhibitor (PPI), misoprostol or an H_2 receptor antagonist may be indicated; of these drugs, the PPI is most potent in the suppression of gastrointestinal bleeding. Patients with cancer are not often given aspirin because of its effect on platelet aggregation and high incidence of gastropathy. The use of paracetamol is limited by its hepatotoxic potential; the daily dose should not exceed 6 g. Visceral pain, e.g.due to peritoneal carcinomatosis, is best treated in the first line with metamizol; serial hemograms are helpful to diagnose drug-related bone marrow toxicity.

Weak Opioid Drugs

On step 2 of the analgesic ladder weak opioids (codeine and related substances) or centrally active analgesics that bind to μ-opioid receptors (tramadol) are administered (Table 2). Patients who do not respond sufficiently to NSAIDs or metamizol but wish to defer treatment with strong opioids are most likely to benefit from tramadol.

Table 1
Step 1 nonopioid analgesics for oral administration

Step 1 analgesic drug	Initial daily dose	Maximum daily dose
Diclofenac	3 × 50 mg	300 mg
Ibuprofen	3 × 400 mg	2400 mg
Paracetamol	4–6 × 500 mg	6000 mg
Metamizol	5 × 20 gtt (=2500 mg)	5 × 40 gtt (=5000 mg)

Table 2
Step 2 weak opioid analgesics for oral administration

Step 2 analgesic drug (slow-release tablets)	Initial daily dose	Maximum daily dose
Dihydrocodeine	2–3 × 60 mg	360 mg
Tilidin-Naloxone	2–3 × 50–100 mg	600 mg
Tramadol	2–3 × 100 mg	600 mg

Table 3

Step 3 strong opioid analgesics for oral or transdermal administration

Step 3 analgesic drug	Initial daily dose	Maximum daily dose
Morphine (slow-release tbl)	$2-3 \times 10-200$ mg	not defined
L-Methadone gtt	$2-3 \times 20$ gtt ($2-3 \times 5$ mg)	not defined
Fentanyl (transdermal patch)	25 µg/h every 72 h	100 µg/h every 72 h
Buprenorphine (sublingual)	$3-4 \times 0.2$ mg	$3-4 \times 0.4$ mg

Strong Opioid Drugs

Morphine, L-methadone, fentanyl, and buprenorphine are commonly prescibed step 3 analgesic drugs suitable for the treatment of moderate to severe cancer pain (Table 3). Slow-release formulations of morphine which can be administered at a dosing interval of 12 h allow the control of severe pain in most patients. Methadone can be used alternatively while pentazocine and pethidine are not recommended for chronic administration. The fentanyl transdermal therapeutic system has gained high acceptance because it is easy to administer and causes less constipation than oral morphine. Sublingual buprenorphine is limited by its low maximum efficiency. A maximum dose cannot be defined for oral morphine; while most patients require 240 mg or less per day, some may need 1200 mg or more.

Adjuvant Analgesics

Adjuvant analgesic drugs enhance the efficacy of opioids and, independently, produce analgesia for specific types of pain. Neuropathic pain (by nerve compression or damage) is a domain for adjuvant analgesics. Corticosteroids are helpful in the treatment of acute nerve compression, visceral distension, or increased intracranial pressure. A high initial dose over a short period of time, followed by a tapering course is advised to optimize benefit and minimize adverse effects. Tricyclic antidepressants (e.g. amitriptyline) are most often prescribed for neuropathic pain; its anticholinergic property is often dose-limiting. Anticonvulsant drugs (e.g. carbamaze-pine, gabapentin), alone or added to a tricyclic antidepressant, may be useful in patients with lancinating or tic-like pain and myoclonic jerks from opioids.

Other Modes of Analgesia

Patients with bone metastases benefit from adjuvant treatment with pamidronate (60–90 mg i.v./3 h, repeat every 3 weeks). This bisphosphonate inhibits osteoclast activity and reduces pain or analgesic requirement significantly. Another mode of analgesia is palliative radiation for bone metastases, hepatic or splenic distension, or soft tissue infiltration by tumors. These options for palliative care should be used in conjunction with pharmacological therapy.

Using these WHO guidelines gastroenterologists should be able to control symptoms sufficiently in the vast majority of their cancer patients. In refractory cases the help of experts from outpatient pain clinics should be sought. Invasive techniques (nerve blocks, spinal administration of local anaesthetics or opioids, spinal cord stimulation, surgical interventions) may be useful if pharmacological pain control is inadequate. All possibilities should be considered to alleviate pain which has such a dramatic negative impact on the quality of life.

Antiemetic Therapy

Synopsis

Chemo- and radiotherapy are the most frequent causes of emesis in cancer patients; however, other conditions (e.g., gastric or small bowel obstruction, gastroenteritis, increased intracranial pressure) have to be ruled out. During chemotherapy, acute emesis is distinguished from delayed and anticipatory emesis. Acute vomiting responds best to 5-hydroxytryptamin-3 receptor antagonists. In delayed vomiting, dexamethasone alone or in combination with metoclopramide is recommended. Anticipatory vomiting is best prevented by aggressive prophylaxis and therapy of acute emesis. A promising new class of antiemetic compounds are the neurokinin-1 antagonists, which in preliminary studies have shown impressive efficacy in the control of acute and delayed vomiting.

Nausea and vomiting are among the most disturbing symptoms which occur during chemotherapy, radiotherapy, or a combination of both. Effective control of these symptoms is essential for the administration of multimodal treatment protocols.

Acute emesis (onset within 24 hours after the start of chemotherapy) is distinguished from delayed (onset on day 2–5) and anticipatory emesis. Acute vomiting is mainly mediated by the 5-hydroxytryptamin-3 receptor ($5-HT_3$) with a high density in the area postrema located on the dorsal surface of the medulla oblongata at the caudal end of the fourth ventricle. The availability of $5-HT_3$ receptor antagonists has improved the patients' tolerance to highly emetogenic regimens significantly. Other targets for specific antagonists are the dopamin D_2 receptors while the histamine H_1, acetylcholine and opioid receptors seem to be of minor importance. In contrast to chemotherapy-induced acute vomiting, delayed and anticipatory vomiting are mediated by serotonin-independent pathways. Results with the $5-HT_3$ antagonists in cisplatin-induced delayed emesis have been disappointing to date. A promising new class of antiemetic compounds are the neurokinin-1 antagonists, which in preliminary studies have shown impressive efficacy in the control of acute and delayed vomiting. Anticipatory nausea and vomiting is a consequence of drug-related side effects during preceding chemotherapies (classical conditioning) and may impair patients' compliance [6].

Although chemotherapy and radiotherapy are the most frequent causes of emesis in cancer patients, other conditions have to be considered (Table 4).

It is the objective of antiemetic treatment to avoid nausea and vomiting from the beginning of emetogenic therapies. Prophylactic treatment is clearly indicated. Table 5 lists groups of antiemetic drugs currently available.

The acute emetogenicity of antineoplastic chemotherapeutic agents has been classified by Hesketh et al. [7] according to the scheme outlined in Table 6. Level 1 agents do not require concomitant antiemetic treatment. For level 2 agents the recommendations are equivocal; the administration of either dexamethasone or metoclopramide seems adequate. $5-HT_3$ receptor antagonists are recommended for level 3 to 4 agents. If highly emetogenic chemotherapeutic regimens (level 5) are used,

Table 4
Differential diagnosis of emesis in cancer patients

Iatrogenic causes	Chemotherapy
	Radiotherapy
Organic causes	Gastric outlet obstruction
	Small bowel obstruction
	Gastroenteritis
	Increased intracranial pressure
Metabolic causes	Diabetic ketoacidosis
	Hypercalcemia
	Uremia
	Liver failure
Other causes	Psychological factors

Table 5
List of frequently used antiemetic drugs

Pharmocologic class	Substance	Dose/interval
5-HT₃ receptor antagonists	Ondansetron	8 mg every 12 h, i.v./p.o.
	Granisetron	3 mg/d i.v., 2 mg/d p.o.
	Tropisetron	5 mg/d, i.v./p.o.
	Dolasetron	100 mg/d i.v., 200 mg/d p.o.
Corticosteroids	Dexamethasone	8–20 mg/d i.v./p.o.
Dopamin D2 receptor antagonists	Metoclopramide	10–20 mg every 6 h, i.v./p.o.
	Alizapride	50–100 mg every 8 h, i.v./p.o.
Benzodiazepines	Lorazepam	1–2 mg every 12 h, i.v./p.o.
Neuroleptic agents	Triflupromazine	5–10 mg every 8 h, i.v./p.o.

Table 6
Acute emetogenic potential of antineoplastic drugs used in the treatment of gastrointestinal tumors

Level of emetogenicity	Agents often used in the treatment of gastrointestinal tumors
Level 1 (<10% of patients symptomatic)	Capecitabine
Level 2 (10–30% of patients symptomatic)	5-Fluorouracil (<1000 mg/m²)
	Gemcitabine
	Paclitaxel
Level 3 (30–60% of patients symptomatic)	5-Fluorouracil (>1000 mg/m²)
Level 4 (60–90% of patients symptomatic)	Cisplatin (<50 mg/m²)
	Irinotecan
	Oxaliplatin
Level 5 (>90% of patients symptomatic)	Cisplatin (>50 mg/m²)

5-HT$_3$ blockers are best combined with dexamethasone. According to the scheme of Hesketh et al, the combination of chemotherapeutic drugs increases the emetogenic potential by 1 to 2 levels.

In delayed vomiting, 5-HT$_3$ receptor antagonists are of little benefit; instead dexamethasone alone or in combination with metoclopramide is recommended. Anticipatory vomiting is best prevented by aggressive prophylaxis and therapy of acute emesis. If anticipatory nausea and vomiting has been conditioned, benzodiazepines should be tried.

The incidence of radiation-induced emesis is dependent on the location of the region irradiated; it may be as high as 80% if the upper abdomen is included in the radiation field. Symptoms respond to 5-HT$_3$ receptor antagonists and/or dexamethasone.

Management of Malignancy-Related Ascites

Synopsis

As malignancy-related ascites is an important cause of suffering in end-stage tumor disease, palliative treatment is mandatory. In patients with peritoneal carcinomatosis, diuretics are ineffective in mobilizing ascitic fluid. On the contrary, patients with massive liver metastases but without peritoneal carcinomatosis, who develop ascites on the basis of portal hypertension, usually respond to diuretics. In the absence of more efficient modes of treatment, the therapeutic mainstay for peritoneal carcinomatosis is periodic paracentesis. The combination of paracentesis with intraperitoneal chemotherapy sounds attractive but controlled data are awaited.

Etiology

Metastases from cancers of adjacent organs are the most frequent cause of malignant ascites. Gastrointestinal tumors that commonly metastasize to the peritoneum include gastric, colonic, pancreatic, and hepatocellular carcinomas. In addition, adenocarcinomas of the ovary, lymphomas, and mesothelial tumors have to be considered. In peritoneal carcinomatosis caused by these malignancies, ascites is due to the presence of tumor cells on the peritoneal surface. This is pathophysiologically important since the treatment response to diuretics is poor. Malignancy-related ascites may also be caused by portal hypertension, e.g. secondary to massive liver metastases or hepatocellular carcinoma superimposed on cirrhosis [8]. In this context the Budd-Chiari syndrome (hepatic venous thrombosis due to a coagulation disorder or tumorous obstruction) has to be mentioned. These conditions are usually characterized by a high serum to ascites albumin gradient and a response to diuretics. Chylous malignant ascites due to the destruction of lymphatic vessels is easily distinguished by its milky appearance on paracentesis.

Symptoms and Clinical Signs

Ascites which occurs in the context of malignancies indicates advanced disease with poor prognosis. Pain due to abdominal wall tension is more likely in patients with peritoneal carcinomatosis than patients with liver cirrhosis and reduced abdominal musculature. Early satiety occurs with tense ascites and contributes significantly to cancer cachexia. In the course of peritoneal carcinomatosis solid tumor tissue accumulates and may lead to mechanical ileus. Tense ascites also impairs diaphragmatic excursions which leads to dyspnea.

Diagnostics

While the physical examination fails to identify mild to moderate degrees of ascites, even small amounts of abdominal fluid are easily detected by transabdominal and endoscopic ultrasound (Fig. 4). The diagnosis of peritoneal carcinomatosis is made by paracentesis and cytologic examination of the aspirate which is highly sensitive (>95%). Contrary to common belief, bloody ascites is an unreliable indicator of malignancy. Patients with peritoneal carcinomatosis but without massive liver metastases have usually a high ascitic fluid protein concentration and a low serum-to-ascites albumin gradient.

Other forms of malignancy-related ascites can be distinguished from peritoneal carcinomatosis by analysis of ascitic fluid. Patients with massive liver metastases but without spread to the peritoneum have a negative cytology, low ascitic protein concentration, and high serum-to-ascites albumin gradient. Analysis of ascitic fluid is similar in patients with hepatocellular carcinoma superimposed on cirrhosis. Chylous ascites is characterized by a negative cytology and an elevated ascitic fluid triglyceride concentration.

Treatment

As malignancy-related ascites is an important cause of suffering in end-stage tumor disease, palliative treatment is mandatory. In patients with peritoneal carcinomatosis, diuretics (e.g. spironolacton, xipamid, furosemid) are ineffective in mobilizing ascitic fluid. A high-dose diuretic therapy may even be complicated by hypotension or renal dysfunction. On the contrary, patients with massive liver metastases but without peritoneal carcinomatosis who develop ascites on the basis of portal hypertension (negative ascitic cytology, high serum-to-ascites albumin gradient) usually respond to diuretics. Thus, the analysis of ascitic fluid may help to direct diuretic therapy according to the pathophysiologic considerations outlined above.

In the absence of more efficient modes of treatment, the therapeutic mainstay for peritoneal carcinomatosis is periodic paracentesis. Symptoms from tense ascites (pain, early satiety, dyspnea) are temporarily relieved. The procedure should be accompanied by intravenous albumin substitution (6–8 g/l ascites removed) as a compensation for ascitic protein loss. In order to avoid unnecessary hospitalizations, paracentesis should be preferentially performed on an outpatient basis.

The combination of paracentesis with intraperitoneal chemotherapy sounds attractive but controlled data are awaited. Chemotherapeutic agents used in gastrointestinal malignancies include mitoxantron, 5-fluorouracil, cisplatin, and mitomycin C. A possible scheme would be total paracentesis, followed by intraperitoneal instillation of 30 mg mitoxantron (dissolved in 1000 ml saline). Although large topical doses might be administered intraperitoneally, systemic toxicities have to be considered. Furthermore it is a disadvantage that the effect is limited to malignant cells which are floating in the ascitic fluid or which adhere superficially to the peritoneal surface.

Following encouraging experiences with aggressive treatment protocols in ovarian cancer, cytoreductive surgery and hyperthermic intraoperative intraperitoneal chemotherapy (HIIC) has been applied in gastrointesti-

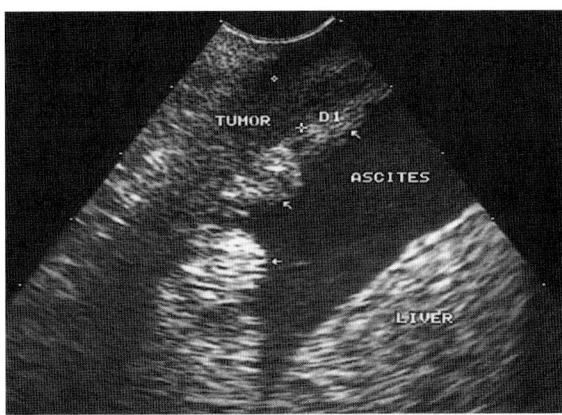

Figure 4
Endoscopic ultrasound (EUS) imaging of gastric carcinoma ("tumor") with peritoneal carcinomatosis (arrows indicate thickening of the parietal peritoneum) and malignant ascites

nal malignancies. In a recent series from the Washington Cancer Institute, the feasibility of this procedure has been demonstrated. HIIC was, however, accompanied by major morbidity in 27% and treatment-related mortality in 1.5% [9]. Peritoneovenous shunting for the control of ascites from peritoneal carcinomatosis is associated with disseminated intravascular coagulation in approximately one third of patients. The systemic dissemination of tumor cells is clinically irrelevant within the short life expectancy of affected patients; however, shunt occlusion due to tumor cells is a major technical problem.

In chylous malignant ascites, a low-fat diet supplemented with MCT (medium-chain triglyceride) fats reduces the substrate flow through the thoracic duct and thus helps to reduce the frequency of paracentesis.

Prognosis

The survival of patients with peritoneal carcinomatosis is in the range of weeks to some months. The clinical course is determined by poor quality of life due to major symptoms (pain, no appetite, dyspnea), progressive wasting, and frequent complications (e.g. bowel obstruction). Palliation for these patients is a real challenge for health care providers and patients' families.

Management of Bowel Obstruction Due to Peritoneal Carcinomatosis

Synopsis

Gastrointestinal as well as other tumors with spread to the peritoneum may cause intestinal obstruction, either by mechanical compression of bowel loops or by impairment of peristalsis. Isolated mechanical stenoses can be managed by palliative surgery; recently self-expanding metallic stents have emerged as an alternative for those parts of the intestine that can be treated endoscopically. Motility disorders due to peritoneal carcinomatosis respond poorly to propulsive agents. In selected cases with intractable bowel obstruction, intestinal decompression by PEG can be combined with permanent parenteral nutrition. The pros and cons of invasive procedures have to be considered with caution in this terminal phase of a malignant disorder.

Symptoms and Clinical Signs

Patients will present with abdominal discomfort due to bowel distension, nausea, vomiting, and inability of passing flatus or stool. Clinical signs include meteorism and tenderness which is, however, less pronounced than in cases with underlying inflammatory conditions. On auscultation, bowel sounds are augmented in early mechanical obstruction and reduced in late mechanical obstruction as well as in paralytic ileus.

Diagnosis

The distribution of intestinal gas on plain abdominal radiograph usually allows the distinction between mechanical and paralytic ileus. In unclear cases radiographic contrast studies (enema, small bowel follow-through) are useful. When administered orally, barium is preferred to aqueous contrast agents; it allows imaging of distal stenoses although it is diluted by large amounts of fluid present in the obstructed intestine. Aqueous (iodine-based) contrast agents are sufficient for use in contrast enemas; they obviate the risk of barium impaction at the site of obstruction. On the basis of these procedures the distinction between circumscript mechanical (amenable to interventional procedures) and non-mechanical obstruction should be possible.

Treatment

As in other cases of ileus, the initial treatment consists of nasogastric aspiration, intravenous hydration, and correction of electrolyte imbalances.

In the case of mechanical obstruction, a decision must be made if the patient is a candidate for palliative surgery. Especially patients with colonic obstruction by a colorectal primary tumor have a chance of prolonged postoperative palliation. On the other hand, patients with non-colorectal primaries, ascites, small bowel involvement and preoperative serum albumin of <3 g/100 ml have an inferior survival. Operative procedures (resections, bypass operations, diverting colostomies) undertaken in patients with advanced cancer carry the risk of high postoperative morbidity (up to 50%) and mortality (up to 15%). These problems will have to be discussed with the patient and family.

Recently, self-expanding metallic stents have come up as a less invasive alternative to surgery. At present, stent placement is feasible in esophageal, gastric, duodenal and proximal jejunal stenoses; the introduction of through-the-scope techniques has facilitated stent placement in the proximal small intestine. Colonic stents have been implanted primarily to provide temporary relief of obstruction so that subsequent colonic resections could be performed electively. However, colonic stents can also be used as a palliative treatment for unresectable advanced tumors; this technique is at present confined to stenoses of the left-sided colon.

Motility disorders due to peritoneal carcinomatosis (in the absence of mechanical obstruction) are difficult to treat. Propulsive agents such as metoclopramide (effective in the upper GI tract) or erythromycin can be tried but no medical treatment modality has reached the stage of a clinical standard. In the case of concomitant ascites, paracentesis may be accompanied by temporary relief. PEG or PEJ tubes can be inserted endoscopically for intestinal decompression; the discomfort of a nasogastric tube is thus avoided. This procedure must be combined with permanent parenteral nutrition via port systems or Hickman / Broviac catheters.

Prognosis

Bowel obstruction due to peritoneal carcinomatosis is a terminal event in malignant disease. As these patients have a short life expectancy, the advantages and possible procedure-related complications of interventions need to be carefully balanced.

End-of-life Care

Synopsis

Palliative end-of-life care focuses on the relief of pain, dyspnea, and other kinds of suffering while the requirement for adequate feeding steps back. Analgesics and sedatives are used in doses sufficient to minimize discomfort; side effects such as impairment of consciousness and breathing are accepted though not intended ("double effect"). When decisions about the withholding or withdrawal of life support are made, the preferences of the patient will have to be respected ("informed consent and informed refusal"). Advance directives are encouraged in which competent patients express their will in the case of incapacitating critical illness. A stable relationship between physician, patient and patient's family is essential to communicate the basis for medical decisions which are intended to make a humane dying process possible.

Towards the end of life, effective control of pain and other causes of suffering becomes most important, while the requirement for adequate nutrition steps back. While there is a widespread intuitive assumption that the physical and emotional well-being of the patient is enhanced by artificial nutrition and hydration, few objective data exist to substantiate these beliefs. In a series of 32 patients terminally ill with cancer, 20 patients never experienced any hunger, while 11 patients had symptoms only initally. Similarly, 20 patients felt no thirst or thirst only initially during their terminal illness. In all patients, symptoms of hunger, thirst, and dry mouth could be alleviated, usually with small amounts of food and fluid. Comfort care included use of narcotics for relief of pain or shortness of breath in 94% of patients. It can be concluded that food and fluid administration beyond the specific requests of patients may play a minimal role in providing comfort to terminally ill patients [10]. Iso-osmotic exsiccation occurs under these circumstances which does not seem to cause suffering.

Palliative end-of-life care focuses on the relief of pain, dyspnea, and other kinds of discomfort. It usually entails the use of analgesics and sedatives in doses suf-ficient to reduce suffering reliably. Side effects, such as impairment of consciousness and breathing, are accepted though not intended ("double effect"). Physicians should document in the patient's records how decisions were made, how informed consent was obtained and how the process of achieving comfort was conducted. Because the goal of palliative care is to provide comfort, measures that do not relieve suffering but merely hasten death should be avoided. If palliative medicine as described above is performed in a humane and compassionate manner, there is no need for physician-assisted suicide (recently legalized in the State of Oregon and the Netherlands). In the view of the author, it is a specific lesson from recent German history that physicians should never cross the dividing line between terminal comfort care and physician-assisted suicide/euthanasia because the potential for criminal misuse is enormous; the National Socialist Euthanasia Program (1939–1941) is mentioned as a deterring example.

End-of-life care of terminally ill patients includes two closely related practices [11]: the withholding or withdrawal of life support, and the provision of palliative care. The withholding/withdrawal of life support defines medical decisions not to give or to remove interventions (e.g., hemodialysis, mechanical ventilation, artificial enteral or parenteral nutrition) with the expectation that the patient will die soon of the underlying illness. There must be unequivocal signs of terminal disease to justify the withholding of life-saving interventions. Cancer patients with a poor overall prognosis who are still in a fair physical condition are entitled to the same extent of treatment as comparable patients with non-malignant conditions. For example, patients with underlying malignancies should not be excluded from admission to intensive care units on principle. When decisions about the withholding or withdrawal of life support are made, the inalienable right of the competent patient to refuse therapy ("informed consent and informed refusal") should prevail. In the incompetent critically ill, the physician will have to find out the presumable wish of the patient, usually by questioning close family members. A solution to this problem might be advance directives in which mentally competent patients express their will concerning medical procedures in the case of incompetence. In the absence of reliable evidence of the patient's desires, a unilateral decision will have to be made by the physician in the patient's best interest; this has to take the benefits and burdens of continued life into account. Unilateral actions, however, carry the risk of disagreement between physician and family members. Thus, to avoid misperceptions, a stable relationship between the physician, the patient and the patient's family will have to be established; communications may be improved by family conferences.

References

1. Shils ME, Shike M (1998) Nutritional support of the cancer patient. In: Shils ME (Ed.): Modern nutrition in health and disease. 9th Edition, Williams & Wilkins, Baltimore
2. Bozzetti F, Gavazzi C, Miceli R, Rossi N, Mariani L, Cozzaglio L, Bonfanti G, Piazenza S (2000) Perioperative total parenteral nutrition in malnourished, gastrointestinal cancer patients: A randomized, clinical trial. J Parenter Enteral Nutr 24:7–14
3. Scheppach W, Bartram HP (1993) Experimental evidence for and clinical implications of fiber and artificial enteral nutrition. Nutrition 9: 399–405
4. WHO Cancer Program Monography: Cancer Pain relief. 2nd Edition, 1996.
5. Levy MH (1996) Pharmacological treatment of cancer pain. N Engl J Med 335:1124–1132
6. Quigley EMM, Hasler WL, Parkman HP (2001) American Gastroenterological Association medical position statement: nausea and vomiting. Gastroenterology 120:261–286
7. Hesketh PJ, Kris MG, Grunberg SM, Beck T, Hainsworth JD, Harker G, Aapro MS, Gandara D, Lindley CM (1997) Proposal for classifying the acute emetogenicity of cancer chemotherapy. J Clin Oncol 15:103–109
8. Pockros PJ, Esrason KT, Nguyen C, Duque J, Woods S (1992) Mobilization of malignant ascites with diuretics is dependent on ascitic fluid characteristics. Gastroenterology 103:1302–1306
9. Stephens AD, Alderman R, Chang D, Edwards GD, Esquivel J, Sebbag G, Steves MA, Sugarbaker PH (1999) Morbidity and mortality analysis of 200 treatments with cytoreductive surgery and hyperthermic intraoperative intraperitoneal chemotherapy using coliseum technique. Ann Surg Oncol 6:790–796
10. McCann RM, Hall WJ, Groth-Juncker A (1994) Comfort care for terminally ill patients. J Am Med Assoc 272:1263–1266
11. Luce JM, Alpers A (2001) End-of-life care: What do the American courts say? Crit Care Med 29 (Suppl):N40-N45

Addendum

XI

Index